LaFleur Brooks'
HEALTH UNIT
Coordinating

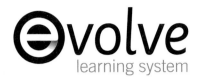 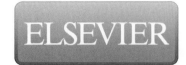
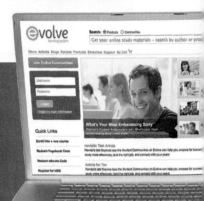

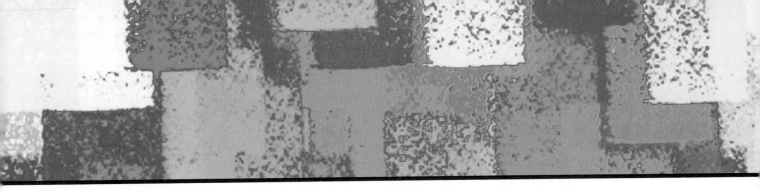

LaFleur Brooks'

HEALTH UNIT
Coordinating

SEVENTH EDITION

Elaine A. Gillingham, AAS, BA, CHUC
Program Director 1993 – 2005 (retired),
Health Unit Coordinating Program,
GateWay Community College,
Phoenix, Arizona

Monica Melzer Wadsworth Seibel, BS, MEd, CHUC
Program Director,
Health Unit Coordinating Program,
GateWay Community College,
Phoenix, Arizona

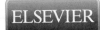

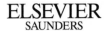

ELSEVIER
SAUNDERS

3251 Riverport Lane
St. Louis, Missouri 63043

Library of Congress Cataloging-in-Publication Data

Gillingham, Elaine Tight.
Lafleur Brooks' health unit coordinating/Elaine A. Gillingham, Monica Wadsworth Seibel. -- 7th ed.
    p. ; cm.
Health unit coordinating
Includes bibliographical references and index.
ISBN 978-1-4557-0720-1 (pbk. : alk. paper)
I. Seibel, Monica Wadsworth. II. LaFleur-Brooks, Myrna. Health unit coordinating. III. Title. IV. Title: Health unit coordinating.
[DNLM: 1. Hospital Units--organization & administration. 2. Personnel, Hospital. 3. Medical Records. 4. Nursing Records. WX 159]
610.1'4--dc23
                                                                            2012045603

Vice President and Publisher: Andrew Allen
Content Manager: Ellen Wurm-Cutter
Publishing Services Manager: Julie Eddy
Senior Project Manager: Celeste Clingan
Design Direction: Karen Pauls

Printed in United States of America

Last digit is the print number: 9   8   7   6   5   4   3   2   1

Reviewers

Jennifer M. Evans, MEd
Faculty/Program Coordinator
South Seattle Community College
Seattle, Washington
Green River Community College
Auburn, Washington

Donna Mary Harper, CHUC, PID
Health Unit Coordinator
Lions Gate Hospital
Royal Columbian Hospital
Instructor
Canadian Health Care Academy
Vancouver, British Columbia
Canada

Anita Mills
Health Unit Coordinator Instructor
Saint Paul College
Saint Paul, Minnesota

Lynn Owen, MSN, RN
Faculty
Lakeshore Technical College
Cleveland, Wisconsin

Thank you to Bill, my loving, brave husband who will always be my inspiration.

Elaine A. Gillingham

Thank you, Myrna and Elaine, for leading me to so many wonderful opportunities.
Thank you Jennifer, Erin, Colin, Aiden Brendan, and Ryan for lighting my life,
and
Thank you, Scott, for love and a lifetime of companionship.

Monica Melzer Wadsworth Seibel

Preface

A CAREER IN HEALTH UNIT COORDINATING

Welcome to the exciting, challenging, and evolving career of Health Unit Coordinating. Individuals practicing as Health Unit Coordinators soon realize that they have far-reaching effects on the delivery of care to patients. Health Unit Coordinators manage all non-clinical tasks on hospital nursing units, making them essential members of the health care team. Responsibilities include monitoring electronic medical records or transcribing physicians' orders for patient treatment, preparing patient charts, (when paper charts are utilized) maintaining statistical reports, dealing with visitors, and much more. The implementation of the electronic medical record (EMR) with computer physician order entry (CPOE) has expanded the HUC responsibilities. Health Unit Coordinators will have a more efficient role of traffic control, coordination of care, and management of the electronic record. When CPOE is implemented, the Health Unit Coordinators will no longer have to interpret and transcribe handwritten physicians' orders.

As a recognized health care profession, Health Unit Coordinating has its own national organization, the National Association of Health Unit Coordinators (NAHUC), which offers certification to individuals who meet certain standards of excellence.

NEW TO THIS EDITION

Instructors and students using the 7th edition of *LaFleur Brooks' Health Unit Coordinating* will benefit from all of the quality pedagogical elements in the previous edition, plus a simulated electronic medical record system that helps students better prepare for their role and responsibilities on the job. Every chapter has been reviewed and updated as needed while maintaining the approach and features that make *LaFleur Brooks' Health Unit Coordinating* a success.

TOTAL EDUCATIONAL PACKAGE

The 7th edition of *LaFleur Brooks' Health Unit Coordinating* is part of a total educational package for health unit coordinating offered by Elsevier. Supplemental materials include the following:

LaFleur Brooks' Skills Practice Manual for Health Unit Coordinating, 7th edition

This printed manual contains practice activities to reinforce skills taught in the text, such as transcribing doctors' orders, communicating with co-workers, assembling a patient's paper chart, and documenting lab values. Generic hospital forms and actual physicians' orders provide hands-on examples of tasks students will need to perform on the job. Also included is a clinical skills evaluation record, designed to help students objectively record and evaluate their performance during hospital rotations.

Practice Activity Simulated Electronic Medical Record System

Simulates a hospital's computer EMR system to be used in the classroom for practice in completing HUC tasks, and contains printable census records, consent forms, laboratory, and diagnostic reports. The simulated EMR includes mock nursing units with lists of patients, doctors' rosters, diagnostic test results, and more, offering realistic practice to enhance students' skills and confidence.

TEACH for LaFleur Brooks' Health Unit Coordinating, 7th edition

This instructor resource is available via Evolve. The **TEACH Lesson Plan Manual** provides instructors with customizable lesson plans and lecture outlines based on learning objectives. With these valuable resources, instructors will save valuable preparation time and create a learning environment that fully engages students in classroom preparation. The lesson plans are organized into easily understandable sections – Instructor Preparation, Student Preparation, the 50-Minute Lesson Plan, an Assessment Plan, and a Laboratory Activities Plan (where applicable).

The content covered in each textbook chapter is divided across several lesson plans, each designed to occupy 50 minutes of class time. The consistent time for each lesson plan allows the instructor to re-sequence them in any order to fit their class calendar.

A 900-question Test Bank, PowerPoint lecture slides, an electronic image collection containing all the images from the textbook, and additional Physician Orders for Student Practice are also included.

EVOLVE Website for *LaFleur Brooks' Health Unit Coordinating*, 7th edition

This feature provides free materials for both students and instructors. Resources for instructors only include the following:
- TEACH Lesson Plans with PowerPoint lecture slides
- Electronic Image Collection
- Additional Images
- 900-question Test Bank
- Physician Orders for Student Practice
  Resources for students include the following:
- Textbook Chapter Exercises and Chapter Review Questions in a downloadable format

- Drag-and-Drop Exercises, Fill-in-the-Blank Exercises, and Vocabulary Flash Cards (**NEW!**)
- Abbreviations Flash Cards (**NEW!**)
- Certification Review Guide
- Mock Certification Exam

MARKET-LEADING TEXTBOOK

LaFleur Brooks' Health Unit Coordinating, 7th edition, by Elaine A. Gillingham and Monica Wadsworth Seibel, is the best-selling textbook of its kind on the market. It provides comprehensive coverage of the theory and practice underpinning the Health Unit Coordinator's responsibilities, introduces students to hospitals and health care, and explains non-clinical management of the nursing unit. It also offers a complete module on anatomy, physiology, and medical terminology, enabling students to learn the language of medicine so they can interact confidently with doctors, nurses, and other health care workers. Exercises in each chapter reinforce newly learned material and test students' retention and critical thinking abilities. Abundant photographs, diagrams, and illustrations further enhance understanding of the material. Students studying in programs using this text will be able to master everything they need to know to begin their career performing at a competent level.

TO THE STUDENT

How to Use This Text

This text is organized to provide theory in conjunction with hands-on activities in the *LaFleur Brooks' Skills Practice Manual for Health Unit Coordinating* to prepare you to work as a Health Unit Coordinator. The text is divided into five sections:

Section 1, *Orientation to Hospitals, Medical Centers, and Health Care,* provides a fundamental understanding of health care, including the Health Unit Coordinator position. Recent *changes in health care,* including the electronic record (EMR) with computer physician order entry (CPOE) and the impact on Health Unit Coordinating are discussed.

Section 2, *Personal and Professional Skills,* presents guidelines to use for effective interpersonal and intercultural communication and management skills. Workplace behavior and appearance, confidentiality as mandated by the Privacy Rule and Security Rule contained the Health Insurance Portability and Accountability Act (HIPAA), and other ethical and legal issues are discussed.

Section 3, *The Patient's Electronic Record or Paper Chart,* provides information needed to understand written doctors' orders and enhances understanding of the various departments that carry out the orders. Activities are included that provide hands-on experience transcribing handwritten doctors' orders by using the *LaFleur Brooks' Skills Practice Manual for Health Unit Coordinating* and the *Simulated Electronic Medical Record System.* Information regarding the Health Unit Coordinators' role when the electronic medical record with computer physician order entry is implemented is outlined.

Section 4, *Health Unit Coordinator Procedures,* provides information regarding emergencies, infection control, recording vital signs, and admission, preoperative, postoperative, discharge, postmortem, and transfer procedures.

Section 5, *Introduction to Anatomic Structures, Medical Terms, and Illnesses,* presents a basic overview of human anatomy and medical terminology.

Working Your Way Through a Chapter
Read the Objectives

The objectives outline what you are expected to know when you have completed all of the exercises for the chapter. When you have read the chapter and completed the exercises, return to the objectives and quiz yourself to ensure that you have mastered the material.

Read the Vocabulary Lists

Each chapter introduces a list of words related to the material covered in that chapter. When reading the chapter, note the words in the vocabulary list to enhance your understanding of their meanings. Return to the vocabulary list after you have read the chapter and complete the exercises to quiz yourself on the definitions of the words.

Complete the Exercises that Follow the Abbreviation Lists

Most chapters include a list of abbreviations that relate to the material covered in that chapter. Exercises are included to assist you in learning those abbreviations. The abbreviations are also used throughout the chapter. It may be helpful to create flash cards for the abbreviations.

Complete the Review Questions

The review questions are written from the objectives and will assist you in learning and understanding the skills necessary to be successful as a Health Unit Coordinator.

High Priority Boxes

Pay special attention to the information provided in the *High Priority* boxes, as this information is especially important in performing your job accurately and efficiently. This information is emphasized to reduce the risk of errors while working as a Health Unit Coordinator.

Surfing For Answers

Websites are provided at the end of each chapter for practice in using search engines and to provide interesting articles and information related to topics discussed in the chapter.

Hands-On Activities

Most chapters in *LaFleur Brooks' Health Unit Coordinating* include references to activities found in *LaFleur Brooks' Skills Practice Manual for Health Unit Coordinating.* Chapters 4 and 7 have activities related to communication and management skills. Chapter 8 has activities that will familiarize you with patient chart forms and chart assembly. Chapters 10 through 19 include doctors' orders that relate to material discussed in each chapter.

Use of Appendixes

Appendix A, *Abbreviations,* helps refresh your memory when you cannot recall the meaning of an abbreviation used in a doctors' order.

Appendix B, *Word Parts,* assists you in finding the definition of a word part while defining or building a medical term. You may need to find a prefix or suffix that you recognize from Chapter 22, but for which you have forgotten the definition.

Answers

Check your answers after completing exercises and review questions to ensure that you have answered them correctly.

FROM THE AUTHORS

Congratulations—you have opened the door to the health care world. By using *LaFleur Brooks' Health Unit Coordinating* as a learning tool, you may obtain a career in health care. Our hope is that you will continue to become a valuable member of the health care field and feel the pride and satisfaction that comes with helping others. Continuous advancement in technology makes working in the health care field an exciting and educational experience.

Acknowledgments

Preparing the 7th edition of *LaFleur Brooks' Health Unit Coordinating* required the expertise of many, since changes in the health care delivery system and advancement in medical technology demand new knowledge for the Health Unit Coordinator and change in the Health Unit Coordinating practice.

We thank the reviewers who helped to ensure that this was the most up-to-date revision it could be. We would also like to express our appreciation for the cooperation we received from Banner Estrella Medical Center, who allowed pictures to be taken of their facility and their employees to participate. We would like to give a special thanks to the Banner Estrella Medical Center employees who shared their knowledge and allowed their pictures to be taken. Thank you to Gateway Community College in Phoenix, Arizona, who allowed access to their various health care programs to obtain information to prepare the manuscript. In addition, we wish to thank the following individuals for their assistance:

Charo Bautista, BSN
Faculty, Health Unit Coordinator Program, GateWay Community College, Phoenix, Arizona

Kathryn Patterson, BS, RRT
Faculty, Respiratory Therapy Program, GateWay Community College, Phoenix, Arizona

Bryan Dodd, MEd, RDMS, RVT(R)RT
Faculty, Diagnostic Medical Sonography Program, GateWay Community College, Phoenix, Arizona

Mary J. Carillo, MBA, HCMRT(R)(M)CDT
Program Director, Medical Radiography Program
GateWay Community College
Phoenix, Arizona

Jennifer M. Phoebe, BSN
Tucson, Arizona

A special thanks to our editors: Ellen Wurm-Cutter, Kristen Mandava, Celeste Clingan, and all the experts from Elsevier for their support and encouragement during the revision of this edition.

About the Authors

Elaine A. Gillingham started her health care career in Sandusky, Ohio, working after school at a local hospital, and was on-the-job-trained as a Health Unit Coordinator. In 1977, she moved to Phoenix, Arizona, met Myrna LaFleur Brooks and Winnie Starr, who encouraged her to obtain a certificate of completion in Health Unit Coordinating and an Associate Degree in Health Services Management from GateWay Community College. She later obtained a Bachelor's degree in education from Ottawa University. Ms. Gillingham served as president of the Phoenix chapter of the National Association of Health Unit Coordinators and sat on the National Board for 2 years. In 1983, she wrote questions for and sat for the first National Certification exam sponsored by the National Association of Health Unit Coordinators. Ms. Gillingham has been teaching in the Health Unit Coordinator Program at GateWay Community College since 1987 and served as Program Director from 1993 to 2005. After retiring, she has been teaching on a part-time basis and traveling. Ms. Gillingham began reviewing, consulting, and writing for the Health Unit Coordinating books in 1993.

Monica Melzer Wadsworth Seibel received her Bachelor of Science degree in Zoology from Arizona State University in 1983 and her Master of Educational Leadership degree from Northern Arizona University in 2002. After working as a Health Unit coordinator in the emergency and cardiovascular intensive care units at Humana Hospital in Phoenix, she acted as the data Coordinator for the Heart/Lung Transplant Program administered by Humana Hospital and the Arizona Heart Institute. She met Myrna LaFleur Brooks while on the job and was given the opportunity to teach as an adjunct instructor with Elaine Gillingham in the Health Unit Coordinating Program at GateWay Community College. After teaching on a part-time basis for 5 years, she was hired as full-time residential faculty in 1992. She has served as the Program Director since the retirement of Ms. Gillingham in 2005, and is currently a member of the GateWay Faculty Senate. Ms. Wadsworth Seibel was a contributing author for the 4th and 6th edition of the Health Unit Coordinating textbook. She is a member of the National Association of Health Unit Coordinators (NAHUC) as well as the American Rock Art Research Association (ARARA).

Contents

CHAPTER 1

Health Unit Coordinating:
An Allied Health Career

OUTLINE

CHAPTER OBJECTIVES

On completion of this chapter, you will be able to:

1. Define the terms in the vocabulary list.
2. Write the meaning of the abbreviations in the abbreviations list.
3. Identify four stages that health professions have traditionally gone through to become a profession.
4. Explain the events that led up to creating the position that eventually became known as *health unit coordinator* (HUC).
5. List five benefits of being a member of the National Association of Health Unit Coordinators.
6. List five benefits of becoming a certified HUC.
7. List three tasks that the HUC would perform related to each of the following: nursing personnel, doctors, hospital departments, patients, and hospital visitors.
8. Discuss the benefits of using the electronic medical record (EMR), computer physician order entry (CPOE) with e-prescribing, and clinical decision support system (CDSS).
9. Identify four ways to prepare for the changing HUC position with the use of EMR and six things that the HUC can do to stay current in the position.
10. Demonstrate use of the Internet and search engines to locate information on the Web.
11. List three positions in which the HUC may be cross-trained.
12. List two possible nonclinical career choices for the health unit coordinator.

VOCABULARY

Browser A computer program that allows one to search for and view (or hear) various kinds of information on the Web, such as websites, videos, and audio files.

Certification The process of testifying that a person has met certain standards, or endorsing him or her as having met them.

Certified Health Unit Coordinator (CHUC) A health unit coordinator who has passed the national certification examination sponsored by the National Association of Health Unit Coordinators (NAHUC).

Clinical Decision Support System (CDSS) An interactive decision support system (DSS) computer program designed to assist physicians at the point of order entry.

Clinical Tasks Tasks performed at the bedside or in direct contact with the patient (direct patient care).

Computer Physician Order Entry (CPOE) A computerized program into which physicians directly enter patient orders; replaces handwritten orders on an order sheet or prescription pad.

Doctor A person licensed to practice medicine (used interchangeably with the term *physician* throughout this textbook).

Doctor's Orders The health care that a doctor prescribes in writing for a hospitalized patient.

Electronic Medical Record (EMR) An electronic record of patient health information generated by one or more encounters in any care delivery setting.

E-Prescribing (electronic prescribing) The electronic transmission of prescription information from the prescriber's computer (hospital or doctor's office) to a pharmacy computer.

Health Unit Coordinator (HUC) The health care team member who performs nonclinical patient care tasks for the nursing unit (also may be called *unit clerk* or *unit secretary*).

Hospital Departments Divisions within the hospital that specialize in services, such as the nutritional care department, which plans and prepares meals for patients, employees, and visitors.

Internet Service Provider A company that provides Internet connections and services to individuals and organizations for a monthly fee.

Meaningful Use (EMR) Use of certified electronic medical record (EMR) technology in ways that can be measured significantly in quality and in quantity.

Nonclinical Tasks Tasks performed away from the bedside (indirect patient care).

Nurses' Station The desk area of a nursing unit.

Nursing Team A group of nursing staff members who care for patients on a nursing unit.

Nursing Unit An area within the hospital that includes equipment and nursing personnel available for the care of a given number of patients (also may be referred to as a *wing, floor, pod, ward,* or *station*).

Patient (pt) A person who receives health care, including preventive, promotional, acute, and chronic, and all other services in the continuum of care.

Policies and Procedures Information such as guidelines for practice and hospital regulations found online or in a manual.

Recertification A process by which certified health unit coordinators exhibit continued personal and professional growth and current competency to practice in the field.

Search Engine A website that collects and organizes content from all over the Web.

Surfing the Web Using different search engines on the Web to locate information.

Transcription A process used to communicate the doctors' orders to the nursing staff and other hospital departments; computers or handwritten requisitions are used.

Web Address (uniform resource locator [URL]) A series of characters (often preceded by "http://www") that, when entered into the address bar of an Internet browser will take the user to a specified location, referred to as a *website*.

ABBREVIATIONS

Abbreviation	Meaning
CDSS	clinical decision support system
CHUC	certified health unit coordinator
CPOE	computer physician order entry
EMR or EHR	electronic medical (health) record
HIMSS	Healthcare Information and Management Systems Society
HUC	health unit coordinator
SHUC	student health unit coordinator
pt	patient
www	World Wide Web

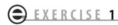 EXERCISE **1**

Note: All exercises in this textbook are provided on the Evolve website. To access your student resources, visit http://evolve.elsevier.com/Gillingham/HUC/.

Write the abbreviation for each term listed.

1. certified health unit coordinator
2. electronic medical (health) record
3. student health unit coordinator
4. patient
5. health unit coordinator
6. clinical decision support system
7. computer physician order entry
8. Healthcare Information and Management Systems Society
9. World Wide Web

EXERCISE **2**

Write the meaning of each abbreviation listed.

1. CHUC
2. EMR or EHR
3. SHUC
4. CDSS
5. HUC
6. pt
7. CPOE
8. HIMSS
9. www

INTRODUCTION TO HEALTH UNIT COORDINATING

The **health unit coordinator (HUC)** is usually the first person encountered when one walks onto a hospital **nursing unit.** The HUC has always been considered essential to the **nursing team** and to the effectiveness of the unit. The HUC coordinates activities on the unit, monitors the **electronic medical record (EMR)**, or transcribes handwritten or preprinted **doctor's orders,** and functions under the direction of the nurse manager or unit manager. The overall job is **nonclinical** in nature, and the work area is the **nurses' station** (Fig. 1-1). Most everyone who works on or visits the nursing unit depends on the HUC for information and assistance.

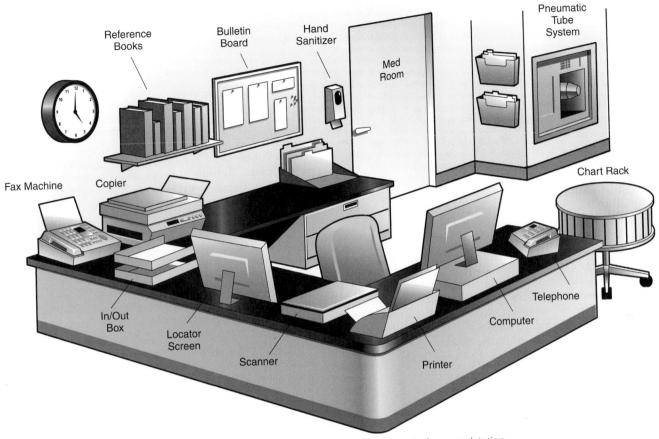

Figure 1-1 The health unit coordinator's work area is the nurses' station.

Comments often heard in the hospital include the following:

- "We are so disorganized if the HUC isn't here."
- "The HUC creates the attitude for the entire unit."
- "The HUC sets the pace for the day's work."
- "Ask the HUC—HUCs usually know everything."

Working on a nursing unit can be very fast paced and stressful; the HUC must possess a calming, pleasant, and professional attitude, because the HUC sets the tone for the unit. Whether an efficient HUC is working on a nursing unit is usually obvious to anyone who walks onto that unit. If the HUC is having a bad day or is in a bad mood, the whole unit is affected because everyone has to interact with the HUC. It is important for staff members to maintain a positive, friendly attitude when working on the nursing unit. The HUC can enhance or inhibit the delivery of health care to patients on the unit. The position involves many responsibilities associated with assisting the nursing staff, **doctors,** hospital departments, patients, and visitors to the nursing unit (Fig. 1-2). Many health care facilities require the HUC to wear scrubs, sometimes in a particular color, whereas other facilities opt for professional, nonclinical dress. In some facilities, HUCs may be cross-trained and may alternate working as HUCs, a nonclinical position—away from the patient bedside—and as certified nursing assistants (CNAs; discussed in Chapter 3), a

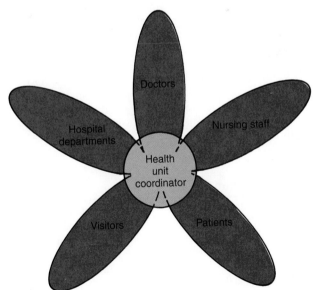

Figure 1-2 The health unit coordinator coordinates the activities of doctors, nursing staff, hospital departments, patients, and visitors on the nursing unit.

clinical position—at the **patient (pt)** bedside. HUCs also may be employed in doctors' offices, clinics, and long-term care facilities to assist with clerical or management duties related to patients' health records.

HISTORY OF HEALTH UNIT COORDINATING

Traditionally, health professions have evolved through four stages: on-the-job training, formal education, formation of a national association, and certification or licensure. Health unit coordinating is no exception to this tradition.

On-the-Job-Training

During World War II, hospitals experienced a drastic shortage of registered nurses. To compensate for this shortage, auxiliary personnel were trained on the job. The HUC was trained to assist the nurse with nonclinical tasks, and the nursing assistant was trained to assist the nurse at the bedside.

After World War II ended, the nursing shortage was not as critical; however, as technology advanced and the workload of the doctor increased, many tasks shifted to the nursing staff (e.g., taking blood pressure and starting intravenous therapy). Hospitals were becoming larger and more complex; there were more specialists, who were ordering newly available tests and treatments. Federally sponsored health programs required more detailed record keeping, and nonclinical demands for every hospitalized patient increased proportionately, so the need to employ HUCs continued. Today HUCs remain valued members of the hospital's health care team, and the role continues to change and expand. HUCs were trained on the job for longer than 20 years (Fig. 1-3, *A* and *B*).

FIRST RECORD OF HEALTH UNIT COORDINATING—1940

An article published in *Modern Hospital* authored by Abraham Oseroff, a hospital administrator, stated, "A new helper was introduced to the nursing unit to take care of the many details of a secretarial nature that formerly made demands on the limited time of the nurse." The title of the new helper was "floor secretary." Oseroff wrote, "The idea of floor secretary was first met with skepticism, but it proved to be worthwhile from the beginning." The hospital was Montefiore Hospital in Pittsburgh, Pennsylvania.

Formal Education

In 1966 a research project led to the implementation of one of the first educational programs for health unit coordinating at a vocational school in Minneapolis (Fig. 1-3, *C*). An article published in *Nursing Outlook* authored by Ruth Stryker described the project and recommended that the title "ward" or "unit clerk" be changed to "station coordinator" because the data showed that the unit clerk did a great deal of managing in the form of coordinating activities. Ruth Stryker later wrote one of the first textbooks for health unit coordinating, *The Hospital Ward Clerk*, which was published by the C.V. Mosby Company in 1970.

Today, before employment, most HUCs are educated in one of the many community colleges or vocational technical schools nationwide that offer HUC educational programs. The individual who completes a program emerges with better preparation for the job and a greater knowledge base on which to build. Educational programs outline the competencies or job skills that students are expected to acquire by the time they have completed the program (Box 1-1, *Example of Competencies for an Educational Program for the Student Health Unit Coordinator*).

Professional Association

The HUC position existed and grew for 40 years without the guidance of a professional association. The purpose of a professional association is to set standards of education and practice for peers to be enforced by peers for the protection of the public. Altruistic in nature, it is designed to enlighten its members and guide the profession to better serve the public. The constitution states the basic laws and principles of the association, and elected officers carry out the purpose listed in the constitution. By 1980, several HUC educational programs were well established across the nation, and educators in these programs began to discuss the possibility of forming a national association.

The first organizational meeting was held in Phoenix, Arizona, on August 23, 1980. This date has since been proclaimed National Health Unit Coordinator Day by the national association. The 10 founding members who represented both education and practice (Box 1-2, *Founding Members of the National Association of Health Unit Coordinators*) declared the formation of a national association for health coordinators to be called the *National Association of Health Unit Coordinators (NAHUC)* (Fig. 1-3, *D*). A new title, Health Unit Clerk/Coordinator, was created for the position; the title would be updated and used consistently nationwide. Because "unit clerk" was the most popular title nationwide in 1980, it was included in the title with the intent that it would be dropped when the term "coordinator" became recognized. In 1990, the national association became the National Association of Health Unit Coordinators, after "clerk" was dropped from its name (Fig. 1-3, *F*).

At the second organizational meeting, held in San Juan Capistrano, California, the constitution was ratified and the officers were elected. Standards of Practice (see Chapter 6), including educational requirements and a code of ethics (see Chapter 6), were adopted.

The NAHUC Board of Directors consists of the President, Vice President, Secretary/Treasurer, Communication Director, Membership Director, Certification Board Director, and Education Board Director. (See Box 1-3, *Five Reasons to Become a Member of the National Association of Health Unit Coordinators*, and Box 1-4, *National Association of Health Unit Coordinators Membership Information*.)

Certification

Certification and/or licensure is the final step in the evolution of a health profession. Certification is the process of testifying or endorsing that a person has met certain standards. The first certification examination was offered by NAHUC in May 1983. American Guidance Service, a professional testing company, was employed to administer the test. Nearly 5000 people took the first examination (Fig. 1-3, *E*). Today this examination is administered nationwide through an electronic system by another testing agency, Applied Measurement Professionals (AMP), at testing sites. Questions are answered

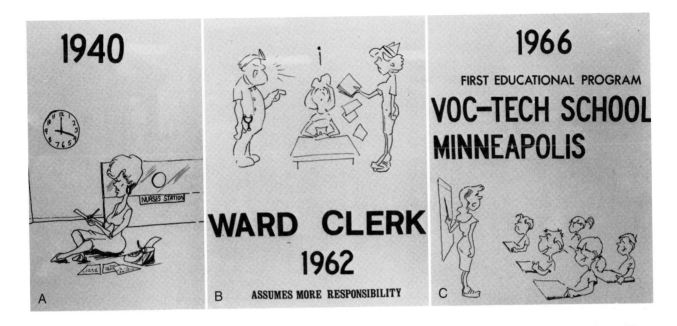

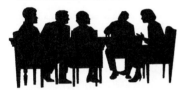

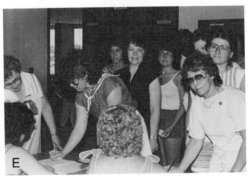

First certification exam

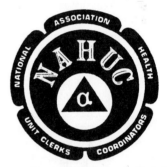

Logo prior to 1990 showing "unit clerk"

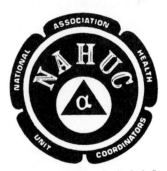

F   Logo as of 1990 — "unit clerks"
dropped

Figure 1-3 History of health unit coordinating. **A,** In 1940, health unit coordinating was first introduced as a health care occupation. The first job title was "floor secretary." **B,** In 1962 the more common title was "ward clerk." More responsibilities were added to the job. **C,** In 1966 the first vocational educational program for health unit coordinating was established. **D,** On August 23, 1980, the first meeting to discuss the formation of the National Association of Health Unit Coordinators/ Clerks was held in Phoenix, Arizona. **E,** In 1983 the first certification examination was offered by the National Association of Health Unit Coordinators/Clerks. **F,** Logo for the National Association of Health Unit Coordinators. The five outer segments represent doctors, nursing staff, patients, visitors, and hospital departments. The circle that connects the segments is symbolic of the health care coordinator's role in coordinating the activities of these five groups. In 1990, "clerk" was dropped from the name of the association, which is now known as the *National Association of Health Unit Coordinators.*

BOX 1-1	**EXAMPLE OF COMPETENCIES FOR AN EDUCATIONAL PROGRAM FOR THE STUDENT HEALTH UNIT COORDINATOR**

On completion of this program, the student demonstrated the ability to:

- perform health unit coordinator (HUC) tasks and provide accountability to nursing personnel, medical staff, other hospital departments, patients, and visitors
- manage and operate the nursing unit communication systems, including Internet, telephone, scanner, fax machine, intercom (patient call lights), locator, mobile wireless devices, and pager systems
- record diagnostic test values, vital signs, and census data; order daily diets and daily laboratory tests (when required)
- scan reports into the patient's electronic medical record (EMR) or send them to Health Information Management (if paper charts are used, insert the reports into the patient's chart)
- transcribe doctors' orders (when paper charts are used) or monitor patient orders (when electronic medical records are used) using basic knowledge of anatomy and physiology, disease processes, medical terminology, and approved abbreviations
- coordinate scheduling of patients' tests and diagnostic procedures (when required)
- prepare patient consent forms (when required)
- transcribe medication orders, incorporating concepts of drug categories, automatic stop dates, time scheduling, and routes of administration (when paper charts are used) (most hospitals have implemented e-prescribing, eliminating the transcription of medications by the HUC)
- schedule radiologic procedures that require patient preparation (when required)
- maintain patients' paper charts, or manage patients' electronic records
- perform nonclinical tasks required for patient admission, transfer, discharge, and preoperative and postoperative procedures
- plan and execute a daily routine for the performance of nonclinical tasks for the nursing unit
- manage the nonclinical functions of the nursing unit and maintain nursing unit equipment and supplies
- distribute wireless mobile devices at the beginning of shift and collect at end of shift
- communicate effectively with patients, visitors, and members of the health care team
- listen to patient and visitor complaints and concerns, and use problem-solving skills
- practice within the professional ethical framework of health unit coordinating

---

BOX 1-2	**FOUNDING MEMBERS OF THE NATIONAL ASSOCIATION OF HEALTH UNIT COORDINATORS**

Kathy Jordan, Winnie Starr, Connie Johnston, Estelle Johnson, and Myrna LaFleur from Arizona
Kay Cox from California
Helga Hegge from Minnesota
Jane Pedersen from Wisconsin
Carolyn Hinken from New Mexico
Velma Kerschner from Texas

BOX 1-3	**FIVE REASONS TO BECOME A MEMBER OF THE NATIONAL ASSOCIATION OF HEALTH UNIT COORDINATORS**

1. Professional representation
2. Forum for sharing ideas and challenges—assistance in being prepared and proactive regarding changes that are taking place in health care and the HUC profession
3. National networking
4. National directory
5. Opportunity to develop leadership skills

BOX 1-4	**NATIONAL ASSOCIATION OF HEALTH UNIT COORDINATORS MEMBERSHIP INFORMATION**

To receive a National Association of Health Unit Coordinators (NAHUC) membership application, contact NAHUC in the following ways:

Phone:
  Toll-free: 888-22-NAHUC (62482)
  Local: 815-633-4351
Address: 1947 Madron Road
             Rockford, IL 61107-1716
Fax: 815-633-4438
Website: www.nahuc.org
E-mail: office@nahuc.org

---

on a touch-sensitive computer screen, and test results are given immediately on completion of the examination. The test is available to anyone with a General Educational Development (GED) certificate or a high school diploma.

It is not necessary to be a member of NAHUC or to have completed an educational program to sit for the examination as some HUCs have been trained on the job and have years of experience. The goal of every HUC or future HUC should be to become a **certified health unit coordinator (CHUC)**. Passing the national certification examination indicates that one has met a standard of excellence and is competent to practice health unit coordinating (Box 1-5, *Five Reasons to Become*

BOX 1-5	FIVE REASONS TO BECOME CERTIFIED

1. Enhanced credibility
2. Broader perspective on health unit coordinating (not just one specialty)—opportunity to be prepared and proactive regarding changes that are taking place in health care and the health unit coordinator profession
3. Increased mobility, geographically and vertically
4. Peer and public recognition and respect
5. Improved self-image

BOX 1-6	TO MAKE A RESERVATION FOR THE CERTIFICATION EXAMINATION FOR HEALTH UNIT COORDINATORS

Reservations may be made online by linking to Applied Measurement Professionals (AMP) from the National Association of Health Unit Coordinators (NAHUC) website: www.nahuc.org. (The current candidate handbook can also be downloaded; Adobe Acrobat Reader is needed to download.)

Alternatively, call NAHUC at 815-633-4351 or 888-22-NAHUC or e-mail the NAHUC office to request information concerning NAHUC certification.

Or call AMP (Applied Measurement Professionals) at 888-519-9901 or e-mail AMP through www.goAMP.com.

Certified, and Box 1-6, *To Make a Reservation for the Certification Examination for Health Unit Coordinators*).

Recertification

Recertification is a process by which CHUCs exhibit continued personal and professional growth and current competency to practice in the field. The NAHUC requires certified HUCs to be recertified to ensure that they stay current in their field of practice. Recertification may be achieved by taking the test every 3 years or by earning continuing education units (CEUs). NAHUC offers various opportunities for acquiring CEUs. Also, employers often offer seminars and workshops that provide CEUs to the HUCs in their health care facility or in the community.

The dedication of HUCs nationwide in developing and implementing these practices (Box 1-7, *For a Group to Become a Profession*) have advanced health unit coordinating to the level of professionalism it deserves.

ROLE OF THE HEALTH UNIT COORDINATOR

Responsibilities and Interactions of the Health Unit Coordinator

Nursing Personnel

Responsibilities of HUCs vary among health care facilities, especially between those that are using paper charts and those using the electronic record. The HUC is a member of the

BOX 1-7	FOR A GROUP TO BECOME A PROFESSION

The following credentials are required:
- A national association
- A formal education
- Certification or licensure
- A code of ethics
- An identified body of systematic knowledge and technical skill
- Members who function with a degree of autonomy and authority under the assumption that they alone have the expertise to make decisions in their area of competence

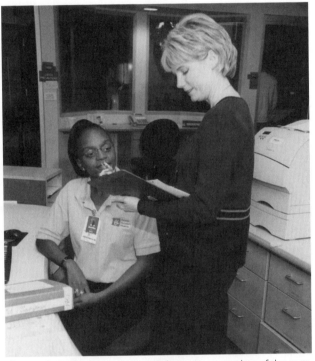

Figure 1-4 The health unit coordinator is a member of the nursing team and usually functions under the direction of the nurse manager or unit manager.

health care team (Fig. 1-4) and usually functions under the direction of the nurse manager or unit manager. Responsibilities include the following:

- Communicate all new doctors' orders or messages to the patient's nurse
- Maintain the patient's paper chart or manage the electronic record
- Communicate information involving new patient arrivals and requests for patient transfers
- Perform the **nonclinical tasks** required for admission, discharge, and transfer of a patient
- Prepare the patient's chart for surgery (if a paper chart is in use)
- Prepare necessary consent forms for patient surgeries or procedures

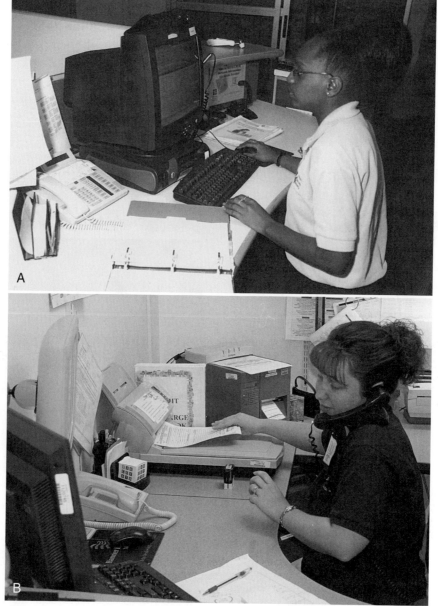

Figure 1-5 A, A major responsibility of the health unit coordinator (HUC) when paper charts are used is to transcribe doctors' orders. **B,** A major responsibility of the HUC when the electronic record is used is to scan reports and documents into the patient's electronic record.

- Handle all telephone communication for the nursing unit
- Maintain nursing unit supplies

Additional responsibilities may include the following:

- Create time schedules for nursing unit staff
- Monitor and maintain documentation required by The Joint Commission (TJC) on licenses and certifications and in-services for nursing unit staff

Doctors

The HUC assists the doctor as necessary in the following ways:

- Assists in finding patients' charts
- Assists as necessary with physician order entry if EMR is used

- Transcribes the doctors' orders (if paper charts are used) (Fig. 1-5, *A*)
- Scans reports or documents into the patient's electronic record (or sends to Health Information Management) (Fig. 1-5, *B*)
- Procures requested equipment for patient examinations
- Places calls to and receive calls from doctors' offices
- Obtains information for the physician regarding whether previously ordered procedures have been completed (Fig. 1-6)

Hospital Departments

The HUC interacts with hospital departments in the following ways:

- Orders, schedules, and coordinates diagnostic procedures and treatments when required

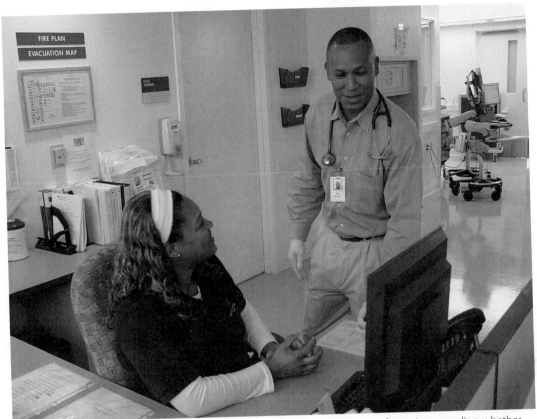

Figure 1-6 The health unit coordinator assists the doctor in obtaining information regarding whether previously ordered procedures have been completed.

- Relays messages and information to appropriate departments as required
- Requests services from maintenance and other service departments
- Works closely with the admitting department to admit, transfer, and discharge patients
- Orders supplies for the nursing unit ranging from food to paper products and patient care supplies

Patients

The HUC greets new patients when they arrive on the nursing unit and may accompany them to their rooms (Fig. 1-7, *A*). Responsibilities may include the following:

- Instruct new patients on how to use the call light (Fig. 1-7, *B*), turn on the television, and operate bed controls
- Relay patient requests to nursing personnel when answering the intercom located in each patient's room
- Greet and listen to concerns or requests of patients who come to the nursing station (the HUC usually has little bedside contact with patients)

The HUC can enhance or inhibit the delivery of health care to patients on the nursing unit. HUCs also may be employed in doctors' offices, clinics, and long-term care facilities to assist the nurse with clerical duties related to patients' health records.

Hospital Visitors

The HUC is usually the first person the visitors encounter when arriving at the nursing station. Responsibilities may include the following:

- Assist visitors looking for a patient by locating the patient on the computer (Fig. 1-8)
- Provide information about the location of bathrooms, visitors' lounge, cafeteria, and so on
- Inform visitors about the rules of visitation, and explain any special precautions that may be required during their visit to a patient's room
- Receive telephone calls from relatives or friends who are inquiring about the patient's condition
- Listen to, document, and handle visitor concerns

Introduction to the Electronic Medical Record and Computer Physician Order Entry

The EMR is a computerized medical record created by a hospital or physician's office. Electronic medical records tend to be a part of a local stand-alone health information system that allows storage, retrieval, and modification of records. **Computer physician order entry (CPOE)** allows physicians to enter orders directly into the computer rather than writing them by hand. The orders are then automatically sent to the appropriate departments. **E-prescribing (electronic prescribing)** is the electronic transmission of medication orders (prescriptions) from the prescriber's computer to the pharmacy computer. E-prescribing eliminates the HUC's responsibility of transcribing medication orders and having to interpret the doctor's handwriting.

A **clinical decision support system (CDSS)** offers assistance to the physician at the point of entering patient orders. A patient's height, weight, and medication history including drug and food allergies is entered (by the patient's admitting

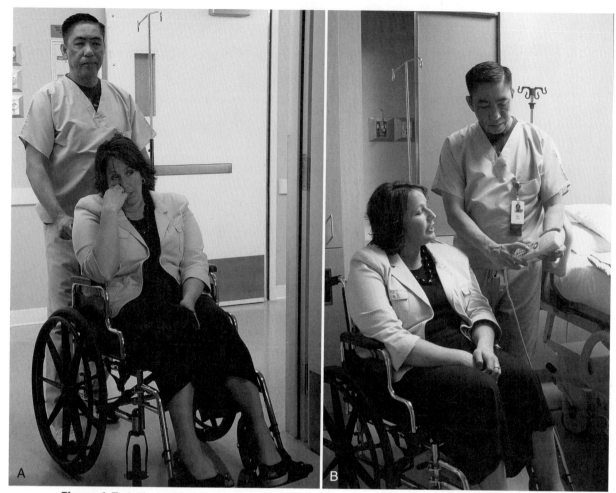

Figure 1-7 A, The health unit coordinator (HUC) may greet the new patient on arrival to the nursing unit and may accompany the patient to the assigned room. **B,** The HUC may instruct new patients on use of the call light, television, computer Internet connection, and so on.

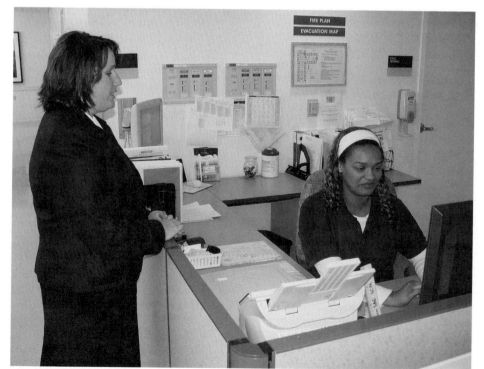

Figure 1-8 The health unit coordinator informs visitors about the location of the patient, visiting hours, and any special precautions that may be required.

nurse or by the pharmacist) into the EMR. When the physician is entering the patient's orders, the CDSS will provide prompts that warn against the possibility of a drug interaction, an incorrect dose, or a patient allergy. The system also may provide reminders to the physician, such as a reminder to order aspirin for a patient who is going home after undergoing heart surgery

Changes in Health Unit Coordinating

Most of the HUC's time has been spent on interpretation and transcription of doctors' hand written orders and paper chart management. With the use of EMRs and CPOE, the HUC's role has become more administrative. Responsibilities include traffic control, coordination of care, and management of the electronic record.

Comments that have been made by experienced HUCs working in hospitals that have implemented the EMR with CPOE include the following:

- "It's awesome! No more trying to decipher a doctor's terrible handwriting!"
- "No more hunting down charts or having them taken away from me before I'm finished with them. More than one person can be viewing and working on a patient's chart at the same time."
- "Patient information is always current and at your fingertips."
- "I can spend more time helping visitors and staff with their needs."
- "I have time to help the nurse manager with administrative work."
- "I'm busy from the time I get here until I leave, but it's a less stressful busy!"

Transitioning to Electronic Medical Records with Computer Physician Order Entry

The use of EMR with CPOE and CDSS and e-prescribing in hospitals as well as in doctors' offices can significantly improve patient care by reducing the risk of human error in interpreting doctors' handwriting. Also, the ability to access all of the patient information, which is organized in one place, at the click of a mouse eliminates the duplication of tests, reduces delays in treatment, and can help doctors collaborate more effectively, as patients often see a variety of specialists. The federal government is encouraging adoption of **meaningful use of EMRs** and other health information technology. Under the American Recovery and Reinvestment Act of 2009 (ARRA), about $20 billion has been appropriated for EMR "incentives" payable to health care providers over a 5-year period.

The Healthcare Information and Management Systems Society (HIMSS) is a nonprofit organization dedicated to improving the quality, safety, and cost-effectiveness of and access to health care through the best use of information technology and management systems. HIMSS Analytics, the authoritative source on EMR adoption trends, devised the EMR Adoption Model to track EMR progress at hospitals and health systems. The EMR Adoption Model consists of eight stages (numbered 0 to 7), with the goal being to reach stage 7. Stage 0 indicates that the key ancillary department systems (e.g., laboratory, pharmacy, radiology) do not have the EMR installed. More capabilities are added with each stage until stage 7, at which the paper chart is no longer used and the physician has the

BOX 1-8	**THREE COMPONENTS OF ELECTRONIC MEDICAL RECORD (EMR) MEANINGFUL USE (AS OUTLINED BY THE AMERICAN RECOVERY AND REINVESTMENT ACT)**

1. The use of a certified EMR in a meaningful manner, such as e-prescribing.
2. The use of certified EMR technology for electronic exchange of health information to improve quality of health care.
3. The use of certified EMR technology to submit clinical quality and other measures. The Medicare and Medicaid EMR Incentive Programs will provide incentive payments to eligible professionals, eligible hospitals, and critical access hospitals as they adopt, implement, upgrade, or demonstrate meaningful use of certified EMR technology.

For more information on the implementation of the EMR, see Chapter 2.

ability to enter orders on the computer into the patient's EMR. At stage 7 there is the ability to share interoperable patient data and analyze clinical data for performance and improvements, and CDSS is implemented. As of the end of the first quarter of 2012 1.2% of hospitals in the United States have been validated by HIMSS Analytics to be at stage 7 (Box 1-8, *Three Components of Electronic Medical Record [EMR] Meaningful Use [as Outlined by the American Recovery and Reinvestment Act]*).

Note: To view the current U.S. EMR Adoption Model go to: www.himssanalytics.org

⭐ HIGH PRIORITY

HealthGrades is the leading health care ratings organization, providing ratings and profiles of hospitals, nursing homes, and physicians to consumers, corporations, health plans, and hospitals. HealthGrades's hospital ratings are independently created; no hospital can opt in or opt out of being rated, and no hospital pays to be rated. Consumers can go to the **Web address** (uniform resource locator [URL]) www.healthgrades.com to see how hospitals or doctors in their area are rated.

The Health Unit Coordinator Position with the Use of Electronic Records and Computer Physician Order Entry

Over the years, with advances in technology, health care has undergone many changes—a trend that will continue into the future. Change can be stressful but is most often an opportunity for growth. Those working in the health care field must be flexible and proactive to deal with these changes. The use of the EMR has had a dramatic effect on the role of the HUC. The main focus of the HUC position has been **transcription** involving the reading of often illegible physicians' handwriting and making sure each order is completed and properly documented. The implementation of the

EMR and CPOE has changed the HUC position to a more administrative, customer service–oriented role. Responsibilities consist of receptionist duties, coordination of the nursing unit, and monitoring of the electronic record, including scheduling, coordinating ordered procedures, arranging consultations, preparing consent forms, and scanning various reports and documents that will become part of the patient's permanent record (in some hospitals documents may be sent to Health Information Management). The HUC will still on occasion be asked to enter an order by a patient's doctor or nurse in an emergency situation. Often health care facilities train the HUC as a "super user" of the EMR in order to be a resource person for doctors and other health care professionals. Other administrative tasks will be explained in future chapters. Internet, other advanced computer database, communication, organization, management, and leadership skills are required for interfacing with health care personnel, visitors, and patients.

Suggestions for Preparing for a Health Unit Coordinator Position

- Complete a HUC program.
- Complete communication and management classes related to health care
- Complete advanced computer classes including advanced computer skills (typing and keyboarding, Microsoft Office [including Word, Excel, PowerPoint, Access, and Outlook]) and, if possible, an electronic medical records class.
- Become a member of NAHUC.
- Become certified by taking the national health unit coordinator certification test.

★ **HIGH PRIORITY**

Internet and advanced computer skills (typing and keyboarding, Microsoft Office [including Word, Excel, PowerPoint, Access, and Outlook]); basic knowledge of electronic medical records; and communication, organization, management, and leadership skills are required for the new health unit coordinator role.

Suggestions for Staying Current in the Health Unit Coordinator Profession

- Attend job-related in-services that are offered through the hospital.
- Take classes that are available at local community colleges (most hospitals have a continuing education program).
- Stay active in the National Association of Health Unit Coordinators.
- Receive and read the NAHUC newsletter and attend conferences.
- Keep certification current by taking the certification test or by obtaining continuing education units.
- Be curious—research new procedures or information on the Web.

★ **HIGH PRIORITY**

Because not all hospitals have yet fully implemented the electronic medical record with computer physician order entry, information will be provided throughout this book for working as a health unit coordinator with and without implementation of the electronic medical record.

Understanding and Using the Internet

The HUC has access to the Internet because the hospital pays a company called an **internet service provider** to supply Internet access. A **browser** is a software application used to locate and display webpages. Currently, the three most popular browsers are *Microsoft Internet Explorer*, *Mozilla Firefox*, and *Google Chrome*. To locate information requires use of an application called a **search engine**—a website that collects and organizes content from all over the Web. When searching or "surfing" for information, the user enters a key word or phrase into a provided text box and presses "enter"; search results (commonly called "hits") containing information that is related to the specified word or phrase are usually presented in a list of websites that may contain articles, blogs, images, videos, and so on (Box 1-9, *Guidelines for Surfing the Web*).

Surfing the Web is much like "channel surfing" the television. In channel surfing the television, information may be found that is old, or the information may not be reliable or worthwhile. The same is true when surfing the Web: information may be old, outdated, or not reliable or worthwhile. When surfing for information on the Web, one should view sites from at least three different reliable sources (e.g., government agencies, universities, hospitals, news outlets, medical journals, national associations such as NAHUC). It is

BOX 1-9	**GUIDELINES FOR SURFING THE WEB**

- Choose words or phrases that accurately describe what you are searching for.
- Enter the words or phrases into the text box provided in a selected search engine.
- Generally, capitalization and punctuation are not needed.
- Choose reliable websites such as those belonging to government agencies, universities, hospitals, news outlets, medical journals, and so on.
- Check the date on which the article or information was written or the site was last updated.
- Change the search words to be more specific if you are unable to find information.

A Few Common Search Engines
www.google.com
www.yahoo.com
www.MSNsearch.com
www.ask.com
www.dogpile.com
www.webopedia.com
  Some websites listed in the Websites of Interest box may be good search options.

important to check the date on which the article or information was written or when the site was last updated. If unable to find wanted information, change the search words to be more specific. For example, if searching for information about the number of hospitals using stage 7 EMR, choose a search engine such as www.google.com and enter "hospitals using stage 7 EMR" in the text box provided by the search engine; to narrow the search to a particular area, change the search words to, for instance, "Arizona hospitals using stage 7 EMR." If a site that would provide the exact information is known, the Web address (uniform resource locator [URL]) (e.g., www.himssanalytics.org) would be entered into the text box.

Employment and Job Description
Hospital Policies and Procedures

Hospital **policies and procedures (found online or in a manual)** contain hospital-specific policies and procedures on topics such as identification badges, medical record training, and pagers. All staff members are responsible for being knowledgeable about and complying with hospital policies and procedures and should review them from time to time, as they are subject to change. The tasks that may be performed by the HUC are many and vary greatly among hospitals and even among units within a hospital. Implementation of the EMR with CPOE has resulted in the elimination of transcribing doctors' orders and the addition of many new tasks to the HUC job description.

Hospitals outline responsibilities for each category of employee in a formal written statement called a *job description*. Because health unit coordinating practices vary, it is important to research and review the hospital's job description before applying for a position. Examples of job descriptions for an HUC with and without implementation of the EMR and the CPOE are provided in the following sections.

Examples of Job Descriptions

A job description for an HUC Using EMR and CPOE may include the following:

- Coordinate administrative functions on the nursing unit.
- Make decisions and take follow-up action to ensure effective communication and information flow throughout the nursing department.
- Perform receptionist or clerical duties on the nursing unit.
- Handle customer problems or collect necessary data and follow through to appropriate person for problem resolution.
- Monitor and maintain the electronic record.
- Manage the maintenance of equipment (notify appropriate department) on the nursing unit, including computers, printers, telephone, fax machines, locators, mobile wireless devices, telemetry, and so on.
- Distribute mobile wireless devices at beginning of shift and collect at end of shift.
- Place requests to the nutritional care department and to the appropriate department for other unit supplies.
- Coordinate patient activities and patient information.
- Assist the nursing staff as needed with processing of medical records related to patient admission, discharge, and transfer.

- Maintain confidentiality of patient information.
- Integrate or scan paper documents created by caregivers into the EMR.
- Send electronic requisitions for clerical, office, nutritional care, and medical supplies, and maintain adequate supply levels on the nursing unit.
- Input data for reports, and assist in the coordination of mandatory education and skill assessment.
- Maintain the nursing bulletin board.
- Assist with staffing and scheduling.
- Compile statistical data and prepare reports.
- Provide assistance in process improvement.
- Be trained and serve as a "super user" of the EMR in order to be a resource for doctors and other health care professionals.
- Manage the maintenance of equipment (notify appropriate department) on the nursing unit including computers, printers, telephones, fax machines, locators, mobile wireless devices, telemetry, and so on.
- Be aware of hospital policies and procedures (and where to locate them) that are relevant to the HUC position.

A job description for an HUC using paper charts may include the following:

- Communicate all new doctors' orders to the patient's nurse.
- Maintain the patient's paper chart.
- Perform nonclinical tasks required for patient admission, discharge, and transfer.
- Prepare the patient's chart for surgery.
- Handle all telephone communication for the nursing unit.
- Greet doctors on their arrival to the nurses' station, and assist them, if necessary, in obtaining patients' charts.
- Obtain information regarding scheduling of tests.
- Locate and print out test results.
- Transcribe the doctors' orders.
- Place phone calls to and receive calls from doctors' offices.
- Schedule diagnostic procedures and treatments.
- Request services from maintenance and other service departments.
- Work closely with the admitting department to admit, transfer, and discharge patients.
- Order all supplies for the nursing unit, ranging from food to paper products and patient care supplies.
- Recapture lost supply purchasing department charges.
- Manage the maintenance of equipment (notify appropriate department) on the nursing unit, including computers, printers, telephones, fax machines, locators, mobile wireless devices, telemetry, and so on.
- Greet new patients when they arrive on the nursing unit and accompany them to their rooms.
- Answer patient call lights on intercom and relay patient requests to the nurse.
- Use the intercom or locators to locate health care personnel and/or to relay patient requests to nursing staff. (The HUC usually has little bedside contact with patients.)
- Distribute mobile wireless devices at beginning of shift and collect at end of shift.

- Locate patients by using the computer and advise visitors of patient location.
- Provide information on the location of bathrooms, visitors' lounge, cafeteria, and so on.
- Inform visitors of the rules of visitation and explain any special precautions required during their visit to a patient's room.
- Receive telephone calls from relatives or friends inquiring about the patient's condition.
- Handle visitor complaints.
- Perform advanced duties, possibly including cardiac monitoring, some coding, or admitting responsibilities.
- Be aware of hospital polices and procedures (found online or manual) (and where to locate them) that are relevant to the HUC position.

(*Note:* Mobile wireless devices are defined and discussed with other communication devices in Chapter 4.)

CROSS-TRAINING OPPORTUNITIES

Some hospitals cross-train hospital employees so that they are qualified to handle more than one position as needed. Examples of positions for which the HUC may be cross-trained include telemetry technician, or case management assistant or secretary. A HUC may also be cross-trained as a CNA and may have a title of Patient Care Assistant or Patient Care Associate (PCA). In a few hospitals, HUCs are also trained to perform electrocardiography and/or phlebotomy.

★ HIGH PRIORITY

For the health unit coordinator to be proactive, more marketable, and prepared for taking on additional responsibilities in case of cross-training, additional classes or programs that could be taken include the following:
- Certified Nursing Assistant (CNA) program
- Billing and coding classes or program
- Patient Care Technician (PCT) program
- Phlebotomy class
- Monitor Technician (electrocardiogram [ECG]) class

CAREER CHOICES FOR THE HEALTH UNIT COORDINATOR

Health unit coordinating can be a fulfilling and rewarding career, and many HUCs have made this their career choice. The HUC program provides a core knowledge base in health care and many of the prerequisites to pursue other careers in health care. Ancillary health care students or student nurses often work as HUCs to gain health care experience, earn a salary, obtain health care benefits, and earn tuition reimbursement, while continuing to participate in educational programs in their chosen profession. Many facilities offer employees opportunities for assisted advancement, such as prepaid on-campus educational programs, college tuition reimbursement, and flexible work schedules. Additional training opportunities for the HUC in areas such as cardiac monitoring, coding, and information processing are often offered.

Nonclinical Career Choices

There are many nonclinical positions available in health care, such as clinical research associate and health information manager. Employment information for both of these positions is provided in Box 1-10, *Possible Nonclinical Career Opportunities for the Health Unit Coordinator.*

KEY CONCEPTS

Management, communication, data entry, and customer service are all part of the HUC position with the use of the EMR with CPOE. It would be impossible for textbooks to stay current with the fast-paced changes to technology and health care. We have all experienced buying a computer or cell phone to find that it is soon obsolete because of advancing technology! It is up to the HUC to be aware of upcoming changes regarding health care (watch related news shows, read newspaper and medical journal articles, research the Web, fact check rumors, attend hospital in-services, join NAHUC, attend conventions, and read the NAHUC newsletters).

Websites of Interest

National Association of Health Unit Coordinators: www.nahuc.org
Institute of Medicine of the National Academies: www.iom.edu
Healthcare Information and Management Systems Society: www.himss.org
HIMSS Analytics: www.himssanalytics.org
Healthcare.gov: www.healthcare.gov
iHealthBeat: www.ihealthbeat.org
U.S. Department of Health and Human Services: www.hhs.gov
HealthGrades: www.healthgrades.com
Centers for Medicare and Medicaid Services: www.cms.gov

⊖ REVIEW QUESTIONS

Note: All review questions in this textbook are provided on the Evolve website. To access your student resources, visit: http://evolve.elsevier.com/Gillingham/HUC/.

1. Define the following terms:
   a. clinical tasks
   b. nonclinical tasks
   c. meaningful use (EMR)
   d. certification
   e. transcription
   f. browser
   g. search engine
   h. Internet service provider
   i. e-prescribing
   j. surfing the Web
   k. Web address (URL)
   l. clinical decision support system

2. Identify the following tasks as clinical or nonclinical:
   a. assisting a patient to the bathroom
   b. transcribing doctors' orders
   c. scanning a report into a patient's EMR
   d. filing reports in patients' charts
   e. feeding a patient

BOX 1-10	POSSIBLE NONCLINICAL CAREER OPPORTUNITIES FOR THE HEALTH UNIT COORDINATOR

For more information about these positions and about community colleges that offer degree programs and classes for these positions, the titles may be searched on the Web.

Position
Health Information Manager

Responsibilities
Responsible for the maintenance and security of all patient electronic records. The health information manager must keep up with current computer and software technology and with legislative requirements and developments regarding the maintenance and security of patient electronic records.

Work Environment
Health information managers work in health care settings such as hospitals, nursing homes, home health care agencies, and health maintenance organizations.

Job Outlook
Rapid employment growth is projected with implementation of the electronic medical record.

Educational Requirement
A bachelor's degree from an accredited program and a Registered Health Information Administrator certificate from the American Health Information Management Association are required.

Position
Clinical Research Associate (CRA)

Responsibilities
A CRA manages day-to-day operations related to a particular research project. The CRA makes sure that all appropriate safety precautions are being taken and is responsible for recording the results of the research experiments. Whenever there are complaints filed by regulatory agencies, the Clinical Research Associate plays a role in rectifying these complaints.

Work Environment
Most CRAs work in hospitals, physicians' offices, biomedical research organizations and institutions, specialty disease centers, and pharmaceutical and medical device companies. Clinical research encompasses many different health care settings and specialties.

Job Outlook
The emerging industry of clinical research has significantly increased the demand for CRAs, especially in the areas of genomics, biomedical technologies, medical device development, and several major disease categories.

Educational Requirement
A Certificate of Completion program is a 16-credit, four-course program achievable within a 12-month period if two classes are taken each semester. There are also associate and bachelor's degree programs available.

f. answering the unit telephone
g. monitoring a patient's EMR
h. changing a patient's dressing
i. answering a patient's request on the intercom

3. Explain the events that led up to creating what eventually became the health unit coordinator position.

4. Identify four stages that health professions have traditionally gone through to evolve into a profession.

5. List five reasons why an HUC should become a member of NAHUC.

6. List five reasons why an HUC should become certified.

7. The date proclaimed to be National Health Unit Coordinator Day is what?

8. List three health unit coordinating tasks that relate to each of the following:
   a. nursing personnel
   b. doctors
   c. hospital departments
   d. patients
   e. hospital visitors

9. Discuss the benefits of:
   a. EMR, CPOE with e-prescribing
   b. CDSS

10. Give an example of how the clinical decision support system could assist the physician at the point of order entry.

11. List four ways to prepare for the changes to the HUC position with the implementation of EMR with CPOE and six ways to stay current in the position.

12. List three positions for which the HUC may be cross-trained.

13. List two possible nonclinical career choices.

SURFING FOR ANSWERS

Following the guidelines for surfing the Web (see Box 1-9), find the following information and list the websites used. (If necessary, use a school computer or go to a library.)

1. Locate the name of your local NAHUC representative.
2. Find and list three websites that discuss electronic medical records.
3. Find and list three hospitals in your area that are using stage 7 electronic medical records.
4. Locate three HUC job openings in your area and copy the job descriptions.

CHAPTER 2

Overview of Health Care Today

CHAPTER OBJECTIVES

On completion of this chapter, you will be able to:

1. Define the terms in the vocabulary list.
2. Write the meaning of the abbreviations in the abbreviations list.
3. List at least five challenges facing today's health care system.
4. List five key elements of the Affordable Care Act.
5. Explain why it is important to stay current with any additional changes made to the Affordable Health Care Act.
6. Explain how the implementation of a national EMR system would assist in a pandemic or national emergency.
7. Identify the challenge a health care provider faces when implementing an EMR system as addressed in the American Health Insurance Portability Act of 1996 (HIPAA).
8. Explain the difference between the client server–based EMR and the cloud- or Web-based EMR.
9. Identify the EMR system used throughout the United States Department of Veterans Affairs (VA) medical systems known as the Veterans Health Administration (VHA).
10. Explain the use of HIPAA-compliant mobile phone apps and patient portals.
11. List three categories of telemedicine and three major advances aided by surgical robots.
12. Explain the main characteristics of indemnity insurance, managed care, and worker's compensation insurance.
13. Identify the federal and state program that provides health care for the indigent.
14. Explain the differences among Medicare Part A, Medicare Part B, and Medicare Part D.
15. List five functions a hospital may perform.

16. List three ways in which hospitals may be classified.
17. Explain what "Magnet status" signifies and at least six benefits a hospital would obtain by achieving Magnet status.
18. Identify two agencies that set hospital operational guidelines.
19. Describe the responsibilities of a hospital CEO and governing board.
20. Identify the main function of each department in a provided list of hospital departments.
21. Identify at least three health care delivery systems that provide long-term or custodial care for patients unable to care for themselves.
22. Explain the basic concept of freestanding, in-home, or hospital-based hospice care.
23. List three resources that may be used for finding health care job opportunities.

VOCABULARY

Accepting Assignment Agreement by which providers of medical services concede that the receipt of payment from Medicare for a professional service will constitute full payment for that service.

Accreditation Recognition that a health care organization has met an official standard.

Capitation Payment method whereby the provider of care receives a set dollar amount per patient, regardless of services rendered.

Case Manager Health care professional and expert in managed care who assists patients in assessing health and social service systems to ensure that all required services are obtained; coordinates care with doctor and insurance companies.

Catastrophic Coverage Coverage a Medicare beneficiary has after paying a certain amount of out-of-pocket monies for their medications during the temporary coverage gap. The beneficiary will pay a coinsurance amount (e.g., 5% of the drug cost) or a copayment ($2.15 or $5.35 for each prescription) for the rest of the calendar year.

Chief Executive Officer (CEO) Individual in direct charge of a hospital who is responsible to the governing board.

Client Server–Based EMR System The software is hosted on the hospital internal server and the licenses are purchased outright.

Cloud- or Web-Based EMR (virtualization of computer function) Use of an Internet site to host data and programs instead of keeping them on an internal computer.

Community Health Field concerned with the members of a community with emphasis on prevention and early detection of disease.

Coverage Gap (donut hole) A temporary coverage gap in Medicare that occurs after the beneficiary and his or her Medicare Part D drug plan have spent a set amount of money in total prescription drug expenses. The beneficiary pays 100% of drug costs while in the donut hole until another set amount is reached, at which point the beneficiary receives catastrophic coverage.

Custodial Care Unskilled care given for the primary purpose of meeting personal needs, such as bathing and dressing.

Diagnosis-Related Groups (DRGs) Classification system used to determine payments from Medicare by assigning a standard flat rate to major diagnostic categories. This flat rate is paid to hospitals regardless of the full cost of the services provided.

Governing Board Group of community citizens at the head of the hospital organizational structure.

Health Maintenance Organization (HMO) Organization that has management responsibility for providing comprehensive health care services on a prepayment basis (capitation) to voluntarily enrolled persons within a designated population.

Health Savings Account (HSA) A tax exempt bank account that is owned by an individual and managed by a financial institution. The individual must have a qualified high-deductible health plan. An individual cannot use the tax benefit of an HSA until the qualified health plan is in place. Also called a *medical savings account (MSA)*.

Home Health Equipment and services provided to patients in their homes to ensure comfort and care.

Hospice Supportive care for terminally ill patients and their families.

Indigent Refers to the state of living in extreme poverty; lacking the necessities of life, such as food and clothing.

International Statistical Classification of Diseases and Related Health Problems (ICD) A detailed description of known diseases and injuries. Each disease (or group of related diseases) is described with its diagnosis and is given a unique code, up to six characters long. Published by the World Health Organization.

Long-Term Care (LTC) A variety of services, often provided in nonhospital settings, that help meet both the medical and the nonmedical needs of people with a chronic illness or disability who cannot care for themselves for long periods of time.

Magnet Status Award given by the American Nurses' Credentialing Center to hospitals that satisfy a set of criteria designed to measure their strength and quality of nursing.

Managed Care The use of a planned and systematic approach to providing health care, with the goal of offering quality care at the lowest possible cost.

Medicaid Federal and state program that provides medical assistance to the indigent.

Medicare Government insurance; enacted in 1965 for individuals older than age 65 and any person with a disability who has received Social Security benefits for 2 years (some disabilities are covered immediately).

Patient Portal An online application that allows a patient to register for an appointment, schedule an appointment, request prescription refills, send and receive secure patient-physician messages, view lab results, or pay bills electronically.

Primary Insurance Insurance coverage that is responsible for paying claims first and protects against medical expenses up to the policy's limit, regardless of whatever other insurance is held.

Proprietary For profit.

Robotic Surgery The use of robots in performing surgery.

Secondary Insurance Insurance coverage used to supplement existing policies or to cover any gaps in insurance coverage; billed after primary insurance has paid (also called *supplemental insurance*).

Skilled Nursing Facility (SNF) A medical institution that provides medical, nursing, or custodial care for an individual over a prolonged period.

Telemedicine The combined use of telecommunications and computer technologies to improve the efficiency and effectiveness of health care services by eliminating the traditional constraints of place and time.

Telepresence (virtual presence) The virtual presence of somebody whose actions are transmitted by electronic signals to a physically remote site.

Voice-Activated Transcription A local, PC-based large-vocabulary voice-recognition engine that generates reports, often using macros and templates to make the process more efficient and reduce recognition errors.

Voluntary Not for profit (nonprofit).

ABBREVIATIONS

Abbreviation	Meaning
AHA	American Hospital Association
app	application; an "app" is a piece of software that can run on the Internet, on a computer, or on a phone or other electronic device
CCM	certified case manager
CEO	chief executive officer
CFO	chief financial officer
COO	chief operating officer
DRG	diagnosis-related groups
ECF	extended care facility
HIMS	health information management system
HMO	health maintenance organization
ICD	International Statistical Classification of Diseases and Related Health Problems
LTC	long-term care
PPO	preferred provider organization
SNF	skilled nursing facility
TJC	The Joint Commission (formerly the Joint Commission on Accreditation of Healthcare Organizations [JCAHO])
WHO	World Health Organization

⊖ EXERCISE 1

Write the abbreviation for each term listed.

1. American Hospital Association
2. application
3. certified case manager
4. chief executive officer
5. chief financial officer
6. chief operating officer
7. diagnosis-related groups
8. extended care facility
9. health information management system
10. health maintenance organization
11. International Statistical Classification of Diseases and Related Health Problems
12. long-term care
13. preferred provider organization
14. skilled nursing facility
15. The Joint Commission
16. World Health Organization

⊖ EXERCISE 2

Write the meaning of each abbreviation listed.

1. AHA		9. HIMS	
2. app		10. HMO	
3. CCM		11. ICD	
4. CEO		12. LTC	
5. CFO		13. PPO	
6. COO		14. SNF	
7. DRG		15. TJC	
8. ECF		16. WHO	

CHALLENGES FACING THE U.S. HEALTH CARE SYSTEM TODAY

1. *More than 50 million people were uninsured in 2010,* almost one in six U.S. residents, the Census Bureau reported (published 9/13/2011). Millions of Americans lost their jobs and their health benefits during the recession and often had no way to regain affordable health coverage.

2. *There is a disparity in care provided to insured people compared with the uninsured or underinsured, many of whom belong to racial and ethnic minorities.*

3. *The staggering cost of advanced technology.* Medical technology discoveries have been a major contributor to rising health care cost, but imposing controls could impede medical innovation.

4. *Increasing insurance costs and out-of-pocket costs continue to soar.* Customers of health insurance are now assuming a greater share of premiums and are paying higher deductibles, higher copayments, and a higher percentage of coinsurance.

5. *Many doctors and health care facilities are refusing or limiting the number of Medicare patients they treat.* The doctors' reasons are that reimbursement rates are too low and the paperwork is too much of a hassle. There is the real possibility of a far worse health crisis than we see today.

6. *Medicaid cuts are expected to cause about 17,000 adults to lose state health coverage and 30,000 more to pay higher premiums.* In April, 2012, the federal government approved state Medicaid cuts. The approved cuts save $28 million, in state money officials said. Other proposed cuts await federal approval.

7. *Medical errors are one of the nation's leading causes of death and injury.* A 1999 report by the Institute of Medicine of the National Academies (IOM), *To Err is Human,* estimated that as many as 44,000 to 98,000 people die in U.S. hospitals each year as a result of medical errors. This means that more people die from medical errors than from motor vehicle accidents, breast cancer, or acquired immunodeficiency syndrome (AIDS). The reaction to this IOM report was swift and positive. Congress launched a series of hearings on patient safety and in 2000 $50 million was appropriated to the Agency for Healthcare Research and Quality to support a variety of efforts targeted to reducing medical errors.

THE AFFORDABLE CARE ACT

The Affordable Care Act, signed into law in 2010, puts in place comprehensive health insurance reform that will roll out over 4 years and beyond; most changes will have taken place by

BOX 2-1	KEY PROVISIONS OF THE AFFORDABLE CARE ACT

2010

- Adults with preexisting conditions who have been uninsured for at least 6 months became eligible to join a temporary high-risk pool.
- Insurers are prohibited from imposing lifetime dollar limits on essential benefits, such as hospital stays, in new policies issued.
- All new plans must cover certain preventive services such as mammograms and colonoscopies without charging a deductible, copay, or coinsurance.
- Dependents (children) are permitted to remain on their parents' insurance plan until their 26th birthday.
- Enhanced methods of Medicare fraud detection are implemented.

2011

- The Centers for Medicare and Medicaid Services is responsible for developing the Center for Medicare and Medicaid Innovation and overseeing the testing of innovative payment and delivery models.

2012

- Employers must disclose the value of the benefits they provided beginning in 2012 for each employee's health insurance coverage on the employees' annual Form W-2's.
- Health plans are required to begin adopting and implementing rules for the secure, confidential, electronic exchange of health information (electronic medical record [EMR]).

2014

- Insurers are prohibited from discriminating against or charging higher rates for any individual based on preexisting medical conditions.
- An annual penalty of $95, or up to 1% of income, whichever is greater, is imposed on individuals who do not secure insurance; this will rise to $695, or 2.5% of income, by 2016. This is an individual limit; families have a limit of $2085. Exemptions to the fine in cases of financial hardship or religious beliefs are permitted.
- Insurers are prohibited from establishing annual spending caps.
- A new health insurance marketplace will offer a choice of health plans that meet certain benefits and cost standards.
- Chain restaurants and food vendors with 20 or more locations are required to display the caloric content of their foods on menus, drive-through menus, and vending machines. Additional information, such as saturated fat, carbohydrate, and sodium content, must also be made available on request.

For more information, go to www.healthcare.gov/law/provisions/index.html.

2014, and other changes have already taken place. Key provisions of the Affordable Care Act are provided in Box 2-1, *Key Provisions of the Affordable Care Act.*

Many Americans have voiced concerns regarding the Affordable Care Act, and several states are challenging the constitutionality of the "individual mandate." In June of 2012, the U.S. Supreme Court ruled that the individual mandate was constitutional as a tax. The individual mandate requires that virtually all legal residents of the United States obtain minimum essential health insurance coverage for each month, starting in 2014, or pay a penalty that will be included with the individual's federal tax return. It is important to stay current with changes made, as the changes may have an impact on health care providers as well as everyone receiving health care. (See Box 2-2, *Concerns Voiced by States and Individuals Regarding the Affordable Health Care Act.*)

IMPLEMENTING A NATIONAL INTERCONNECTED ELECTRONIC MEDICAL RECORD SYSTEM

A national electronic medical record (EMR) system will allow the federal government to track the course and impact of a pandemic in real time. A spokesperson from the Center for Health Transformation reported that a national EMR system would provide local, state, and federal governments with the necessary data to direct therapies, medical personnel, and supplies during an emergency. Studies conducted by the

BOX 2-2	CONCERNS VOICED BY STATES AND INDIVIDUALS REGARDING THE AFFORDABLE HEALTH CARE ACT

- The mandate that individuals purchase coverage or face penalties is contrary to the Tenth Amendment of the United States Constitution. The individual mandate was upheld by the U.S. Supreme Court in June of 2012.
- Government is too big; health care makes up one fifth of the U.S. economy.
- Higher costs than predicted will be incurred (e.g., taxes will be raised).
- Individuals will have to give up high-quality health care to pay for this legislation.
- There will be rationing of health care, and panels will turn down needed procedures for cheaper options.
- Electronic medical record (EMR) systems have a high cost, ranging from 20 million to 100 million dollars.

Leapfrog Group have shown that computer physician order entry (CPOE) with clinical decision support system (CDSS), if implemented in all urban hospitals in the United States, could prevent as many as 907,600 serious medication errors each year. Studies have also shown that the EMR and CPOE reduce length of stay and reduce retesting and turnaround times for laboratory, pharmacy, and radiology requests while delivering cost savings.

Hospitals and practices that are not using "meaningful use" EMR by the federally set goal of 2014 will be penalized by a cut in the percentage of their Medicare payments starting in 2015. Once the provisions of the law are fully phased in, the penalties could amount to a loss of $3.2 million annually in Medicare funding for the average 500-bed hospital.

ADVANCING ELECTRONIC MEDICAL RECORD TECHNOLOGIES

Confidentiality and Security

Health care is in the midst of an information technology (IT) revolution. One cannot have confidentiality without information security. There is a balancing act between ease of access for prompt medical care and the maintenance of confidentiality. The American Health Insurance Portability and Accountability Act of 1996 (HIPAA) (detailed in Chapter 6) protects private individual health information from being disclosed to anyone without the consent of the individual. The Health Information Technology for Economic and Clinical Health (HITECH) Act (detailed in Chapter 6), enacted as part of the American Recovery and Reinvestment Act, was signed into law in 2009, to promote the adoption and meaningful use of health IT. Subtitle D of the HITECH Act addresses the privacy and security concerns associated with the electronic transmission of health information, in part, through several provisions that strengthen the civil and criminal enforcement of the HIPAA rules.

See Chapter 6 for complete information on HIPAA and the HITECH Act.

Health care providers must make sure their EMR system is HIPAA compliant and that the EMR systems installed take care of all the privacy and information security issues. Physicians and nurses have unlimited access to the patient's electronic chart, and other health care providers may have limited access to it, in accordance with their area of expertise. A patient's chart may be opened and viewed or used by more than one person at a time. If someone who is viewing the record steps away from the computer, it will turn off automatically, and when the person returns and signs onto the computer again with his or her code, the screen will be at the same place.

Client Server–Based Electronic Medical Record System

A **client server–based EMR system** is software that is hosted on the hospital internal server and licenses that are purchased outright. Challenges include the following:

- A certain amount of local IT expertise is required to support the local server.
- Backups are required.
- Client software needs to be installed on each computer.
- Upgrades are required to the software (usually two or three times a year).

There are many client server–based EMR systems. Some of the more common examples are Cerner Solutions, EpicCare, and PrognoCIS.

VistA (Veterans Health Information Systems and Technology Architecture) is an EMR application ("app") throughout the United States Department of Veterans Affairs (VA) medical systems known as the Veterans Health Administration (VHA). VistA is one of the most widely used EHRs in the world. Nearly half of all US hospitals that have a full implementation of an EMR are VA hospitals using VistA.

Cloud- or Web-Based Electronic Medical Record

Cloud or Web-Based EMR (virtualization of computer function) is use of an Internet site to host data and programs instead of keeping them on an internal computer. Services include software from e-mail to entire IT platforms, which are hosted in the cloud, meaning that someone else makes them available when needed. The need to store an expanding archive of medical images is driving some health care providers to turn to cloud services. Many hospitals' data centers are already crowded; advances in scanning technologies mean they will have an ever-mounting volume of data to maintain. Major EMR vendors provide a host of conventional client-server offerings, but more cloud-based health IT options are becoming available. A public cloud provides IT resources that are provisioned remotely from the consumer and operated by a third party. In a private cloud, the infrastructure policies are governed by a single organization; workloads and data can be moved to and from internal and external data centers.

Cloud computing would cut costs significantly because fewer servers are needed, there is less need for support, and power consumption is reduced. There is hesitancy to use cloud computing in health care owing to security and HIPAA regulations. The health care industry and technology providers are working to ensure that cloud computing is secure and meets the regulations of the HITECH Act in the way data are stored and transferred in the cloud. It is important for health care providers to determine if cloud computing can provide them a secure, reliable, inexpensive, and HIPAA-compliant EMR system.

Electronic Medical Record Applications for Mobile Phones

Canvas has developed HIPAA-HITECH–compliant mobile applications that are available for Android, BlackBerry, and Windows Mobile smartphones. iSALUS Healthcare, one of the top U.S. Web-based EMR and practice management software companies that exclusively focuses on small and medium-sized physician practices, has developed an iPhone mobile application. The new HIPAA-compliant mobile EMR-EHR service allows doctors to access critical patient records and office information from their iPhones. The new iSALUS mobile EMR-EHR application enables physicians to securely access real-time patient information such as progress notes, medical images, and contact and insurance information. It also provides doctors and practice managers with access to office items such as schedules, rounds, task lists, dictations, patient charges, and office communications.

Patient Portal

A **patient portal** is an online application that allows a patient to interact and communicate with his or her health care provider, increasing efficiency and productivity. Patient portal applications might allow patients to register and complete forms online, which can streamline and shorten visits to clinics and hospitals. Many portal applications also allow patients to request prescription refills online, order eyeglasses and contacts, access medical records, pay bills, review lab results, and schedule necessary medical appointments. Some patient portal applications exist as a standalone website that is purchased by the health care provider. Other portal applications are integrated into the existing website of the health care provider, and others are modules added onto an existing EMR system.

INCREASING RECENT TRENDS AND TECHNOLOGIES IN HEALTH CARE

Telemedicine

Telemedicine is the combined use of telecommunications and computer technologies to improve the efficiency and effectiveness of health care services by eliminating the traditional constraints of place and time.

Three Categories of Telemedicine

1. *Acquiring medical data* such as medical images or biosignals (e.g., electrocardiogram [ECG] tracings) and then transmitting these data to a doctor or medical specialist at a remote site. It does not require the presence of both parties at the same time.
2. *Remote monitoring*, which enables medical professionals to monitor a patient remotely using various technologic devices. This is primarily used for managing chronic diseases or conditions such as heart disease, diabetes, mellitus, or asthma.
3. *Interactive real-time interactions* between patient and provider, provided through telephone conversations, online communication, and home visits. Polycom is a company that manufactures and sells **telepresence (virtual presence)** and voice communications solutions that enable medical professionals to provide patients access to care regardless of time or distance constraints. See Chapters 3 and 4 for more information on telemedicine.

Robotic Surgery

Three major advances aided by surgical robots are remote surgery, minimally invasive surgery, and unmanned surgery. Major advantages of **robotic surgery** include precision, miniaturization, articulation beyond normal manipulation, and three-dimensional magnification.

Types of Robotic Surgery

Currently there are three types of robotic surgery systems:

1. *Supervisory-controlled systems* (computer-assisted surgery) such as the RoboDoc system (developed by Integrated Surgical Systems) are commonly used in orthopedic surgeries.
2. *Telesurgical systems* such as the da Vinci robotic surgical system enhance surgery by providing three-dimensional visualization deep within hard-to-reach places such as the heart, as well as enhancing wrist dexterity and control of tiny instruments.
3. *Shared-control systems* monitor the surgeon, providing stability and support during the procedure; the human does the bulk of the work. Before getting started, the surgeons program the robots to recognize safe, close, boundary, and forbidden territories within the human body. Safe regions are the main focus of the surgery. When the forbidden zone is reached, the robotic system actually locks up to prevent any further injury. Shared-control systems might work best for brain surgeries, in which the surgeon provides the action but the robot arm steadies the hand.

An article in *Science Daily* (February 3, 2011) stated that surgeons of the future might use a system that recognizes hand gestures as commands to control a robotic scrub nurse or tell a computer to display medical images of the patient during an operation. This might help to reduce the length of surgeries and the potential for infection. See Chapter 4 for other uses of robots in health care.

TYPES OF HEALTH INSURANCE

Indemnity

Indemnity insurance, also known as fee-for-service insurance, provides individuals the freedom and flexibility to control their own health decisions concerning doctor choices and medical treatments. However, premiums are higher and there are deductibles and other out-of-pocket expenses. Most plans come with an annual coinsurance maximum, and once the insured has met this amount (which varies depending on the plan), the insurance company will pay 100% of the medical costs for the rest of the calendar year. Indemnity plans generally do not pay for preventive care. Examples of types of preventive care that are typically not covered by indemnity plans include annual physical examinations, birth control, and flu shots. Indemnity insurance covers accidents and illnesses.

Managed Care

Managed care usually has a lower deductible and smaller copayment than an indemnity plan. There are limited choices when it comes to doctors or hospitals. Physicians must be authorized by the managed care provider. Permission must be obtained from the primary doctor to see a specialized doctor. Managed care systems most often are associated with a **health maintenance organization (HMO)** which has management responsibility for providing comprehensive health care services on a prepayment basis **(capitation)** to voluntarily enrolled persons within a designated population.

Types of Health Maintenance Organizations

- The *staff model HMO:* a multispecialty group of physicians who practice at an HMO and who are salaried employees.
- The *group model HMO:* no specific facility called an HMO; physicians contract with the HMO to provide nearly all services to members.
- The *individual practice association (IPA) model:* HMO contracts with an association of individual physicians to provide services for members in their private offices.
- The *preferred provider organization (PPO):* an independent group of physicians or hospitals that provide health care for fees that are 15% to 20% lower than customary rates; there is a "participating physician list," and patients usually do not need referrals.

Medical Savings Account

A *medical savings account (MSA)* or **health savings account (HSA)** is a tax-free savings account that allows the individual to pay current medical expenses while saving for future health care. According to the U.S. Department of Treasury (www.treas.gov), an HSA has two components. The first is an insurance plan: the individual must have a high-deductible insurance plan to cover significant health concerns. High-deductible plans are relatively inexpensive. The second part is a savings account to spend as one pleases on health care. The benefits are in the tax savings and investment options. Taxpayers can invest pretax income. Annual increases in the contribution limits are based on inflation. In 2011 a family could contribute $6250 ($520.83 per month) to an HSA. (If the owner of the plan was older than age 55 years, that limit increased to $7250.) A single person could contribute $3100 (if over 55 years old, $4100). Any money not used during a calendar year is rolled over to the following year, so the account balance can grow over time.

Worker's Compensation

Worker's compensation pays the medical bills and a significant portion of the lost wages when an on-the-job accident or illness results in injury or disability. The employer pays a premium to an insurance carrier for the worker's compensation policy. The injured worker must fill out a claim form and send it to the insurance carrier. The injured worker receives no bill, pays no deductible, and is covered 100% for medical expenses related to that injury or illness.

Medicaid and Medicare

Medicaid and **Medicare** are two governmental programs that provide medical and health-related services to specific groups of people in the United States. They are very different but both are managed by the Centers for Medicare and Medicaid Services, a division of the U.S. Department of Health and Human Services.

Medicaid

Medicaid is a federal and state program that provides medical assistance for the **indigent.** It has no entitlement features; recipients must prove their eligibility. Funds come from federal grants and are administered by the state; benefits are closely associated with the economic status of the beneficiary.

The benefits cover *inpatient* care, *outpatient* and diagnostic services, skilled nursing facility (SNF) costs, physician services, and **home health** care.

Medicare

Medicare is health insurance for people age 65 or older, people under 65 with certain disabilities, or people of any age with end-stage renal disease (ESRD) (permanent kidney failure necessitating dialysis or a kidney transplant). In 1983, Congress authorized the creation of Medicare's prospective payment system (PPS) for hospitals. This changed the way physicians and hospitals receive payment: they no longer establish their own prices. Instead, providers of medical services agree that the receipt of payment from Medicare for a professional service will constitute full payment for that service—called **accepting assignment.** The policy requires Medicare to fix prices in advance on a cost-per-case basis, with the use of 500 *diagnosis-related groups(DRGs)* as a measure.

The different parts of Medicare are as follows:

- *Medicare Part A (hospital insurance):* helps cover inpatient care in hospitals and helps cover SNF care, hospice, and home health care.
- *Medicare Part B (medical insurance):* helps cover doctors' services, hospital outpatient care, and home health care and helps cover some preventive services to help maintain health and to keep certain illnesses from getting worse.
- *Medicare Part D (Medicare prescription drug coverage):* a prescription drug option run by Medicare-approved private insurance companies; helps cover the cost of prescription drugs until a preset amount of money is reached. Then the Medicare beneficiary is in a temporary **coverage gap** (donut hole). After paying a certain amount of out-of-pocket monies for medications, the beneficiary can receive **catastrophic coverage.**

★ HIGH PRIORITY

Many individuals are covered by more than one health insurance policy to assist in paying for medical expenses. The **primary insurance** is billed and pays first, and then the **secondary insurance** is billed and pays some or the entire amount of the charges that the primary insurance does not pay.

HEALTH CARE DELIVERY SYSTEMS AND SERVICES

History of Hospitals

The histories of early Egyptian and Indian civilizations indicate that crude hospitals were in existence in the 6th century bce. The early Greeks and Romans used their temples to the gods as refuges for the sick. During the Crusades, *hospitia* were established, at which pilgrims could rest from their travels. The word *hospital* comes to us originally from the Latin noun *hospes,* which means "guest" or "host." The term *hospice,* which relates to family-centered care for the terminally ill, also is derived from *hospes.*

During the 12th and 13th centuries, great hospital growth occurred in England and France.

The earliest hospital in what is now the United States served sick soldiers on Manhattan Island in 1663. However, the first established hospitals were founded in Philadelphia in the early 18th century. The middle 19th and early 20th centuries were important for hospital growth because during this period the foundations of modern biology were laid and books on the subject were written. The education of nurses and doctors increased in the early 20th century.

The hospital of today continues to serve those in need during illness or injury with modern technologies, improved medical knowledge, and compassion.

Hospital Functions

The primary functions of the hospital are the care and treatment of the sick. This is true of all hospitals, regardless of size. Other functions include the education of physicians and other health care personnel, research, and prevention of disease. Especially in smaller communities, the hospital also serves as a local health center.

Only large hospitals may find it possible to perform all these functions. The functions the hospital performs depend on many factors, including the hospital's location, the population it serves, and the size of the facility. The care and treatment of the sick or injured necessitate proper accommodations for the patient, along with adequate medical and nursing care. The care and treatment of each patient call for a team effort. Each department that is involved with the patient plays an important role in assisting the patient to return to a better state of health.

Some hospitals maintain schools in various health services, such as radiology, clinical laboratory, and respiratory care. Other hospitals provide practical experience for students enrolled in university or community college educational programs in all levels of nursing, diet therapy, hospital administration, health unit coordinating, and other hospital-related fields. A hospital may have a residency program for doctors, and it may provide additional experiences for medical students.

The type of research conducted in hospitals may depend on specific services rendered by the hospital. A hospital that specializes in the care of patients with cancer would do research in cancer. The trend today is toward the prevention of disease. The hospital may serve as a **community health** center, providing low-cost or free clinics for the early detection of symptoms of disease conditions and for administration of immunization programs. Doctors and other health care personnel also provide counseling and instruction in health care.

Hospital Classifications

Hospitals can be classified in many ways. The three most common classifications are (1) the type of patient service offered, (2) the ownership of the hospital, and (3) the type of accreditation the hospital has been given.

Type of service offered refers to the distinction between general hospitals and specialized hospitals. General hospitals render various services for patients with many disease conditions and injuries. Not all general hospitals in a community offer identical services because this would prove too costly.

Specialized hospitals provide services to a particular body part (e.g., an eye hospital), to a particular segment of the population (e.g., a children's hospital), or for a particular type of care (e.g., a psychiatric or rehabilitation hospital).

Ownership of the hospital is the second type of classification. The federal government maintains hospitals for veterans and for personnel in the U.S. Navy and Air Force. The government also provides health services in hospitals for Native Americans. States, counties, and cities are also owners of hospitals. Churches and fraternal organizations may own and control general or specialized hospitals, which are usually nonprofit agencies. **Proprietary** hospitals are operated for profit and are owned by a group of individuals or corporations.

The hospital of today is often part of a health care system that usually has a "parent" corporation that oversees the companies within the system. The hospital is one of the subsidiary companies. Subsidiaries are designated as profit or nonprofit, and each has its own board of directors. Aside from the hospital, the system may include a company that provides durable medical equipment, another that provides home care in the community, another that operates parking facilities or linen services, and so forth. Most health care systems have a component called a *foundation*, whose purpose is to focus on donations and fundraising activities that benefit the entire system.

Accreditation refers to recognition that a hospital has met an official standard. For example, a *TJC-accredited hospital* has been surveyed, graded, and approved by The Joint Commission (TJC). Participation in TJC accreditation is **voluntary**. Several other accrediting agencies also conduct surveys, according to the services provided by the hospital. All facilities that are receiving Medicare reimbursement must receive TJC accreditation.

The hospital's license to operate usually is granted by the Department of Health Services of the individual state.

Magnet Recognition Program

The Magnet Recognition Program was developed by the American Nurses Credentialing Center (ANCC), an affiliate of the American Nurses Association (ANA). **Magnet status** is an award given by the ANCC to hospitals that satisfy a set of criteria designed to measure the strength and quality of their nursing. Magnet evaluation criteria are based on quality indicators and standards of nursing practice as defined in *Scope and Standards for Nurse Administrators* by the ANA (1996). These criteria are similar to TJC standards. Currently, no registered nurse (RN)–to-patient ratios are required for achievement of Magnet status. To obtain Magnet status, health care organizations must apply to the ANCC, must submit extensive documentation that demonstrates their adherence to ANA standards, and must undergo an on-site evaluation to verify the information provided in the submitted documentation and to assess for the presence of the "forces of magnetism" within the organization. The ANCC collects a fee from hospitals for its Magnet recognition process. Magnet status is awarded for a 4-year period, after which time the organization must reapply.

This program is marketed by ANCC as a vehicle that can provide to hospitals the following benefits: enhanced nursing care, increased staff morale, appeal to high-quality physicians, reinforced positive collaborative relationships, creation of a "Magnet culture," improved patient quality outcomes, enhanced nursing recruitment and retention, and a competitive advantage. The premise is that staff nurses are more valued and more involved in data collection and decision making in patient care delivery. Nurses are rewarded for advancing in nursing practice, and open communication between nurses and other members of the health care team is encouraged. Hospitals may use their Magnet status as a promotional tool.

Operational Guidelines

The American Hospital Association (AHA) and TJC determine hospital operational guidelines. AHA guidelines address confidentiality, privacy, informed consent, patient rights, and the like. TJC guidelines promote quality of care and dimensions of performance. TJC-required annual in-services for all health care employees include cardiopulmonary resuscitation (CPR) (if working in a clinical position), infectious disease control, fire and safety training, universal (standard) precautions, and HIPAA training. TJC also requires a preemployment tuberculosis skin test. Hospitals may have additional preemployment requirements. For detailed information regarding preemployment requirements, see Chapter 6.

Hospital Organization
Administrative Personnel

The **governing board,** which is at the top of the organizational structure of a hospital, also may be referred to as the *board of* *trustees* or *board of directors.* Three of the main responsibilities of the board include establishing policy, providing adequate financing, and overseeing personnel standards. The board is composed of persons from the business and professional communities, as well as concerned citizens from all socioeconomic groups. The number of hospital board members varies with the size of the hospital. In hospitals that are part of a health care system, the hospital's governing board is responsible to the board of the parent corporation of the system.

In direct charge of the hospital and responsible to the governing board is the **chief executive officer (CEO)**. The CEO plans the implementation of policies set forth by the governing board. The *chief operating officer (COO)* is responsible for the day-to-day operation of the hospital and reports directly to the CEO. The chief financial officer (CFO) is responsible for the fiscal aspects of the hospital administration and reports directly to the CEO. A vice president or a director supervises each service within the hospital. Vice presidents report to the hospital COO. Figure 2-1 is an example of a typical hospital structure.

The board delegates the supervision of patient care quality and of the conduct of physicians who practice in the hospital to a committee that is representative of the medical staff. The hospital governing board has a duty to the community to exercise care in the selection of doctors appointed to the medical staff. A doctor who has submitted credentials to the state medical board and who has a license to practice in the state may submit an application for appointment to the staff of a hospital or hospitals.

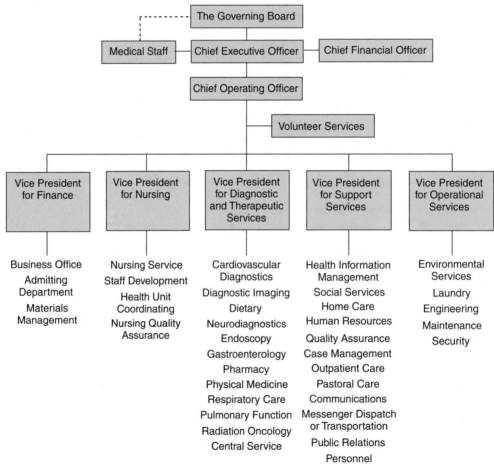

Figure 2-1 An example of a typical hospital organizational structure.

See Chapter 3 for information regarding the medical staff and a list of common medical specialties.

Hospital Departments and Services

The HUC interacts daily with many hospital departments during the transcription or scheduling of doctors' orders or when requesting services provided by the department. Therefore it is important to have an overall view of the departments and their functions as they relate to the role of the HUC. See Table 2-1 for a brief description of their services. These services are divided into business services, diagnostic and therapeutic services, support services, and operational services. It is important to remember that not all hospitals have each of the

TABLE 2-1 **Hospital Departments**

Department	Service
Business	
Business office	Patient accounts.
Admitting	Admission of new patients.
Diagnostic and Therapeutic	
Cardiovascular diagnostics	Tests related to heart and blood vessels.
Diagnostic imaging	Radiographs, nuclear medicine, and ultrasound studies.
Nutritional care	Meals.
Neurology	Studies of the nervous system.
Endoscopy	Diagnostic procedures performed with the use of endoscopes.
Gastroenterology or GI lab	Studies related to the digestive system.
Pathology or clinical laboratory	Diagnostic procedures on specimens from the body.
Pharmacy	Medications.
Physical medicine	Rehabilitation.
Cardiopulmonary or respiratory care department	Treatment related to respiratory function.
Radiation oncology or radiation treatment department	Treatment of cancer growths.
Support Services	
Case management	Monitors a patient's progress while exploring and suggesting alternative and cost-effective options; coordinates care with the patient, patient's family, doctor, and insurance company.
Central supply department, materials management, or supply purchasing department	Obtains, stores, and distributes supplies and equipment used for patient care.
Health information management systems or medical records department	Manages the patient's EMR or stores and manages patient's paper records.
Quality assurance	Quality care.
Social services	Assistance to patients and families.
Home care or discharge planning	Transition from hospital to home.
Patient advocate services	Acts as a support structure and if legally contracted to do so may act as a liaison between a patient and his or her health care provider(s). A patient advocate may accompany a patient to appointments, monitor the patient at the bedside in a hospital, or be a good choice for a health care proxy.
Patient advocate patient representative ombudsman	
Outpatient	Services to patients outside the hospital.
Pastoral care	Spiritual support.
Communications	Switchboard.
Transportation department	Delivery.
Public relations	Provides information to the public.
Volunteer services	A variety of services provided by volunteers.
Operational Services	
Housekeeping or environmental services	Housekeeping duties.
Mechanical	Keeps equipment in working condition.
Information technology (IT) department (often referred to as the "help desk")	Installation and repair of telephones and electronic equipment, including computers, printers, and software.
Laundry, or linens department	Maintains linens.
Human resources	Recruitment, records, and benefits.
Security	Protection.

departments listed, nor must the department in each hospital use the same name as is used in this text. The use of the EMR may change the way some of the listed department responsibilities are carried out and by whom. Some hospitals participate in an internship program for college students enrolled in a health care career curriculum. Most hospitals provide clinical experiences for students in various departments.

Business Services

The business services department deals with the financial aspects of the hospital. The HUC works closely with the admitting department during the patient's admission to, transfer within, and discharge from the hospital. The HUC orders all the unit supplies from the purchasing department.

The *business office* is in charge of patient accounts, budget planning, and payment of bills incurred by the hospital. This office determines the ability of the patient to pay through hospitalization insurance and Medicare or Medicaid. The business office also provides a place for safekeeping of patient valuables. Each department is issued a cost control number to be included on all requisitions for purchases, maintenance fees, and other expenses for record-keeping purposes. The EMR makes this process more efficient.

The *admitting department*, sometimes called *patient services*, admits new patients to the hospital, transfers patients within the hospital, and discharges patients from the hospital. On admission, the admitting department obtains pertinent information from patients or their relatives. If the EMR is implemented, the admitting department will enter demographic information into the EMR. Admitting department personnel witness the signing of the admission agreement by the patient or his or her representative, ask if the patient has an advanced directive or if one is desired, and prepares the identification bracelet.

Diagnostic and Therapeutic Services

The following departments relate to the direct care of the hospitalized patient. During the transcription process, the HUC orders procedures, tests, treatments, or supplies from these departments, according to doctors' orders. If the EMR is in use, the HUC may need to coordinate the orders and may or may not need to order the supplies.

The *cardiovascular diagnostics department* performs tests related to cardiac (heart) and blood vessel function. The diagnostic procedures ordered may be performed at the patient's bedside (e.g., ECGs and echocardiograms). Other diagnostic procedures such as a cardiac catheterization are performed in the cardiovascular department.

The *diagnostic imaging department* includes the radiology, nuclear medicine, and ultrasound departments. Diagnostic studies are performed with the use of radiography, ultrasound, computed tomography, magnetic resonance imaging, and radioactive element scanners. A radiologist—a medical doctor qualified in the use of x-ray and other imaging devices—is in charge of this department. The radiographer, a graduate of a 2- or 4-year educational program, performs many of the technical procedures.

The *nutritional care department* plans and prepares meals for patients, employees, and visitors and works under the direction of a registered dietitian (a graduate of a 4-year college program). Personnel within the department deliver meals and nourishment to nursing care units. The doctor may order a dietician consultation or diabetic education for a patient.

The *neurology department* performs diagnostic studies of the brain. An electroencephalogram (EEG) is a recording of the electrical impulses of brain waves. An EEG technician performs the test, and a physician, usually a neurologist, interprets the brain wave tracings.

The *endoscopy department* performs diagnostic procedures with the use of endoscopes that permit the visual examination of a body cavity or hollow organ, such as the stomach. A specialist employed by the hospital or in private practice may perform endoscopies.

The *gastroenterology department* or *gastrointestinal (GI) laboratory* performs studies to diagnose disease conditions of the digestive system. Tests, which are usually performed on an outpatient basis, are related to problems of the esophagus, stomach, pancreas, gallbladder, and small intestine. A gastroenterologist, a doctor with additional education related to diseases of the GI system, is in charge of the department.

The *pathology department* or *clinical laboratory* is concerned with diagnostic procedures performed on specimens from the body, such as blood, tissues, urine, stools, sputum, and bone marrow. This department may be separated into several divisions that are named for the tests or substances to be examined, such as hematology, urinalysis, microbiology, chemistry, and blood bank. The pathologist also examines specimens removed during surgery. Autopsies are performed under the direction of this department. The laboratory functions under the direction of a pathologist and employs medical technologists and medical laboratory technicians who have graduated from a recognized school for laboratory personnel.

The *pharmacy* provides the medications used within the hospital or in the clinics and may be involved in instructing patients regarding the proper use of medications. The pharmacist fills the prescription ordered by the doctor. Intravenous solutions to which medications have been added are prepared in the pharmacy under sterile conditions. A registered pharmacist is in charge of the pharmacy.

The *physical medicine department* is composed of several smaller departments related to the rehabilitation of the patient. The physical medicine department works under the direction of a physiatrist. *Physical therapy* and *occupational therapy* are the two most common therapeutic areas within the physical medicine department. Small hospitals may have only a physical therapy department. The physical therapy department provides treatment through the use of exercise, massage, heat, light, water, and other methods. Registered physical therapists (graduates of a 4-year college program) and physical therapy technicians (graduates of a 2-year community college program) carry out prescribed evaluations and treatments.

The *occupational therapy department* provides patients with purposeful activities that are designed to evaluate and treat those who are impaired physically, mentally, and developmentally. These activities help prevent deformities, restore function to affected body parts, and preserve morale. Registered occupational therapists, graduates of a 4-year college program, are employed in the occupational therapy department.

The *cardiopulmonary* or *respiratory care department* performs diagnostic tests to determine lung function, provides treatment related to respiratory function, and assists in maintaining patients on ventilators (breathing machines). The respiratory care therapist and the respiratory care technician, graduates of 1- to 4-year educational programs, are employed in this department.

The *radiation oncology department* or *radiation therapy department* may be a division within the diagnostic imaging department or a separate department. Its primary purpose is to treat cancerous growths. Cobalt beam units and linear accelerators are examples of equipment used in these departments. The radiation oncologist, a physician with additional education in the use of radiation for the treatment of disease, is the head of the radiation oncology department.

Support Services

The following departments are also very important in the concept of caring for all patients' needs. The HUC interacts with most of the following departments by requesting services, supplies, and/or equipment for patients on the nursing unit.

The *central service department (CSD)*, *materials management department*, or *supply purchasing department (SPD)*, is responsible for obtaining and distributing all supplies and equipment to be used by nursing personnel to perform treatments on patients. Sometimes, small hospitals band together to have greater purchasing power and to save money. Enema kits, dressing trays, bandages, and other supplies used most frequently by nursing unit personnel may be kept on the nursing unit. When a nurse takes an item from floor stock for patient use, the item is charged (by use of computer) to the appropriate patient by scanning the bar code on the item into the patient's account. CSD technicians replenish the unit supply daily. Figure 2-2, *A*, shows an example of a CSD or SPD supply room (also called *C-locker*); Figure 2-2, *B*, shows examples of

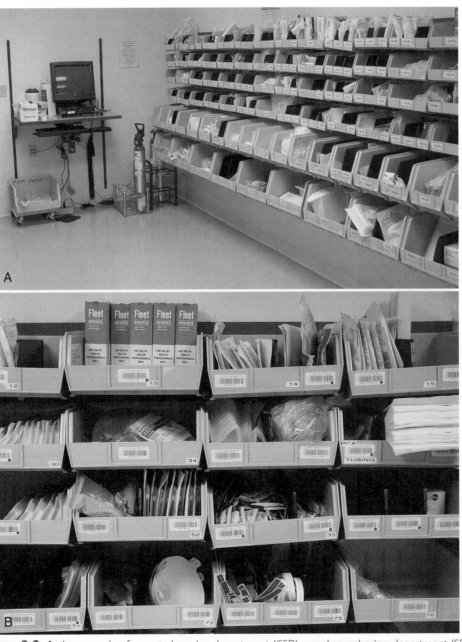

Figure 2-2 A, An example of a central service department (CSD), supply purchasing department (SPD) supply room, or C-locker located on the nursing unit. **B,** An example of floor stock found in the CSD, SPD supply room, or C-locker.

floor stock. Packs of supplies used by the operating and delivery rooms may be processed and sterilized by CSD personnel.

The *health information management system (HIMS)* or *medical records department* manages the patient's EMR or cares for the patient's paper record after the patient has been discharged from the hospital. Records are stored in this department and may be retrieved for the doctor if the patient is readmitted. These records (electronic and paper) also may be used for research. This department is also responsible for coding medical and surgical conditions of patients on discharge.

Coding is related to the system of Medicare reimbursement and involves **diagnosis-related groups (DRG)**, whereby payment is based on the type of illness. Accurate coding of the patient's diagnosis that is based on the **International Statistical Classification of Diseases and Related Health Problems (ICD)** is a critical function within the department. If coding is not exact, the direct result can be financial loss for the hospital. The ICD is used worldwide for morbidity and mortality statistics, reimbursement systems, and automated decision support in medicine. The **World Health Organization (WHO)** publishes three major and other minor updates annually.

Medical transcription (not related to transcription as used in the transcription of a doctor's orders) is another service of the health records department that is available to doctors for the dictation of patient history and physical examination findings, consultations, and various reports. The transcriptionist prepares typewritten reports from dictated tapes. These reports are placed or entered into the patient's EMR or chart. Some hospitals are using **voice-activated transcription,** by which the doctor speaks into the computer and the voice recognition software turns the dictation into accurate, formatted documents for final review and editing by medical transcriptionists. Because the drafts are formatted according to set standards, transcriptionists focus on checking primarily for important medical corrections.

The *quality assurance department* provides information to various departments within the hospital for the purpose of assisting those departments in providing high-quality care. Through analysis of actual occurrences and practices against standards set by various departments, quality assurance continuously uses ongoing activities to suggest improvements. Individual departments, such as nursing, may have their own quality assurance component, which coordinates with the hospital-wide quality assurance department. *Risk management,* a system of ensuring appropriate nursing care, can be part of the quality assurance manager's responsibilities. Risk management includes identifying possible risks, analyzing them, acting to reduce them, and evaluating the steps taken.

The *social services department* provides services to patients and to their families when emotional and environmental difficulties impede the patient's recovery. The social worker's knowledge of the community and of the agencies that provide a variety of services aids in lifting emotional and financial burdens caused by the illness. This department arranges nursing home and extended care facility placement and when necessary prepares patients for the transition from hospital to home. The department head holds an advanced degree in social work. This department may also be responsible for preparing patient health care directives when requested.

The *case management department* consists of individuals who work in health care facilities to coordinate patient care with insurance companies. The **case manager,** who is usually an RN and an expert in managed care, acts as an advocate for the patient to most appropriately enforce the benefits and coverage of his or her health policy and may also assist patients in preparing for the transition from hospital to home. A case manager may be certified as a *CCM (certified case manager),* as a nursing case manager through the ANCC, or in a specialty area, such as rehabilitation or disability. The case manager may have assistants or a secretary to assist with the workload.

The *home care department* identifies the needs of the patient who is returning to the home environment, plans for care by the visiting nurse service, and arranges the rental of needed equipment before the patient is discharged. Follow-up studies also are provided for the doctor. An RN with a public health background usually heads the department.

The *outpatient department* or clinic provides services to patients outside the hospital. Clinics for various disease conditions, such as diabetes, allergies, and gynecologic problems, may be open weekly. Prenatal care and dental care also may be offered. Visits are usually scheduled by appointment. The outpatient area provides clinical experience for resident doctors.

The *patient advocate, patient representative, or ombudsman* provides patient support in various capacities: communicating with physicians and insurance providers, identifying the best treatment options, clarifying doctors' instructions, and ensuring that a patient's rights aren't overlooked. Patients navigating the health care system are disadvantaged by a lack of medical and insurance knowledge. With the help of an advocate, a patient can be sure that his or her interests are being considered throughout the process

The *pastoral care department* provides spiritual support to the patient and family in time of need. Some hospitals maintain a chaplaincy program for members of the clergy who are interested in becoming hospital chaplains.

The *communications department* may be called the *telephone switchboard* or *hospital operator;* this department may serve as an information station for visitors to the hospital. Telephone operators process incoming and outgoing telephone calls and operate the doctor paging system. In emergencies, such as fire, disaster, or cardiac arrest, communications personnel alert hospital personnel in code, such as code 1000 to announce a fire. Again, there is advanced technology that has greatly improved the emergency alert process. Area hospitals are developing emergency communications plans that include mass communication devices that allow immediate worldwide communication and data capability. One person has the ability to communicate critical emergency information to tens, hundreds, or thousands of individuals, anywhere, anytime, and on any device within minutes. See Chapter 4 for more information on mass communication alert systems.

The *transportation department* performs multiple tasks throughout the hospital. Delivery of interdepartmental mail, carrying of specimens to the laboratory, assisting with the discharge or admission of patients, and transporting of patients from one area of the hospital to another are all carried out by personnel of this department.

The *public relations department* serves to provide the public with information concerning the hospital's activities. This may be accomplished by means of the community newspaper. Many hospitals publish a weekly, bimonthly, or monthly newspaper for patients and/or employees.

The *volunteer services department* is made up of people from the community. Members of the women's auxiliary or its counterpart, the men's auxiliary, give generously of their time and talents to staff the patient library or gift shop. Many perform tasks for the various hospital departments or on the nursing unit. High school students also may have an auxiliary organization.

Operational Services

The following services are not related to the direct care of the hospitalized patient but are concerned with the patient's hospital environment. It is the task of the HUC to request services from these departments as needed by the nursing unit.

The main responsibility of *environmental services* or the *housekeeping department* is to maintain a clean hospital through proper cleaning methods aimed at preventing the spread of infection. The environmental service department is responsible for daily cleaning and cleaning the individual patient unit after a patient has been discharged.

The *mechanical services department* responsibilities include keeping the hospital and its surroundings, equipment, and furnishings in good condition. In a large hospital, this department may be divided into various branches, such as engineering (heating, lighting, air conditioning, power systems, water, and sewage) and maintenance (painting, maintenance of televisions, carpentry, and pneumatic tube systems repair). Gardeners and groundskeepers are also members of this department.

The *hospital IT department* performs a variety of technical tasks involving the installation, diagnosis, repair, and maintenance of telephones, computers, network job entry stations, and related equipment within the computer network. Also, IT resolves network communications problems to ensure users' access to hospital networks. An IT manager and IT technicians are employed.

The *laundry department* or *linens department* maintains the hospital's linen supply; tasks may include the washing, drying, and repairing of linens. Many hospitals send the laundry out to a commercial laundry under the coordination of the hospital laundry department. Some hospitals may join together in ownership of a laundry service if this more economically serves the needs of all. Laundry personnel may deliver the linen to nursing care units.

The *human resources department* is responsible for employee payroll, organizes recruitment programs, interviews new employees, conducts employee termination interviews, and maintains records for all employees. Employee benefits and retirement records are also the responsibility of the human resource department. An employee fitness center is available in many hospitals to assist employees with their own health maintenance. Some hospitals may provide counseling services to employees to assist them in coping with personal and employment problems.

The *security department* is responsible for protecting the hospital, patients, visitors, and employees. Thefts and disturbances on the premises should be reported to this department. Whenever a threat of violence is perceived by the HUC, it must be immediately reported to security and to the nurse in charge. Most hospitals are using wireless mobile devices that enable instant two-way voice conversation without the need to remember a phone number or use a handset. See Chapter 4 for more information regarding communication and emergency alert devices.

Other Health Care Delivery Systems

Health care services such as **long-term care (LTC)** are often provided in nonhospital settings. Extended care facilities (ECFs) provide skilled or intermediate levels of care for patients who are not acutely ill and cannot be cared for at home.

Nursing homes, also called *health care centers*, provide **custodial care** for those who are so sick or functionally disabled that they require ongoing nursing and support services provided in a formal health care institution. Nursing homes are licensed by the state and may be classified by ownership and accreditation. Many hospitals also operate a SNF.

Physical medicine and rehabilitation facilities may be classified as ECFs, although such care may be given to outpatients as well. Individuals who receive care in such facilities primarily require special support services, in addition to varying levels of nursing care.

LTC also may be provided in the home through a home health agency. These agencies provide such services as skilled nursing, rehabilitation (for such problems as speech or language pathology or for physical or occupational therapy), pharmacy, and medical social work.

Hospice is a concept of providing long-term health care services wherever necessary. It provides palliative and supportive care for terminally ill patients and their families. Emphasis is placed on control of symptoms and preparation for and support before and after death. The hospice can be freestanding, hospital based, or home based.

EMPLOYMENT IN THE HEALTH CARE FIELD

The Bureau of Labor Statistics website states that health care will generate 3.2 million new wage and salary jobs between 2008 and 2018 (more than any other industry). This is largely in response to rapid growth in the elderly population. Ten of the 20 fastest-growing occupations are related to health care. Many job openings should arise in all health care employment settings as a result of employment growth and the need to replace workers who retire or leave their jobs for other reasons. Wage and salary employment in the health care industry is projected to increase 22% through 2018, compared with 11% for all industries combined. Employment growth is expected to account for about 22% of all wage and salary jobs added to the economy over the 2008-to-2018 period. (See Box 2-3, *Current Health Care Professionals*, and Box 2-4, *Health Care Employment Resources*.)

KEY CONCEPTS

Health care reform is a work in progress with many issues to be resolved. The HUC needs to be aware of changes and be prepared to meet the challenges. Working as an HUC provides an insight into what other health care careers are available and whether such a career is one that should be investigated further. Health care careers often involve very long and irregular hours but can be very rewarding, both personally and financially.

Websites of Interest

State Legislation and Actions Challenging Certain Health Reforms, 2011-2012: www.ncsl.org

GoHealth—Health insurance quotes for individuals and families: http://gohealthinsurance.com

Kaiser Health News: www.kaiserhealthnews.org

The Medicare and Medicaid Center: http://medicare-medicaid.com

The Free Medical Dictionary: http://medicaldictionary.thefreedictionary.com

Pros and cons of internet based EMR: www.electronic-medicalrecords.com/pros-and-cons-of-internet-based-electronic-medical-records-platforms/

BOX 2-3	CURRENT HEALTH CARE PROFESSIONALS

- Ambulance attendant
- Animal health technologist
- Art therapist
- Athletic trainer
- Audiologist or speech-language pathologist
- Cardiovascular technologist
- Chiropractor
- Clinical laboratory scientist
- Clinical laboratory technician
- Counselor
- Cytotechnologist
- Dental assistant
- Dental hygienist
- Dentist
- Diagnostic medical sonographer
- Dialysis technician
- Dietetic technician
- Dietitian or nutritionist
- Electrocardiograph technician
- Electroneurodiagnostic technician
- Emergency medical technician, paramedic
- Health information (medical records) administrator
- Health information specialist
- Health information technician
- Health unit coordinator
- Histotechnologist
- Home health aide
- Homeopath
- Hospital admitting clerk
- Hospital central service worker
- Licensed practical nurse
- Medical assistant
- Medical biller
- Medical coder
- Medical and health services manager
- Medical illustrator
- Medical radiation technologist
- Medical transcriptionist
- Midwife
- Music therapist
- Naturopath

- Nuclear medicine technologist
- Nurse anesthetist
- Nurse practitioner
- Nursing assistant
- Occupational therapist
- Occupational therapist assistant
- Ophthalmic dispensing optician
- Ophthalmic laboratory technician
- Ophthalmic medical technician
- Optician
- Optometrist
- Orthotist
- Patient advocate
- Patient care technician
- Perfusionist
- Perioperative nurse
- Pharmacist
- Pharmacist assistant
- Phlebotomist
- Physical therapist
- Physical therapist assistant
- Physician
- Physician assistant
- Physician specialist
- Physiotherapist
- Podiatrist
- Prosthetist
- Psychologist
- Psychology technician
- Radiology technician
- Radiology technologist
- Registered nurse
- Rehabilitation counselor
- Respiratory therapist
- Respiratory therapy technician
- Surgical technician first assistant
- Surgical technologist
- Therapeutic recreation specialist
- Ultrasonographer
- Veterinarian

Internet Evolution—Macrosite for news, analysis, and opinion about the future of the Internet: www.internetevolution.com

Careers in Healthcare American Medical Association: www.ama-assn.org/ama/pub/education-careers/careers-health-care.page

Occupational Outlook Handbook: www.bls.gov/oco

 REVIEW QUESTIONS

Visit the Evolve website to download and complete the following questions.

1. Define the following terms:
   a. diagnosis-related group
   b. primary insurance
   c. indigent
   d. secondary insurance
   e. telemedicine
   f. voice-activated transcription
   g. accreditation
   h. capitation
   i. coverage gap
   j. home health
   k. hospice
   l. voluntary
   m. catastrophic coverage
   n. custodial care
   o. proprietary
   p. patient portal

2. List five challenges facing today's health care system.

3. List four key elements of the Affordable Care Act.

BOX 2-4 **HEALTH CARE EMPLOYMENT RESOURCES**

Web listings of local job openings
Newspaper classifieds
School job placement center, career counselors, or instructors
Health care hotlines
Employment agencies
Library resources
Health care facility websites and bulletin boards
Networking with professionals in the field
Networking with NAHUC members
Local NAHUC representative

Useful Web Sites
www.jobsearch.monster.com
www.careerbuilder.com
www.beyond.com
www.hound.com
www.job.com
www.simplyhired.com

---

4. Explain why it is important to stay current with additional changes to the Affordable Care Act.

5. Explain how the implementation of a national EMR system would assist in a pandemic or national emergency.

6. Identify the challenge a health care provider faces when implementing an EMR system that is addressed in the U.S. Health Insurance Portability and Accountability Act of 1996 (HIPAA).

7. Explain the difference between client server–based EMR and cloud- or Web-based EMR.

8. Identify the EMR system used throughout the U.S. Department of Veterans Affairs (VA).

9. Explain the use of HIPAA-compliant mobile phones and patient portals.

10. List three categories of telemedicine and three major advances aided by surgical robots.

11. Explain the main characteristics of indemnity insurance, managed care, and worker's compensation insurance.

12. Identify the federal and state program that provides health care for the indigent.

13. Define the coverage of each of the following parts of Medicare: Medicare Part A, Medicare Part B, and Medicare Part D.

14. Identify at least three health care delivery systems that provide long-term or custodial care for patients unable to care for themselves.

15. Explain the basic concept of freestanding, in-home, or hospital-based hospice care.

16. List five functions a hospital may perform.

17. List three ways in which hospitals may be classified.

18. Explain what Magnet status signifies, and identify at least six benefits a hospital would obtain by achieving Magnet status.

19. Identify two agencies that set hospital operational guidelines.

20. Name the citizens' group that is at the head of the hospital's organizational structure, and describe its responsibilities.

21. Identify the individual in direct charge of a hospital, and explain his or her responsibilities.

22. Name the main function of the following hospital departments:
    a. business office
    b. admitting
    c. pathology or clinical laboratory
    d. diagnostic imaging
    e. radiation oncology
    f. pharmacy
    g. physical medicine
    h. cardiopulmonary or respiratory
    i. nutritional care
    j. endoscopy
    k. gastroenterology (GI lab)
    l. cardiovascular diagnostics
    m. neurology
    n. health information management system
    o. central supply
    p. social services
    q. environmental services
    r. security
    s. IT services
    t. mechanical
    u. human resources

23. List three resources used to access employment opportunities.

SURFING FOR ANSWERS

Following the guidelines for **surfing the Web** (see Box 1-9 provided in Chapter 1), find the following information and list the websites used. If necessary, use a school computer or go to a library.

1. Locate the government website for the Affordable Health Care Act, and identify two changes that will have a direct impact on you or a family member.
2. Find three websites that discuss cloud- or Web-based EMR versus server client–based EMR, list the websites, and write a one-paragraph opinion based on the facts presented.
3. Locate three health care careers (other than health unit coordinating) that are of interest, and copy the job descriptions.

CHAPTER 3

The Nursing Department and Medical Staff

OUTLINE

CHAPTER OBJECTIVES

On completion of this chapter, you will be able to:

1. Define the terms in the vocabulary list.
2. Write the meaning of the abbreviations in the abbreviations list.
3. Identify the respective roles of each of the provided medical staff.
4. Identify the titles of physicians who serve in a provided list of specialties.
5. List two common examples of physician extenders.
6. List and describe two complementary or alternative medicine options.
7. Describe the responsibilities of the nursing service department.
8. Identify the title of the person responsible for the overall administration of the nursing service and the person responsible for nursing unit administration.
9. Identify the services provided by each of the regular (floor) nursing units and intensive care units in provided lists.
10. List five telecommunication services and explain the benefits of an eICU.
11. Explain what is required for an outpatient to become an inpatient.
12. Describe the purpose of the following specialty units: emergency department, hospice inpatient, and the chronic pain management unit.
13. List three services that come under the general heading of perioperative services, and provide a description of each.
14. List four personnel commonly employed in nursing units, and briefly describe the role of each.
15. Describe the team patient care model and the total patient care model.
16. List six benefits of interdisciplinary teamwork.
17. Explain the philosophy of holistic nursing care.
18. Explain the purpose of a clinical pathway, and list four goals to be met when developing a clinical pathway.
19. Describe information that would be included on an assignment sheet.

VOCABULARY

Acuity Level of care patients would require on the basis of their medical condition; used to evaluate staffing needs.

Acupuncture Field that originated in China more than 5000 years ago; based on a belief that all living things have a vital energy, called *qi*.

Acute Care Level of health care generally provided in hospitals or emergency departments for sudden, serious illnesses or trauma.

Alternative Medicine Any practice not generally recognized by the medical community as a standard or conventional medical approach and used instead of standard treatments.

American Nurses Association (ANA) The national professional association of registered nurses in the United States, founded in 1896 to improve standards of health and the availability of health care.

Assignment Sheet A form completed at the beginning of each work shift that indicates the nursing staff member(s) assigned to each patient on that nursing unit.

Assistant Nurse Manager A registered nurse who assists the nurse manager in coordinating activities on the nursing unit.

Attending Physician Term applied to a physician who admits and is responsible for a hospital patient.

Certified Nursing Assistant A certified health care giver who performs basic nursing tasks.

Chiropractic Medicine Complementary and alternative health care profession with the purpose of diagnosing and treating mechanical disorders of the spine and musculoskeletal system with the intention of affecting the nervous system and improving health.

Chronic Long-lasting: describes an illness or medical condition that lasts over a long period and sometimes causes a long-term change in the body.

Clinical Pathway A method of outlining a patient's path of treatment for a specific diagnosis, procedure, or symptom.

Complementary Medicine Nonstandard treatments that may be used along with standard treatments.

Director of Nursing A registered nurse in charge of nursing services (may be called *director of patient services, nursing administrator, vice president of nursing services,* or *chief nursing officer* [CNO]).

Electronic Intensive Care Unit (eICU) An intensive care unit with a highly advanced electronic clinical information system and a consolidated treatment unit (also called *Advanced Intensive Care Unit* or *tele-ICU*).

Holistic Nursing Care A modern nursing practice that expresses the philosophy of total patient care that considers the physical, emotional, social, economic, and spiritual needs of the patient. Also called *comprehensive care.*

Homeopathy A natural form of medicine that treats the whole person with natural medicines. It is good therapy for mood swings, depression, anxiety, obsessive-compulsive disorder, and also attention-deficit/hyperactivity disorder.

Hospitalist Full-time, acute care specialist who focuses exclusively on hospitalized patients.

Inpatient Patient to receive medical or surgical care whose doctor has written an admission order.

Intensivist Specializes in the care of critically ill patients, usually in an intensive care unit (ICU).

Interdisciplinary Teamwork Well-coordinated collaboration among health care professionals toward a common goal (improved, efficient patient care).

Licensed Practical Nurse A graduate of a 1-year school of nursing program who is licensed in the state in which he or she is practicing; provides direct care and functions under the direction of the registered nurse.

Native American Healing The practices and healing beliefs of hundreds of indigenous tribes of North America. Native American healing is a combination of religion, spirituality, herbal medicine, and rituals.

Naturopathic Medicine Alternative medical system that proposes that there is a healing power in the body that establishes, maintains, and restores health. Treatments include nutrition and lifestyle counseling, nutritional supplements, medicinal plants, exercise, homeopathy, and treatments from traditional Chinese medicine.

Nurse Manager A registered nurse who assists the director of nursing in carrying out administrative responsibilities and is in charge of one or more nursing units (may also be called *unit manager, clinical manager,* or *patient care manager*).

Nurse Practitioner (NP) A registered nurse (RN) who has completed advanced education (a minimum of a master's degree) and training in the diagnosis and management of common medical conditions, including chronic illnesses.

Nursing Intervention Actions undertaken by a nurse to further the course of treatment for a patient.

Nursing Service Department Hospital department responsible for all nursing care administered to patients.

Nursing Unit Administration Division within the hospital responsible for nonclinical patient care.

Outpatient A patient receiving medical or surgical care while registered as an outpatient and whose doctor has not written an admission order. The patient's doctor may order the patient to stay overnight for observation without writing an admitting order.

Patient Care Conference Meeting of a patient's doctor or resident, primary nurse, case manager or social worker, and other health care professionals for the purpose of planning the patient's care.

Patient Support Associate Nursing unit staff member whose duties may include some patient-admitting responsibilities, coding, or stocking of nursing units; job description and title may vary among hospitals.

Perioperative Services Department of the hospital that provides care before (preoperative), during (intraoperative), and after (postoperative) surgery. It encompasses total care of the patient during the surgical experience.

Physician Assistant (PA) One who practices medicine under the supervision of physicians and surgeons.

Physician Extender A health care provider who is not a physician but who performs medical activities typically performed by a physician (includes nurse practitioners and physician assistants).

Primary Care Physician (PCP) A general practitioner or internist, chosen by an individual to serve as his or her health care professional. Sometimes referred to as *gatekeepers.*

Registered Nurse Graduate of a 2- or 4-year college-based nursing program or a 3-year hospital-based program who is licensed in the state in which he or she is practicing; may provide direct patient care or may supervise patient care given by others.

Remote Patient Monitoring Use of wireless technologies to remotely collect and send data to medical professionals for interpretation.

Resident A graduate of a medical school who is gaining experience in a hospital.

Shift Manager Registered nurse who is responsible for one or more units during his or her assigned shift. Also may be called *nursing coordinator* or *charge nurse.*

Staff Development Department responsible for orientation of new employees and continuing education of employed nursing service personnel. Also may be called *educational services.*

SWAT HUC, SWAT Nurse, or SWAT Team A health unit coordinator, a nurse, or a group of health care workers who are on call for all units in the hospital to provide assistance as needed.

Note: the definition of "SWAT" is special weapons and tactics and is usually associated with specially trained policeman; when used in the context of health care it means "SWAT like, meaning that trained personnel are able to respond quickly when needed or called upon"

Team Leader Registered nurse who is in charge of a nursing team. Also may be called *pod leader* or *charge nurse.*

Team Patient Care Model Model of care involving a team that consists of a charge nurse and two or three team leaders, along with four or five team members who work under the supervision of each team leader.

Telecommunication The transmission, emission, or reception of data or other information in the form of signs, signals, writings, images, and sounds or any other form, via wire, radio, visual, or other electromagnetic systems (from the ANA).

Total Patient Care Model Model of care in which one nurse provides total care to assigned patients (also called *Primary Care Model* or *Case Nursing Model*).

Triage Nursing interventions. Classification defined as establishing priorities of patient care, usually according to a three-level model: emergent, urgent, and nonurgent.

ABBREVIATIONS

Abbreviation	Meaning
ANA	American Nurses Association
ANCC	American Nurses Credentialing Center
CNA	certified nursing assistant
DO	doctor of osteopathy
DSU	day surgery unit
ED or ER	emergency department, emergency room
eICU	electronic intensive care unit
ENT	ear, nose, and throat doctor (otorhinolaryngologist)
HO	house officer
LPN	licensed practical nurse
MD	medical doctor
MDA	medical doctor of anesthesia
ND or NMD	naturopathic doctor, doctor of naturopathic medicine, naturopathic medical doctor
NP	nurse practitioner
OR	operating room
PA	physician assistant
PACU	postanesthesia care unit
PCP	primary care physician
PSA	patient support associate
RN	registered nurse
SAD or SDS	save-a-day (surgery), same-day surgery (patient admitted on the day of surgery)

EXERCISE 1

Write the abbreviation for each term listed.

1. American Nurses Association
2. American Nurses Credentialing Center
3. certified nursing assistant
4. doctor of osteopathy
5. day surgery unit
6. ear, nose, and throat doctor (otorhinolaryngologist)
7. electronic intensive care unit
8. emergency department or emergency room
9. house officer
10. licensed practical nurse
11. medical doctor of anesthesia
12. medical doctor
13. doctor of naturopathic medicine or naturopathic medical doctor
14. nurse practitioner
15. operating room
16. primary care physician
17. patient support associate
18. physician assistant
19. postanesthesia care unit
20. registered nurse
21. save-a-day (surgery) or same-day surgery

EXERCISE 2

Write the meaning of each abbreviation listed.

1. ANA
2. ANCC
3. CNA
4. DO
5. DSU
6. eICU
7. ED or ER
8. ENT
9. HO
10. LPN
11. MD
12. MDA
13. ND or NMD
14. NP
15. OR
16. PA
17. PACU
18. PCP
19. PSA
20. RN
21. SAD (surgery) or SDS

THE MEDICAL STAFF

Often doctors and especially residents refer to the health unit coordinator (HUC) as their best friend. The HUC gives and receives messages for the doctors and residents, assists with the use of the electronic medical record (EMR), transcribes orders, locates charts and information, and is generally helpful.

A physician who has been appointed to the medical staff and who sends a patient to the hospital for admission is known as the patient's **attending physician**. The attending physician may also be the patient's **primary care physician (PCP)**, a general practitioner or internist who has been chosen by an individual to serve as his or her health care professional and who is capable of handling a variety of health-related problems. The attending physician or PCP prescribes care and treatment (doctor's orders) during the patient's hospital stay and may be a medical doctor (MD) or a doctor of osteopathy (DO). Both pursue identical approved programs of study, but colleges of osteopathic medicine place special emphasis on the relationship of organs to the musculoskeletal system. Structural problems are corrected by manipulation. Attending physicians are not hospital employees and receive no salary from the hospital. A **hospitalist** is a hospital-based general physician who is usually an internist, family practice physician, or pediatrician. Hospitalists assume the care of hospitalized patients in place of patients' PCPs. This position was created in 1991 to enable family physicians to effectively manage their inpatient practices and treat more people in their outpatient practices. Hospitalists are employed by and receive a salary from the hospital. There may be other doctors on the staff (such as the director of medical education, the hospital pathologist, an infection disease doctor, or the director of radiation oncology) who are salaried hospital employees.

Large hospitals may offer an educational program in which medical school graduates can apply their knowledge to the practice of medicine. The term **resident** is applied to all medical school graduates who are gaining hospital experience. Such a graduate is frequently referred to as a *postgraduate year 1 (PGY-1)* or *first-year resident*. A resident may be referred to as *house staff* or a *house officer (HO)*.

Physicians who specialize in a particular aspect of medicine, such as pediatrics, internal medicine, or general surgery, spend 3 to 5 years in a specific residency program. After completing the residency and passing a specific examination, the physician is acknowledged as certified. Often after residency, a 1- to 2-year fellowship period provides the opportunity for the clinician to become more familiar with a specific area, such as cardiology. These practitioners are referred to as *fellows*. Some attending physicians serve as teachers of hospital residents.

Many physicians have chosen to practice in special fields and are known by their specialties. It is common to refer to a doctor by his or her specialty, as in the terms *cardiologist, gynecologist,* and *pediatrician*. In the course of work at the hospital, medical specialty terms may be required when one is referring to doctors (Table 3-1).

Physician Extenders

Physician extenders are in high demand with the expansion of health care. Examples of physician extenders include; A **physician assistant (PA)** practices medicine under the supervision of physicians and surgeons. A PA may be the principal care provider in rural or inner-city clinics where a physician is present for only 1 or 2 days each week and would confer with the supervising physician and other medical professionals as needed and as required by law. PAs also may make house calls or go to hospitals and nursing care facilities to check on patients, after which they report back to the physician. PAs also may prescribe certain medications.

A **nurse practitioner (NP)** is a **registered nurse (RN)** who has completed advanced education (a minimum of a master's degree) and training in the diagnosis and management of common medical conditions, including **chronic illnesses**. NPs provide some of the same care provided by physicians and maintain close working relationships with physicians. An NP can serve as a patient's regular health care provider.

COMPLEMENTARY AND ALTERNATIVE MEDICINE

Alternative medicine is any practice not generally recognized by the medical community as a standard or conventional medical approach and that is used instead of standard treatments. Some alternative therapies have dangerous or even life-threatening side effects. With others, the main danger is that the patient may lose the opportunity to benefit from standard therapy. **Complementary medicine** refers to nonstandard treatments that are used along with standard ones. Some of the complementary and alternative medicine options include the following:

- **Chiropractic medicine** is a complementary and alternative health care profession with the purpose of diagnosing and treating mechanical disorders of the spine and musculoskeletal system with the intention of affecting the nervous system and improving health.
- **Acupuncture** originated in China more than 5000 years ago and is based on a belief that all living things have a vital energy, called *qi*. Acupuncture is a popular alternative therapy.
- **Homeopathy** is a natural medicine that treats the whole person with natural medicines. It is good therapy for mood swings, depression, anxiety, obsessive-compulsive disorder, and attention-deficit/hyperactivity disorder.
- **Native American healing** is the practices and healing beliefs of hundreds of indigenous tribes of North America. Native American healing is a combination of religion, spirituality, herbal medicine, and rituals. Sacred traditions in healing are passed from one healer to the next on through generations and are more about healing the person than curing a particular illness.
- **Naturopathic medicine** is based on the belief that the human body has an innate healing ability. A *naturopathic doctor (ND or NMD)* uses diet, exercise, lifestyle changes, and cutting-edge natural therapies to enhance a patient's body's ability to ward off and combat disease. Naturopathic physicians craft comprehensive treatment plans that blend the best of modern medical science and traditional natural medical approaches not only to treat disease, but also to restore health.

TABLE 3-1 Common Medical Specialties

Physician's Specialty	Specialty Description
Allergist	Treats patients who have hypersensitivity to pollens, foods, medications, and other substances.
Anesthesiologist (Medical Doctor of Anesthesia [MDA])	Administers drugs or gases to produce loss of consciousness or sensation in the patient; care during surgery and recovery from an anesthetic is included.
Cardiologist	Diagnoses and treats diseases of the heart and blood vessels.
Dermatologist	Diagnoses and treats disorders of the skin.
Emergency room physician	Diagnoses and treats patients in trauma and emergency situations.
Endocrinologist	Diagnoses and treats diseases of the internal glands that secrete hormones.
Family practitioner	Specializes in primary health care for all family members.
Gastroenterologist	Diagnoses and treats diseases of the digestive tract.
Geriatrist	Diagnoses and treats diseases and problems of aging.
Gynecologist	Diagnoses and treats disorders and diseases of the female reproductive tract.
Hospitalist	Assumes the care of hospitalized patients in the place of patients' primary care physician.
Intensivist	Specializes in the care of critically ill patients, usually in an intensive care unit (ICU).
Internist	Diagnoses and medically treats diseases and disorders of the internal organs of adults.
Interventional radiologist	A board-certified physician who specializes in minimally invasive, targeted treatments.
Neonatologist	Diagnoses and treats disorders of the newborn.
Neurologist	Diagnoses and treats diseases of the nervous system.
Obstetrician	Cares for women during pregnancy, labor, and delivery, and after delivery.
Oncologist	Diagnoses and treats cancerous conditions.
Ophthalmologist	Diagnoses and treats diseases and defects of the eye.
Orthopedist	Diagnoses and treats diseases or fractures of the musculoskeletal system.
Otolaryngologist	Diagnoses and treats diseases of the ear, nose, and throat (ENT)
Pathologist	Studies cell changes and other alterations of the body caused by disease.
Pediatrician	Provides preventive care and diagnoses and treats diseases of children.
Physiatrist	Diagnoses and treats diseases of the neuromusculoskeletal system with physical elements to restore the individual to participation in society.
Proctologist	Diagnoses and treats diseases of the rectum and anus.
Psychiatrist	Diagnoses and treats mental illness.
Pulmonologist	Diagnoses and treats pulmonary (lung) conditions and diseases.
Radiation oncologist	Treats cancer through the use of radiation.
Radiologist	Diagnoses and treats diseases with the use of various methods of imaging such as radiography, ultrasound, scanning with radioactive materials, and magnetic resonance imaging.
Surgeon	Treats diseases and injuries through operative methods; may specialize in a particular area, such as heart, eye, or pediatric surgery.
Urologist	Diagnoses and treats diseases of the male and female urinary tracts and of the male reproductive system.

NURSING SERVICE ORGANIZATION

The Nursing Service Department

The **nursing service department** is basically responsible for ensuring the physical and emotional care of the hospitalized patient. The **American Nurses Association (ANA)** definition of nursing is as follows: "Nursing is the protection, promotion, and optimization of health and abilities, prevention of illness and injury, alleviation of suffering through the diagnosis and treatment of human response, and advocacy in the care of individuals, families, communities, and populations." Other responsibilities include patient assessment and recording, planning and implementing patient care plans, and patient teaching. Implementation of the EMR requires the nurse to enter documentation directly into the patient's record at the bedside via computer. The nurse enters documentation on electronic flow sheets packed with an array of drop-down menus. There are required pieces of documentation that address the concern of different health care agencies. In 2005 The Joint Commission (TJC; formerly the Joint Commission on Accreditation of Healthcare Organizations) put "falls" on its national patient safety list, so charting now has to detail a commitment to fall prevention. The Centers for Medicare and Medicaid Services will not reimburse the cost of treating bedsores that develop during a hospital stay, so a new drop-down menu charts whether a patient is at risk and whether he or she has pressure ulcers already.

The nursing service department is usually the single largest component of the hospital. Often 50% or more of all hospital personnel are employed in the nursing service department. More than a quarter million nurses have been certified by the American Nurses Credentialing Center (ANCC) since 1990. More than 80,000 advanced practice nurses are currently certified by ANCC.

NURSING SERVICE ADMINISTRATIVE PERSONNEL

The **director of nursing**, also called the *vice president of nursing*, is responsible for the overall administration of nursing service. Setting nursing practice standards and staffing are two examples of the responsibilities of the director of nursing. The director of nursing is responsible to the chief executive officer of the health care facility.

The **nurse manager** (also called *clinical manager, patient care manager,* or *unit manager*) is a registered nurse (RN) who usually is responsible for the patients and nursing personnel on the unit for 24 hours a day. The nurse manager reports to the director of nursing. Managerial responsibilities include the planning and coordinating of high-quality nursing care for patients hospitalized on the unit. Selecting, supervising, scheduling, and evaluating personnel employed on the unit are other managerial responsibilities of the nurse manager. The nurse manager works closely with physicians to coordinate nursing care with the care prescribed by the physician. Usually, an RN titled charge nurse, **shift manager**, nursing care manager, or **assistant nurse manager** oversees the nursing unit in the absence of the nurse manager.

The director of **staff development** is responsible for the orientation and evaluation of new nursing service employees and for the continuing education, including TJC requirements, of all employed nursing service personnel. The person in this position usually reports to the director of nursing.

Nursing Unit Administration

Some hospitals have a division of **nursing unit administration** that is responsible for nonclinical patient care functions. In this model, the nursing unit administration is made up of two categories of workers: the HUC and the health unit manager. The HUC is supervised by the health unit manager rather than by the nurse manager. The HUC continues to work very closely with the nursing unit team.

The *health unit manager* performs supervisory and administrative nonclinical functions, such as budgeting, research, and training of new employees, possibly for several nursing units. Health unit managers also may be RNs or may hold degrees in other disciplines. Unit management usually functions under administration rather than under the nursing services department. See Figure 3-1 for an organizational chart that includes nursing unit administration.

HOSPITAL NURSING UNITS

The HUC works at the nurses' station on the nursing unit. The hospital is divided into nursing units according to the types of services provided to patients. The HUC usually has a computer that is used for transcribing orders and for entering and retrieving information. Additional computers, including portable computers and notebooks that may be taken into the patients' rooms, are available on the unit for the use of doctors, nurses, and other health care personnel. The area where the HUC sits may be a much smaller and partially enclosed area with a computer, a scanner, and a fax machine.

Many methods are used to name the nursing units within the hospital. Sometimes units are named according to the service offered, such as pediatrics, or the name may be derived from the floor level and direction of the hospital wing (e.g., 4 East).

Regular (Floor) Nursing Units

Most nursing units are designed to accommodate 18 to 50 hospitalized patients. A nursing unit may provide one of the following services:
- *Behavioral health:* Includes *psychiatry ("Psych"),* which is the care of patients hospitalized for treatment of disorders of the mind or having difficulty coping with life situations; also may include programs for treatment of alcohol and drug abuse and programs related to changing destructive behaviors such as eating disorders.

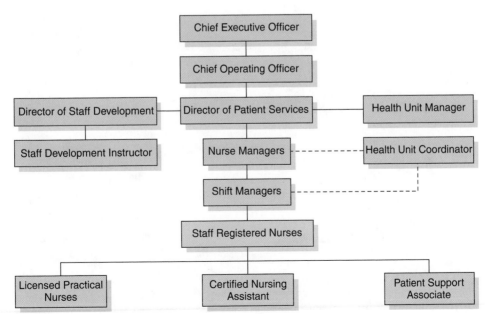

Figure 3-1 Organizational structure of the nursing services department and nursing unit administration.

- *Cardiovascular:* Care of patients who are hospitalized for the treatment of diseases of the circulatory system.
- *Gynecologic surgery ("Gyn"):* Care of women who are hospitalized for surgery of the female reproductive tract.
- *Intermediate or step-down care unit:* Care of patients who require more specialized care than that given on floor nursing units but who do not require intensive care (also called *intermediate* or *transitional care unit*).
- *Medical ("Med"):* Care of patients who are hospitalized for medical treatment.
- *Neurology ("Neuro"):* Care of patients who are hospitalized for treatment of diseases of the nervous system. Some hospitals have Parkinson and epilepsy units.
- *Obstetrics ("OB"), labor and delivery ("L&D"), and nursery:* Care of mothers before, during, and after labor and care of newborn infants.
- *Oncology:* Care of patients who are hospitalized for treatment of cancer.
- *Orthopedics ("Ortho"):* Care of patients who are hospitalized for treatment of diseases or fractures of the musculoskeletal system.
- *Pediatrics ("Peds"):* Care of children (12 and younger) who are hospitalized for medical or surgical treatment.
- *Rehabilitation ("Rehab"):* Care of patients who have had a stroke, head injury, amputation, multiple trauma, neuromuscular disorders, and other conditions. The goal is to improve the patient's function and maximize the potential for return to home, school, work, and the community.
- *Surgical ("Surg"):* Care of patients who are hospitalized for general surgical treatment.
- *Telemetry ("Tele"):* Care of patients with cardiac arrhythmias and other heart problems. Electrocardiogram (ECG) readings are monitored at the nurses' station. An example of telemetry screens on a telemetry unit is shown in Figure 3-2.

- *Urology:* Care of patients who are hospitalized for treatment of diseases of the male reproductive or urinary system or of the female urinary system.

Intensive Care Units

Specialized *intensive care units* (ICUs) contain the equipment, medical and nursing staff, and monitoring devices necessary to provide intensive-care medicine. The ICU (also called *critical care unit [CCU]*) provides constant specialized **acute care** to critically ill patients. As the condition of the critically ill patient improves (but not enough to go to a floor unit), the patient is transferred to the *intermediate care (IMC)* or *step-down unit* for less intensive nursing care. ICUs are usually identified by the type of care they provide to a particular population of patients. For example, the *surgical intensive care unit (SICU)* cares for critically ill surgical patients, the *medical intensive care unit (MICU)* cares for critically ill medical patients, the *coronary care unit* cares for patients with acute heart disease, the *trauma intensive care unit (TICU)* cares for patients involved in trauma such as a car accident whose condition is considered critical, the *neonatal intensive care unit (NICU)* cares for premature and ill newborns, and the *pediatric intensive care unit (PICU)* cares for critically ill pediatric patients.

Personnel employed in an ICU are specially qualified for acute nursing care. An **intensivist** specializes in the care of critically ill patients and usually works in an ICU.

Telecommunication Services

Telecommunication is not a new role for nurses, who have made follow-up calls to patients after outpatient procedures or surgery and have provided guidance, education, and lab results over the telephone for more than 25 years. In recent years, telecommunication has come to include more sophisticated systems than the telephone, such as two-way audio and

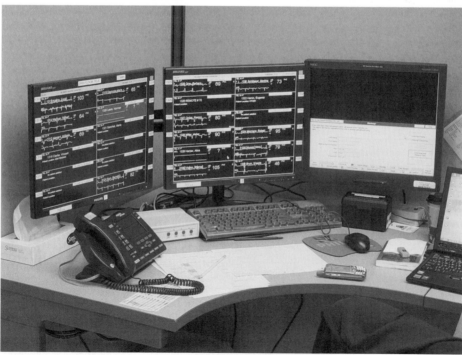

Figure 3-2 An example of telemetry screens on a telemetry unit.

video systems, the Internet (including social networks), and other communication systems. Telecommunication services include the following:

- *Specialist referral services* involve a specialist assisting a general practitioner in making a diagnosis and may involve a patient and/or nurse "seeing" a specialist via a live, remote consultation or the transmission of health records and diagnostic images and/or video.
- *Interactive telemedicine services* provide real-time interactions between the patient and the doctor and/or nurse. Nurses may visit and assist homebound patients via videoconferencing, the Internet, social networking, videophone conferencing, and so on. "Clinician-interactive" telemedicine services may be less costly than in-person visits—one nurse can "visit" 12 to 16 patients per day. *Call centers* operated by managed care organizations are staffed by RNs who act as case managers, perform patient **triage,** or provide information, education, and counseling as a means of regulating patient access and decreasing the use of emergency rooms.
- *Remote patient monitoring* uses wireless technologies to remotely collect and send data to medical professionals for interpretation. These data may include blood glucose levels, pulse oximetry results, ECGs, or a variety of indicators for homebound patients. Such services can be used to supplement the use of visiting nurses.
- *Medical education* provides continuing medical education credits for health professionals and special medical education seminars for targeted groups in remote locations.
- *Consumer medical and health information* includes the use of the Internet and social networks for consumers to obtain specialized health information and have access to online discussion groups for peer-to-peer support.

Electronic Intensive Care Unit

The **electronic intensive care unit (eICU)** was developed by Philips VISICU to address the intensivist shortage. The advanced or electronic ICU uses telemedicine technology that combines clinical management software with patient data and real-time video feeds to allow intensivists and critical care nurses to care and monitor the ICU 24 hours a day, 7 days a week. The technology used includes a dashboard view of key patient information such as vital signs, physiologic data, medications, lab results, and more. Telemedicine care tools include a high-definition, remote-controlled camera located in the ceiling that is so sensitive that one can tell if the patient's eyes are reactive and dilated. Videoconferencing allows tele-ICU physicians and nurses to see and communicate directly with patients, families, and on-site clinicians from a central control station. The system also provides automated alerts that can identify trends in the patient's condition before an on-site caregiver might notice. For example, a patient's blood pressure may seem stable each time it is checked, when in actuality it could vary considerably between those checks.

The advanced ICU intensivist-led program helps hospitals improve patient outcomes and support continuous quality improvements. It is perfect for understaffed hospitals, as it acts as an extra set of eyes to help support nurses and physicians— nurses can't be everywhere at once! Hospitals using the advanced ICU have reported a 40% reduction in ICU mortality on average.

Patients have lower risks of death and shorter ICU and hospital stays when an intensivist physician is on duty. The advanced ICU intensivist-led program is presently implemented at 22 hospitals in 10 states.

⭐ **HIGH PRIORITY**

Tele-intensivists have privileges at all of the hospitals to which they are providing supplemental care and therefore are able to prescribe treatments and enter notes into the chart. The orders and notes are electronically signed using a unique personal identification number (PIN) and transmitted to a printer or transferred electronically for inclusion in the chart.

Outpatient Care

Day surgery or *outpatient surgery unit* or *ambulatory surgery* involves the care of patients who are having surgery or examinations but who do not require overnight hospitalization. Nearly six of every 10 surgeries performed at hospitals (usually in a day surgery unit [DSU]) are outpatient procedures. Outpatient surgeries may be performed in the hospital or at a surgicenter (surgical center).

Inpatient versus Outpatient Surgery

A patient having surgery may be admitted on the day of surgery rather than the day before, to reduce the cost of the hospital stay; this is called *save-a-day (SAD) surgery* or *same-day surgery (SDS).* A patient who is to receive medical or surgical care that has been preapproved by the insurance company is considered an **inpatient** when a doctor formally writes an admission order. A patient receiving medical or surgical care is considered an **outpatient** when registered on hospital records as an outpatient even if his or her doctor has ordered overnight observation (but has not written an admission order). Being an inpatient or an outpatient affects the patient's out-of-pocket costs.

Specialty Units
Emergency Department or Emergency Room

The emergency department (ED or emergency room (ER) involves care of patients who need emergency treatment. After emergency treatment has been administered, the patient is admitted to the hospital or is discharged to home, according to his or her medical needs.

Hospice Inpatient Unit

Some hospitals have hospice units for terminally ill patients who need more care than can be managed at home or whose symptoms require more intense management than a family caregiver can provide. Admissions to and from the unit are coordinated with the patient's physicians and the hospice team. Inpatient services are usually reimbursed by Medicare and private insurance providers once specific clinical criteria have been met.

Chronic Pain Management Unit

Some hospitals have a *chronic pain management unit (CPMU),* which offers treatment of individuals in chronic pain. *Chronic pain* can be defined as pain that lasts for more than 3 months despite medical intervention and treatment. The pain management unit provides a specialist service including assessment, treatment, and management planning, as well as group and individual therapy for patients and their families.

Perioperative Services

Perioperative services include the following:

- *Preoperative area:* Area in the hospital where patients are prepared for surgery
- *Intraoperative area:* Operating room (OR); area in the hospital where surgery is performed
- *Postoperative area:* Postanesthesia care unit (PACU) or recovery room; area in the hospital where patients are cared for immediately after surgery until they have recovered from the effects of the anesthesia

NURSING UNIT PERSONNEL

To maintain 24-hour coverage, nursing service personnel usually are scheduled in two shifts. An example would be one shift from 7:00 AM to 7:30 PM (day shift) and one from 7:00 PM to 7:30 AM (night shift). Three shifts also may be used; these shifts are usually 7:00 AM to 3:30 PM, 3:00 PM to 11:30 PM, and 11:00 PM to 7:30 AM. Shifts overlap by half an hour to allow communication between personnel.

Nursing personnel other than the HUC, who may be employed on the nursing unit and functioning under the supervision of the nurse manager, are discussed in the following paragraphs.

The registered nurse is a graduate of a 2- to 4-year college-based program or a 3-year hospital-based program and is licensed to practice in the state of employment. The RN performs all types of treatments, and it is usually hospital policy that only the RN can perform complex procedures, such as administering intravenous (IV) medication. The RN is responsible for applying the nursing process. This encompasses assessment, nursing diagnosis, planning, implementation, and evaluation of patient care, as well as participating in educating patients and family and teaching staff members. When the EMR is in use, the RN is responsible for reading doctors' orders from the patient's electronic record, carrying them out, and entering his or her notes directly into the computer to become part of the patient's permanent record.

The **licensed practical nurse (LPN)** is a graduate of a 1-year school of nursing program and is licensed to practice in the state of employment. The LPN functions under the direction of the RN and provides direct patient care; performs technical skills, such as discontinuing an IV injection; and administers medication to patients as prescribed by physicians.

The **certified nursing assistant (CNA)** has completed a short training course (6 to 12 weeks in length) at a vocational school. A state examination is required for the nursing assistant to be certified. Nursing assistants perform bedside tasks, such as bathing and feeding patients. They also provide basic treatments, such as taking vital signs and giving enemas. The CNA functions under the supervision of the RN or LPN.

The **patient support associate (PSA)** is a staff member whose duties may include some patient admitting responsibilities, coding, or stocking supplies on nursing units. This job description may vary among hospitals.

When help is needed on a nursing unit owing to new admissions, medical emergencies, or a shortage of help, most hospitals employ a **SWAT HUC, SWAT nurse,** or **SWAT team** that can be called on to assist.

NURSING CARE DELIVERY MODELS

The two most common nursing care delivery models used in hospitals today are the team and total or patient care models, as described in the following sections.

Team Patient Care Model

In the **team patient care model,** the charge nurse oversees the nursing unit, with two or three teams, each led by a **team leader** (RN) and three or four team members working under the supervision of each team leader. Members of the team may be RNs, LPNs, and/or CNAs. The team leader assigns patients to each team member on the basis of patient **acuity** for care during a shift. Team members perform the particular tasks for their patients that they are qualified to perform. The team leader is responsible for the patients and for the members of his or her team. A team usually cares for 15 or fewer patients; thus a nursing unit may have one to three teams. Many hospitals use modified forms of the team patient care method. An example of a team patient care model is shown in Figure 3-3.

Total Patient Care Model

The **total patient care model** sometimes is referred to as *primary care* or *case nursing.* In total patient care, the RN assigned to a group of patients is responsible for planning, organizing, and performing all care, including providing personal hygiene, medications, treatments, emotional support, and education, required for that group of patients during an assigned shift. An example of a total patient care model is shown in Figure 3-4.

INTERDISCIPLINARY TEAMWORK

Interdisciplinary teamwork is the well coordinated collaboration across health care professions toward a common goal (improved, efficient patient care). Planning of nursing care involves consultation with other members of the health care team. Consultations are most advantageous during planning

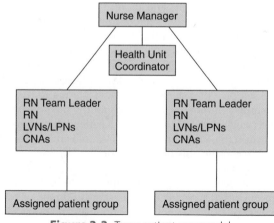

Figure 3-3 Team patient care model.

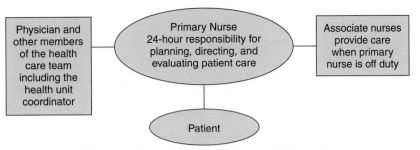

Figure 3-4 Total patient care (case nursing) model.

and implementation and are based on problem solving. Often, a **patient care conference** is held with members of the health care team, which may include the patient's doctor or resident, primary nurse, and case worker or social worker, as well as any other health care professional who is caring for the patient and can provide input. Benefits of interdisciplinary teamwork include the following:

- Facilitates continuous quality improvement
- Improves patient care
- Decreases errors
- Provides total patient care
- Maximizes resources
- Increases professional satisfaction for health care givers

There is no team without personal accountability. The HUC is a member of the health care team who plays an important role in maximizing efficiency in patient care and treatment.

Holistic Nursing Care

Holistic nursing care is defined as "all nursing practice that has healing the whole person as its goal" (American Holistic Nurses Association, 1998, Description of Holistic Nursing). Holistic nursing care is the modern nursing practice that expresses the philosophy of comprehensive patient care (total patient care) and considers the physical, emotional, social, economic, and spiritual needs of the patient, his or her response to illness, and the effect of the illness on ability to meet self-care needs. Holistic health is the concept that concern for health requires the perspective of the individual as an integrated system; rather than treating specific symptoms, practitioners consider all factors when completing a patient's clinical pathway.

CLINICAL PATHWAY

A **clinical pathway**, also called a *critical path*, is used as a method of outlining a patient's path of treatment for a specific diagnosis, procedure, or symptom. A **nursing intervention** is any action undertaken by a nurse to further the course of treatment for a patient. Nursing interventions include assessment, development of an intervention plan, and evaluation of the patient to determine the outcome of the intervention. The doctor's predetermined orders are entered into the patient's EMR. The doctor may enter any modifications to the orders in the patient's EMR, and the orders will automatically be sent to the appropriate departments. If paper charts are used, the preprinted orders will be inserted into the patient's paper chart with options from which

the doctor may choose to meet the patient's specific needs. After the doctor has signed the orders, the HUC transcribes the orders. Examples of preprinted or stored doctors' orders include surgical and medical orders. See Figure 3-5 for an example of a clinical pathway for a patient with a diagnosis of pneumonia. Each physician develops a protocol that is incorporated into the orders.

Goals for developing and using clinical pathways include the following: (1) identify patient and family needs, (2) determine realistic patient outcomes and time frames required to achieve those outcomes, (3) reduce length of stay and inappropriate use of resources, and (4) clarify the appropriate care setting, providers, and timelines for intervention. The pathway can be viewed as an organizational structure for nursing services, a road map for the patient, and a guide for the health care team to follow to enhance the patient's care, management, and recovery. As the patient progresses along the path, specified goals should be accomplished. If a patient's progress deviates or leaves the planned path, a variance has occurred. A positive variance occurs when the patient's progress is ahead of schedule, and a negative variance is noted when a predicted goal is not accomplished.

ASSIGNMENT SHEET

An **assignment sheet** is a form completed at the beginning of each work shift that indicates the nursing staff assigned to each patient on that nursing unit. The form also may include lunch times and break times for nursing personnel. The HUC keeps the assignment sheet close at hand to refer to when necessary to locate the nurse who is caring for a particular patient. If a locator system (discussed in Chapter 4) is used, the HUC can look at a computer screen to locate nursing unit personnel. Information on the assignment sheet may vary depending on the nursing delivery system used. Refer to Figure 3-6 for an example of an assignment sheet used for the total patient care and team patient care models.

KEY CONCEPTS

The HUC, being the most visible person on the nursing station, is often the first person to hear the complaints, concerns, and sometimes anger of patients, family members, and others. Anger may be a result of worry about diagnosis, loss of wages, insurance coverage, or long-term care, or there may be a legitimate complaint regarding care. The HUC can make a difference by actively listening, not taking the anger personally, and showing concern. The HUC should document what is said and refer the complaints or concerns to the appropriate person (usually the patient's nurse).

Diagnosis: _____

Comorbidities: ☐Angina ☐Atrial Fibrillation ☐Cardiomyopathy ☐COPD ☐CHF ☐Dehydration ☐Malnutrition
☐ Diabetes w/ Manifestations ☐ Diabetes, Insulin Dependent ☐ Diabetes, Uncontrolled
☐ Other: _____

Condition:

Consults:

Treatments:
O2 via nasal prongs, titrate to maintain sats ≥ 90%, decrease as tolerated.
Vital signs q 4hrs. x 24hrs., then routine.
I&O
Incentive spirometer q 2hrs. while awake, cough and deep breathe.

Activity:
Ambulate QID, if possible.

Diet:
☐4gm Na, Low in Saturated Fat.
☐If patient is diabetic, 1800-2400 ADA.
☐Regular

Laboratory Requests: (Do not repeat if done in ER)
Stat blood culture x 2
Sputum culture
CBC, CMP, UA
☐Other:

Diagnostics: (Do not repeat if done in ER)
☐ Chest x-ray
☐ Other:

IV Fluids:
IV lock

Medications:
Antibiotics for community-acquired pneumonia (give first dose within 2hrs. of orders being noted, even if blood or sputum cultures not done). Antibiotic recommendations per updated Infectious Disease Society of America guidelines, 2000. *Please use choices from either one column or the other, not both.*

For those with low risk for complications or resistant organisms:
☐ Ceftriaxone (Rocephin) 1gm IV q 24hrs.
☐ Doxycycline (Vibramycin) 100mg IV q 12hrs.
(Combination therapy optimal for streptococcal and atypical organism coverage).
☐ MD aware of Penicillin allergy, OK to give Rocephin.

For those with frequent hospitalizations where resistant organisms are suspected:
☐ Levofloxacin (Levaquin) 500mg IV q 24hrs.
(monotherapy)

If patient taking **scheduled oral medications**, will **receive oral Levaquin starting on Day 2** (per P&T decision, May 2001)

☐ Albuterol inhaler with spacer _____ puffs q _____hours.
☐ Atrovent inhaler with spacer _____ puffs q _____hours.
☐ Medication/inhaler/spacer teaching per Respiratory if on metered-dose inhaler (MDI)
SVN's with Albuterol 2.5mg/3ml unit dose q 4hrs.
☐ Include Atrovent in SVN 500mcg/2.5ml unit dose q 4hrs.
☐ Self administer SVN's
☐ Other:

Discharge Planning:

Physician signature to activate per path: **Date:**

Opportunity Medical Center

**PNEUMONIA
ORDER SET**

Figure 3-5 Clinical pathway for a diagnosis of pneumonia.

ASSIGNMENT SHEET

Nursing Unit _3 West_   Date _00/00/00_   Shift _7 A – 7 P_

Nurse	Pager #	Lunch	Breaks
Sara	17–8234	12:30	9A & 4P

Patient Name	Rm #
Tony Garcia	321–1
Frank Gerod	321–2
Pat Smith	322
Jody Hackenheimer	327–1

Nurse	Pager #	Lunch	Breaks
Cheryl	17–8222	1:00	10A & 4:30P

Patient Name	Rm #
Carl Patell	318–1
Frances Conners	319–1
Penny Packer	319–2

	Name	Office ext	Pager #
Nurse Manager	Pat Lawson	3249	17–6000
Residents on call	Julie		17–2244
	David		17–2238
Case Managers	Jan	3245	17–5525
	Stan	3245	17–5528

A

Figure 3-6 A, An example of an assignment sheet for the total care nursing delivery model.

ASSIGNMENT SHEET

Nursing Unit _3 West_   **Date** _00/00/00_   **Shift** _7 A D-7 P_

Team 1		Pager #	Lunch	Breaks	Assignment	Rm #
TL	Sara	17D-8234	12:30	9A & 4P		321D-327
LPN	Elaine	17D-3749	1:30	10A & 3:30P	medications	318D-327
CNA	John		2:00	9A & 4P	T. Garcia	321D-1
					F. Gerod	321D-2
					P. Smith	322
					J. Hackenheimer	327D-1
CNA	Julie		2:30	11A & 4:30P	C. Patell	318D-1
					F. Conners	319D-1
					P. Packer	319D-2

Team 2		Pager #	Lunch	Breaks	Assignment	Rm #
Peter		17D-8222	2:30	10A & 5P	TL	316D-320
CNA	Jane		1:00	9A & 4P	T. Johns	316D-1
					T. Pratt	317D-2
					P. Smith	318D-1
					C. Luctzu	318D-2
CNA	Cynthia		2:30	11A & 4:30P	M. Peterson	318D-1
					I. Hayes	319D-1
					M. Baker	319D-2

	Name	Office ext	Pager #
Nurse Manager	Pat Lawson	3249	17D-6000
Resident on call	Julie		17D-2244
Case Manager	Jan	3245	17D-5525

B

Figure 3-6, cont'd **B**, An example of an assignment sheet for the team nursing delivery model.

Websites of Interest

Official U.S. Government site for Medicare: www.medicare.gov
American Association of Retired Persons: www.aarp.org
Health and medical information produced by doctors:
    www.medicinenet.com
Alternative medicine: http://altmedicine.about.com
American Telemedicine Association: www.americantelemed.org
Overview telepresence technology:
    www.telepresencetech.com

 REVIEW QUESTIONS

Visit the Evolve website to download and complete the following questions.

1. Define the following terms:
    a. acuity
    b. acute care
    c. chronic
    d. hospitalist
    e. inpatient
    f. intensivist
    g. nursing intervention
    h. outpatient
    i. patient care conference
    j. primary care physician
    k. resident

2. Match a specialist from the following list with his or her area of expertise.

    internist
    cardiologist
    gynecologist
    dermatologist
    allergist
    neonatologist
    pediatrician
    endocrinologist

    anesthesiologist
    otolaryngologist
    geriatrist
    pathologist
    hospitalist
    pulmonologist
    psychiatrist

    a. disorders of the newborn
    b. treatment of mental disorders
    c. diseases of ear, nose, and throat
    d. study of cell changes and other alterations in the body caused by disease
    e. administration of drugs or gases that cause loss of feeling or sensation
    f. glandular diseases
    g. hypersensitivity to foods, pollens, or medicines
    h. focuses exclusively on hospitalized patients
    i. problems and diseases of the aged
    j. diseases and disorders of internal organs of adults
    k. diseases of children
    l. diseases of the female reproductive tract
    m. diseases of heart and blood vessels
    n. diseases of the skin
    o. diseases of the lungs

3. Match a specialist from the following list with his or her area of expertise.

    surgeon
    urologist
    orthopedist
    neurologist
    physiatrist

    radiologist
    oncologist
    obstetrician
    radiation oncologist
    proctologist

    ophthalmologist
    intensivist

    emergency room doctor
    interventional radiologist

    a. use of x-rays, ultrasound, and radioactive element scanners
    b. diseases of the nervous system
    c. diagnosis and treatment of cancerous conditions
    d. treats trauma patients
    e. eye diseases
    f. treatment of cancer by radiation
    g. diseases of the male and female urinary tracts and of the male reproductive tract
    h. diseases of the rectum
    i. use of operative methods
    j. diseases of the skeletal system
    k. care of pregnant women
    l. treatment of diseases of the neuromusculoskeletal system with the use of physical elements
    m. specializes in the care of critically ill patients, usually in an intensive care unit
    n. a board-certified physician who specializes in minimally invasive, targeted treatments

4. List and describe two complementary or alternative medicine options.

5. From the following list, choose the nursing unit to which a patient with the condition listed should be admitted.

    GYN
    urology
    behavioral health
    surgical
    telemetry
    neurology
    cardiovascular

    pediatrics
    orthopedics
    oncology
    obstetrics
    medical
    rehab
    L&D

    a. cardiac arrhythmia
    b. drug abuse
    c. surgical treatment
    d. disease of the circulatory system
    e. disease of the urinary system
    f. 10 years old
    g. treatment and care to return to independence if possible after stroke
    h. cancer
    i. fractured hip
    j. surgery on the female reproductive tract
    k. diabetes
    l. disease of the nervous system
    m. pregnant and about to deliver
    n. high-risk pregnancy

6. Give two examples of physician extenders.

7. List and give a brief description of two complementary or alternative medicine options.

8. Briefly describe the responsibilities of the nursing service department.

9. Define the roles of a director of nursing and a nurse or clinical manager.

10. List five telecommunication services.

11. Explain the benefits of an eICU.

12. List four nursing personnel commonly employed on a nursing unit, and briefly describe the role of each.

13. List three services that come under the general heading of perioperative services, and give a brief description of each.

14. Explain why a patient would be admitted to an ICU and why a patient would be transferred to an intermediate or step-down unit.

15. Describe the type of patients who would be in need of the following specialty units:
    a. emergency department
    b. hospice inpatient
    c. chronic pain management

16. Explain what is required for an outpatient to become an inpatient.

17. Describe the team patient care model and the total patient care model.

18. Explain the purpose of a clinical pathway, and list four goals to be met when developing a clinical pathway.

19. Identify the information that would be included on an assignment sheet.

20. Explain what is involved in holistic nursing care.

21. List six benefits of interdisciplinary teamwork.

SURFING FOR ANSWERS

Following the guidelines for surfing the Web (see Box 1-9) provided in Chapter 1, find the following information and list the websites used. If necessary, use a school computer or go to a library.

1. Search the Web for information about patient advocacy. Write a paragraph describing what a patient advocate does and any other information found from at least three different websites.

2. Enter the phrase "questions a patient should ask" into a browser, and document information found from three different websites.

CHAPTER 4

Communication Devices and Their Uses

CHAPTER OBJECTIVES

On completion of this chapter, you will be able to:

1. Define the terms in the vocabulary list.
2. Write the meaning of the abbreviations in the abbreviation list.
3. List and apply eight rules of telephone etiquette.
4. Identify circumstances in which it would be necessary to use the hold and transfer buttons on the telephone, and demonstrate the use of each button.
5. List six items to be recorded when taking a telephone message, and explain why it is important to accurately record and communicate messages.
6. Explain the steps required when receiving a critical (panic) value message.
7. Describe briefly how to plan a telephone call to a doctor's office regarding a patient.
8. Identify two methods of leaving messages for hospital personnel and doctors, and provide guidelines for each method.

9. List the information that would be found in the hospital telephone directories, including the doctors' roster.
10. Describe three uses of robots in the hospital setting.
11. Identify at least five capabilities and benefits of using wireless communication systems in the hospital setting, and list three wireless communication systems used in hospitals.
12. Explain what is meant by "mass communication," and identify what events would require its use.
13. List four uses of GPS tracking systems.
14. Identify three biometric authentication methods for patient identification, and list three benefits of its use.
15. Explain the use of common equipment and communication devices that may be used on a nursing unit.
16. Identify three supply transportation systems for transporting supplies such as some laboratory specimens, some medications, and other items to and from nursing units and hospital departments.

17. Discuss possible repercussions of using the redial button on a fax machine on the nursing unit.
18. List four basic types of computers that may be used in the hospital.
19. Explain the main difference in the HUC role when the EMR is in use versus paper charts.
20. Discuss how the health unit coordinator may be notified when an HUC task needs to be performed, when the electronic record has been implemented.
21. Discuss the possible consequences of an employee's inappropriate use of e-mail and/or social networks on hospital computers.
22. List three types of documents or items that the HUC would scan to be entered into the patient's electronic record.
23. Discuss the uses of and the HUC's responsibilities in the maintenance of the nursing unit census and bulletin boards.

VOCABULARY

Ascom 914T Pocket Receiver A wireless voice and message transmission system with customized alarm and positioning applications.

Biometric Authentication Methods for uniquely recognizing humans based on one or more intrinsic physical or behavioral traits.

Bulletin Boards Two or more boards that may be present on a nursing unit, including one for education and policy changes and one for personal information for nursing staff.

Census Board Whiteboard, usually in the nurses' station area, on which to record census information including unit room numbers, admitting doctors' names, and the name of the nurse assigned to each patient.

Critical (Panic) Value Messages Messages usually involving laboratory values of such variance from normal values as to be life-threatening unless some intervention is performed by the physician and for which there are interventions possible.

Desktop A nonmobile personal computer (PC) intended to be used at the same dedicated location day after day for use by one computer operator at any given moment.

Doctors' Roster Alphabetic listing of names, telephone numbers, and directory telephone numbers of physicians on staff (most hospitals have made this available via computer).

Document Management System Computer system (or set of computer programs) used to track and store electronic documents and/or images of paper documents.

Document Scanner Device used to transmit images of paper documents or images to be entered into the patient's electronic record.

Document Shredder A machine located in hospitals that shreds confidential material. Most hospitals have bins located in each nursing unit that are emptied periodically; the contents are taken to an area where they are shredded in the shredder.

Downtime Requisition A paper order form (requisition) that is used to process information when the computer is not available for use.

Dumbwaiter A mechanical device for transporting food or supplies from one hospital floor to another.

E-Mail (electronic mail) System used to send and receive messages; frequently used for communication between the HUC and hospital personnel and departments within the hospital.

Fax Machine A telecommunication device that transmits copies of written material over a telephone wire from one site to another.

GPS Tracking Systems Systems used for tracking patients, hospital personnel, and equipment; controlling temperatures; reducing or preventing hospital theft; and identifying people.

Handheld Computers Portable computers that are intended to be held and used in a hand.

Hospital Robots Devices used to make up for nursing and staff shortages. Robots are used to dispense medication, make deliveries, visit patients, and help doctors reach patients across distances.

Label Printer Machine that prints patient labels from information entered into the computer; located near the health unit coordinator's area.

Laptop or Notebook A portable computer. Some laptops are actually in a tablet form. Tablets are essentially just laptops with a touchscreen and possibly a pen for input.

Locator Communication Tracking System Use of devices that are worn by nursing personnel, including health unit coordinators, so their location may be detected on the interactive console display when necessary; also used for communication between nursing unit personnel and the nursing station.

Mass Communication System A system that in an emergency can quickly and efficiently deliver messages to tens, hundreds, or thousands of recipients.

Patient Call System Intercom Device used to communicate between the nurses' station and patient rooms on the nursing unit.

Pen Tablet or Tablet PC Computer that may be removed from its base, or a portable computer that can be taken into patient rooms. A stylus is used to enter information directly into a patient's electronic record, as in a notebook.

Personal Data Assistant (PDA) A handheld mobile device that functions as a personal information manager. Also called a *personal digital assistant* or *palmtop computer.*

Pneumatic Tube System System in which air pressure transports tubes carrying supplies, some lab specimens, and some medications to and from hospital units or departments.

Pocket Pager Small electronic device that when activated by entering a series of numbers into a telephone delivers a digital or voice message to the carrier of the pager.

Polycom SpectraLink A wireless telephone system that allows hospital workers to have immediate access to one another and, more important, to patients.

Server or Application Server Device that provides network services to other computers on a network.

Smartphone A high-end mobile phone built on a mobile computing platform with more advanced computing ability.

Social Network An online community of people with a common interest who use a website or other technologies to communicate with one another and share information, resources, and so on.

Telelift A small boxcar that is carried on a conveyor belt to designated locations. Usually located in a small room between nursing units. A keypad is used to program the car to go to a specific unit or department.

Toughbook A brand of laptop designed to withstand vibration, drops, spills, extreme temperatures, and other rough handling that occurs in many hospitals.

Vocera 802.11 Voice Devices Devices that can be integrated with data event notification and escalation applications, critical alert and alarm systems, and patient monitoring.

Vocera B2000 Communications Badge A wearable device that weighs less than 2 ounces and can easily be clipped to a shirt pocket or worn on a lanyard. It enables instant two-way voice conversation without the need to remember a phone number or use a handset.

Vocera Mobile Applications Allow users to leverage the benefits of Vocera instant voice communication anytime, anywhere, on any device (e.g., Apple iPhone, BlackBerry, or Android).

Vocera Smartphone Smartphone that supports traditional phone dialing as well as the Vocera badge capabilities with one-touch instant communication and voice-system interface; is compatible with the Vocera system.

Voice Paging System System by which the hospital telephone operator pages a message for a doctor or makes other announcements; the system reaches all hospital areas (used only when absolutely necessary to keep noise level down).

Workstation A relatively powerful kind of desktop with a faster processor, more memory, and other advanced features than a more basic desktop.

Workstation on Wheels (WOW) A mobile computer that can be taken to a patient's bedside, allowing nurses and other health care providers the ability to access and enter information into patient records.

⭐ HIGH PRIORITY

Some of the most common of the many electronic medical record programs and wireless communication systems currently used in hospitals nationwide are discussed in this chapter. Some of the communication devices discussed may not be used in all areas because they are too new or are outdated. All are included because the book is used nationwide.

ABBREVIATIONS

Abbreviation	Meaning
CRP	critical response performance
DMS	document management system
GPS	Global Positioning System
PC	personal computer
PCTS	Patient care technology systems
PDA	personal data assistant
WOW	workstation on wheels

⊝ EXERCISE **1**

Write the abbreviation for each term listed.

1. critical response performance
2. document management system
3. Global Positioning System
4. personal computer
5. Patient care technology systems
6. personal data assistant
7. workstation on wheels

⊝ EXERCISE **2**

Write the meaning of each abbreviation listed.

1. CRP   5. PCTS
2. DMS   6. PDA
3. GPS   7. WOW
4. PC

Communication, organization, and operating and monitoring the communication systems and devices are the main responsibilities of the health unit coordinator (HUC). Another part of the HUC position is to maintain the equipment on the nursing unit by knowing the appropriate department to call when repair is needed. The HUC monitors the patients' electronic medical records (EMR) and is a resource for doctors, nurses, and ancillary personnel in the use of the EMR. If the EMR has not been fully implemented, the HUC is responsible for transcribing doctors' orders.

USING THE TELEPHONE

The telephone is probably the most used communication device at the nurses' station (Fig. 4-1). Because we are so familiar with using the telephone, often we fail to use it in a professional manner. Speaking on the telephone requires a different

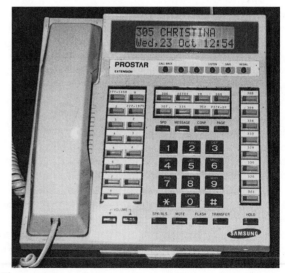

Figure 4-1 A telephone with several lines and a hold button.

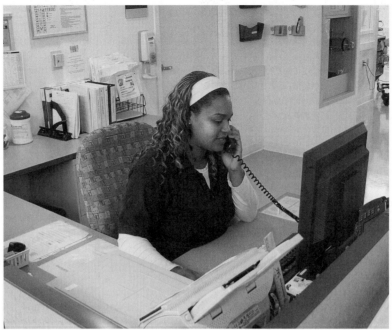

Figure 4-2 The health unit coordinator handles telephone communication for the nursing unit.

interaction than occurs with face-to-face speaking (Fig. 4-2). A good attitude about telephone transactions will result in positive customer and co-worker relationships, so proper telephone etiquette is essential in the health care setting to promote effective communication and workflow.

Telephone Etiquette

1. Answer the telephone promptly and professionally, preferably before the third ring. If engaged in a conversation at the nurses' station, excuse yourself to answer the telephone.
2. Identify yourself properly by stating location, name, and status—for example, "4 East, Stacey, Health Unit Coordinator." The manner in which you identify yourself and address the caller is the caller's first clue about your professional identity, self-esteem, mood, expectations, and willingness to continue the communication. At this time, you are conveying to the caller an image of the hospital. If you identify yourself correctly, the caller is saved time and confusion.
3. Speak into the telephone receiver. Be sure the mouthpiece is not under your chin, making it difficult for the caller to hear.
4. Give the caller your undivided attention. It is difficult to focus on the telephone conversation while attempting to do something else.
5. Speak clearly and distinctly. *Do not eat food or chew gum while talking on the telephone.*
6. Always be courteous. Say "Please" and "Thank you."
7. When you do not know the answer, state that you will locate someone who can help the caller.
8. If necessary to step away or answer another call, place the caller on hold *after asking permission to do so and waiting for an answer*—for example, "May I put you on hold, Mr. Phillips, while I find Jenny to speak to you?"

 HIGH PRIORITY

When the telephone is used for communication, an image of the hospital and/or the nursing unit is created for the caller. Realize this, and handle each caller and conversation with care.

Use of the Hold Button

Telephones on hospital nursing units may have several incoming telephone lines plus a hold button. The hold button allows a caller to stay on the line while other calls are answered.

Use the hold button for the following purposes:

1. To locate information or a person for the caller. Always return to the person on hold every 30 to 60 seconds to ask if he or she wishes to remain on hold or prefers to leave a number for a return call.
2. To answer other phone lines. Return to the first caller after asking the second caller if he or she will hold, or offer that caller an option to be called back.
3. To protect patient confidentiality. Conversations held in the nursing station often involve confidential patient information and should not be overheard.

When communicating a message regarding a call on hold, include the name of the caller, the nature of the call if possible, and which line the call is on. The message may be as

 SKILLS CHALLENGE

To practice answering the telephone and placing a caller on hold, complete Activities 4-1 and 4-2 in the *Skills Practice Manual.*

follows: "Colleen, Dr. Sanchez is on line 1 regarding Mr. Lingren's sedation order."

Use of the Transfer Button

It is often necessary for the HUC to transfer a phone call to another person or department. Reasons may include that the caller reached the wrong department or wrong extension or the caller has questions that only another person or department can answer.

To transfer a call:

1. Always explain to the caller why it is necessary to transfer the call, and provide the name of the person or department along with the direct number in case the call is disconnected.
2. Place the caller on hold.
3. Press the transfer button, and dial the correct person or department.
4. Advise the person answering the phone that you are transferring the call (provide the caller's name), and when it is certain that the connection is complete, quietly hang up.

Taking Messages

When taking messages over the telephone or in person, be sure to get all the information needed for the person for whom the call is intended. Record the following:

1. Who the message is for
2. The caller's name
3. The date and time of the call
4. The purpose of the call
5. The number to call if a return call is expected
6. Your name

Most messages received on the nursing unit need to be communicated immediately—for instance, notifying a patient's nurse that the surgery department is ready to pick up the patient, who is scheduled for surgery. Not relaying this message in a timely manner can cause delays in the surgery department, causing stress for the patient, the patient's nurse, and the surgeon. Other messages may include the surgery department notifying the nurse that a patient is returning from surgery and requesting specific equipment to be in the room. The HUC would need to notify the patient's nurse and may also need to order the equipment. The nursing unit can be hectic with constant interruptions so that even these messages can be forgotten. Always write the information down; if necessary to clarify, repeat the message back to the person leaving the message. As a student or a newly employed HUC, gaining the trust and confidence of medical staff and nursing team members is important. Putting messages in writing may be the first important step toward gaining that confidence while guaranteeing accuracy during the communication process. Always have a notepad and pencil or a pen near each telephone. Deliver messages promptly

Critical (Panic) Value Messages

A critical (panic) value message is one usually involving a laboratory value of such variance from normal as to be life-threatening unless some intervention is performed by the physician, and for which there are interventions possible. All hospitals have a protocol for handling **critical (panic) value messages** that includes the lab technician verifying the value and immediately calling the results to the licensed provider or the designated responsible personnel (nurse or nursing unit). A read-back of the critical value by the person taking the message is required, and the name of the person providing the message and the person taking the message should be documented.

SKILLS CHALLENGE

To practice recording messages, complete Activity 4-3 in the *Skills Practice Manual.*

Placing Telephone Calls

When asked to place a call to a doctor, to another department, or to someone outside of the health care facility, *plan the call.* If it concerns a patient, have the information or the patient's chart handy, so that facts will be available when questions are asked. Also, write down the main facts that need to be discussed and the telephone number to be called, should the line be busy and the call need to be placed later.

When someone requests a call to be placed regarding a patient, write down the name of the person to be called, the name of the person requesting the call, the name of the patient, and the reason for the call. Before placing a call requested by a nurse to a doctor, alert the nurse that the call is being placed, and ask that he or she stay on the unit or designate someone else to take the call in his or her place.

SKILLS CHALLENGE

To practice placing a telephone call, complete Activity 4-4 in the *Skills Practice Manual.*

Voice Mail

Voice mail on a telephone answering machine, voice pocket pager, or wireless device is sometimes used for messages for hospital department personnel, physicians' offices, and homes of hospital personnel or patients. To use voice mail effectively, follow these guidelines.

After listening to the recorded greeting and/or indicated tone, do the following:

1. Speak slowly and distinctly so the person listening to the message can hear and understand what is being communicated.
2. If leaving a message, include the name of the patient and/or the doctor. Give the first and last names, and spell the last name.
3. If the message includes a telephone number or laboratory values, speak slowly and repeat the numbers twice, allowing time for the listener to record the information.

4. Always leave your name and telephone number, and repeat both twice (at the beginning of the message and at the end of the message) so the listener can call for clarification if necessary.

Text Messages

Texting to a telephone or pocket pager is another way of leaving messages for doctors or off-duty personnel. Keep texts brief and to the point, and do not use abbreviations that may not be understood. Use of texting for personal messages is prohibited while at the nursing station. All personal telephone calls and texting when at work should be limited to when one is on a break or at lunch.

HIGH PRIORITY

When leaving a telephone number, it is helpful to say it in units—for example, "589" followed by a 2-second pause, then "932" and a 2-second pause, then "5867."

SKILLS CHALLENGE

To practice leaving a voice-mail message, complete Activity 4-5 in the *Skills Practice Manual*.

Telephone Directories

Health care facilities provide an easy-to-use alphabetized directory of extension numbers for telephones in the hospital. Both department numbers and key personnel are listed. Hospitals using the individual pocket pager also may publish a directory of pocket pager numbers. This information may be available on the computer or in hard copy.

The **doctors' roster** (usually available on the computer) is a directory including the names of the doctors (in alphabetic order) with an indication of who has admitting or visiting privileges, medical specialties, office telephone numbers, and answering service telephone numbers. When placing a telephone call, select the doctor's number with care because often several doctors are listed with the same first and last name. If two doctors have the same names, refer to their specialties to select the correct telephone number. Some hospitals may have the doctors' roster in hard copy.

USE OF HOSPITAL ROBOTS

Hospital robots are the newest members of the hospital support and nursing staff and are used to dispense medication, make deliveries, and visit patients. The RobotWorx transports materials such as food, x-ray films, and linens throughout the hospital and travels a set path and prevents collisions by using sonar. The HelpMate and Aethon TUG are other mechanized couriers. McKesson's ROBOT-Rx is an automated system that stores and dispenses single doses of drugs for entire hospitals. Pharmacists enter prescriptions into the computer, and the robot collects the doses by scanning the bar codes on the medications and bags them, all while keeping track of the medication and

ensuring that the right medicine reaches the right patient. (See Chapter 13 for more information on the ROBOT-Rx.)

Robot doctors are used by doctors to examine patients from continents away with interactive robotic devices and hi-tech visuals. Mobile robots such as the InTouch Health Remote Presence (RP-6 and RP-7) are facilitating faster service and doctor-patient face time. These robots have computer screens for heads, real-time video cameras for eyes and audio sensors for ears, and are completely mobile. Doctors operate them using a joystick and wireless technology. These robots are also saving staff from cross-infection. The use of robots to examine patients from a remote location is a form of telemedicine that is discussed in more detail in Chapter 11.

WIRELESS COMMUNICATION SYSTEMS

Wireless communication systems can help doctors, nurses, and health care facilities improve the quality and efficiency of patient care by meeting their normal and emergency response communication needs. Capabilities and advantages include the following:

- Hospital workers are able to quickly reach area law enforcement as well as one another for help.
- The nurses' stations are quieter and less hectic, as calls are made directly to caregivers.
- They can be integrated with third-party applications such as nurse call systems and in-building private branch exchange PBX systems The nurse call system integration allows nurses to respond faster to patient needs.
- Patients and families have the ability to contact the nurse directly from both inside and outside the hospital.
- When paged, health care professionals do not have to waste time finding a phone, and they do not have to leave whatever they are doing at the moment. Now they can take the call directly without leaving the bedside, even in the intensive care unit.
- They are easy to use with naturally spoken commands and hands-free conversations.
- There is no need to memorize telephone or extension numbers.
- They save money by lowering or eliminating phone and pager costs.

Examples of Wireless Communication Systems

The Vocera communication system includes the following:

The **Vocera B2000 Communications Badge** is a wearable device that weighs less than 2 ounces and can easily be clipped to a shirt pocket or worn on a lanyard. The badge has all the capabilities listed earlier. To locate and initiate a conversation with a staff nurse named Kate, for example, the user would push a button of the badge and would simply say, "Find Kate." In addition, when a live conversation is not necessary, text messages and alerts can be sent to the high-contrast organic light-emitting diode (OLED) display on the back of the badge. The exterior surfaces of the Vocera badge incorporate a silver-ion technology from BioCote that inhibits the growth of bacteria, fungi, and algae.

Note: The HUC may have the responsibility of distributing the Vocera badges at the beginning of the shift and collecting them at the end of the shift.

The **Vocera Smartphone** supports traditional phone dialing as well as the Vocera badge capabilities with one-touch instant communication and voice user interface and is compatible with the Vocera system. The smartphone is designed to allow users to retain a fixed phone number with permissions and group affiliations attached to the system profile, not the device.

Vocera mobile applications allow users to leverage the benefits of Vocera instant voice communication anytime, anywhere, on any device. Vocera mobile applications are available for Apple iPhone, BlackBerry, and Android. Benefits include device choice (the right device is paired with the right job function based on the tasks that are performed); combination of the Vocera one-button, instant voice communication capability with mission-critical data applications such as inventory status, positive patient identification, and medication administration; and provision of instant alerts and communication to the appropriate Vocera user for faster response to patient needs.

Locator communication tracking system includes small devices worn by nursing unit personnel, including HUCs (clipped on uniforms). Figure 4-3 shows an example of a

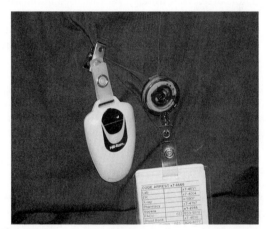

Figure 4-3 A locator device clipped to a nurse's uniform.

locator clipped on a nurse's uniform. A display screen displays a list of the nursing unit personnel who wear the locators, along with their locations. Figure 4-4 shows a HUC who is locating and communicating with a nurse using the locator system. If the locator is flipped over or obstructed, it may not show the nurse's location. The locator system is used for communication between nursing unit personnel and the nursing station. If the person who is wearing the locator needs help, a button on the locator may be pushed to call the nursing station. The HUC may also call into a patient's room to speak to the nurse. This system is also very helpful when personnel are covering more than one unit or are working as SWAT HUCs, nurses, or team members—meaning on call for all units in the hospital. Some hospitals use pagers or cell phones for this purpose.

Locator display systems are often interactive with a device on the patient's bed. A small box with a display screen may also be located on the wall at each end of the nurses' station; when pushed, this box displays the location of nursing personnel.

Note: The HUC may have the responsibility of distributing the locators at the beginning of the shift and collecting them at the end of the shift.

The **Polycom SpectraLink** wireless telephone has all of the capabilities listed previously, as does the **Ascom 914T Pocket Receiver.**

MASS COMMUNICATION SYSTEMS

All hospitals in the United States have developed disaster or emergency preparedness plans that outline chains of command, communication procedures, and other important protocols to keep the hospital running in a crisis. When an event occurs such as a multiple-injury car, train, or airplane accident; a bombing; an earthquake; or an infectious disease outbreak, rapid access to information is critical. It can sometimes mean the difference between life and death. **Mass communication systems** are becoming part of hospital disaster preparedness plans.

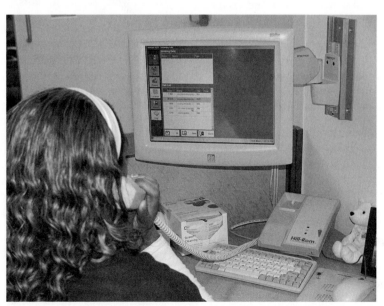

Figure 4-4 A health unit coordinator locating and communicating with a nurse using the locator system. This system may be used to answer patients' call lights and to communicate with patients in their rooms.

Common mass communications systems include the following:

- The Ascom Mobile Monitoring Gateway, which was developed in cooperation with General Electric's GE Healthcare division and provides an interface between the GE Healthcare CARESCAPE Network and Ascom Unite. It enables hospitals to customize, filter, and send secondary alarms to inform health care professionals of particular medical-related events captured by the GE Healthcare CARESCAPE Network. The alarm is forwarded to Ascom handsets or a wide variety of display devices, including pagers, mobile handsets, and light-emitting diode (LED) signs.
- **Vocera 802.11 voice devices,** which can be integrated with data event notification and escalation applications and critical alert and alarm systems.
- Everbridge Aware allows one person to communicate critical information to tens, hundreds, or thousands of individuals, anywhere, anytime, and on any device. The Aware emergency notification system contacts individuals based on their preferences and stops sending messages after a recipient has confirmed receipt.
- The REACT Critical Response Notification System, which provides mass notification and emergency management solutions that enable organizations to communicate and organize response during critical events. REACT dramatically improves critical response performance (CRP) by notifying first responders and those at risk anywhere in the world, within seconds, delivering targeted video, audio, and voice- and text-based information via any mode of communication.
- The AtHoc IWSAlerts system, which allows hospitals and clinics to reach staff via personal computer (PC), **personal data assistants (PDA)**, land or cell phone, pager, BlackBerry, social media (Twitter, Facebook), or public address system in real time. AtHoc's unified alert management console allows authorized managers to trigger and control alerts through a single Web-based console. AtHoc connects to external sources of alerts, such as the Centers for Disease Control and Prevention (CDC), to automate the dissemination of local or national CDC information.

PATIENT CARE TECHNOLOGY (TRACKING) SYSTEMS

GPS Tracking Systems

Hospitals can now account for equipment, patients, personnel, and processes throughout the facility, as well as understanding resource status, usage, and availability with the use of patient care technology systems (PCTS). The Awarepoint real-time location system (RTLS) is a Global Positioning System (GPS)–style system that affects all aspects of the health care enterprise—workflow, revenue, costs, compliance, safety—allowing hospital staff to ensure that the right equipment, the right skilled staff resources, and the right patient are in the right place at the right time. RadarFind is another GPS-style system that uses tags on every item, and readers that track the tags; to locate something, a nurse can go to any computer and check a map. Icons show where the item (such as an infusion

pump) is and how many of them there are. Each icon is also color-coded to show whether the item is available, in use, or needs cleaning.

Uses of **GPS tracking systems** include the following:

- Locate key equipment (such as crash carts, infusion pumps, and wheelchairs)
- Maintain inventory and provide immediate, real-time information regarding the location and condition of equipment.
- Track patients and personnel (to improve workflow and track exposure to infection).
- Provide the status of bed availability and the nearest skilled staff resources needed to care for patients.
- Improve efficiency of transport and order turnaround times to departments such as pharmacy, laboratory, and radiology.
- Provide the information needed to effectively move patients to appropriate levels of care, or discharge them, in a timely, safe, and cost-effective way.
- Monitor conditions such as temperature (e.g., of refrigerators, freezers, warmers). Tags are used in pharmacies, blood banks, laboratories, operating rooms, and nursing units, where proper temperature conditions are critical.
- Monitor the temperature of warming blankets in the operating room and on nursing units. Temperature-monitoring tags can be placed into any temperature-controlling device and be programmed to record temperature as frequently as desired. Corrective action documentation and logging are accessible from any computer throughout the facility, and reports are easily retrieved to comply with regulatory agency requirements.

⭐ **HIGH PRIORITY**

Locators may also be used to track nursing personnel. A display screen displays a list of the nursing unit personnel who wear the locators, along with their locations.

Biometric Authentication

Most people have heard horror stories about surgeons operating on the wrong limb or medical errors in which a medical professional has administered the wrong medication or a medication to the wrong patient. The Institute of Medicine of the National Academies recently reported that similar medication errors harm at least 1.5 million people each year, and that medical costs of treating drug-related injuries amount to $3.5 billion per year. Records are mixed up, medical charts are confused for one another, or someone who should not have access to medical information obtains it.

⭐ **HIGH PRIORITY**

To avoid errors of operating on the wrong body part, most hospitals now require doctors to see the patient in the preoperative area and mark the body part to be operated on with a marking pen after confirming with the patient.

According to the 2012 HIMSS Analytics Report: Security of Patient Data, a bi-annual survey of healthcare providers nationwide, shows a steady rise in data breaches over the last six years. Doctors have dealt with increasing cases of identity theft in which patients seeking a prescription to fuel an addiction or habit will pose as someone else in order to obtain pills. **Biometric Authentication** is making it possible for patients and health care professionals to feel secure that patient information is being kept confidential and being released only to those who have the right to see it. Errors resulting from confusing one patient's chart with another's can be deadly if the wrong medication is given or if a diagnosis is incorrect because the physician is looking at the wrong information. Even the problem of sending a baby home with the wrong mother can be eliminated if the baby's and mother's physical characteristics can be matched with certainty.

Ultra-Scan Corporation's fingerprint technology is used in some hospitals when a patient enters the hospital admissions area. Fingerprint registration is voluntary. The process involves taking fingerprints from two or three fingers on the left and right hands; scanning two or three pieces of identification, including a driver's license; taking a photo; scanning health insurance information; and getting an electronic version of the patient's signature. All this is accomplished through an Ultra-Scan unit that incorporates a fingerprint unit, scanner, and Web camera and signature block. When a patient is already in the system and returns, admissions staff identifies him or her using a fingerprint and date of birth.

Fujitsu PalmSecure (vascular biometrics) is a biometric reader that noninvasively scans the venous structure of a patient's palm, making a key image from the scan that is used for identification and future admittance. Vascular biometrics saves time and reduces clerical errors and is often chosen by health care facilities because it does not require any contact with the device for authentication and would not create an issue with germs or bacteria. The palm key is stored in an encrypted SQL database and entered into the hospital's registration system, accurately identifying patients more than 99.99% of the time. Patients are also asked for personal information such as their birth date to provide additional layers of identity protection. Often patients are unconscious or not alert enough to identify themselves, and in such cases a simple palm scan is most effective.

Iris recognition systems may also be used to ensure patients' identities and keep charting and medical diagnostics and procedures accurate. SafeMatch (Eye Controls) is a handheld device that uses a webcam-type imager with a low-energy light to illuminate a patient's iris. The iris scanner has improved issues of potential patient fraud, has lowered the risk of writing in the wrong medical record, and has improved workflow, reducing registration time for patients by about 10 seconds each.

COMMON EQUIPMENT AND COMMUNICATION DEVICES THAT MAY BE USED ON A NURSING UNIT

Patient Call System Intercom

The **patient call system intercom** is another method that is used to communicate between the nurses' station and patient rooms on a nursing unit (see Fig. 4-4). The intercom provides a method of hearing patients' requests without going into their rooms. On admission, the patient should be given directions regarding use of the call light and intercom by the HUC or another member of the nursing staff.

A buzzer and/or a light on the intercom alerts the HUC or nurse at the nurses' station that someone has activated the call system. The room number button lights up on the intercom console to designate the caller's room. By pressing the appropriate button, one may converse with the patient. Always identify yourself and your location. For example, "This is Kimberly at the nurses' station. May I help you?" When two or more patients are assigned to the room, ask the patient's name.

The HUC may also use the intercom to locate nursing personnel. To page personnel on the intercom, depress the button that allows the message to be heard in each of the rooms. A simple message, such as "Susan, please call the nurses' station," is all that is needed. One should be selective about information communicated over the intercom because some types of messages may prove embarrassing to the patient. For example, do not use the intercom to ask a patient whether he has had a bowel movement. Try to keep the message as brief as possible, and do not communicate any confidential patient information to a nurse over the intercom because other patients may hear the message.

Note: If the Vocera system is used, the system can be integrated with the nurse call systems so that the patient can communicate directly with his or her nurse.

Pocket Pager

The **pocket pager** (Fig. 4-5) is a small electronic device that is activated by dialing a series of numbers on a telephone to deliver a message to the carrier of the pager. The pocket pager may be digital or voice activated. When using a voice pager, dial the pager number and state the message. Always say the message, including name and extension number, twice. A digital pager is similar in appearance to a voice pager. To contact a person by digital pager, dial the pager number from a touch-tone phone. Listen for a ring followed by a series of beeps. Dial the nursing unit telephone number followed by the pound sign (#). A series of fast beeps indicates a completed page. The number appears on the pager display. The receiver then calls back to the provided number for the message. Allow at least 5 minutes before paging a second time, unless it is a stat (emergency) situation.

Some nursing units use a number code entered at the end of the callback number: number 1 indicates "stat," number 2

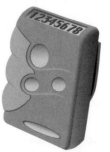

Figure 4-5 A pocket pager. (Courtesy Motorola Communications and Electronics, Schaumburg, Illinois.)

indicates "as soon as possible," and number 3 indicates "when convenient." Residents, ancillary personnel, and instructors usually carry pocket pagers.

Note: Although rare, pocket pagers may still be used in some areas.

SKILLS CHALLENGE

To practice contacting a person using a digital pager, complete Activity 4-6 in the *Skills Practice Manual*.

Voice Paging System

The **voice paging system** is a communication system by which the hospital switchboard operator, on request, pages someone on a speaker that is heard in every area of the hospital. To locate a doctor with this system, dial the hospital switchboard operator, indicate the name of the doctor who is needed, and give the telephone extension number of the nursing unit. The operator announces the name of the doctor who is needed and the extension number to call.

The operator also uses the voice paging system to locate a doctor for calls received from outside the hospital. The HUC frequently is asked by doctors to listen for their pages, especially when they are in patients' rooms. When a page for a doctor is announced, the HUC may contact the operator for the message and deliver it to the doctor. The voice paging system may also be used to call a code (discussed in Chapter 21).

Note: Use of the voice paging system is also becoming obsolete with newer technologies.

Copiers and Document Shredders

Copy machines are usually available on or near nursing units for making copies of written or typed materials. The fax machine also can be used to make a minimal number of copies.

Photocopying of patient records is discussed in Chapter 6.

Document shredders or bins for materials to be picked up and taken to be shredded are placed on nursing units. Patient forms that contain confidential information cannot be thrown into the wastebasket. Chart forms that have labels with patient name, patient account number, and health record identification number without documentation on them must be shredded.

Label Printer

A label printer is a machine that prints patient labels from information entered into the computer. The **label printer** is located near the work area of the HUC. Patient labels usually contain the name of the patient, age, and date of birth; the doctor's name; and patient identification numbers. When electronic records are implemented, labels with bar codes are used to identify types of documents. Labels are placed on forms or documents for identification purposes. In many hospitals, commonly used chart forms can be printed with all the patient information (that would be on labels) on them.

Supply Transportation Systems

With a **pneumatic tube system,** air pressure transports tubes carrying supplies, some laboratory specimens, and some medications to and from hospital units or departments (Fig. 4-6). These items are placed into a special carrying tube, which then is inserted into the pneumatic tube system; a keypad is used to enter the location to which the item is to be sent. Medications that do not break or spill are transported in this manner. Do *not* place specimens obtained via a painful or difficult procedure into the pneumatic tube. When a tube carrying supplies or other items arrives at the nursing unit, it is the responsibility of the HUC to remove the tube from the pneumatic tube system as soon as possible and disperse the items appropriately. Easy-to-understand instructions (including what should and should not be sent via tube system) for the operation of the hospital's pneumatic tube system are posted next to the tube system on each unit and will also be provided during hospital orientation.

Some health care facilities have a **telelift system** that is operated in much the same way and for the same purposes as the tube system. It is usually located in a small room between nursing units and consists of a small boxcar that is carried on a conveyor belt to designated locations. A keypad is used to program the car to go to a specific unit or department.

Some older hospitals have a **dumbwaiter,** a mechanical device (a miniature elevator car) used for transporting food trays or supplies from one hospital floor to another.

Fax Machine

A **fax machine** is a telecommunication device that transmits copies of written material over a telephone wire from one site to another (Fig. 4-7). Reports and other documents are

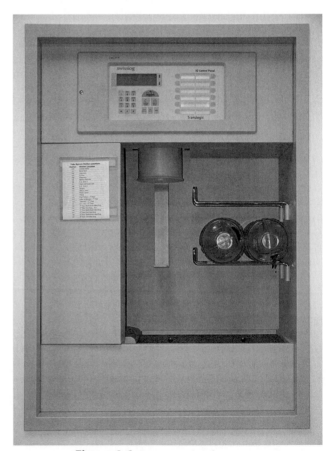

Figure 4-6 A pneumatic tube system.

faxed to and from health care institutions and doctors' offices. Often the HUC has the responsibility of faxing medical record requests, signed by the patient, to another health care facility and will receive faxed records at the nurses' station.

Many hospitals are moving toward a paperless system but have not yet implemented the electronic record. Physician order sheets are faxed to the pharmacy when paper charts are used. When faxing the physicians' orders, the HUC can use the fax machine to make a copy of the orders to give to the appropriate nurse. Fax machines have a redial option, allowing a document to be sent to the location last programmed into the machine. Many health care workers in the nurses' station use the fax machine. Therefore it is important not to use the redial option if it may send a document to the wrong location. Patient information is extremely confidential, and if it is sent to the wrong location, an employee may be disciplined or terminated. The fax machine is not for personal use, such as sending jokes to coworkers or entries to contests.

> ⭐ **HIGH PRIORITY**
>
> Do not use the redial option when using the fax machine. It may result in confidential patient information being sent to the wrong location. This could result in an employee losing his or her job.

Computers

There are four basic types of computers:

- **Desktop** computer—a nonmobile PC intended to be used at the same dedicated location day after day by one computer operator at any given moment. A computer known as a **workstation** is a relatively powerful kind of desktop computer with a faster processor, more memory, and other advanced features, when compared with a more basic desktop.
- **Laptop or notebook** computer—a portable computer. Some laptops are actually in a tablet form. Tablets are essentially just laptops with a touchscreen and possibly a pen for input. A **Toughbook** is a laptop designed to withstand vibration, drops, spills, extreme temperatures, and other rough handling; it can be taken into patient rooms for bedside documentation.
- **Handheld computer**—a kind of portable computer that is intended to be held and used in a hand. This category includes various kinds of PDAs such as those running Palm OS or Windows Mobile applications. Mobile phones have slowly begun to be replaced by the **smartphone**and similar handhelds with mobile phone capabilities. Phones such as those running Google Android, Windows Mobile, and iPhones are actually handheld computers that also function as mobile phones.
- **Server or application server**—provides network services to other computers on a network. One kind of server is known as a file server on a network and provides files to computers that request them. The servers used for serving Web pages are actually a kind of file server. Another kind of server is an application server.

The health care facility's server computer system contains a great deal of confidential information that must be protected; therefore a security system is used. When hired, each employee is assigned an identification code and a password. When the computer is used, a password is required to gain entry into the system. Employees are asked to sign a confidentiality statement. Never share the identification code and password with anyone. It is imperative for patient confidentiality and employee protection that employees sign off of the computer when leaving the nursing unit for a break or when going home. When someone

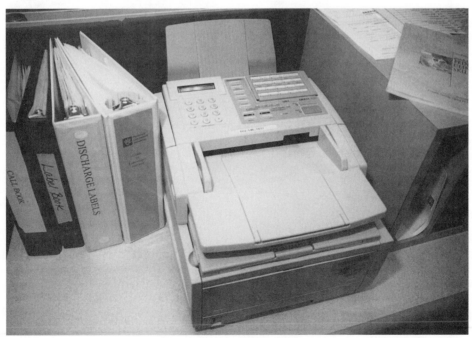

Figure 4-7 A facsimile (fax) machine.

is signed onto the computer with his or her personal identification code, any misuse will be tracked back to that individual.

Computer Use in Hospitals with the Electronic Medical Record

When the EMR system is implemented, multiple computers are made available on the nursing unit, including a workstation for the HUC to use; additional desktops for doctors, nurses, and authorized ancillary health care workers to use (Fig. 4-8); **workstation on wheels (WOW)** (Fig. 4-9); laptops (including **toughbooks**, and **pen tablet or tablet PC** (Fig. 4-10), which may be used at the patient's bedside. The doctor can enter orders directly into the patient's EMR, access computerized reports, access diagnostic images, access diagnostic test results, and access nurses' notes for review. Nurses can also enter documentation and notes directly into the patient's medical record, access the doctor's orders, access diagnostic test results and diagnostic images for evaluation, and access computerized reports. (Many nurses use a PDA, which contains software that has been downloaded into it, such as a nurse's drug reference, a medical dictionary, and other nursing reference books. Nurses use this information to calculate drug doses and to research information.)

The HUC monitors the patient's EMR for tasks that need to be performed. Icons appear on the computer screen next to the patient's name on the census screen when there is an HUC task that must be performed to complete the doctor's order. This could be a telephone icon, meaning a call is to be made to schedule a consultation or to obtain medical records from another facility. Other icons and tasks are discussed in later chapters. E-mail may also be used to notify the HUC of tasks to be performed. The HUC accesses doctors' telephone numbers and locates patients for visitors or doctors on the computer. Most health care facilities are or soon will be using EMRs. Practice will be provided using the Internet and the *Skills Practice Manual*. Computer training usually is provided for new employees, and some facilities allow HUC students to sit in on these classes.

HUCs often receive advanced training on the EMR program so they can be a resource for medical staff and nursing staff as well as other health care professionals. Students will be instructed in the specifics of the hospital computer program by an experienced working HUC during their clinical experience. Applications of the EMR will be introduced in later chapters. Practice using an EMR system is also provided on the Evolve website.

Computer Use in Hospitals with the Paper Chart

Usually there are several computers available on the nursing unit for doctors, nurses, and other health care professionals to use. The HUC usually has a workstation for ordering diagnostic tests, supplies, and equipment and for entering discharges, transfers, and admissions. Computer knowledge and typing skills are essential to perform the ordering and data entry tasks required.

A menu can be brought up on the screen so that an item or a test to be ordered can be selected, or a menu can be recalled for informational purposes only, such as a census (list of room numbers with patients' names and their admitting physicians' names). The HUC should be alert to printed material being sent via the printer and should remove the printed documents as soon as possible. Printed documents such as dictated patient history and physical examination findings, dictated consultation notes, or other reports should be placed in the appropriate patient's chart. At times the computer is shut down for scheduled routine servicing (usually at night) or because of mechanical failure. During these times, a **downtime requisition** is used to process information. When computer function

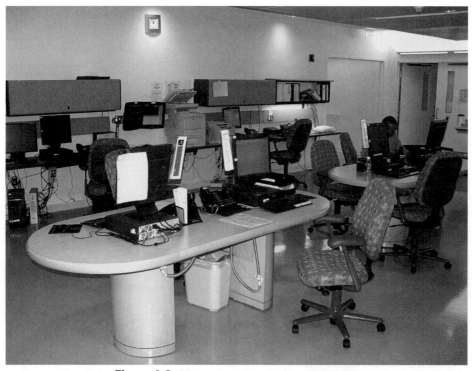

Figure 4-8 Computer stations on the nursing unit.

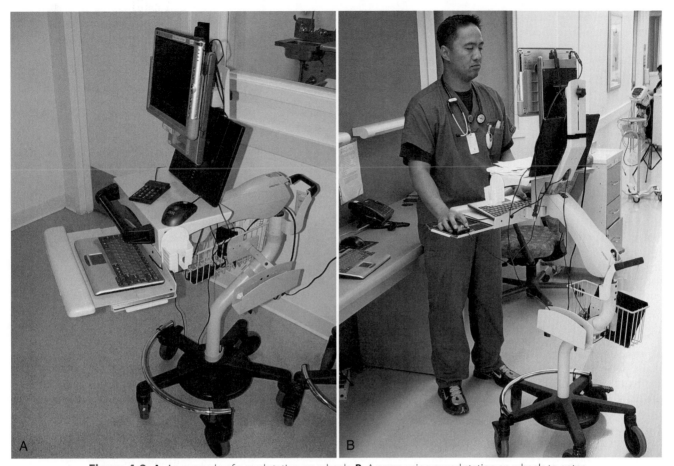

Figure 4-9 A, An example of a workstation on wheels. **B,** A nurse using a workstation on wheels to enter documentation into a patient's electronic record.

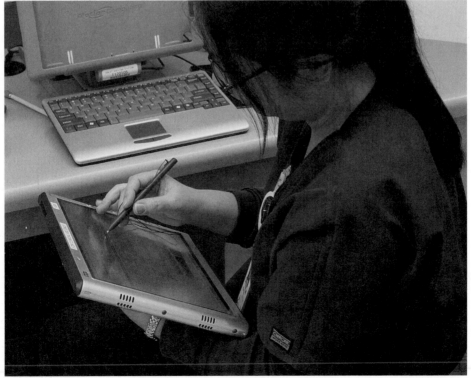

Figure 4-10 A nurse using a pen tablet.

returns, the information processed by the paper method must be entered into the computer. Handwritten and printed orders and requisitions as well as a computerized program are provided for transcription practice in the *HUC Skills Manual* and on the Evolve website.

E-Mail

E-mail (electronic mail) is used to send and receive messages and is frequently used for communication between the HUC and hospital personnel and departments within the hospital. In some hospitals using the EMR, e-mail may be used to communicate HUC tasks that need to be performed, so it is important for the HUC to check e-mail frequently. Guidelines to be followed when using e-mail in the workplace include the following: (1) Do not use for personal messages; (2) do not send inappropriate material such as jokes; and (3) send or respond to the necessary person or department only—refrain from "sending to all" or using "reply to all" unless necessary. E-mail is not to be used for personal communication; such usage can be easily tracked and could be grounds for dismissal.

Social Networks

More hospital and health care systems are using a **social network** such as Facebook or Twitter because of the high visibility: blogging, social networking, and social bookmarking are highly—and some would say more—effective in reaching online users versus reaching them solely through the hospital's website. Social media tools are a powerful way to listen to patients and obtain a better understanding of them, as well as an easier way to reach the media for news stories and press releases. The cost is lower, and causes, events, health fairs, and support groups can be publicized and promoted. It may be easier to monitor how people really perceive the hospital, hear

what they say, accept criticism (if criticism is offered), and respond honestly. Social media help users engage and interact with several different communities internally and externally. Social networks are not to be used for personal communication; such usage can be easily tracked and could cause one to lose his or her job.

Document Scanner

A **document scanner** is a device used to transmit images of documents or pictures into a computer system (or set of computer programs) used to track and store electronic documents and/or images of paper documents. This **document management system (DMS)** uses bar codes to identify types of documents. The HUC scans documents such as printed reports, handwritten doctors' progress notes, and electrocardiograms (ECGs) into the patient's EMR (Fig. 4-11). These documents are sent to the health information management systems (HIMS) department and are certified by the health information technician before they become a part of the patient's permanent EMR.

Bundles of up to 14 documents may be placed in the scanner at a time; documents containing color (e.g., ECGs) have to be scanned alone. After documents have been scanned, the originals should be rubber-banded and placed in a bin to be picked up by someone from the HIMS department. Documents are then stored for a specified length of time before being shredded.

Nursing Unit Census Board

Many nursing units have whiteboards in the nurses' station area on which to record census information. These boards show unit room numbers, admitting doctors' names, and

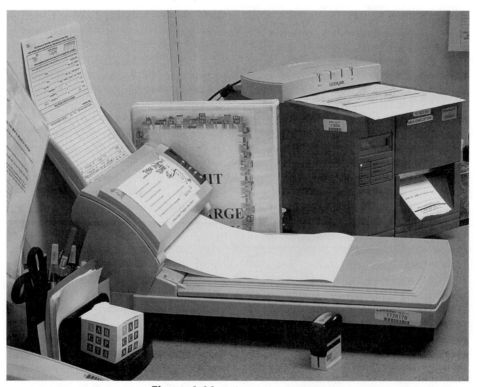

Figure 4-11 A document scanner.

the name of the nurse assigned to each patient. The HUC has the responsibility of maintaining the **census board.** New Health Insurance Portability and Accountability Act (HIPAA) laws (see Chapter 6) have changed usage of census boards. The patient's name may be omitted intentionally, or just the patient's initials may be used to maintain patient confidentiality.

Nursing Unit Bulletin Boards

There may be two or more **bulletin boards** located on a nursing station, usually including one for policy changes, education updates, schedules of staff development classes, workshops, in-services, meetings, and computer updates and one for personal events such as weddings, showers, birthdays, and holiday parties. Some hospitals may send group e-mails for policy changes, education updates, schedules of staff development classes, workshops, in-services, meetings, and computer updates. The HUC may be given the responsibility of maintaining the nursing unit education bulletin board. This includes posting material in an attractive manner and keeping posted material current. The material to be posted on the bulletin board may be determined by the nurse manager or may be set forth by administration policy.

If the date is not indicated on the bulletin, the HUC should indicate the date posted. Policy changes are very important. It may be requested that each person initial the notice after reading it so the nurse manager will know that all unit employees have read it. The HUC then would place the initialed notice on the nurse manager's desk when it is removed from the bulletin board. A neat board with up-to-date notices prompts unit personnel to read what is posted.

KEY CONCEPTS

The ability to use and maintain all the communication devices and systems efficiently and effectively contributes to the smooth operation of the nursing unit. Accuracy in taking telephone messages and in communicating them in a timely manner to the appropriate person is a must for an efficiently run nursing unit. It is imperative that the HUC demonstrate professionalism, especially when using communication devices. One can lose one's job for inappropriately using the telephone (making personal calls or texting) or the computer (visiting inappropriate websites, sending personal e-mails, or using social networks for personal use). Computer use can be tracked; there is no expectation of privacy when using a computer at work.

Websites of Interest

Vocera www.vocera.com
Ascom: www.ascomwireless.com .com
Polycom video conferencing: : www.polycom.com
Awarepoint equipment tracking system:
    www.awarepoint.com/our-solutions/rtls React Systems:
    www.reactsystemsinc.com/about/vision.php
Emergency Notification Systems: www.everbridge.com
    Biometrics—Global Identity Management:
    www.findbiometrics.com/health-care/
Stanford University Medical Center—Laboratory Critical/Panic
    Value List: www.stanfordlab.com/pages/panicvalues.htm

REVIEW QUESTIONS

Visit the Evolve website to download and complete the following questions.

1. Define the following terms:
   a. biometric authentication
   b. workstation on wheels
   c. doctors' roster
   d. desktop
   e. document management system
   f. downtime requisition
   g. dumbwaiter
   h. critical (panic) value messages
   i. laptop or notebook
   j. personal data assistant (PDA)
   k. hospital robots
   l. pen tablet or tablet PC
   m. Server or application Server
   n. workstation on wheels (WOW)
   o. Toughbook

2. List eight rules of telephone etiquette.

3. Identify circumstances in which it would be necessary to use the hold and transfer buttons on the telephone.

4. List six items to be recorded when taking a telephone message.

5. Explain why it is important to accurately record and communicate telephone messages.

6. Explain the steps required when receiving a value or panic message.

7. Briefly describe how the HUC would plan a call to a doctor's office regarding a patient.

8. Identify two methods of leaving a message for hospital personnel or a doctor, and list guidelines for each method.

9. List the information that would be located in the hospital telephone directories including the doctors' roster

10. List three ways in which supplies, some laboratory specimens, and some medications could be transported to and from nursing units and hospital departments.

11. Describe three uses of robots in the hospital setting.

12. List three wireless communication systems used in hospitals.

13. Identify at least five capabilities and benefits of using wireless communication systems in the hospital setting.

14. Explain what is meant by "mass communication."

15. List three events that would require the use of mass communication.

16. List four uses of GPS tracking systems in hospitals.

17. Identify three biometric authentication methods used for patient identification.

18. List three benefits of using biometrics for patient identification.

19. Describe the use of each of the following.
    a. document shredder
    b. census board
    c. bulletin board
    d. document scanner
    e. Vocera B2000 badges
    f. patient call system intercom
    g. pneumatic tube system
    h. label printer
    i. locators
    j. pocket pagers
    k. fax machine
    l. copier

20. Discuss possible repercussions of using the redial button on a fax machine on the nursing unit.

21. List the four basic types of computers that may be used in the hospital.

22. List three guidelines to follow with regard to e-mail in the workplace.

23. Discuss the possible consequence of inappropriate use of e-mail and/or social networks on hospital computers.

24. Discuss how the HUC may be notified when an HUC task needs to be done when the EMR is in use.

25. List three types of documents or items that the HUC would scan to be entered into the patient's EMR.

26. Explain the main difference in the HUC role when EMR is in use versus paper charts.

SURFING FOR ANSWERS

1. Go to the website www.vocera.com. Click on "Products," watch demonstrations of the Vocera wireless communication devices, and discuss the scenarios demonstrated.
2. Research biometric authentication methods used in health care, and list uses and benefits. Document three websites used.
3. Find three websites that discuss GPS tracking systems. List uses and benefits. Document websites used.

CHAPTER 5

Communication and Interpersonal Skills

OUTLINE

CHAPTER OBJECTIVES

On completion of this chapter, you will be able to:

1. Define the terms in the vocabulary list.
2. Explain why implementation of the electronic medical record is requiring advanced communication and skills for the health unit coordinator (HUC).
3. Give instances that exemplify human needs, classify each according to Maslow's hierarchy of human needs, and give appropriate responses to meet the listed needs.
4. List four components of the communication process.
5. Interpret and apply the communication model.
6. Explain how unsuccessful communication can occur during the encoding and decoding process.
7. Discuss two types of nonverbal communication.
8. List five levels of listening and nine ways to improve listening skills.
9. List five ways to improve feedback skills.
10. Define and explain the importance of culturally sensitive care in the health care setting.
11. List five guidelines to follow that could improve intercultural communication.
12. Identify assertive, nonassertive, and aggressive behaviors, and evaluate your assertiveness; and respond to situations using assertiveness skills.
13. List six steps to follow when dealing on the telephone with a person who is angry.
14. Identify five ways that communication and interpersonal skills are used in the health care setting.
15. List 12 preceptor guidelines for training a HUC student or a new employee.
16. List 10 student guidelines for completing the clinical experience.

VOCABULARY

Ageism (age discrimination) Stereotyping of and discrimination against individuals or groups because of their age.

Aggressive A behavioral style in which a person attempts to be the dominant force in an interaction. Aggressive behavior may escalate into a physical and/or verbal act.

Assertive A behavioral style in which a person stands up for his or her own rights and feelings without violating the rights and feelings of others.

Broken Record Technique An assertiveness technique that consists of just repeating one's requests or refusals every time he or she is met with resistance.

Communication The process of transmitting feelings, images, and ideas from the mind of one person to the mind of another person or persons by the use of speech, signals, writing, or behavior.

Conflict A disagreement or clash among ideas, values, principles, or people.

Cultural Differences Factors such as age, gender, race, religion, and socioeconomic status that vary among groups of people.

Culturally Sensitive Care Care that involves understanding and being sensitive to a patient's cultural background. Also called *cultural competence.*

Culture A set of values, beliefs, and traditions that are held by a specific social group.

Decoding The process of translating verbal and nonverbal symbols received from the sender to determine the message.

Diversity Social inclusiveness: ethnic variety, as well as socioeconomic and gender variety, in a group, society, or institution.

Elitism A belief or attitude that a selected group of persons have personal abilities, specialized training, or other attributes that place them at the top of any field and that these people's views on a matter are to be taken most seriously.

Empathy The ability to understand and to experience other people's feelings, or the ability to put oneself "into their shoes."

Encoding Translating mental images, feelings, and ideas into verbal and nonverbal symbols to communicate them to the receiver.

Esteem Needs A person's need for self-respect and for the respect of others.

Ethnocentrism The inability to accept other cultures, or an assumption of cultural superiority.

Feedback Verbal or nonverbal response to a message.

Fogging Assertive skill in which a person responds to a criticism by making noncommittal statements that cannot be argued against.

HUC Clinical Experience The time the HUC student spends on a nursing unit (after having completed the classroom portion of an educational program) with a working HUC to acquire hands-on work experience.

HUC Preceptor An experienced working HUC who is selected to train or teach a HUC student or a new employee.

Interpreter A person who facilitates oral communication between or among parties who are conversing in different languages.

Love and Belonging Needs A person's need to have affectionate relationships with people and to have a place in a group.

Manipulation Attempts at influencing or controlling others' actions or behaviors to one's own advantage.

Message Images, feelings, and ideas transmitted from one person to another.

Negative Assertion An assertive skill in which a person verbally accepts having made an error without letting it reflect on his or her worth as a human being.

Negative Inquiry An assertive skill in which a person requests clarification of a criticism to get to the real issue.

Nonassertive (passive) A behavioral style in which a person allows others to dictate her or his self-worth.

Nonverbal Communication Communication that is not written or spoken but creates a message between two or more people through eye contact, body language, or symbolic and facial expression.

Paraphrase Repeating a message back to the sender in one's own words to clarify meaning.

Passive Aggressive A type of aggressive behavior characterized by an indirect expression of negative feelings, resentment, and aggression in an unassertive way (as through sullenness, obstructionism, stubbornness, and unwillingness to communicate).

Physiologic Needs A person's physical needs, such as the need for food and water.

Precept To train or teach (a student or a new employee).

Receiver The person who receives a message.

Safety and Security Needs The need to be sheltered, to be clothed, to feel safe from danger, and to feel secure about one's job and financial future.

Self-Actualization Needs The need to maximize one's potential.

Self-Esteem Confidence in and respect for oneself.

Sender The person who transmits a message.

Stereotyping The assumption that all members of a culture or ethnic group act in the same way (generalizations that may be inaccurate).

Subcultures Subgroups within a culture; people with distinct identities but who have specific ethnic, occupational, or physical characteristics found in a larger culture.

Verbal Communication The use of language or actual spoken words.

Workable Compromise Dealing with conflict in such a way that the solution is satisfactory to all parties.

EXPANDING COMMUNICATION ROLE FOR THE HEALTH UNIT COORDINATOR

The health unit coordinator (HUC) is the liaison among the doctor, the nursing staff, ancillary departments, visitors, and patients. The main responsibility of the HUC is to keep the nursing unit running effectively and smoothly. With the implementation of the electronic medical record (EMR), the HUC has expanded responsibilities and is often the "go-to" person to assist doctors, nurses, and ancillary personnel in use of the EMR system. The HUC also has a larger role in listening to visitor, patient, and nursing unit personnel complaints and also in problem solving. The nursing unit can become very hectic, and tensions can build easily. If communication breaks down and tempers become short, chaos most likely will result, and the risk of errors being made becomes higher. Hospitals are rated by The Joint Commission (TJC) on patient safety goals that include the **communication** process. The HUC as well as all health care professionals need to stay proactive to meet the requirements placed on the hospital. Many hospitals provide computer-based learning (including communication and other topics) for employees that can be completed on their own time.

INTERPERSONAL BEHAVIOR

To develop effective communication and interpersonal skills, one must first attain an understanding of interpersonal behavior. *Interpersonal* refers to between persons; involving personal relationships. Behavior is how people act—what they say or do. We have many different relationships with people. Some researchers say that our definition of interpersonal communication must account for these differences; for instance, interactions with a sales clerk in a store are different from the relationship we have with our friends and family members. Research indicates that in conversation a person behaves according to who the other person is and how he or she behaves. An understanding of interpersonal behavior assists us in understanding our own behavior and in understanding the behavior of others.

Although several models may be used to study interpersonal behavior, we have chosen Maslow's hierarchy of needs, developed by the late Abraham Maslow, a famous psychologist. Maslow's human needs model emphasizes that all people have the same basic needs and that these needs motivate and influence a person's behavior, consciously or unconsciously. The needs are arranged in a pyramid, with the most basic or immediate needs at the bottom of the pyramid and less critical needs at the top of the pyramid (Fig. 5-1). Needs that are lower on the pyramid have the greatest influence on

a person's behavior. For instance, a person will work harder to meet the need for water to drink than to meet the need for **self-esteem.**

As lower level needs are satisfied to an adequate degree, we become increasingly concerned about satisfying the next or a higher-level need. Most people find that all their needs are both partially satisfied and partially unsatisfied at the same time. Unsatisfied needs influence an individual's behavior in terms of motivation, priorities, or action taken. According to Maslow, the average person is satisfied perhaps 85% in their physical needs, 70% in their safety needs, 50% in their love needs, 40% in their self-esteem needs, and 10% in their self-actualization needs.

Maslow's Hierarchy of Needs
Physiologic Needs

Each person needs food, fluids, oxygen, physical activity, sleep, and freedom from pain. These needs are the most basic and the most dominant of all human needs. They are the first to develop in the human organism. The normal adult probably has satisfied his or her **physiologic needs.**

What about the person who is ill or hospitalized? The illness itself, diagnostic testing, or surgery may interrupt a person's normal eating and drinking habits. Diseases such as emphysema make it impossible for the body to receive the amount of oxygen needed to function normally. Physical activity is decreased on the patient's admission to the hospital, affecting the body's need for exercise.

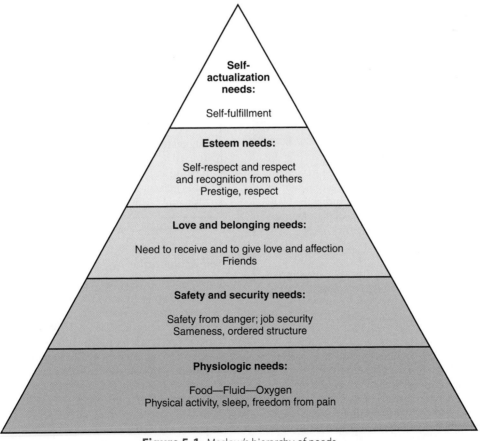

Figure 5-1   Maslow's hierarchy of needs.

Bill, a patient, has been fasting since midnight for a diagnostic imaging procedure. It's now 10:45 AM, the test has been completed, and Bill is ready for his breakfast. When the HUC informs him that his tray will not arrive from the nutritional care department until lunch time (12:00), Bill becomes angry. Bill's behavior is influenced by his unsatisfied physiologic need.

Suggested Resolution
The HUC would (after checking Bill's diet) give him a snack from the nursing unit diet kitchen and/or call the nutritional care department and request that his tray be sent early.

Safety and Security Needs

Everyone has **safety and security needs**—the need to be sheltered, to be clothed, to feel safe from danger, and to feel secure about one's job and financial future. Each person has a need for a certain degree of sameness, familiarity, order, structure, and consistency in life. Freedom from fear, anxiety, and chaos is also important.

The normal healthy person probably has met these basic needs; however, illness or hospitalization may interrupt a person's ability to continue to satisfy them. What about the patient who is waiting for test results to learn a diagnosis, the unpredictable course of a lengthy illness, the fear of death, the cost of medical care, or the unfamiliarity of hospital routines and medical procedures? Many obstacles may interfere with efforts to meet the safety and security needs of a person who is ill or hospitalized.

Note: Hospital employees who are new on the job feel insecure and may make more mistakes during this stressful time. In addition, rumors about layoffs, true or not, can affect the security needs of employees and often send them scurrying to apply elsewhere for employment.

Donna, a patient, has just been told by her surgeon that the test results show she has a tumor that may be malignant. The surgeon has recommended she have surgery as soon as possible. Donna is very upset and demands that the HUC put a call in to her family physician immediately. Donna's behavior is motivated by unsatisfied security needs.

Suggested Resolution
The HUC would advise Donna's nurse. After speaking to Donna's nurse, and upon the nurse's request, the HUC would place the call.

Love and Belonging Needs

Once physiologic and safety needs have been relatively well met, **love and belonging needs** surface. Now, the person has a desire for affectionate relationships with others and is motivated to belong to or be a part of a group. Patients who are hospitalized, especially for a long time, may be cut off from their family, friends, or group.

Sarah, a 76-year-old woman, has been hospitalized for 2 weeks. During this time, she has been visited only once by her daughter. In an attempt to meet her belonging needs, she has been turning on her call light hourly for minor requests.

Suggested Resolution
The HUC would ask a volunteer to visit with Sarah. The volunteer could read to her, comb her hair, or just talk with her for a time.

Esteem Needs

As a person develops satisfying relationships with others, **esteem needs** and the need for self-respect and for the respect of others emerge. Esteem needs may be met by seeking special status within a group, excelling at a job, obtaining a promotion, learning a skill very well, or developing a talent to be performed for others. Attainment of self-respect leads to feelings of adequacy, self-confidence, and strength. These qualities result in prestige, recognition, and dignity for the individual.

Hospitalization frequently interferes with the ability to meet esteem needs. Many aspects of hospitalization such as wearing hospital gowns, sharing a room with others, having side rails on the bed, and being referred to as a room number or a disease instead of by name serve to depersonalize the patient. Often, busy hospital personnel overlook a patient's past accomplishments and status.

Tom has been hospitalized for longer than a week. He is walking past the nurses' station and stops to read the name tag of the HUC. "You're Jenny Mason. That's a nice name. You know, since I've been in the hospital, no one has called me by my name. I feel like I've lost my identity."

Suggested Resolution
The HUC would advise Tom's nurse and the certified nursing assistant (CNA) of Tom's comment and if applicable make a note on Tom's Kardex to please call him by his name.* This should be addressed at the staff meeting.

*All patients should be called by name.

Self-Actualization Needs

Once a person feels basic satisfaction of the first four needs, the next step is for him or her to become "self-actualized." **Self-actualization needs** are met with the development of a personality to its full potential. Contentment, self-fulfillment, creativity, originality, independence, and acceptance of other people all characterize the self-actualized person. Self-actualization is growth motivated from within an individual. As Maslow expressed it, "What a man can be, he must be." Thus, self-actualization is the desire to become what one is capable of becoming. It is growing and changing because you feel it is important. A self-actualized person has taken steps to make this happen.

SCENARIO

Mahatma Gandhi is an example of a self-actualized person. This Indian leader frequently sacrificed his physiologic and safety needs for the satisfaction of other needs when India was striving for independence from Great Britain. In his historic fasts, Gandhi went weeks without nourishment to protest governmental injustices. He was operating at the self-actualization level.

Examples of Different Needs in a Conversation

The human needs model can be used to demonstrate interpersonal behavior between HUCs and hospital personnel or between HUCs and patients or visitors.

HUC: "Mary is in isolation. You will need to put this gown on before going into her room." *(No dominant need expressed.)*

Husband: "Mary is in isolation? What are you talking about? What for? I want to know exactly what is going on here!" *(Safety need expressed. Mary's husband is concerned about her safety and is also concerned that he may contract what Mary has.)*

HUC (defensively): "Look, if you don't want to wear the gown, don't go in. I don't make the rules here." *(Esteem need expressed. The HUC interprets the husband's request for information as an attack on her competence; self-esteem is at stake. Fighting back is used to try to satisfy self-esteem needs.)*

In this example, if the HUC had perceived that the husband's question was motivated by *safety* needs, she could have responded with understanding rather than with defensiveness and aggression.

⊜ EXERCISE 1

Match the level of need from Maslow's hierarchy of human needs listed in Column 2 with the human needs listed in Column 1.

Column 1
1. The need for oxygen
2. The need for shelter
3. The need to be safe from danger
4. The need to be loved
5. The need for respect
6. The need to feel self-confident
7. The need for acceptance within a group
8. The need to belong
9. The need for exercise
10. The need for the feeling of security

Column 2
a. Physiologic needs
b. Safety and security needs
c. Belonging and love needs
d. Esteem needs
e. Self-actualization needs

UNDERSTANDING PATIENT NEEDS

Many hospitals have developed programs (Buddy Program, Pairs Program, and Pediatric Stars Program) that pair first-year medical students with individuals with early- to moderate-stage Alzheimer disease, children with sickle cell anemia, and children with cancer. The programs provide the students an "up-close and personal" experience of the impact and challenges patients with these diseases and their families face every day. The students also gain **empathy** and learn to see the patients as human beings and not just a disease. Often the friendships formed last beyond the end of the program.

COMMUNICATION SKILLS

Most of us spend much of our time communicating, but few of us communicate as effectively as we should. Many factors contribute to communication difficulties. For instance, the English language has grown considerably throughout its history, and the language now consists of approximately 750,000 words. It is impossible to know how many words an individual may have in his or her vocabulary, but it is believed that an average educated person comprehends about 20,000 words. How does the speaker know which of the 750,000 words are included in the receiver's 20,000-word vocabulary? The medical world also has a growing language of its own, which is made up of abbreviations and medical terms. "Remember now, Sidney is NPO" or "Your doctor feels that you may have diverticulitis, so she has scheduled you for a BE tomorrow" may have little meaning to those not familiar with the medical terms. Some words have more than one meaning. For instance, a *chip* in the computer world has a much different meaning than a *chip* used in a poker game.

Communication is 55% visual, including facial body language and symbolism; 38% vocal qualities, including tone, loudness, firmness, hesitations, and pauses; and 7% verbal, meaning actual words (Fig. 5-2). There is often inconsistency between what a person is saying and how he or she appears.

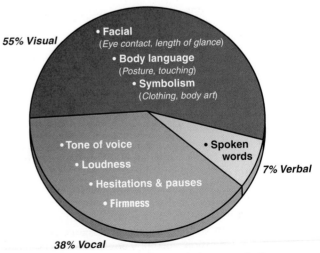

Communication is:

Figure 5-2 Verbal and nonverbal communication.

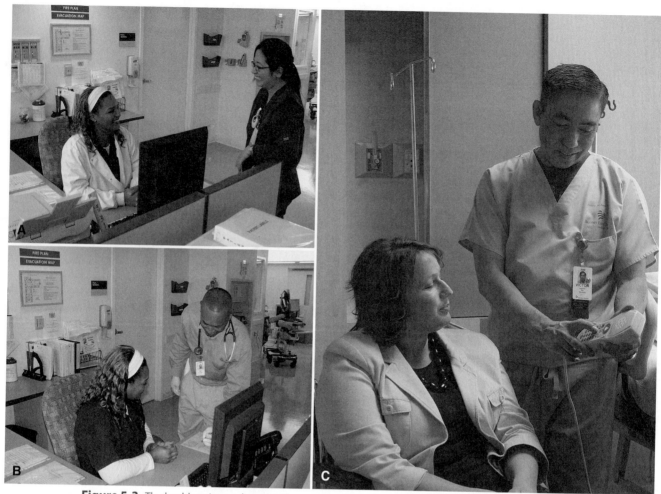

Figure 5-3 The health unit coordinator is the communicator for the nursing unit. **A,** Communicating with a nurse. **B,** Assisting a doctor. **C,** Answering a patient's questions regarding visiting hours, operation of call light, and so on.

("Of course I'm listening to you, Mother," says the 9-year-old boy as he sits glued to the television set, leaving the mother wondering whether the child is indeed listening to her.)

Another major weakness in the communication process involves poor listening skills. Often we are thinking of something else while the speaker is talking to us; we are formulating a response or prejudging what is being said.

> *Daughter:* I've stopped eating breakfast meats.
> *Mother:* But breakfast is the most important meal of the day. You should not give it up.

Instead of listening to what is being said, the mother has prejudged that the daughter is skipping breakfast altogether rather than just breakfast meats.

Because the HUC is the communicator for the nursing unit, effective communication is vital for job success and for proficient operation of the nursing unit.

Communication takes place daily with nurses (Fig. 5-3, *A*), physicians (Fig. 5-3, *B*), allied health professionals, patients (Fig. 5-3, *C*), visitors, and administrators. The HUC is often the first person seen by the new patient and visitors. The words, gestures, facial expression, and body posture that are used can suggest that one is opinionated, supportive, thoughtful, or insecure. The tone of voice, the words spoken, and the facial expressions used during the patient's or the visitor's initial contact with the nursing unit leave a lasting impression.

Components of Communication

Communication is the process of transmitting images, feelings, and ideas from the mind of one person to the mind(s) of one or more other people for the purpose of obtaining a response. The communication process consists of four components:

> **Sender:** the person transmitting (sending) the message
> **Message:** the images, feelings, and ideas transmitted (sent)
> **Receiver:** the person receiving the message
> **Feedback:** the response to the message

Communication seems like a simple process; however, the act of communicating does not guarantee that effective communication has taken place, nor that the message sent was the same as the message received. For example, a program was developed for a computer to translate one language into another. The computer translated the English phrase "out of sight, out of mind" into Russian, and then translated it back into English as "invisible idiot."

Sender   Receiver

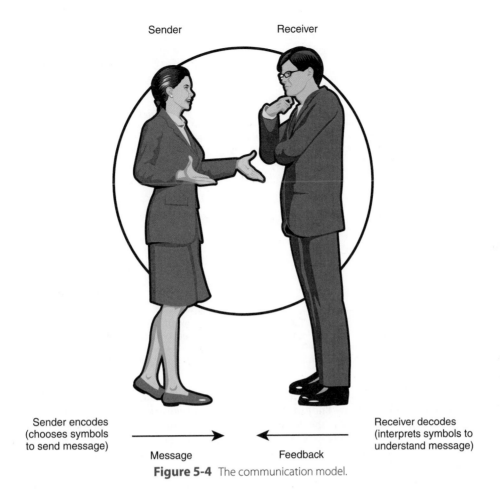

Sender encodes
(chooses symbols
to send message)   Receiver decodes
                                        (interprets symbols to
                                        understand message)

Message   Feedback

Figure 5-4 The communication model.

Communication Model

A model is a representation of a process—a map, for instance. We will use a model to take a closer look at the communication process, to identify why so many of us communicate poorly, and to find ways to improve our ability to communicate with others (Fig. 5-4).

Sender

The sender must translate mental images, feelings, and ideas into symbols to communicate them to the receiver. This process is called **encoding**. When encoding, the sender decides whether to send the message in verbal symbols or in nonverbal symbols (Fig. 5-5). What are the right words to use so the receiver will understand the message? Different words are used if you are speaking to a child, to an adult, or to another health care professional. Nonverbal symbols, such as facial expressions, may be used to communicate the message. Encoding occurs each time we communicate. A poor choice of words or an inconsistency between verbal and nonverbal messages may result in unsuccessful communication.

Message

Once the idea, feeling, or image is encoded, it is sent to the receiver. This step of the communication process is called the **message.**

Receiver

As the message reaches the receiver, the verbal and nonverbal symbols are decoded. **Decoding** is the process of translating

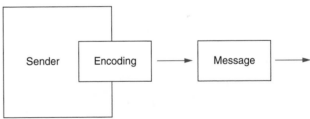

Figure 5-5 The communication process: message sending.

symbols received from the sender to determine the message. Unsuccessful decoding can be caused by inconsistency in the verbal and nonverbal symbols received from the sender. For instance, "Of course I love you" said harshly may be difficult to decode correctly. Lifestyle, age, cultural background, environment, and poor listening habits are other reasons for incorrect decoding. In successful communication, the ideas, feelings, and images of the sender match those of the receiver (Fig. 5-6, *A*). In unsuccessful communication, errors occur in encoding or in decoding the message (Fig. 5-6, *B*).

Verbal and Nonverbal Communication

Two methods of communication are verbal and nonverbal. **Verbal communication** is the use of language or the actual words spoken, whereas **nonverbal communication** is the use of eye contact, body language, facial expression, or symbolic expressions such as clothing that communicate a message. Sometimes our verbal and nonverbal communications

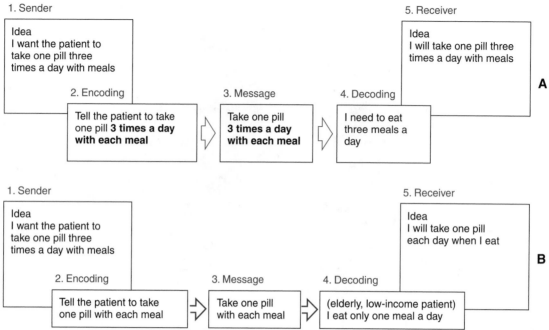

Figure 5-6 **A,** An example of successful communication. **B,** An example of unsuccessful communication.

contradict each other. For example, when a person is asked, "What is wrong?" and responds, "Oh nothing, I'm just fine" and shrugs his shoulders, frowns, and turns away, the dejected body language is more believable than the words spoken.

Types of Nonverbal Communication

Nonverbal communication can be separated into two types: symbolic and body language.

Symbolic	Body Language
Clothing	Posture
Hair	Ambulation
Jewelry	Touching
Body art	Personal distance
Cosmetics	Eye contact
Automobile	Breathing
House	Hand gestures
Perfume or cologne	Facial expressions

Listening Skills

Listening is something we have done all our lives, but most of us have had little or no training in how to do it effectively. We take it for granted. Many of us think of communication as the sender giving us a message, but for successful communication to occur, the sender and the receiver both must participate actively in the communication process. Hearing is a physical ability, whereas listening is a skill. Active participation for the receiver requires effective listening skills.

Five Levels of Listening

According to Dr. Stephen R. Covey in his bestselling book, *The Seven Habits of Highly Effective People,* we listen at five different levels, depending on our interest in what is being said or what we might be doing while we are listening.

1. *Ignoring:* making no effort to listen
2. *Pretend listening:* giving the appearance that you are listening

3. *Selective listening:* hearing only the parts that interest you
4. *Attentive listening* (also called *active listening*): paying attention and focusing on what the speaker says and comparing it with your own experience
5. *Empathic listening:* listening and responding with both the heart and the mind to truly understand, realizing that all persons have the right to feel as they do

Guidelines for Improving Listening Skills

1. *Stop talking.* The first step toward improving listening skills is to stop talking. "We have two ears and one mouth so that we can listen twice as much as we speak" (Epictetus—a Roman [Greek-born] slave and Stoic philosopher).
2. *Teach yourself to concentrate.* The average person speaks 100 to 200 words a minute. The listener can process up to 400 words a minute. Often we find ourselves pretending to listen, listening selectively to the speaker, not listening for meaning in the message, or hearing only what interests us; in so doing, we miss important cues or even words. "We cannot send you any help" has a much different meaning from "We cannot send you any help *right now.*"
3. *Take time to listen.* When someone talks to you, stop what you are doing and look at the speaker. Practice attentive listening by focusing on the meaning of the words and watching for the nonverbal symbols. "I wish I were dead" spoken by an elderly patient may mean "I'm lonely."
4. *Listen with your eyes.* Practice empathetic listening by looking into the eyes of the sender. What is the sender saying? A visitor standing at the desk saying, "My mother is not back from surgery yet" may really be saying, "I'm frightened. She's been in surgery so long there must be complications."
5. *Listen to what is being said, not only to how it is being said.* Use both attentive and empathetic listening to fully understand what is being said. Avoid being distracted by a lisp, by how fast the sender is talking, or by what the sender is wearing, for instance. Concentrate on the verbal and nonverbal communication symbols used by the sender.

6. *Suspend judgment.* Often we react emotionally to what is said or what we think is being said. We prejudge what the speaker is saying and unconsciously tune out ideas or beliefs that do not match our own.

7. *Do not interrupt the speaker.* Interrupting the speaker or finishing the sentence discourages the sender and breaks down communication. To break this habit, try apologizing each time you interrupt the sender.

8. *Remove distractions.* Noise, a ringing telephone, and conversations of others are types of distractions that interfere with effective listening.

9. *Listen for both feeling and content* (seek to understand). Use empathetic listening by keeping in mind that all persons have the right to feel as they do.

Feedback

Feedback, the verbal and nonverbal response to the message sent, is the final component in the communication process. Effective communication is virtually impossible without it. Feedback tells the sender how much of the message was understood, indicates whether the receiver agrees or disagrees with the message, and helps the sender correct confusing or vague language. Feedback can be as simple as a nod, it may be an answer to a question, or it may be used to encourage further communication and to assist the sender in developing ideas or sharing feelings.

Guidelines for Improving Feedback Skills

1. *Paraphrase* (repeat the message to the sender in your own words). Phrases such as "Let me see if I have this right…" and "This is what you want…" are acceptable as lines leading into paraphrasing. For example, "Let me repeat that to you. For the dressing change tomorrow, you want a dressing tray, size 7 gloves, and three packages of 4 × 4's."

2. *Repeat the last word or words of the message* (to allow the speaker to more fully develop the thought). Be careful not to parrot the whole message, or the speaker may respond with "That's what I just said."

   Patient: I'm not sure I want to have the myelogram.
   HUC: Myelogram?
   Patient: Yes, I'm scheduled for one this afternoon, and frankly I'm scared stiff. My neighbor had one…

3. *Use specific rather than general feedback.* "Your idea has merit" is more meaningful than "You are so bright."

4. *Use constructive feedback rather than destructive feedback.* Do not use feedback that makes a person feel worse. "Moving your workstation to the other counter may work" is better than saying, "That's a dumb idea, it won't work there!"

5. *Do not deny senders' feelings.* The use of statements such as "Don't worry" or "You shouldn't feel that way" to someone who is frightened that he has cancer is of no help. Feedback that encourages the person to expound on his or her fears is much more helpful to the person.

Intercultural Communication Skills

The United States often is referred to as a "melting pot" because of its culturally diverse society. Valuing **diversity** means creating an environment that respects and includes differences, recognizing the unique contributions that individuals with many types of differences can make, and creating an environment that maximizes the potential of all individuals. Cultures are developed when groups of people spend an extended time together. Each of us has values, beliefs, habits, and customs as a result of the backgrounds that make up our **culture**. **Subcultures** are smaller groups of people with certain ethnic, occupational, religious, or physical characteristics within the larger culture (e.g., elderly people, teens, nurses, Christians, athletes). It is essential for health care workers to understand and evaluate their own values, beliefs, and customs before working with and caring for people of varying cultures in health care. A **conflict** may occur in the health care delivery system because of cultural misunderstandings (e.g., verbal and nonverbal language miscues, lack of courtesy, lack of objectivity). **Culturally sensitive care** or *cultural competence* involves taking the time to learn about the cultural backgrounds of patients and may require incorporating their beliefs and practices into their care plan. Refer to Table 5-1 to learn about the cultural backgrounds of African Americans, Asians, Hispanics, and Native Americans.

Often people judge others by the standards of their own values and beliefs and find it difficult to accept other cultures. This is referred to as **ethnocentrism.** HUCs may have attitudes regarding a patient's refusal of treatment because of religious beliefs, a patient who is admitted for sex change surgery, or a patient who is a former alcoholic who is receiving a liver transplant. These attitudes are based on ethnocentrism and must not affect the care given to these patients. It is also very important to avoid **stereotyping** and to refrain from making assumptions or drawing conclusions about a patient or a co-worker on the basis of race or ethnicity. **Ageism (age discrimination)** is stereotyping of individuals or groups based on age. **Elitism** is a belief or attitude that a selected group of persons have personal abilities, specialized training, or other attributes that place them at the top of any field and that these people's views on a matter are to be taken most seriously.

Patients and co-workers deserve to be treated and respected as unique individuals, regardless of their **cultural differences** including gender, age, economic status, religion, sexual status, education, occupation, physical makeup or limitations, and command of the English language.

★ HIGH PRIORITY

Guidelines for Improving Intercultural Communication

- Understand and evaluate your own values, beliefs, and customs before working with and caring for people of varying cultures.
- Take the time to learn about the cultural backgrounds of patients; this may involve incorporating their beliefs and practices into their care.
- Do not judge others by the standards of your own values and beliefs.
- Avoid stereotyping or making assumptions about a patient or a coworker on the basis of race or ethnicity.
- Treat all people with respect as unique individuals, regardless of their gender, age, economic status, religion, sexual status, education, occupation, physical makeup or limitations, or command of the English language.

TABLE 5-1 Variations among Selected Cultural Groups

	African Americans	Asians	Hispanics	Native Americans
Verbal communication	Asking personal questions of someone met for the first time is seen as improper and intrusive.	High respect for others, especially those in positions of authority.	Expression of negative feelings is considered impolite.	Speak in a low tone of voice and expect that the listener will be attentive.
Nonverbal communication	Direct eye contact in conversation often is considered rude.	Direct eye contact with superiors may be considered disrespectful.	Avoidance of eye contact usually is a sign of attentiveness and respect.	Direct eye contact often is considered disrespectful.
Touch	Touching another's hair often is considered offensive.	It is not customary to shake hands with persons of the opposite sex.	Touching often is observed between two persons in conversation.	A light touch of the person's hand instead of a firm handshake often is used when greeting a person.
Family organization	Usually have close, extended family networks. Women play key roles in health care decisions.	Usually have close, extended family ties. Emphasis may be on family needs rather than on individual needs.	Usually have close, extended family ties. All members of the family may be involved in health care decisions.	Usually have close, extended family ties. Emphasis tends to be on the family rather than on individual needs.
Time	Often present oriented.	Often present oriented.	Often present oriented.	Often present oriented.
Alternative healers	"Granny," "root doctor," voodoo priest, spiritualist.	Acupuncturist, acupressurist, herbalist.	Curandero, espiritualista, yerbo.	Medicine man, shaman.
Self-care practices	Poultices, herbs, oils, roots.	Hot and cold foods, herbs, teas, soups, cupping, burning, rubbing, pinching.	Hot and cold foods, herbs.	Herbs, corn meal, medicine bundle.

Data from Giger JN, Davidhizar, RE: *Transcultural nursing*, ed 3, St Louis, 1999, Mosby; Spector RE: *Cultural diversity in health and illness*, ed 5, Upper Saddle River, NJ, 2000, Prentice Hall; Payne KT: In Taylor OL, editor: *Nature of communication disorders in culturally and linguistically diverse populations*, San Diego, 1986, College Hill Press.

Guidelines for Speaking to Someone Who Does Not Speak English Well

While working as a HUC, you may need to speak to someone from a different culture who does not speak English well.

Use the following guidelines in this process:

- Do not speak loudly.
- Talk distinctly and slowly.
- Emphasize key words.
- Let the listener read your lips.
- Use printed words (after determining the reading ability of the listener) and pictures.
- Do not use slang or jargon.
- Organize your thoughts.
- Choose your words carefully.
- Construct your sentences to say exactly what you want to say.
- Observe body language carefully.
- Try to pronounce names correctly.
- Ask for feedback to assess understanding.
- Ask how the person wishes to be addressed.
- Call for an **interpreter** if necessary and if available.
- Speak directly to the person, even if an interpreter is present.

⭐ **HIGH PRIORITY**

Most hospitals provide a list of interpreters who speak and understand various languages and may be called when necessary to provide assistance in communicating with patients or visitors.

ASSERTIVENESS FOR THE HEALTH UNIT COORDINATOR

Have you ever said "Yes" to a request but really wanted to say "No," or left a conversation wishing you had "stood up for yourself"? If your answer is "Yes," then you responded to the request in a **nonassertive** behavioral style.

Have you ever allowed a situation to get out of control, then "blown up" and later wished you had handled the situation better? If your answer is "Yes," then you responded to the situation in an **aggressive** behavioral style. Have you hidden your displeasure and anger at assigned tasks at work and deliberately failed to complete the tasks? This is **passive aggressive** behavior.

A third type of response is an **assertive** behavioral style, in which an individual expresses her or his wants and desires in an honest and appropriate way, while respecting other people's rights.

As a HUC, you may have to ask patients or visitors to change their behavior to conform to safety regulations and hospital rules, or to allow for the comfort of others. For example, you may have to ask a patient's relative not to smoke in the hospital, or you may have to ask a patient to turn down the television volume at the request of the patient's roommate. Asking another person to change a behavior can provoke a defensive reaction. Knowing you have a choice of behavioral styles and choosing the best way to handle a given situation assists you in communicating more effectively. The following list of adjectives and feelings will assist in understanding the nonassertive, aggressive, and assertive behaviors.

Adjectives and feelings that describe behaviors include the following:

- *Nonassertive:* Shy, helpless, needy, afraid, cowardly, anxious, dependent, self-pitying, apologetic, timid, doormat, martyr, poor me, feels inferior, disrespects self, others' needs come first. *You win, I lose.*
- *Aggressive:* Overbearing, dominating, demanding, angry, disturbed, cruel, combative, uncooperative, disagreeable, tense, controlling, abusive, disrespectful of others, feels superior, my needs come first. *I win, You lose.*
- *Assertive:* Confident, fair, compromising, calm, comfortable, unbiased, kind, cooperative, agreeable, independent, self-assured, respectful of others as well as self, everyone's needs are important. *I win, You win.*

★ HIGH PRIORITY

Both nonassertive and aggressive behaviors can be manipulative and frustrating to others. Someone with a *nonassertive personality* finds everything unfair and falls to pieces, attempting to gain sympathy and cause guilt in the other person in order to use it to further their own needs. Someone with an *aggressive personality* will cause an argument to make the other person feel terrible or guilty over something that was said or done, to gain sympathy and to use as a manipulation tool.

As a HUC, you may have encounters that could lead to conflict each day that you are on the job. Using assertiveness, the art of expressing yourself clearly and concisely; being able to clarify when necessary; and being able to explain and communicate in an open, honest manner are techniques that enable you to cope effectively with problems and conflicts as they arise (Box 5-1, A *Bill of Assertive Rights*).

Behavioral Styles
Nonassertive Behavioral Style

A nonassertive response is typically self-denying and does not express true feelings. The person does not stand up for his or her rights and allows others to choose for him or her. Because of an inadequate response to the situation, the individual feels hurt and anxious. Nonassertive HUCs may have strong opinions about things that are going on at the nurses' station but may keep those feelings to themselves.

BOX 5-1	BILL OF ASSERTIVE RIGHTS

Manuel J Smith's book, *When I Say No, I Feel Guilty*, published in 1975, provided a "Bill of Assertive Rights," which center around the principle that assertiveness is largely about expressing oneself clearly and resisting manipulation. The ideas in his book provide a basis for current assertiveness training.

Smith asserts that you have the right to:

- ...judge your own behavior, thoughts, and emotions, and to take responsibility upon yourself for their initiation and consequences.
- ...offer no reasons or excuses to justify your behavior.
- ...judge whether you are responsible for finding solutions to other people's problems.
- ...change your mind.
- ...make mistakes—and be responsible for them.
- ...say "I don't know."
- ...be independent of the goodwill of others before coping with them.
- ...be illogical in making decisions.
- ...say "I don't understand." "I don't care." "No" without feeling guilty.

SCENARIO

Kim feels that she is scheduled to work more weekends and holidays than the other HUCs on the unit. Instead of saying anything to the nurse manager, she gets upset every time she looks at the new work schedule.

A nonassertive choice avoids conflict; therefore feelings of frustration or anger are not expressed to the person responsible.

SCENARIO

Robert spent 15 minutes in the unit lounge complaining to co-workers about how Betsy, a nurse, is condescending toward him and makes disparaging remarks in conversations with him. She expects him to leave what he is working on to run special errands for her. He is angry and frustrated but refuses to talk to her directly about these problems.

A nonassertive choice avoids conflict; therefore feelings of frustration or anger are not expressed to the person responsible.

SCENARIO

Two visitors are relaxing in a visitors' lounge near the nursing station. They both light cigarettes. A "No smoking" sign is posted nearby. Mary approaches the visitors and says, "I'm sorry, but I have to ask a little favor. This is not my rule, but smoking is not allowed here."

A nonassertive approach to requesting a behavioral change is to use general or apologetic statements or to use words that minimize the message. This low-key approach allows others to easily ignore the request.

> ### SCENARIO
>
> An EMR system has been implemented at the hospital where Tammy works, and she has been told that absolutely no handwritten physicians' orders should be accepted. Dr. Jamison has admitted a new patient and hands Tammy a sheet of handwritten orders. Tammy accepts the order sheet and says, "I was told that we were not to accept any handwritten orders. Would you mind entering the orders into the computer for me?" Dr. Jameson replies, "You can enter them into the computer for me, can't you?" Tammy replies, "Yes, sir."

A nonassertive approach and response often result when one is intimidated by someone in a higher position.

Aggressive Behavioral Style

An aggressive response is typically self-enhancing at the expense of others. The person may express feelings but hurts others in the process. Verbal attacks, disparaging remarks, and **manipulation** indicate aggressive behavior.

> ### SCENARIO
>
> Kim feels that she is scheduled to work more weekends and holidays than the other HUCs. Kim approaches the nurse manager and says, "You're so unfair. You don't care about me or my life. I have to work more weekends and holidays than the others."

An aggressive HUC uses "you" statements, often followed by personal judgments. Use of "you" statements provokes greater defensiveness than is aroused by the use of "I" statements.

> ### SCENARIO
>
> Robert is upset with the nurse, Betsy, because she expects him to leave what he is doing to run errands for her. Robert responds aggressively, "You *always* expect me to stop my work for you; you think what you want is so important and you *never* think about anyone else."

Statements that use *always* and *never* are often part of aggressive communication.

> ### SCENARIO
>
> An aggressive HUC would ask visitors to stop smoking by saying, "Put out your cigarettes. You can't smoke here. Can't you see the big 'No smoking' sign?"

An aggressive HUC makes demands instead of requests. Demanding does not elicit another's cooperation and generates defensiveness. Disparaging remarks result in the receiver feeling humiliated.

> ### SCENARIO
>
> Dr. Jamison has admitted a new patient and hands Tammy a sheet of handwritten orders. Tammy refuses the order sheet and says, "I know you and all doctors on staff have been told that all orders have to be entered into the computer. You need to enter them into the computer, and don't think about asking me to do it!"

An aggressive approach may result when one feels intimidated by someone in a higher position.

Assertive Behavioral Style

An assertive response includes standing up for your rights without violating the rights of others. Assertive behavior is self-enhancing but not at the expense of others. It involves open, honest communication and the ability to express needs, expectations, and feelings. Being assertive also means being able to accept compliments with ease and to admit errors. It means taking responsibility for your actions. It is common for a person to assert himself or herself verbally only after frustration builds. At that point, it is too late to communicate assertively, and an aggressive response is used instead. It is useful to use assertiveness in all interactions before frustration builds. It is sometimes easy to confuse assertive behavior with aggressive behavior. To distinguish the difference, remember that with assertive behavior, the rights of another are not violated.

> ### SCENARIO
>
> Kim, as an assertive HUC, chooses to talk to the nurse manager about her feelings. "I feel that I'm working more weekends and holidays than the other HUCs. I had to work two-and-a-half weekends last month, and I'm scheduled to work Christmas and New Year's day this year. I would like to share working weekends and holidays equally with the others. I would be glad to work every third weekend, and our family celebrates Christmas on Christmas Eve, so I would be happy to work Christmas day and have New Year's day off. It would allow me more time to spend with my family."

An assertive HUC uses concise statements and specific behavioral descriptions.

> ### SCENARIO
>
> Robert is being assertive in dealing with Betsy when he chooses to talk to her. He begins by using an "I" statement and then describes the incident in which he felt Betsy was condescending. "I felt you were condescending toward me when you said, 'Even *you* should have been able to see that I needed help.'" He also mentions the specific remark that she made that he found disparaging. Depending on the discussion that follows, it also may be appropriate for him to ask Betsy for a behavior change. Robert also describes an incident in which Betsy asked him to interrupt his work to run errands for her. He describes how he could be more productive if he is allowed to do the task for her when it is convenient for his work schedule.

TABLE 5-2 Comparison of Nonassertive, Aggressive, and Assertive Behavioral Styles

Components	Nonassertive	Aggressive	Assertive
Rights	Does not stand up for rights	Stands up for rights but violates the rights of others	Stands up for rights without violating rights of others
Choice	Allows others to choose (to avoid conflict)	Chooses for others	Chooses for self
Belief	I'm not OK, you're OK; lose/win	I'm OK, you're not OK; win/lose	I'm OK, you're OK; win/win
Responsibility	Holds others responsible for behavior; blames self for poor results; may blame others for feelings	Feels responsible for others' behavior; blames others for poor results; feelings are not important	Feels responsible for own behavior; assumes responsibility for own errors; assumes responsibility for feelings
Traits	Self-denying, apologetic, timid, emotionally dishonest; difficult to say, "No"; guilty, whining, "poor me"	Dominates, humiliates, uses sarcasm; self-enhancing at the expense of others; opinionated	Expresses feelings, feels good about self; candid, diplomatic; listens; makes eye contact
Goals	Does not achieve goals	Achieves goals at the expense of others	May achieve goals
Word choices	Minimizing words, such as: "I'm sorry" "I believe" "I think" "A little," "sort of" General instead of specific statements; statements disguised as questions	"You" statements Always and never statements Demands instead of requests	"I understand…" "I feel…" "I apologize…" Neutral language Concise statements
Body language	Lack of eye contact; slumping, downtrodden posture; words and nonverbal messages that do not match	"Looking-through-you" eye contact; tense, impatient posture	Erect, relaxed posture; eye contact; verbal and nonverbal messages match

An assertive HUC is able to use clear, direct, nonapologetic expressions of feelings and expectations. Descriptive rather than judgmental criticisms and "I" rather than "you" statements are used.

SCENARIO

Mary, as an assertive HUC, approaches the visitors and says, "Please do not smoke in the hospital. Smoking is not allowed anywhere in the hospital, but there are designated smoking areas located outside the cafeteria on the back patio, where you can sit down and have a cigarette."

An assertive HUC uses requests instead of demands and personalizes statements of concern.

SCENARIO

Dr. Jamison has admitted a new patient and hands Tammy a sheet of handwritten orders. Tammy hands the order sheet back to him and says, "I know it is difficult to get used to the EMR; if you need any assistance in entering these orders into the computer, let me know."

Assertive behavior is the most effective way to communicate no matter what an individual's status is in comparison with yours.

Assertiveness is based on the belief that each individual has the same fundamental human rights; therefore the doctor is not better than the HUC, and the teacher is not better than the students. In becoming assertive, you need to focus not on changing your personality but rather on changing your behavior in specific situations. It is highly unlikely that anyone is always assertive; however, once assertiveness is learned, it can be one of your behavioral choices.

Table 5-2 compares nonassertive, aggressive, and assertive behavioral styles.

EXERCISE 2

Identify the behavioral style shown in each of the following statements by writing AG for aggressive, AS for assertive, or NA for nonassertive.

1. "I would like to have Monday off."

2. "You should know how to use the phone system! You've been here long enough."

3. "I'm sorry. I'm so forgetful. I won't let it happen again."

4. "I would kind of like to go on my break now if it's all right."

5. "The next NAHUC chapter meeting is tomorrow at 6:00 PM. I'm going. Would you like to go with me?"

6. "I know nothing about it. You were here yesterday—you should know."

7. "I would like to finish scanning these pathology reports into the EMRs before I take this specimen to the lab."

8. "I wish somebody else around here would answer the phone once in a while."

9. "The results are right here, Dr. James. I would think you could find them on your own."

10. "I apologize; I didn't call in that consultation request. I will call Dr. Foster's office immediately."

11. "You're always late and never care that I have to stay over and cover for you."

12. "I really hate to ask you this and you don't have to do it, but would you switch days with me so I can go to my daughter's dance recital?"

13. "May I help you find a stethoscope, Dr. Gomez?"

14. "I don't know what the nurse manager thinks I am—a machine or something. We need more help around here."

15. "You certainly should know how to locate diagnostic reports without my help by now!"

16. "I know I'm not supposed to enter these orders into the computer for you, but if you don't tell anyone, I'll enter them for you."

17. "Mrs. Lukas, I would like you to turn your light off so Mrs. Jones can rest."

18. "Maddie, I would like to switch nursing units with you next week."

Evaluating Your Assertiveness

Table 5-3 is an assertiveness inventory that has been developed by Alberti and Emmons. These authors state that "the inventory provides a list of questions which should be useful in increasing your awareness of your own behavior in situations that call for assertiveness. The inventory is not a standardized psychological test. No one is nonassertive all the time, aggressive all the time or assertive all the time. Each person behaves in each of the three ways at various times, depending on the situation and person(s) involved in the situation." Answer the questions honestly and maybe there will be some self-discovery. There are no right answers. The only "score" is your own evaluation of how you measure up to what you would like to be able to do. Take time now to respond to the questions in the inventory.

Questions 1, 2, 4 to 7, 9 to 12, 14 to 19, 21, 22, 24, 25, 27, 28, 30, and 35 are oriented toward nonassertive behavior. Are you speaking up for yourself? Questions 3, 8, 13, 20, 23, 26, 29, and 31 to 34 are oriented toward aggressive behavior. Are you more aggressive than you realized? Are there some situations or some individuals that give you trouble?

Assertiveness Skills

The goal of using assertiveness in communication is to arrive at an "I win, you win" conclusion—in other words, a **workable compromise.** A workable compromise involves dealing with a conflict in such a way that the solution is satisfactory to all involved parties. Four assertiveness skills that may be used to reach a workable compromise are the broken record technique, fogging, negative assertion, and negative inquiry.

Broken Record

The **broken record technique** is an assertiveness skill that allows you to say "no" over and over again without raising your voice or getting irritated or angry. You must be persistent and not give reasons, excuses, or explanations for not doing what the other person wants you to do. By doing this, you can ignore manipulative traps and argumentative baiting.

> Jane: "Let's go to lunch."
> Sue: "Thanks for asking; However, *I can't go, I just started a new diet.*"
> Jane: "So what! You start a new diet every week. It has never stopped you from going before."
> Sue: "Well, thanks anyway, but *I just started a new diet, I can't go to lunch.*"
> Jane: "Well, you don't have to eat anything fattening."
> Sue: "Thanks anyway. *I can't go. I just started a new diet.*"

Fogging

Fogging is an assertiveness skill that allows you to accept manipulative criticism and anxiety-producing statements by offering no resistance and by using a noncommittal reply, while calmly acknowledging that there may be some truth in what the critic is saying, yet retaining the right to remain your own judge. When you use fogging, it is hard for the other person to see exactly what you are saying.

> John: "You are really too slow to do this job!"
> Bill: "I can see it may appear that I'm a slow worker; however, I've only been here a month. I'll speed up once I know the procedures better."

Negative Assertion

Negative assertion is an assertiveness skill that allows you to accept your errors and faults without becoming defensive or resorting to anger. It is a technique of admitting errors without affecting your worth as a human being. It includes not using self-depreciating language, such as "That was so stupid of me."

> Dr. Smith: "You didn't scan my progress notes from this morning into Mr. Jones's chart as I requested!"
> Sue: "You're right. I didn't scan them. I apologize. I'll scan them now."

Negative Inquiry

Negative inquiry is an assertiveness skill that allows you to actively prompt criticism to use the information or, if manipulative, to exhaust it. By doing this, you obtain clarification about the criticism and hopefully bring out possible hidden issues that may really be the point.

> Nurse manager: "Your work isn't what I expect of a HUC. If you want to stay on this unit, you'll have to improve."
> Unit coordinator: "When you say my work isn't what you expect, what is it about my work that isn't up to your expectations?"

TABLE 5-3 **The Assertiveness Inventory**

The following questions will be helpful in assessing your assertiveness. Be honest with your responses. All you have to do is draw a circle around the number that best describes you. For some questions, the assertive end of the scale is at 0; for others, it is at 3.

Key: 0 means *no* or *never;* 1 means *somewhat* or *sometimes;* 2 means *usually* or *a good deal;* and 3 means *practically always* or *entirely.*

1.	When a person is highly unfair, do you call it to his or her attention?	0	1	2	3
2.	Do you find it difficult to make decisions?	0	1	2	3
3.	Are you openly critical of others' ideas, opinions, or behaviors?	0	1	2	3
4.	Do you speak out in protest when someone takes your place in line?	0	1	2	3
5.	Do you often avoid people or situations for fear of embarrassment?	0	1	2	3
6.	Do you usually have confidence in your own judgment?	0	1	2	3
7.	Do you insist that your spouse or roommate take on a fair share of household chores?	0	1	2	3
8.	Are you prone to "flying off the handle"?	0	1	2	3
9.	When a salesperson makes an effort to sell you something, do you find it hard to say "No," even though the merchandise is not really what you want?	0	1	2	3
10.	When a latecomer is waited on before you, do you call attention to the situation?	0	1	2	3
11.	Are you reluctant to speak up in a discussion or a debate?	0	1	2	3
12.	If a person has borrowed money (or a book, a garment, or something else of value) and is overdue in returning it, do you mention it?	0	1	2	3
13.	Do you continue to pursue an argument after the other person has had enough?	0	1	2	3
14.	Do you generally express what you feel?	0	1	2	3
15.	Are you disturbed if someone watches you at work?	0	1	2	3
16.	If someone keeps kicking or bumping your chair in a movie or at a lecture, do you ask the person to stop?	0	1	2	3
17.	Do you find it difficult to keep eye contact when talking to another person?	0	1	2	3
18.	In a good restaurant, when your meal is improperly prepared or served, do you ask the waiter or waitress to correct the situation?	0	1	2	3
19.	When you discover that merchandise is faulty, do you return it for an adjustment?	0	1	2	3
20.	Do you show your anger by name-calling or using obscenities?	0	1	2	3
21.	Do you try to be a wallflower or a piece of furniture in social situations?	0	1	2	3
22.	Do you insist that your property manager (e.g., mechanic, repairman) make repairs, adjustments, or replacements that are his or her responsibility?	0	1	2	3
23.	Do you often step in and make decisions for others?	0	1	2	3
24.	Are you able to express love and affection openly?	0	1	2	3
25.	Are you able to ask your friends for small favors or help?	0	1	2	3
26.	Do you think you always have the right answer?	0	1	2	3
27.	When you have a difference of opinion with a person you respect, are you able to speak up for your own viewpoint?	0	1	2	3
28.	Are you able to refuse unreasonable requests made by friends?	0	1	2	3
29.	Do you have difficulty complimenting or praising others?	0	1	2	3
30.	If you are disturbed by someone who is smoking near you, can you say so?	0	1	2	3
31.	Do you shout or use bullying tactics to get others to do as you wish?	0	1	2	3
32.	Do you finish other people's sentences for them?	0	1	2	3
33.	Do you get into physical fights with others, especially with strangers?	0	1	2	3
34.	At family meals, do you control the conversation?	0	1	2	3
35.	When you meet a stranger, are you the first to introduce yourself and begin a conversation?	0	1	2	3

⊜ **E X E R C I S E 3**

Practice writing verbal responses to the situations described in the following exercise. Provide examples using assertive, nonassertive, and aggressive behavioral styles for each situation. Practice using assertiveness skills when giving answers.

1. A co-worker comes in at 3:00 PM and finds that the routine tasks have not been done. She asks, "Do you even know what you're supposed to do?" There were several nursing staff members at the nurses' station at the time. You did not have time to do the routine tasks because it was an extremely busy day.

2. You have been asked to float to pediatrics. You have always worked on the orthopedics unit. When you arrive on Peds, a nurse says to you, "It would really be nice to get someone who knows what they're doing."

3. You forgot to order a CBC this morning while transcribing Mr. Barrett's orders. When the error is discovered by the patient's nurse, she says, "You didn't order the CBC on Mr. Barrett this morning!"

4. A local celebrity is a patient on your unit. The doctor has left strict instructions that only relatives can visit the patient and for only short periods. A visitor has just approached the nursing station. He claims he is the local celebrity's manager and must see the patient about some financial matters today.

5. Your immediate supervisor has just told you that your work is just not acceptable and to improve it or else.

6. It is 9:00 AM, and Dr. Frank has asked you to please locate the reports from an outside facility that she requested yesterday on one of her patients. You find them in the basket of documents to be scanned. When you tell this to Dr. Frank, she responds angrily, "What in the hell is going on here? Can't anybody do anything right on this unit?"

DEALING WITH AN ANGRY TELEPHONE CALLER

At times the HUC is confronted with angry or disgruntled telephone callers. Following the few helpful steps outlined here will assist you in handling the situation effectively.

1. *When answering the telephone, always identify yourself by nursing unit, name, and status* (Fig. 5-7). Doing this puts you on a more personal level with the caller. Also, callers may become even more upset if they need to ask questions to determine to whom they are talking.

2. *Avoid putting the person on hold.* Placing an angry person on hold may escalate the anger.

3. *Listen to what the caller is saying.* Do not become defensive. Keep in mind that the caller is not really angry with you.

4. *Write down what the caller is saying.* The notes may come in handy, and they help you control your own anger.

5. *Acknowledge the anger.* Use phrases such as, "I understand that you're angry" and "I hear your frustration."

6. *Do not allow the caller to become abusive.* Say, "I feel you're becoming abusive" or "Please call me back in a few minutes so we can talk about this calmly."

COMMUNICATION AND INTERPERSONAL SKILLS USED IN THE HEALTH CARE SETTING

Following are five major areas in which the HUC may use communication and interpersonal skills discussed in this chapter in the health care setting:

1. *Obtaining information.* Often the HUC must obtain information to communicate a message in a correct and timely manner. Applying assertiveness skills to ask a question correctly, using appropriate listening skills when receiving the response and when the situation calls for it, and using the guidelines for speaking to a person who does not speak English well will be useful.

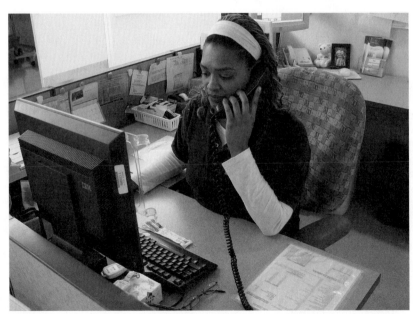

Figure 5-7 When you answer the telephone, always identify yourself by nursing unit, name, and status.

2. *Providing information.* The HUC will be providing information to visitors, doctors, nursing staff, and other hospital departments, as well as to institutions outside the hospital. Being aware of verbal and nonverbal use of language will be helpful in doing this.

3. *Developing trust.* Trust is vital to a healthy work environment, and assertive communication plays a big role in establishing and maintaining this trust.

4. *Showing understanding.* Understanding the needs of patients, families, and co-workers will foster successful communication in the work environment. Using Maslow's hierarchy of needs and intercultural communication skills will be helpful in this area.

5. *Relieving stress.* Stress in the workplace is a constant; how we manage it makes a difference. Recognizing the three behavioral types and using assertiveness skills can be helpful in this area. Using the communication model of selecting words carefully for communication and using effective listening skills may help avoid or alleviate stressful situations.

TRAINING AND BEING TRAINED

When given the opportunity to **precept** (to train or instruct) a student or to orient a new employee to your nursing unit or hospital, keep in mind what it was like when you were new and inexperienced. Were you made to feel welcome, or were you made to feel that you were in the way? How did it affect your clinical or orientation experience? When you are selected to be a *preceptor* (trainer or teacher), your nurse manager is indicating that she or he has confidence in your expertise and your knowledge and ability to teach students or new employees what they need to know. To provide the best learning experience, it is important to make the new employee feel comfortable enough to ask questions, if necessary, to fully understand what you are teaching. Every person learns at a different pace; some will remember what you have told them the first time, some will need to write it down, and others will need to actually perform the task before mastering it. The following guidelines should assist you in becoming an efficient preceptor and in providing a successful clinical experience or orientation.

Guidelines for the Health Unit Coordinating Preceptor

- Provide a copy of dates and times the student or new employee is to be on the nursing unit to complete the clinical experience (provide a copy of your schedule to the student and the student's instructor or to the new employee).
- Obtain a list of objectives (provided by the hospital or by the school), so all are clear on what is to be accomplished by the end of the clinical experience.
- Take the student or new employee on a tour of the nursing unit and hospital, so that he or she can become aware of where restrooms, cafeteria, and hospital departments are located.
- Set a positive example: be on time each day, return on time from appropriate breaks, and maintain a positive attitude regarding your job, the hospital, the administration, and nursing unit personnel.
- If the student or new employee does not call before being late or absent, it is the preceptor's responsibility to notify the instructor or nurse manager.

- Notify the student and your nursing unit or the new employee and the nurse manager if you are going to be tardy, absent, or transferred to another unit (preferably an hour before the start of the shift).
- Stay with the student or new employee to monitor progress and check off objectives as completed with competence, as instructed in the clinical or orientation packet.
- Provide feedback to the student or new employee, and offer suggestions for improvement.
- Notify the student's instructor or the new employee's nurse manager if the student or new employee is not dressed according to hospital or school dress code (the student may have a more strict dress code), is not performing in an appropriate and professional manner, or is having difficulty completing objectives.
- Notify the student's instructor or the new employee's nurse manager if you have questions or concerns.
- Notify the student's instructor or the new employee's nurse manager immediately if you have serious concerns.
- Complete an evaluation form regarding the student's clinical experience.

Guidelines for the Health Unit Coordinating Student or New Employee

- Be sure you know when and where you are to complete your **HUC clinical experience**, and know the name of your **HUC preceptor.**
- If you are a student, provide your preceptor with a list of objectives and the instructor's telephone and/or pager number.
- The student or new employee should notify the nursing unit, the preceptor, and the instructor or nurse manager an hour before the start of the shift (except in the case of an emergency) if he or she is going to be tardy or absent.
- The student must notify the instructor if he or she leaves the hospital before the end of the shift.
- It is the student's responsibility to notify the instructor if the preceptor is going to be late, absent, or transferred to another unit.
- The student or new employee should arrive dressed appropriately and prepared to learn and work each day and should be accountable for his or her learning.
- The student needs to be flexible and should refrain from saying, "That's not the way we were taught in class" or "That's not the way we did it at Previous Community Hospital."
- The student or new employee should communicate openly with the preceptor and instructor or nurse manager regarding any problems with his or her clinical performance.
- The student or new employee should have the preceptor complete and sign off on the list of objectives or evaluation forms 2 days before the last clinical day.
- The student or new employee should complete an evaluation form regarding the clinical experience or orientation.

KEY CONCEPTS

Effective communication is essential in the health care setting. High-quality patient care requires an efficient, professional, and culturally sensitive team. It is vital that personnel remain calm, exercise assertiveness skills, and have empathy for patients and co-workers. Each member of a health care team is important and necessary, and it is imperative that staff members maintain a positive attitude regarding the job, hospital, administration, and nursing unit personnel. About a third of one's time is spent on the job, so why not make it a pleasant experience?

Websites of Interest

The Joint Commission—About Our Standards: www.jointcommi
  ssion.org/standards
Institute of Healthcare Communication:
  www.healthcarecommunication.org
Livestrong.com—improving assertiveness skills:
  www.livestrong.com/article/14699-improving-
  assertive-behavior

⊖ REVIEW QUESTIONS

Visit the Evolve website to download and complete the following questions.

1. Define the following terms:
   a. communication
   b. encoding
   c. decoding
   d. conflict
   e. interpreter
   f. manipulation
   g. paraphrase
   h. passive aggressive
   i. culture
   j. cultural differences
   k. workable compromise
   l. subculture

2. Write the term from the list below that best describes the following statements.
   ageism
   diversity
   elitism
   empathy
   ethnocentrism
   stereotyping
   a. There are nine countries represented among our employees.
   b. She is too old to handle the work on this unit.
   c. Our unit has the best, most educated employees and should be paid more.
   d. Beth has a special relationship with the patients on the oncology unit because her mother is a cancer survivor.
   e. People from Germany do not have a good sense of humor.
   f. I only want American nurses to take care of my mother.

3. Write an example of a hospitalized patient's situation that exemplifies each of the first four needs outlined in Maslow's hierarchy of needs.
   a. physiologic
   b. safety and security
   c. belonging and love
   d. esteem

4. Name four components of the communication process.

5. Explain how unsuccessful communication can occur during the encoding and decoding process.

6. Using the communication model, demonstrate a successful communication process and an unsuccessful communication process (think of personal experiences). Identify at which step of the process the errors occurred.
   a. successful communication
   b. unsuccessful communication
   c. step of the communication process at which error(s) occurred

7. List two common errors in encoding a message.

8. List two common errors in decoding a message.

9. List three examples of *symbolic* nonverbal communication.

10. List three examples of body language used in nonverbal communication.

11. Fill in the percentage used of each of the following verbal and nonverbal types of communication during the process of communicating messages:
    a. Facial expression and eye contact, including the length of glance _____%
    b. Vocal qualities, including tone, loudness, firmness, hesitations, and pauses _____%
    c. Verbal, actual words _____%

12. Identify the cause(s) of unsuccessful communication in each of the following situations:
    a. A nurse interviewing an Asian patient sits on the side of his bed while making direct eye contact. The patient looks away, avoiding eye contact. The nurse thinks the patient is despondent or is being rude. (Refer to Table 5-1.)
    b. Mrs. Fredrick, an elderly female patient who has never been ill before, is admitted to the hospital. Joe, a young male CNA, is assisting her into bed. Joe tells Mrs. Fredrick, "OK, honey, your doctor has ordered that you be NPO because you're going to have a UGI this morning." Mrs. Fredrick begins to cry.
    c. Dr. James asks Sue, the HUC, to answer her calls while she is in the treatment room performing a procedure. Sue leaves the nurses' station for a short break and doesn't hear the operator paging Dr. James. When Dr. James returns to the nursing station and asks for her message, Sue says, "What message?" Dr. James angrily walks away.
    d. Cindi, the registered nurse who is caring for Stan Potter, a homeless man, does not spend the usual amount of time with him on admission because he is dirty and doesn't have any social skills.

13. List five levels of listening,

14. List nine listening skills that would most help you improve your interpersonal communication.

15. List the five feedback skills that you feel would help you improve your interpersonal communication.

16. Define and explain the importance of "culturally sensitive care" in the health care setting.

17. List five guidelines to follow that could improve intercultural communication.

18. Label the following behaviors as assertive, nonassertive, or aggressive.
    a. self-denying
    b. self-enhancing at the expense of others
    c. open, honest, and respectful of others' rights

19. Explain the following assertiveness techniques.
    a. Broken record
    b. Fogging
    c. Negative assertion
    d. Negative inquiry

20. List six steps that you should follow when dealing with an angry caller.

21. List twelve preceptor guidelines for training a HUC student or a new employee.

22. List ten student guidelines for completing the clinical experience.

23. Identify five ways that communication and interpersonal skills are used in the health care setting.

24. Explain why the implementation of the EMR is requiring even greater communication skills of the HUC.

SURFING FOR ANSWERS

1. Conduct a search for *barriers to communication in health care,* and document what barriers you find from at least three websites.
2. Locate three websites that discuss *the importance of effective communication in health care.*
Write a short paragraph explaining the importance of effective communication, and list the websites quoted.
3. Search *culturally sensitive health care,* and document five facts that you did not know before.

CHAPTER 6

Workplace Behavior
Ethics and Legal Concepts

CHAPTER OBJECTIVES

On completion of this chapter, you will be able to:

1. Define the terms in the vocabulary list.
2. Write the meaning of the abbreviations in the abbreviations list.
3. List seven factors that may influence a worker's behavior.
4. Define personal values, and explain how personal values could affect one's interactions in the health care setting.
5. List six behavioral traits that make up one's work ethic.
6. Explain the purposes of the Privacy Rule and the Security Rule contained in the Health Insurance Portability and Accountability Act (HIPAA).

7. List six patient rights as outlined in HIPAA.
8. Identify seven patient identifiers (individually identifiable health information [IIHI]).
9. Explain two purposes of the Health Information Technology for Economic and Clinical Health (HITECH) Act.
10. Explain two main responsibilities the health unit coordinator (HUC) has for HIPAA compliance.
11. Discuss how the HUC can protect patient confidentiality, including electronic and paper medical records.
12. Explain the importance of professional appearance.
13. List three preclinical or preemployment screenings or requirements and four requirements of The Joint Commission.
14. Explain why a supervisor or clinical instructor would request a drug test for cause and what the consequences would be if a clinical student were to refuse the test or were to test positive for drug use.
15. Discuss five guidelines for cell phone use and four rules of elevator etiquette to adhere to when in the hospital setting.
16. Explain where guidelines regarding attendance, punctuality, and breaks would be found, and discuss the importance of employees and potential employees knowing and following those guidelines.
17. Discuss the first step to take when encountering sexual harassment.
18. Describe five signs of impending violence, and explain what action the HUC should take when recognizing signs of or an act of violence.
19. Discuss two purposes of an employee performance evaluation.
20. Discuss the benefits of collecting information and writing out a fact sheet for reference before completing a job application or writing a résumé.
21. Discuss the purpose of a résumé, and list 10 guidelines to follow and items to include when writing a résumé.
22. Explain how one would prepare for a phone interview and for an in-person interview.
23. List seven ethical principles for patient care on which the Code of Ethics for each health care profession and the Patients' Bill of Rights are based.
24. List the three sources from which laws are derived.
25. Define *medical malpractice* and describe how "standard of care" is determined.
26. Identify six preventive measures that can be taken to minimize the risk of medical malpractice within the HUC practice.

VOCABULARY

Accountability Taking responsibility for one's actions; being answerable to someone for something one has done.

American Recovery and Reinvestment Act (ARRA) Commonly referred to as *the Stimulus* or *the Recovery Act*, ARRA is an economic stimulus package enacted in 2009. The act significantly expanded HIPAA requirements affecting group health plans.

Attitude A manner of thought or feeling expressed in a person's behavior.

Autonomy State of functioning independently; personal liberty.

Cardiopulmonary Resuscitation (CPR) The basic lifesaving procedure of artificial ventilation and chest compressions performed in the event of a cardiac arrest. The Joint Commission (TJC) requires that all health care workers be certified in CPR.

Code of Ethics A set of rules and procedures for professional conduct based on the values and ethical standards of an organization or profession.

Confidence Belief in oneself and one's abilities; self-confidence, self-reliance, self-assurance—usually comes with knowledge.

Confidentiality The legally protected right afforded to all patients of having personal and medical information (written or spoken) be protected.

Damages Monetary compensation awarded by a court for an injury caused by the act of another.

Defendant The person against whom a civil or criminal action is brought.

Deposition Pretrial statement of a witness under oath, taken in question-and-answer form, as it would be in court, with opportunity given to the adversary to be present to cross-examine.

Ethics A system of moral principles (beliefs) that determine how we make judgments in regard to right and wrong.

Evidence All the means by which any alleged matter of fact, the truth of which is submitted to investigation at trial, is established or disproved; evidence includes the testimony of witnesses and the introduction of records, documents, exhibits, objects, or any other substantiating matter offered for the purpose of inducing belief in the party's contention by the judge or jury.

Expert Witness A person who has special knowledge of the subject about which he or she is to testify; this knowledge must generally be such as is not normally possessed by the average person.

Fidelity Reliability, trustworthiness, dependability; doing what one promises.

Health Information Technology for Economic and Clinical Health (HITECH) Act Law that stimulates the adoption of electronic health records (EHRs) and widens the scope of privacy and security protections available under HIPAA.

Health Insurance Portability and Accountability Act (HIPAA) A U.S. law designed to provide privacy standards to protect patients' medical records and other health information provided to health plans, doctors, hospitals, and other health care providers.

Hostile Working Environment A threatening or sexually oriented atmosphere or pattern of behavior that is determined to be a form of harassment.

Informed Consent Doctrine that states that before patients are asked to consent to a risky or invasive diagnostic or treatment procedure, they are entitled to receive certain information: (1) a description of the procedure, (2) any alternatives to it and their risks, (3) risks of death or serious bodily disability from the procedure, (4) probable results of the procedure, including any problems with recuperation and anticipated time of recuperation, and (5) anything else that is generally disclosed to patients who are asked to consent to a procedure.

Liability Condition of being responsible for damages resulting from an injurious act or from discharging an obligation or debt.

Medical Malpractice Professional negligence of a health care professional; failure to meet a professional standard of care, resulting in harm to another—for example, failure to provide "good and accepted medical care."

Negligence Failure to satisfactorily perform one's legal duty, such that another person incurs some injury.

Philosophy Guiding or underlying principles; attitude toward life.

Plaintiff Person who brings a lawsuit against another.

Principles Basic truths; moral code of conduct.

Quid pro Quo (Latin) With regard to employment, situation in which conditions of employment (hiring, promotion, retention) are made contingent on the victim's providing sexual or other favors.

Respect Holding a person in esteem or honor; having appreciation and regard for another.

Respondeat Superior (Latin) "Let the master answer"; legal doctrine that imposes liability on the employer as a result of the action of an employee. *Note:* The employee is also liable for his or her own actions.

Retaliation Revenge; payback.

Role Fidelity Requires that health care professionals remain within their scope of legitimate practice.

Scope of Practice Legal description of what a specific health professional may and may not do.

Sexual Harassment Unwanted, unwelcome behavior that is sexual in nature.

Standard of Care The legal duty one owes to another according to the circumstances of a particular case; it is the care that a reasonable and prudent person would have exercised in a given situation.

Statutes Laws passed by the legislature and signed by the governor at the state level and the president at the federal level.

Statute of Limitations Time within which a plaintiff must bring a civil suit; this limit varies with the type of suit, and it is set by the various state legislatures.

Tactfulness Sensitivity to what is proper and appropriate in dealing with others; use of discretion regarding the feelings of others.

Values Personal beliefs about the worth of a principle, standard, or quality; what one holds as most important; values reflect a person's sense of right and wrong.

Values Clarification A method of determining and accessing one's values and how those values affect personal decision making.

Work Ethic Moral values regarding work.

Workplace Behavior A pattern of actions and interactions of an individual that directly or indirectly affects his or her effectiveness while at work; the attitude and amount of enthusiasm that one brings to the job.

ABBREVIATIONS

Abbreviation	Meaning
APS	Adult Protective Services
ARRA	American Recovery and Reinvestment Act (of 2009)
CE	covered entity
CPR	cardiopulmonary resuscitation
CPS	Child Protective Services
EPHI	electronic protected health information
HIPAA	Health Insurance Portability and Accountability Act
HITECH	Health Information Technology for Economic and Clinical Health Act
IIHI	individually identifiable health information
NINP	no information, no publication
PHI	protected health information
SNAT	suspected nonaccidental trauma

⊖ EXERCISE 1

Write the abbreviation for each term listed.

1. Adult Protective Services
2. American Recovery and Reinvestment Act
3. Child Protective Services
4. no information, no publication
5. suspected nonaccidental trauma
6. Health Insurance Portability and Accountability Act
7. Health Information Technology for Economic and Clinical Health Act
8. protected health information
9. covered entity
10. cardiopulmonary resuscitation
11. electronic protected health information
12. individually identifiable health information

⊖ EXERCISE 2

Write the meaning of each abbreviation listed.

1. APS
2. ARRA
3. CPS
4. NINP
5. SNAT
6. HIPAA
7. HITECH
8. PHI
9. CE
10. CPR
11. EPHI
12. IIHI

WORKPLACE BEHAVIOR

Workplace behavior may be described as a pattern of actions and interactions of an individual that directly or indirectly affects their effectiveness while at work. It reflects the **attitude** and amount of enthusiasm that the employee brings to the job. Today's health care employees must perform their jobs efficiently and effectively while showing patients respect, patience, and empathy. We have all made decisions to buy or not buy a product or service based on the salesperson's attitude or behavior. Patient survey responses that assess satisfaction with care are greatly influenced by the caregivers' and other hospital employees' attitudes or "workplace behavior." Patient satisfaction may impact the patient's choice of hospital for their health care or whether they submit a complaint. A variety of factors can influence a person's workplace behavior.

Factors that Influence Workplace Behavior

1. Philosophy and standards of the organization
2. Leadership style of supervisors
3. Meaningfulness or importance of the work
4. How challenging the work is
5. Relationships with co-workers
6. Personal characteristics such as abilities, interests, aptitudes, values, and expectations
7. External factors such as family life, health, and recreational habits

Job satisfaction has a direct correlation to workplace behavior. It is important to choose a career and a position that will best meet one's personal needs and aspirations. Many job options exist for a health unit coordinator (HUC) in the health care field. If one loves to be around children, pediatrics may be ideal, or if an individual wants to be challenged, the emergency room or an intensive care unit may be the best choice. If a job that will provide solitude is wanted, the recovery room may be an option, or if a more social setting is preferred, a medical-surgical unit may be a better choice. Consider options carefully.

PERSONAL VALUES

Personal values reflect the beliefs or culture of an individual; that evolve from circumstances with the external world and can change over time. According to Morris Massey, a sociologist and producer of training videos, values are formed during three significant periods:

1. *Imprint period* from birth to 7 years of age—Like sponges, children absorb everything around them, especially from their parents, and accept much of it as true.
2. *Modeling period* from 8 to 14 years—Youths copy people, often their parents, but also other people such as teachers and religious leaders, and no longer have blind acceptance.
3. *Socialization period* from 15 to 21 years—Young adults are very largely influenced by their peers and by media that seem to resonate with the values of their peer groups. As young adults develop as individuals and look for ways to get away from their earlier programming, it is natural to turn to people who seem more like them.

Significant emotional events in our lives and other life experiences may change our values. For example, losing a loved one may cause one to treasure family and to value life in a way one had not before. Life experiences can change what we view as most important and can also help us gain *empathy* for others. Our values can have a major impact on how we relate to others and on the choices and decisions that we make. Diann B. Uustal, EdD, a well-known nurse and ethicist, describes **values** as being "a basis for what a person thinks about, chooses, feels, and acts on" (Uustal: *Orthoped Nurs* 11(3):11-15, 1992). The HUC position requires communication that is provided in a nonjudgmental way. Personal values may cause problems in certain interactions. Examining one's value system is important in preparing to work in the health care setting.

SCENARIO

Joan, a HUC, has a father who was an abusive alcoholic. Joan is adamant about her feelings regarding alcoholics and is very much against drinking. Mr. Thomas is admitted because he was in a car accident that was caused by his drunkenness. Whenever Mr. Thomas approaches the desk to talk to Joan, she is very rude to him. Joan is allowing her personal values to influence her behavior. It is important to remain nonjudgmental when dealing with patients and their families and to not allow personal values to affect communication with others. At times this may be difficult, especially when one is communicating with a person who has been identified as an abuser of a child, a spouse, or an elderly person.

Influence of Personal Values in the Health Care Setting

A patient's values can also influence a health care professional's behavior when those values conflict with the health professional's values.

SCENARIO

A patient is admitted with internal bleeding; his religion prohibits him from receiving a blood transfusion. Janet, a HUC, states aloud that she cannot understand how anyone could risk his or her life because of a silly religious belief.

The patient has a right to his own values and the right to refuse treatment.

Conversation and statements made at the nursing station or anywhere in the hospital may be overheard. Health care professionals must be aware of what they say and judgments that they make.

SCENARIO

Susan, a HUC working in the pediatric intensive care unit, says to John, a registered nurse (RN) who is taking care of a 5-year-old girl on life support after a near drowning, "Why don't her parents take her off life support? Who'd want to live like a vegetable?" The little girl's father overhears the comment, approaches Susan, and says, "Young lady, I hope you never have to make that decision." Susan is devastated.

Values Clarification

Values clarification is an important tool for HUCs to use in preparing to become competent professionals. Either consciously or unconsciously, values guide personal and professional thinking. It is essential for HUCs to understand and be aware of their values and to remain nonjudgmental of the values others hold that differ from their own. Value conflicts include cultural, spiritual, social, and ethnic differences. There are times when it is difficult to remain nonjudgmental, especially when a child or elderly patient is admitted because of abuse and it is necessary to communicate with the probable abuser. One is entitled to one's feelings, but it is important to remain professional and allow the doctors, nurses, and protective services personnel to do their jobs.

 E X E R C I S E **3**

This exercise is intended to guide you in examining your feelings and values related to future employment in health care. Complete the following sentences:

1. A patient has the right to
2. The health care team works best when
3. I fail to show respect for others' values when
4. The most difficult situation to deal with would be
5. When communicating with patients and families, it is important to

WORK ETHIC

One's **work ethic** refers to a person's moral values regarding work. It is essential that the HUC demonstrate the work ethic traits discussed in the following sections.

Behavioral Traits that Make Up a Person's Work Ethic
Behavioral Traits for "You" as a Health Unit Coordinator

Dependability: Patients and members of the health care team rely on *you* to report to work when scheduled and to be on time. *You* are also depended on to perform duties and tasks as assigned and to keep obligations and promises. Adequate sleep and abstinence from drugs are essential to maintain your dependability. Lack of sleep, use of illegal drugs, or misuse of prescription drugs would clearly endanger patients.

Accountability: Part of being dependable is being accountable. Accountability is taking responsibility for *your* own actions (i.e., being answerable to someone for something *you* have done). HUCs must be aware of and never exceed their **scope of practice.** If *you* are unable to report to work or to do *your* job, it is *your* responsibility to communicate this to the staffing office at least 2 hours before the scheduled shift.

Consideration: Be considerate of the physical condition and emotional state of the patients and *your* co-workers.

Cheerfulness: Greet and converse with patients and others in a pleasant manner. HUCs cannot bring personal problems to work. Sarcasm, moodiness, and bad tempers are inappropriate in the workplace.

Empathy: Make every attempt to see things from the viewpoint of patients, families, and co-workers. Keep in mind that stress and worry can affect people's behavior, so refrain from treating a display of anger or frustration as a personal attack.

Trustworthiness: Your employer, patients, and co-workers have placed their confidence in *you* to keep patient information confidential. HUCs have access to a lot of information and must not engage in gossip regarding patients, co-workers, physicians, or the hospital.

Respectfulness: **Respect** is a primary value in health care and can be shown in many ways, including tone of voice, body language, attitude toward others, and attitude about work. All life is worthy of respect. We all have a right to our own value system and must respect that others have a right to theirs. Make every attempt to understand the values and beliefs of the patients and your co-workers that may differ from your own.

Courtesy: Be polite and courteous to patients, families, visitors, co-workers, and supervisors. Address people by name (e.g., Mrs. Johnson, Dr. Smith). Other courteous acts include saying "please" and "thank you" and not interrupting when others are speaking.

Tactfulness: Be sensitive to the problems and needs of others. Be aware of what you say and how you say it.

Conscientiousness: Be careful, alert, and accurate in following orders and instructions. Never attempt to perform a procedure or a task that you have not been trained or licensed to perform.

Honesty: Be sincere, truthful, and genuine, and show a true interest in your relationships with patients, families, visitors, and co-workers. If you make an error, bring it to the attention of the appropriate person(s). Never attempt to cover up an error!

Cooperation: Be willing to work with others, especially in the team-oriented climate of health care. When co-workers work as a team, everyone involved benefits.

Attitude: Attitude is a manner of thought or feeling that can be seen by others when they are observing your behavior. The tone of your voice and your body language can change the message you are trying to send. Your attitude will be reflected in your work. Be positive about your job and the contribution that you are making.

OVERVIEW OF THE HEALTH INSURANCE PORTABILITY AND ACCOUNTABILITY ACT

HIPAA is an acronym for the Health Insurance Portability and Accountability Act of 1996. Health providers and health plans are legally required to follow this act.

The act is composed of five sections. Components of HIPAA and changes to the original HIPAA legislation have gone into effect several times since 1996, including in 2003, 2005, 2006, and 2007. Additional changes to HIPAA included in the **American Recovery and Reinvestment Act (ARRA)** of 2009 significantly expand HIPAA's privacy and security regulations.

Title I of HIPAA protects health insurance coverage for workers and their families when they change or lose their jobs. It establishes rules on how a group plan handles a preexisting condition.

Title II includes the Privacy Rule and the Security Rule—both enacted in 2003. The Privacy Rule establishes regulations for the use and disclosure of protected health information (PHI). The rule also gives patients rights over their health information, including rights to examine and obtain a copy of their health records and to request corrections (Box 6-1, *Patient Rights as Outlined in the Health Insurance Portability and Accountability Act*). The Security Rule applies to electronic protected health information (EPHI) or individually identifiable health information (IIHI) in electronic form. IIHI relates to (1) an individual's past, present, or future physical or mental health or condition, (2) an individual's provision of health care, and (3) past, present, or future payments provided for provision of health care to an individual; IIHI is information that identifies the individual or with respect to which there is a reasonable basis to believe the information can be used to identify the individual.

The primary objective of the Security Rule is to protect the confidentiality, integrity, and availability of IIHI that is created, received, transmitted, used, or maintained by a covered entity

(Box 6-2, *Health Insurance Portability and Accountability Act Individually Identifiable Health Information (IIHI) and Patient Identifiers*).

Title III gives employees the ability to set up health savings and flexible spending accounts. Health savings accounts allow employees to take out a set amount from their paycheck, pre-taxed, to be used for copays, deductibles, and other approved out-of-pocket expenses.

BOX 6-1	**PATIENT RIGHTS AS OUTLINED IN THE HEALTH INSURANCE PORTABILITY AND ACCOUNTABILITY ACT**

1. Right to receive Notice of Privacy Practices and notice of the uses and disclosures of protected health information (PHI) that may be made by the covered entity.
2. Right to request restrictions on use and disclosure of PHI—The health care provider is not required to agree to a restriction.
3. Right to receive confidential communication—The health care provider must accommodate reasonable requests from individuals to receive communications of PHI by alternative means or at alternative locations and cannot require a reason for the request.
4. Right to not be listed in hospital directory when admitted to hospital.
5. Right to access, inspect, and copy PHI—The health care provider can deny a request under certain conditions, and the requesting individual may appeal a denial of his or her right to access PHI.
6. Right to amend PHI—The health care provider can deny a request and must provide a timely denial in plain language and include the basis for the denial.
7. Right to receive an accounting of disclosures of PHI—Required by law.

Title IV ensures that patient health information is being properly protected and that all health plan requirements are followed. It specifies conditions for group health plans regarding coverage of persons with preexisting conditions, and modifies continuation of coverage requirements.

Title V includes provisions related to company-owned life insurance plans and treatment of individuals who lose U.S. citizenship for income tax purposes.

The **Health Information Technology for Economic and Clinical Health (HITECH) Act**, enacted as part of ARRA of 2009, became effective on February 18, 2009. The HITECH Act provides over $30 billion for health care infrastructure and the adoption and meaningful use of health information technology. According to the Act, physicians are eligible to receive up to $44,000 per physician from Medicare for "meaningful use" of a certified electronic health record (EHR) system (started in 2011). Physicians that do not adopt an EHR by 2015 will be penalized through % decreases in Medicare reimbursement rates. The Act widens the scope of privacy and security protections available under HIPAA, applies the same HIPAA privacy and security requirements (and penalties) for covered entities to business associates, increases the potential legal liability for noncompliance, and provides for more enforcement.

HIPAA Health Care Provider Requirements

- Establish formal policies regarding who has the right to access IIHI.
- Develop formal methods to safeguard the integrity, confidentiality, and availability of paper and electronic data.
- Institute a complaint process to investigate complaints.
- Provide adequate training for staff regarding HIPAA rules and regulations.
- Comply with state privacy laws, which may be even stricter.
- For employers, discipline any employee who disregards or disobeys HIPAA privacy requirements.

BOX 6-2	**HEALTH INSURANCE PORTABILITY AND ACCOUNTABILITY ACT INDIVIDUALLY IDENTIFIABLE HEALTH INFORMATION (IIHI) AND PATIENT IDENTIFIERS**

IIHI relates to (1) an individual's past, present, or future physical or mental health or condition, (2) an individual's provision of health care, and (3) past, present, or future payments provided for provision of health care to an individual; IIHI identifies the individual or is information about which there is a reasonable basis to believe that the information can be used to identify the individual.

List of 18 Patient Identifiers
1. Names
2. All geographical subdivisions smaller than a state, including street address, city, county, precinct, and ZIP code
3. All elements of dates (except year) for dates directly related to an individual, including birth date, admission date, discharge date, date of death; and all ages over 89 and all elements of dates (including year) indicative of such age, except that such ages and elements may be aggregated into a single category of age 90 or older
4. Phone numbers
5. Fax numbers
6. Electronic mail addresses
7. Social Security numbers
8. Medical record numbers
9. Health plan beneficiary numbers
10. Account numbers
11. Certificate or license numbers
12. Vehicle identifiers and serial numbers, including license plate numbers
13. Device identifiers and serial numbers
14. Web Universal Resource Locators (URLs)
15. Internet Protocol (IP) address numbers
16. Biometric identifiers, including fingerprints and voice prints
17. Full face photographic images and any comparable images
18. Any other unique identifying number, characteristic, or code (*Note:* This does not mean the unique code assigned by the investigator to code the data.)

HIPAA COMPLIANCE FOR THE HEALTH UNIT COORDINATOR

The HUC has access to a great deal of PHI and IIHI because of the very nature of the job; this information must be treated with absolute confidentiality. The HUC is required (as are all health care personnel) to sign a confidentiality agreement on initiation of employment or clinical placement.

A HUC has two responsibilities to be in HIPAA compliance and to ensure the confidentiality of patient information: (1) avoid verbally repeating confidential information, and (2) manage the patient's electronic record in a manner that ensures confidentiality of its contents, or control the patient's paper chart.

When admitted to the hospital, patients will be given a facility directory opt-out form to sign that indicates whether they wish to be listed in the hospital directory (Fig. 6-1). Hospitals have different methods of listing or labeling (e.g., name tag outside patient's room, charts) when a patient chooses not to be listed, such as "no information, no publication (NINP)," using a fictitious name, or using the nurse manager's name. Whatever method is used, no information will be provided to anyone who calls, including any statement that the patient is even in the hospital.

Protecting Patient Confidentiality

- *Do not discuss patient information* (other than what is necessary to care for the patient). All patient information is confidential. Some information, such as a patient's sexual preferences, sexually transmitted diseases, or diagnosis, is so confidential that it is obvious to treat it as such. It is important to realize that *all* information, including the patient's name, age, weight, and test results, is confidential per HIPAA regulations. Often, hospital personnel, other patients, visitors, or your own friends, relatives, or neighbors may ask you questions regarding a specific patient (especially if the patient is a celebrity) out of curiosity. Politely refuse to give out the information, and then quickly change the subject. Never discuss any patient information except when necessary for treatment reasons.

FACILITY DIRECTORY OPT OUT FORM

☐ I hereby request that my name, location, general condition, and religious affiliation NOT BE INCLUDED in the facility directory. By invoking this right, I understand that people inquiring by phone or in person will be told, "*I have no information about this patient.*" No deliveries, except U.S. Mail, will be forwarded to me (e.g., flowers).

- -

☐ I hereby request that my name, location, and general condition be released ONLY to those persons listed below. No deliveries, except U.S. Mail, will be forwarded to me (e.g., flowers). (Religious affiliation, if any, will only be provided to clergy.)

_____   _____

_____   _____

- -

☐ I hereby request that my name, location, and general condition be released to anyone EXCEPT those persons listed below. No deliveries, except U.S. Mail, will be forwarded to me (e.g., flowers). (Religious affiliation, if any, will only be provided to clergy.)

_____   _____

_____   _____

- -

☐ I hereby request that my name, location, general condition and religious affiliation BE PLACED in the facility directory.

PRINT PATIENT NAME: _____ DATE: _____

PATIENT SIGNATURE: _____ DATE: _____

WITNESS SIGNATURE: _____

Form to be forwarded or faxed to Admitting Department.

File original in permanent medical record.

Figure 6-1 Facility directory opt-out form.

- *Conduct necessary conversations with other health care personnel outside of the hearing distance of patients and visitors.* Do not hold conversations about patient information in the hallways, in the cafeteria, on the elevator, or away from the hospital. Be aware of the identity of others who are at the nurses' station during necessary discussions regarding patients. Often, overheard bits of information may be misconstrued by patients or visitors, and this could result in unnecessary concern. Even if the medical information is factual, it can produce unnecessary worry, anxiety, or even panic in a patient, family member, or visitor.
- *Do not discuss medical treatment with the patient or relatives* (unless specifically instructed to do so by the doctor or the nurse).
- *Do not discuss hospital incidents away from the nursing unit.* Discussing code arrest procedures, unexpected death, and similar information with persons other than health professionals or within hearing distance of others may instill fear in them regarding health care and is a violation of HIPAA regulations.
- *Refer all telephone calls from reporters, police personnel, legal agencies, and other investigative sources to the nurse manager or public relations department.* If in doubt about the authenticity of a telephone caller, obtain information from the caller so the call may be returned. After the caller's identity has been confirmed, the person may be called back.

Maintaining Confidentiality of the Patient's Electronic Medical Record

Access to the patient's electronic medical record (EMR) is limited. The HUC is privy to demographic protected patient information and is responsible for scanning reports, hand written progress notes, and so on.

- Be aware of who is in the nursing station looking over your shoulder.
- Be aware of who could be eavesdropping on conversations.
- Follow the hospital policy for duplication of patient documents.
- *Ask outside agency personnel for picture identification.* Reviewers for insurance companies have the responsibility of examining patient charts to ensure that tests, procedures, and hospital days will be paid for by the patients' insurance. Social workers from protective services also need to review patient charts when investigating possible abuse. It is the responsibility of outside agency personnel to show the HUC picture identification; if they fail to do this, the HUC must ask to see identification.

Maintaining Confidentiality of the Patient's Paper Chart

- *Follow the hospital policy for duplicating portions of the patient's chart.* Duplication of the patient's chart forms may be the responsibility of the HUC or the health records department of the hospital. (Read the hospital policy and procedures manual to determine policy regarding copying a patient's chart.) Never copy a record for a patient's friend or family member.
- *Control access to the patient's chart.* Only authorized persons, such as doctors and hospital personnel, should have access to the chart. Always know the status of the person who is using the chart at the nurses' station. Do not give a chart to someone on request because they "look like a doctor." Should relatives or friends of a patient request to see the chart, do not give it to them under any circumstance. If a patient requests to see his or her chart, advise the patient that you will notify the nurse and/or doctor. A patient has a legal right to see his or her own chart, but the doctor may need to write an order, and the doctor or the nurse will go over the information in the chart with the patient.
- *Ask outside agency personnel for picture identification* as described when EMR is implemented. *Control transportation of the patient's chart.* Never send the patient's chart to another department through the pneumatic tube system. Do not give patients their charts to hold while they are being transported from one area of the hospital to another.

WORKPLACE APPEARANCE

Professional appearance will earn the trust, respect, and confidence of one's employer, co-workers, patients, and others. A professional appearance also demonstrates **confidence** and sends a message that one has self-respect and respects his or her position. Hospitals have a dress code that is usually outlined in the orientation packet that employees receive when hired. Employees represent the facility for which they work; patients and visitors gain their first impressions of a facility through the appearance of its employees (Fig. 6-2).

Guidelines for Workplace Appearance
Women

- Clothes or uniforms should fit well, should be modest in length and style, and above all should be clean, mended, and wrinkle free. Color and design of undergarments should not be visible through one's clothes or uniform. When business dress is called for, slacks or skirts are appropriate with a blouse or sweater. Denim is usually not acceptable.
- Socks or stockings should be worn, especially with a skirt or dress.
- Sculptured nails and nail polish are not acceptable for health care workers. Sculptured nails and chipped nail polish provide a place for microorganisms to grow.
- Makeup should be modest in amount and color.
- Perfumes, colognes, and hair spray should be applied very lightly or not worn at all.

Men

- Slacks and shirt or sweater should fit well, and they should be clean and pressed.
- Socks should be worn.
- Aftershave, colognes, and hair spray should be applied very lightly or not worn at all.

Women and Men

- Shoes should be clean and appropriate, as defined in the dress code. Most facilities do not allow open-toed or open-heeled shoes. Most nursing personnel wear white tennis shoes (not high-tops) for comfort.

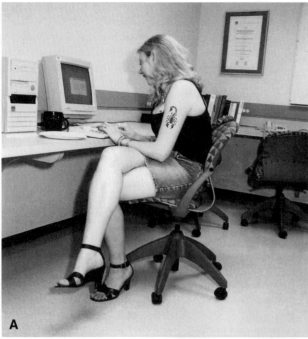

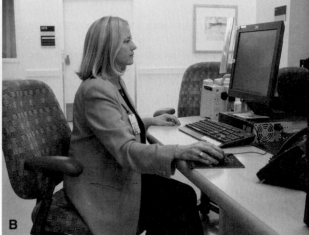

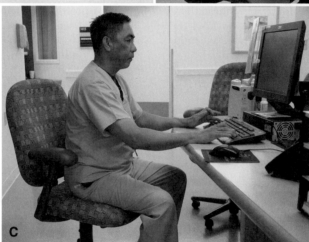

Figure 6-2 A, This health unit coordinator (HUC) is inappropriately dressed. **B,** This HUC is appropriately dressed in business attire. **C,** This HUC is appropriately dressed in scrubs.

- Jewelry worn should be modest. Body piercing may or may not be acceptable in your chosen place of employment. Some earrings will interfere with talking on the telephone. Good taste is the key.
- Tattoos may or may not be acceptable in your chosen place of employment. Many hospital dress codes require that tattoos be covered.
- Hair should be clean and well groomed. Control long hair to keep it out of your face and off of the collar.

★ HIGH PRIORITY

Patients with respiratory problems, allergies, or nausea could experience ill effects from perfumes, colognes, aftershave, or hairspray.

EMPLOYMENT ISSUES

Preclinical or Preemployment Prerequisites, Screenings, and In-Services Required by The Joint Commission/Health Care Facility

Drug Testing

Drug testing is more stringent for health care professionals. Most hospitals require students and new employees to have a urine drug test before starting a clinical experience or employment. Notify the testing agency if you are taking any prescribed medication for pain or sleep that may be detected on the drug screen. Do not drink an excessive amount of water before the urine drug test because when the urine is diluted, you may need to repeat the test at your expense. An employer will likely require a physical assessment and another drug test before hire, and many perform random drug tests after hire.

Recently, the metabolites of nicotine (tobacco) are included in the pre-employment/pre-clinical drug test if the facility is a "non-smoking" one.

Fingerprinting and Background Check

Most health care agencies require a fingerprinting card and a background check before a clinical experience and/or employment. Always be honest about any convictions, because any past convictions will be discovered in the background check, and not disclosing would be viewed as dishonest. If there is a problem in one's background, one may add to the application, "Will discuss during the interview."

Immunizations

Immunizations and screenings are required before a clinical experience or employment; these usually include MMR (measles, mumps, and rubella), tuberculosis (TB) skin tests or blood test, tetanus and diphtheria, varicella, and a hepatitis screen.

If you have a positive TB skin test result, a chest x-ray examination will be required. If a patient tests positive for TB, all employees working on that unit will be required to have a TB skin test.

Signed HIPAA Confidentiality Statement

In compliance with the HIPAA laws, all health care students and employees are required to sign a confidentiality statement before beginning a clinical experience or employment. By signing this statement, the student or employee agrees not to discuss or review any information regarding a patient unless the discussion or review is part of the assignment. Students or employees also state that they understand that they are obligated to know and adhere to the privacy policies and procedures of the health care facility. Signing the confidentiality statement is an acknowledgment that medical records, accounting information, patient information, and conversations between or among health care professionals about patients are confidential under law and this agreement.

Before a clinical experience or employment, The Joint Commission (TJC) requires the following;

- Certification in **cardiopulmonary resuscitation (CPR)**
- Fire and safety in-service
- Infectious disease in-service
- HIPAA in-service

Health care facilities provide classes, handouts, or videos with posttests for the in-services.

Drug Test for Cause

If an odor of alcohol (a drug) is detected on a student's or employee's breath, or if inappropriate behavior is observed, a drug test may be requested by the supervisor or the instructor. If the student or employee refuses the drug test or tests positive for drug use, she or he will be sent home and most likely will be terminated from the HUC program or employment.

Cell Phone Use

Almost everyone owns a cell phone, and some people find it difficult to be without their cell phone. We have all encountered the rudeness of people talking loudly or texting on their cell phones while standing in the middle of the walkway at the mall, blocking doorways, in cubicles in restrooms, or in restaurants while others are trying to have a quiet meal or who are talking or texting while driving—which is dangerous and illegal in many places. Cell phones are heard ringing in hospitals, in movie theaters, in school classes, on airplanes, and even at funerals. Some often forget about others' personal space and boundaries. Cell phones are banned for personal use on most hospital units, and some hospitals do not allow clinical students to bring a cell phone to the unit. Ringing cell phones and conversations are annoying and distracting to nursing unit personnel, as well as to patients in nearby rooms.

Personal cell phones should be turned off while one is working on the nursing unit. Calls recorded on voice mail may be listened to during breaks. If an important call is expected, phones may be placed on vibrate and the call taken off of the nursing unit. Text messaging is also banned while one is working on the nursing unit. Full attention is expected and should be given to your work responsibilities.

General Guidelines for Using a Cell Phone

- Respect people in close proximity (speak more softly, turn cell phone off when appropriate to do so, and pay attention to your surroundings).
- When in a public place, keep conversations brief. Remember you are a professional.
- When out to dinner, spend time with who you are with, not with a phone.
- Follow rules for cell phone use in hospitals, schools, and airplanes and while pumping gas.
- Do not drive while using a cell phone.

Elevator Etiquette

Hospital elevators are very busy places. It is important to know appropriate elevator etiquette, especially in hospitals.

- When the elevator button light is lit, it is not necessary to continue to push the button; this may be causing the door to close on someone on another floor who is trying to enter or exit the elevator.
- When the elevator does arrive, stand aside and allow people to exit before you try to enter.
- When you are riding on an elevator and are going to a high floor in the building, stand to the side or in the back, so others may exit on their floors.
- Patients who are being transported on stretchers and personnel who are pushing hospital equipment have priority for using elevators.

Attendance, Punctuality, and Appropriate Breaks

Guidelines regarding attendance, punctuality, and breaks are usually provided by the employer in an employment packet during orientation. It is essential that nursing unit personnel work as a team and that each member of the team be reliable and act in a responsible, professional manner. When a student is completing a clinical experience on a nursing unit, this should be viewed as an extended evaluation or appraisal period. A student's preceptor and the other nursing unit personnel will be continually appraising the student's knowledge, attendance, punctuality, and professionalism. Often a facility will hire a HUC student before the end of the required clinical hours.

Smoking

Many hospitals have become "non-smoking" facilities and do not allow cigarette use at any location on the hospital campus. Cigarette use may be part of the consideration for employment, and currently smokers are not part of a legally "protected class." Many hospitals offer tobacco cessation opportunities for their current employees who do smoke. The use of tobacco for the clinical student may be problematic.

> ★ **HIGH PRIORITY**
>
> The clinical experience can also be used by the health unit coordinating student to evaluate the health care facility and nursing units to make an employment decision.

Sexual Harassment

Sexual harassment is defined as unwanted and unwelcome behavior that is sexual in nature. There are two forms of sexual harassment: (1) *quid pro quo*, which involves making conditions of employment (e.g., hiring, promotion, retention) contingent on the victim's providing sexual favors, and (2) a **hostile working environment,** which is an environment that a reasonable person would find hostile and abusive.

Victims of harassment may feel intimidated, anxious, angry, ashamed, and/or helpless. Often, sexual harassment is not reported because the victim believes "no action would be taken" against the perpetrator, fears **retaliation,** or has concern for the abuser.

If feeling harassed, health care workers should (1) tell the person to stop and say that they do not like or welcome the behavior, (2) document the comments and behavior of the person, and (3) file a complaint with the supervisor or with management.

Violence in the Workplace

Violence has increased in our society and in the workplace—perhaps because of unemployment, loss of insurance, economic difficulties, political and social differences, and other issues. Workplace violence may be defined as violent acts (including physical assaults and threats of assault) directed toward persons at work or on duty. Physical assaults include attacks ranging from slapping and beating to the use of weapons. Threats are expressions of intent to cause harm; these include verbal threats, threatening body language, and written threats.

When a patient is admitted to the hospital as a victim of gang-related or domestic violence, a restraining order is often put in place to prohibit individuals responsible for the violence from having any contact with the patient. Often, the patient has an NINP order written on the chart. This would require the HUC or anyone who answers the phone to deny any information about that patient, including the patient's presence in the hospital. The patient's name would not be listed on the census board, would not be posted outside the room, and would not be written on the outside of the chart. Usually an alias would be used to avoid visitor suspicion. A code word or phrase is given to the patient's family so the health care worker can know that a person is authorized to visit the patient. All telephone calls from reporters, police personnel, legal agencies, and other investigative sources should be referred to the nurse manager.

The HUC is able to see most of what is happening on the nursing unit from his or her location at the nurses' station. The HUC must be alert to signals that may be associated with impending violence.

Signals of impending violence may include the following:

- Verbally expressed anger and frustration
- Body language such as threatening gestures
- Signs of drug or alcohol use
- Presence of a weapon
- The presence of someone who has a restraining order that prohibits him or her from being there

The HUC should not approach the threatening person but should present a calm attitude and should call security immediately.

Agencies that Investigate Abuse

All states have mandatory reporting laws for suspected child or elder abuse. Some states have mandatory reporting laws for domestic abuse. Child Protective Services (CPS) will be called to investigate suspected child abuse (SNAT, suspected nonaccidental trauma). Adult Protective Services (APS) will be called in to investigate elder or domestic abuse. Social workers from these agencies must show picture identification to the HUC before looking at a patient's chart. If the social worker fails to do this, it is the responsibility of the HUC to ask for identification. It is important to keep this information strictly confidential and to remain nonjudgmental when interacting with family members.

Employee Performance Evaluations

After an employee has been hired, during and after training they must be evaluated. The performance evaluation (also called a *performance appraisal*) is the ongoing process of evaluating the employee's job performance. This process should provide both positive feedback and suggestions on how to improve in areas where improvement is needed. The basic purposes of the evaluation process are to provide feedback and to make compensation decisions (concerning salary increases). Keeping a written record of accomplishments, classes taken, and in-services attended during the evaluation period would be mutually beneficial to the individual (HUC) being evaluated as well as the evaluator (nurse manager). Often employee evaluations are based only on the most recent work history; keeping a record or diary will produce a more accurate work history.

Often supervisors ask their employees to complete an evaluation form to assess their own performance. This provides an opportunity for you to let your supervisors know how valuable you are to the organization. Do not be modest, but do be honest regarding your contributions and accomplishments. Performance evaluations are placed in the employee's file.

JOB APPLICATIONS, RÉSUMÉS, AND INTERVIEWS

Completing a Job Application

Before completing a job application, assemble information and make a fact sheet, or have your résumé available so it can be used as a reference. Most hospitals have a website and accept applications online. It is important to enter accurate information, including correct dates. Have a list of work-related references (check with references to make sure they are comfortable with being called) with you in case you are asked to provide them.

⭐ **HIGH PRIORITY**

Many employers check social networks to screen job candidates. When applying for a position, be mindful of what you post on social networks.

Guidelines for Completing a Job Application

- Follow directions carefully.
- Be neat, and be sure of dates and spelling.
- When there are gaps in employment, explain (e.g., "raising children," "returned to school"). If you were doing anything for pay during this time, write "self-employed."
- When stating a reason for leaving your last job, make it sound positive (e.g., "returned to school," "decided on a career change").
- If you have little work experience, emphasize other strengths. List volunteer jobs.
- List the most recent work or educational experience first, not last.
- When asked the pay that you desire, do not identify a specific amount. It is often best to write "open" or "negotiable."
- If you did not graduate, write "attended" and list the institutions.
- Be honest; deliberately skipping a question is dishonest

Spaces left blank may cause concern. Be honest regarding any misdemeanor or felony convictions. Write, "Will discuss in interview." If a discrepancy is discovered, this will most likely result in your not being granted a job interview.

Writing a Résumé

The purpose of a résumé is to get an interview; it is hoped that the interview will result in your getting a job. The résumé is a marketing tool intended to create interest in one's abilities and potential. A résumé does its job successfully if it does not exclude one from consideration. Read time for a résumé (time spent by human resources when deciding whether or not to interview) is about 10 seconds. A good résumé should be short, simple, and easy to read while gaining the reader's interest and revealing your value to the potential employer. Before writing a résumé, take time to do a self-assessment on paper. Outline skills and abilities, as well as work experiences and extracurricular activities. This will make it easier for you to prepare a thorough résumé. A résumé may be dropped off (dress appropriately in case there is an interview), faxed, or scanned and e-mailed.

Guidelines for Creating a Résumé

Follow these guidelines when creating a résumé:

- Type using a simple font such as Times New Roman, 12 point (avoid using fancy effects such as outline, shadow, script, or other difficult to read styles).
- Use standard 8½ × 11–inch paper in white, ivory, or gray (avoid flashy colors).
- Keep a 1-inch margin on all four sides.
- Limit résumé to one page, if possible.
- Use single space within sections.
- Use double space between sections.
- Bold, underline, or capitalize section headings to make them stand out.
- Use everyday language; be specific. Give examples.
- Do a spelling and grammar check.
- Produce good-quality photocopies.

A résumé should include the following:

- Name, address, telephone number, e-mail address, website address.
- Objective. Be specific about the job wanted—for example, "To obtain a HUC position within a health care facility to apply my organizational skills and medical knowledge."
- Education. New graduates without a lot of work experience should list their educational information first. List the most recent education first; include the grade point average (GPA) if higher than 3.0.
- List National Association of Health Unit Coordinators (NAHUC) certification, if applicable.
- Work experience. Briefly describe work experience, including specific duties performed. List most recent work experience first. Be accurate with dates of employment.
- Other information. This may include special skills or competencies, such as being bilingual or having leadership experience in volunteer organizations. Your instructor can advise you on other information to add to your résumé.
- "References furnished on request." Ask people if they are willing to serve as references before giving their names to a potential employer. Do not include reference information on your résumé.

Preparing for an Interview

Interviews may be conducted in person or over the telephone. Either type of interview can be very stressful. Take three deep breaths to relax before starting an interview. Think positively about your skills and abilities, and do some positive imagery; imagine *you* working in the position. First impressions are lasting ones. During a telephone interview, be sure to speak clearly and with confidence. For an in-person interview, make sure your appearance and posture demonstrate professionalism. Do not give the interviewer a reason to rule you out because you did not take the time to do your best.

Guidelines for Successful Interviews

For an in-person interview:

- Arrive on time (at least one-half hour early).
- Stand until you are asked to sit down.
- Make eye contact with interviewer.

- Give a firm handshake.
- Use body language to show interest: smile, nod, and give nonverbal feedback to the interviewer.

For a telephone interview:

- Be ready to answer the phone or to call in. Employers usually call candidates, but employers may ask a candidate to call them to test how serious the candidate is.
- If expecting a phone call from an employer, be sure that the answering message on your telephone is appropriate and understandable.
- Stand during the telephone interview. This allows one's voice to project and sound more confident.
- Choose a location and time so that there will be no distractions.
- Relax and speak clearly and slowly. Do not sound rushed or anxious (the HUC position requires excellent telephone skills).

For both in-person and telephone interviews:

- Think in advance of work situations and how you would handle them (see review question 11 for examples).
- Role-play: rehearse responses to difficult or uncomfortable issues that may come up.
- Project a positive attitude and confidence.
- Listen attentively to questions.
- Keep answers brief and to the point.
- Never criticize a former employer.
- Be prepared to give a positive summary of your education, work history, and interests.
- Be aware of the job description for the position for which you are applying.
- Ask questions. Avoid yes-or-no answers. Avoid long silences.
- Ask about the next step in the process.
- Thank the interviewer.
- Write a thank-you letter to anyone to whom you have spoken.
- Follow up with a telephone call if you do not hear back from the interviewer in 3 days.

★ HIGH PRIORITY

The interviewer is seeking to fill the open position with a person who is confident that he or she is prepared for and can do the job. Confidence comes with knowledge. One should prepare for the desired career by completing the required education and, if possible, additional job-related education.

HEALTH CARE ETHICS

Ethics is that part of **philosophy** that deals with judgments about what is right or wrong in given situations. Each health care profession has a **code of ethics** that has been derived from a set of basic **principles** that define the concepts of right or wrong for that profession. NAHUC has an established code of ethics (Box 6-3, *National Association of Health Unit Coordinators Code of Ethics*).

BOX 6-3	**NATIONAL ASSOCIATION OF HEALTH UNIT COORDINATORS CODE OF ETHICS**

1. Members shall conduct themselves in such a manner as to gain the respect and confidence of patients, health care personnel, and the community and shall respect the human dignity of each individual.
2. Members shall protect patients' rights, including their right to privacy.
3. Members shall strive to achieve and maintain a high level of competency.
4. Members shall strive to improve their knowledge and skills by participating in educational and professional activities and sharing the benefits of their attainments with their colleagues.
5. Unethical and illegal professional activities shall be reported to the appropriate authorities.

Patient Care Partnership and Patients' Bill of Rights

The American Hospital Association (AHA) approved the first patients' bill of rights in 1973. The expectation was that observance of these rights would result in more effective patient care and greater satisfaction for the patient, the patient's physician, and the health care organization. The AHA has since published *The Patient Care Partnership*, which includes "Understanding Expectations and Rights and Responsibilities." In summary, patient expectations and rights include high-quality hospital care, a clean and safe environment, involvement in care, protection of privacy, help when leaving the hospital, and help with billing claims. The patients' bill of rights has been adopted and modified many times. In 1998, an Advisory Commission on Consumer Protection and Quality in the Health Care Industry appointed by the President of the United States issued a Patients' Bill of Rights (see the box, *Patients' Rights as Outlined in the Health Insurance Portability and Accountability Act*). TJC now requires that all hospitals have a bill of rights and a notice of the facility's privacy practices. Copies must be given to each patient or parent of the patient on admission. In addition, a copy of the bill of rights should be posted at entrances and in other prominent places throughout the hospital. The patients' bill of rights varies in wording among hospitals, but all are based on the basic ethical principles discussed in the following sections.

Ethical Principles for Patient Care
Respect

The principle of respect declares that the patient has the right to considerate and respectful care. *Respect* means to hold in esteem or honor and to show a feeling of appreciation and regard. Health care workers must provide services with respect for human dignity and the uniqueness of each patient, unrestricted by considerations of social or economic status, personal attributes, or the nature of health problems.

Autonomy

The principle of autonomy means that an individual is free to choose and implement his or her own decisions. From this basic principle, we have derived the rule involved in **informed consent**.

The patients' bill of rights states that a patient has the right to refuse treatment to the extent permitted by law and to be informed of the medical consequences of that choice. This right does not judge the quality of a decision by a patient to refuse treatment; it states only that the patient has the right to make the decision. This is the process of **autonomy** at work.

Veracity

The principle of veracity requires both the health care professional and the patient to tell the truth. The health care professional must disclose the truth so the patient can practice autonomy; the patient must be truthful so that appropriate care can be given. Although in some situations health care professionals may feel justified in lying to a patient to avoid some greater harm, other alternatives must be sought. Lying will almost always harm patient autonomy and cause the potential loss of credibility of the provider.

Beneficence

Beneficence is the principle that any action a health care professional takes should benefit the patient. This principle creates an ethical dilemma for clinical practitioners more than it does for HUCs. The dilemma arises because of the advanced technology that is available to practitioners today. In cases in which a patient is maintained on life support machines and is in a coma or a vegetative state, is it of benefit to maintain the patient on the machines?

Nonmaleficence

The principle of nonmaleficence, which comes from the Hippocratic oath, means that a health care professional will never inflict harm on the patient. Although similar to the principle of beneficence, it differs in that beneficence indicates a positive action promoting good. In nonmaleficence, the principle is to refrain from inflicting harm. HUCs should always be aware of the seriousness of transcribing doctors' orders because an error may result in harm to the patient.

Role Fidelity

Health care is a team effort, as no single individual can be solely responsible for providing all of a patient's health care needs. There are currently 100 specialties under the heading of allied health. Practitioners have a duty to understand the limits of their role and practice with **fidelity.** As an example, because of differences in role duty, an allied health professional might be ethically obliged not to tell a patient or a patient's family how critical the situation is, instead having the attending physician do so.

Confidentiality

Principle 2 of the NAHUC Code of Ethics and the AHA's Patients' Bill of Rights outline the individual's right to privacy in health care. HUCs that breach the **confidentiality** of a patient's medical record have not only violated ethical standards but may well have violated the law (Box 6-4, *Consumer Bill of Rights and Responsibilities*).

Interconnection between Ethical and Legal Issues

Ethical issues and legal issues often become intertwined in the health care context. An ethical dilemma is a situation that presents a conflicting moral claim—a situation that is at odds with one's personal system of values. Sometimes conflicts can occur between what is legal and what is ethical. For example, assume you are working in a gynecology clinic and a patient comes in for an abortion. You may believe that abortions should not be performed and are unethical. However, abortions are legal in our country.

To deal with these situations as a HUC, you must learn to examine your values and be aware of how they affect your work. All health care professionals must learn methods of reasoning through ethical dilemmas rather than reacting to them emotionally. Issues that may arise and cause conflict are usually situations involving the privacy rights of patients or the unprofessional conduct of a fellow health care worker.

In any of the potential problem areas you may encounter as a HUC, you must apply good judgment, honesty, and reasoning to come up with a moral and ethical way to resolve the conflict.

LEGAL CONCEPTS

The law is derived from three sources: (1) the constitution—both federal and state constitutions: (2) **statutes**—written laws drawn up by the legislature: and (3) common law—a case-by-case determination by a judge of what is fair under a given set of facts. Laws are subject to change, but common law is especially changeable because each case presented to a judge is different. Judges look to cases that have been decided previously for guidance on how to rule in a particular situation. However, a judge is free to interpret the law in cases where no precedent exists, or to interpret against precedent. Most medical **negligence** or **medical malpractice** law is derived from common law. This means that medical negligence law, similar to other forms of common law, is constantly in a state of change. When a patient brings a medical practice lawsuit against a medical facility and/or personnel, the patient is known as the *plaintiff* and the medical facility and/or personnel would be known as the *defendant.* The attorneys will take a **deposition** under oath from all employees or witnesses involved in the incident or in the patient's care. The **statute of limitations** for bringing a medical malpractice lawsuit varies from state to state.

Standard of Practice for the Health Unit Coordinator

While working as a HUC, one is responsible for performing at the level of competence of other HUCs who work under similar circumstances. This responsibility is one's legal duty as a health care professional and is the standard of practice to which this professional will be held. If one does not carry out this duty and a patient is injured as a result, the HUC may have been negligent of his or her duty and may be held liable for these actions (Box 6-5, *Standards of Practice for the Health Unit Coordinator*). The Standard of Practice may be used much like the Scope of Practice is for licensed health care personnel in delineating what tasks can and cannot be performed.

The standard of practice is established by **expert witness** testimony. For our purposes, an expert is a person who is trained in the HUC profession and who testifies at trial as to what a reasonably prudent HUC would have done under the circumstances in question. **Evidence** of the **standard of care**

BOX 6-4 **CONSUMER BILL OF RIGHTS AND RESPONSIBILITIES**

I Information Disclosure
Consumers have the right to receive accurate, easily understood information, and some require assistance in making informed health care decisions about their health plans, professionals, and facilities.

II Choice of Providers and Plans
Consumers have the right to a choice of health care providers that is sufficient to ensure access to appropriate high-quality health care.

III Access to Emergency Services
Consumers have the right to access emergency health care services when and where the need arises. Health plans should provide payment when a consumer visits an emergency department with acute symptoms of sufficient severity—including severe pain—that a "prudent layperson" could reasonably expect the absence of medical attention to result in placing that consumer's health in serious jeopardy, serious impairment to bodily functions, or serious dysfunction of any bodily organ or part.

IV Participation in Treatment Decisions
Consumers have the right and responsibility to fully participate in all decisions related to their health care. Consumers who are unable to fully participate in treatment decisions have the right to be represented by parents, guardians, family members, or other conservators.

V Respect and Nondiscrimination
Consumers have the right to considerate, respectful care from all members of the health care system at all times and under all circumstances. An environment of mutual respect is essential to maintain a high-quality health care system.

VI Confidentiality of Health Information
Consumers have the right to communicate with health care providers in confidence and to have the confidentiality of their individually identifiable health care information protected. Consumers also have the right to review and copy their own medical records and request amendments to their records.

VII Complaints and Appeals
All consumers have the right to a fair and efficient process for resolving differences with their health plans, health care providers, and the institutions that serve them, including a rigorous system of internal review and an independent system of external review.

VIII Consumer Responsibilities
In a health care system that protects consumers' rights, it is reasonable to expect and encourage consumers to assume reasonable responsibilities. Greater individual involvement by consumers in their care increases the likelihood of achieving the best outcomes and helps support a quality improvement, cost-conscious environment. Take responsibility for maximizing healthy habits, such as exercising, not smoking, and eating a healthy diet.

A summary of the eight areas of consumer rights and responsibilities adopted by the President's Advisory Commission on Consumer Protection and Quality in the Health Care Industry. Last update: July 1998. Available at: www.hcqualitycommission.gov

---

BOX 6-5 **STANDARDS OF PRACTICE FOR THE HEALTH UNIT COORDINATOR (HUC)**

Standard 1: Education
HUC personnel shall be prepared through appropriate education and training programs for their responsibility in the provision of nondirect patient care and nonclinical services.

Standard 2: Policies and Procedures
Written standards of HUCs' practice and related policies and procedures shall define and describe the scope and conduct of nonclinical services provided by the HUC. These standards, policies, and procedures shall be reviewed annually and revised as necessary. These revisions will be dated to indicate the last review, will be signed by the responsible authority, and will be implemented.

Standard 3: Standards of Performance
Written evaluation of HUCs shall be criteria based and related to the standards of performance as defined by the health care organization.

Standard 4: Communication
The HUC shall appropriately and effectively communicate with nursing and medical staff, all ancillary departments, visitors, guests, and patients.

Standard 5: Professionalism and Ethics
The HUC shall take all possible measures to ensure the optimal quality of nondirect, nonclinical patient care. Optimal professional and ethical conduct and practice of members of the National Association of Health Unit Coordinators shall be maintained at all times.

Standard 6: Leadership
The HUC shall be organized to meet and maintain established standards of nonclinical services.

may also be found in textbooks, standards from NAHUC, policy and procedures manuals, or standards of TJC. This means that one must keep up with current practices in the profession, read current literature, be familiar with hospital policies and procedures that affect the HUC job, and know the current job description and the duties it details.

The standard of care for which the HUC is responsible becomes higher with increased experience and education. The actions of a HUC will be compared with those of a reasonably prudent HUC with the same experience and education under the same circumstances.

The role of the HUC has expanded broadly over the past 5 years. You are now recognized as an essential member of the health care team. Incidental to this greater recognition and expanding responsibility is an increased accountability. There is a **liability** dimension to accountability. The HUC may be held legally responsible for judgments made and actions taken in the course of practice.

MEDICAL MALPRACTICE

Medical malpractice is the professional negligence of a health care professional; the failure to meet a professional standard of care, resulting in harm to another; or the failure to provide, for example, "good and accepted medical care." According to the National Academy of Sciences, approximately 98,000 Americans die from "medical mistakes" each year. Each member of the nursing team is responsible for his or her actions. If the HUC is not sure about what the doctor has written because the handwriting is illegible, the doctor's orders must be clarified before they are transcribed. It may be necessary to call the doctor for clarification.

Negligence

Negligence is a legal term that means that someone failed to perform a legal duty satisfactorily, and another person was injured in some way because of that failure. This breach of duty is said to have occurred when something was done that should not have been done, or when something should have been done but was not. Either way, the person responsible for the duty is liable for whatever injury was sustained by the innocent party. For instance, one of the duties of a HUC is to transcribe doctors' orders accurately and promptly. If negligent in doing so—that is, if the orders are not transcribed properly or are not transcribed at all—the HUC may be responsible for a patient's injury that results from negligence.

Liability

Legally, each person is responsible for his or her own acts. When those acts are negligent and are performed during the course and scope of employment as a HUC, they have special ramifications.

The hospital is also liable for an employee's negligence on the job because of the legal doctrine *respondeat superior* (which means "let the master respond"). This means that the employee and the hospital are held responsible for negligent acts of employees while on the job. Remember that the hospital is liable for the employee's actions only when they occur within the course and scope of employment. If the negligent act is a result of conduct outside the scope of employment (i.e., outside of the job description), the employee alone is held responsible.

The *respondeat superior* doctrine does not take away one's personal liability but rather creates an additional party for the injured person to hold responsible for the **damages** incurred.

LEGAL DOCUMENTS

A patient's EMR or chart contains permanent legal documents. All handwritten documents (such as consent forms) are written in ink or are printed from computer, and no erasures are allowed. Because the patient's medical forms and EMR are legal records of the patient's medical course, the HUC must treat them with special care and confidentiality. Only authorized persons may have access to a patient's EMR or chart. This protection of the legal record is part of one's duty as a HUC.

Informed Consent

An informed consent documents that the person signing it has been informed of the risks and characteristics of a planned procedure and understands them. The witness of the signing of the consent by the patient or guardian must date and sign the consent. Telephone consents require that two health care personnel listen to the verbal consent given via the telephone and that those personnel sign as witnesses. Preparation of informed consents and other types of consents is discussed in Chapter 8.

WHAT THE HEALTH UNIT COORDINATOR CAN DO TO AVOID LEGAL PROBLEMS

Following are some tips to help one avoid legal problems while working as a HUC:

- *Know the HUC job description.* Do not engage in activities outside the job description.
- *Keep current with the facility's policies and procedures.* If the policies and procedures are outdated, bring them to the employer's attention and participate in the revisions.
- *Keep current in the HUC practice.* If called on to do something that you are not qualified to do, get help and find out how to do it. Remember, a standard of care can be set by medical literature and periodicals. Continued education is a must for all health care workers. Of course, obtain proper training before assuming any professional position.
- *Do not assume anything.* Question orders, policies, and procedures that do not seem appropriate. Do not do something unless you are sure you know how to do it. The biggest safeguard is to ask questions.
- *Do not perform nursing tasks, even as favors.*
- *Be aware of relationships with patients.* Patients who truly feel that you care and have tried to help them to the best of your abilities are less likely to see a lawyer if a problem arises.

KEY CONCEPTS

The modern health care professional is called on to display professional behavior and judgment in many complex situations. By understanding confidentiality, legal duty, and ethical responsibility, one will be able to legally and morally fulfill his or her professional obligations.

Websites of Interest

Department of Health and Human Services (HHS): www.hhs.gov
HIPAA 101 Guide to Compliance Rules and Laws: www.hipaa-101.com
World Privacy Forum: www.worldprivacyforum.org/whatsnew
UNT Libraries Government Information Connection: www.library.unt.edu/govinfo
The Joint Commission: www.jointcommission.org

REVIEW QUESTIONS

Visit the Evolve website to download and complete the following questions.

1. Match the term from those listed below with the definition:
   accountability
   attitude
   autonomy
   confidence
   code of ethics
   confidentiality
   philosophy
   ethics
   fidelity
   respect
   workplace behavior
   a. a manner of thought or feeling expressed in a person's behavior
   b. state of functioning independently; personal liberty
   c. a pattern of actions and interactions of an individual that directly or indirectly affects his or herr effectiveness while at work; the attitude and amount of enthusiasm that one brings to the job
   d. taking responsibility for one's actions; being answerable to someone for something one has done
   e. a system of moral principles (beliefs) that determine how we make judgments with regard to right and wrong
   f. reliability, trustworthiness, dependability, doing what one promises
   g. a set of rules and procedures for professional conduct based on the values and ethical standards of an organization or profession
   h. belief in oneself and one's abilities; self-confidence, self-reliance, self-assurance; usually comes with knowledge
   i. the legally protected right afforded to all patients of having personal and medical information (written or spoken) protected
   j. holding a person in esteem or honor; having appreciation and regard for another
   k. guiding or underlying principles; attitude toward life

2. Match the legal term from those listed below with the definition:
   damages
   defendant
   deposition
   expert witness
   liability
   negligence
   plaintiff
   statute
   statute of limitations
   a. a person who has special knowledge of the subject about which he or she is to testify; this knowledge must generally be such as is not normally possessed by the average person
   b. condition of being responsible for damages resulting from an injurious act or from discharging an obligation or debt
   c. monetary compensation awarded by a court for an injury caused by the act of another
   d. the person against whom a civil or criminal action is brought
   e. time within which a plaintiff must bring a civil suit; this limit varies with the type of suit and is set by the various state legislatures
   f. pretrial statement of a witness under oath, taken in question-and-answer form, as it would be in court, with opportunity given to the adversary to be present to cross-examine
   g. failure to satisfactorily perform one's legal duty, such that another person incurs some injury
   h. person who brings a lawsuit against another
   i. law passed by the legislature and signed by the governor at the state level and the president at the federal level

3. List seven factors that may influence a worker's behavior.

4. Define "personal values," and describe a situation in which an HUC's personal values could influence her or his interactions on the job.

5. List six behavior traits that make up one's work ethic.

6. Explain the purposes of the Privacy Rule and the Security Rule contained in the Health Insurance Portability and Accountability Act (HIPAA).

7. Explain two purposes of the HITECH Act.

8. Identify seven individually identifiable health information (IIHI) identifiers.

9. List six patient rights as outlined in HIPAA.

10. Explain two main responsibilities of the HUC to achieve HIPAA compliance.

11. Describe how you as the HUC may practice confidentiality in the following situations.
    a. You are having dinner in the cafeteria with several other health care workers. A famous television star was admitted to your unit yesterday. The talk turns to the patient. You are asked, "Is she really only 35?" "Why was she admitted?" and other personal questions. What would be your response?
    b. You are working at the nurses' station and you notice a patient's wife approaching your desk. At the

same time, two other members of the hospital staff, unaware of the wife's presence, begin talking about her husband's condition. What would you do?

c. A visitor is standing at the nurses' station and is obviously listening to two doctors discuss a patient's condition. You notice that this is what is happening. What do you do?

d. A telephone caller says that he is a reporter from the local newspaper and wants to know if a car accident victim was admitted to your nursing unit. What do you tell him?

e. You answer the telephone on the nursing unit. The caller states that he is a relative of the patient and then asks for personal patient information. The patient is hospitalized for a gunshot wound received during a fight and has "NINP" written in his chart. You are somewhat doubtful about the identity of the caller. How do you handle the situation?

f. You are riding home on the bus after work. Another hospital employee sits down beside you and states, "That was quite a code you had on your unit today. Was that Mr. Perez that was transferred from ICU the other day?" How do you respond?

g. You notice a girl that you don't recognize standing behind a nurse watching while a nurse is entering information into a patient's EMR. What do you do?

12. Explain the importance of professional appearance.

13. List four preclinical or preemployment screenings or requirements and four TJC requirements.

14. a. Explain why a supervisor or clinical instructor would require a drug test for cause.
b. What would the consequences be if a clinical student refused the test or tested positive for drugs?

15. Discuss five guidelines for cell phone use and four rules of elevator etiquette to adhere to when in the hospital setting.

16. Explain where guidelines regarding attendance, punctuality, and breaks would be found, and discuss the importance of employees and potential employees knowing and following those guidelines.

17. Describe five signs of impending violence.

18. Explain what action the HUC should take when recognizing signs or an act of violence.

19. Discuss three steps to take when encountering sexual harassment.

20. Discuss two purposes of an employee performance evaluation.

21. Discuss the benefits of collecting information and writing out a fact sheet for reference before completing a job application or writing a résumé.

22. Discuss the purpose of a résumé, and list 10 guidelines to follow and items to include when writing a résumé.

23. Explain how one would prepare for an in-person and for a phone interview.

24. The Patients' Bill of Rights and health care professionals' codes of ethics are based on seven ethical principles. List them.

25. List three sources from which laws are derived.

26. Define *malpractice* and describe how standard of care is determined.

27. Identify six preventive measures that you as a HUC can take to minimize the risk of malpractice within the HUC practice.

28. Make a list of what is inappropriate in terms of the appearance of the HUC pictured in Figure 6-2, *A.*

SURFING FOR ANSWERS

1. Search the Internet, find and list three advantages and three disadvantages of HIPAA, and document at least two websites used.
2. Search for qualifications and job descriptions for both a "health unit coordinator" and a "health unit secretary" in your area. Print at least three of each, and document the websites used.
3. Find a current article involving a malpractice lawsuit, and discuss ways the incident could have been prevented by the health care providers.

CHAPTER 7

Management Techniques and Problem-Solving Skills for Health Unit Coordinating

CHAPTER OBJECTIVES

On completion of this chapter, you will be able to:

1. Define the terms in the vocabulary list.
2. Write the meaning of the abbreviations in the abbreviations list.
3. List five areas of management responsibilities related to the hospital unit coordinator (HUC) position.
4. Name five hospital departments that provide supplies to the nursing unit, identify the department that would provide each supply from a list of supplies, and describe the systems used for restocking supplies.
5. Identify the appropriate hospital department that the HUC would notify, using a list of nursing unit equipment needing repair and problems that need to be resolved.
6. Identify the emergency equipment that is located on a nursing unit, and give an example of reusable patient equipment that would require a daily charge.
7. Explain the importance of the change-of-shift report, and list five items that would be recorded on the census worksheet for quick reference.
8. Briefly explain a method used to record the location of patients and patients' charts, and discuss why it is necessary to keep a record of this information.

9. Describe the HUC's responsibilities regarding the admission, discharge, and transfer (ADT) sheet, the ADT log book, and the patient labels, and identify daily nursing forms that the HUC may prepare when using paper charts.
10. List seven steps to follow when dealing with visitors' complaints.
11. Describe the process for sending and receiving medical records; list five guidelines for scanning medical records into the patient's electronic medical record (EMR) and seven guidelines for filing medical records in the patient's paper chart.
12. Explain the process of retrieving diagnostic test results with and without the EMR.
13. Given a list of several HUC tasks, identify those that would have a higher priority and those that would be of lower priority.
14. List 12 time management tips for the HUC.
15. Define two types of stress, and provide an example of each.
16. List five techniques for dealing with stress on the job.
17. Identify two common work-related injuries and five guidelines for preventing workplace injuries.
18. List four items that should be within reaching distance of the HUC's desk area and at least six reference materials that would be located on the computer or in hard copy on the nursing unit.
19. Discuss the purpose of continuous quality improvement (CQI).
20. Identify and apply the five-step problem-solving model.

VOCABULARY

Admission, Discharge, and Transfer Log Book (ADT log book) Book used to record all admissions, discharges, and transfers on a nursing unit for future reference.

Admission, Discharge, and Transfer Sheet (ADT Sheet) Form used to record daily admissions, discharges, and transfers for quick reference and to assist in tracking empty beds.

Brainstorming Structured group activity that allows three to 10 people to tap into the creativity of the group to identify new ideas. Typically in quality improvement, the technique is used to identify probable causes and possible solutions for quality problems.

Census Sheet A list of patients including room and bed numbers and other relevant information that may be printed from a computer menu.

Census Worksheet Form used on a nursing unit that includes a list of patients' names and room and bed numbers, with blank spaces next to each name. This may be used by the HUC to record patient activities. (May also be called a *patient information sheet* or a *patient activity sheet*).

Central Service Department (CSD) Charge Slip Form that is initiated to charge a discharged patient for any items used during the hospital stay that were not charged to the patient at the time of use.

Central Service Department (CSD) Credit Slip Form that is used to credit a patient for items found in the room unused after the patient's discharge or when a patient was mistakenly charged for an item that was not used.

Central Service Discrepancy Report List of items that are missing from the nursing unit patient supply cupboard or closet that were not charged to a patient. A discrepancy report is sent to the nursing unit each day from the central service department.

Change-of-Shift Report A communication process between shifts, in which nursing personnel who are going off duty report nursing unit activities to personnel coming on duty (report may be provided in person or may be tape-recorded). HUCs may give the report to each other or may listen to the nurse's report.

Continuous Quality Improvement (CQI) The practice of continuously improving quality of each function at each level of every department of the health care organization (also called *total quality management [TQM]*).

Crisis Stress A profound effect experienced by individuals and resulting from common, uncontrollable, often unpredictable life experiences.

Ergonomics Scientific field that is concerned with human factors in the design and operation of machines and the physical environment.

Five-Step Problem-Solving Model A step-by-step process designed to solve problems.

Memory Sheet A notepad kept by the telephone and used to write down messages that need to be relayed and tasks that need to be completed.

Patient Label Book Book used to store labels for patients when computer physician order entry (CPOE) has been implemented; it is also used to store labels for discharged patients for a short time after the time of their discharge.

Perennial Stress The wear and tear of day-to-day living, with the feeling that one is a square peg trying to fit into a round hole.

React Saying or doing the first thing that comes to mind and allowing negative emotions to take over in response to another person or event (a negative choice).

Respond A positive approach to a person or event that puts distance between you and the event (a positive choice).

Standard Supply List A computerized or written record of the quantity of each item that the nursing unit currently needs to last until the next supply order date (separate lists are found inside cabinet doors, in supply drawers, and on the code or crash cart).

Stress A physical, chemical, or emotional factor that causes bodily or mental tension and may cause disease.

Supply Needs List A sheet of paper used by all nursing unit personnel to jot down items that need reordering.

ABBREVIATIONS

Abbreviation	Meaning
ADT log book	book used to record all admissions, discharges, and transfers on a nursing unit
ADT sheet	form used to record admissions, discharges, and transfers on a nursing unit on a daily basis
CQI	continuous quality improvement

⊜ EXERCISE 1

Write the abbreviation for each term listed.

1. admission, discharge, and transfer log book
2. admission, discharge, and transfer sheet
3. continuous quality improvement

⊜ EXERCISE 2

Write the meaning of each abbreviation listed.

1. ADT log book
2. ADT sheet
3. CQI

Merriam-Webster's Collegiate Dictionary, Eleventh Edition, defines *manage* as "to handle or direct with a degree of skill." The health unit coordinator (HUC) who learns to handle or direct with a degree of skill certain facets of the job is able to realize the full potential of health unit coordinating.

To implement the management techniques discussed in this chapter, it is important to (1) understand the philosophy of the health care facility, and (2) know and understand the health unit coordinating job description for the nursing unit. When hired, study these areas carefully. Implementation of the electronic medical record (EMR) and computer physician order entry (CPOE) has resulted in increased managerial responsibilities for the HUC. It is important to remember that the nursing unit will function more efficiently when unit personnel work as a team. The HUC is an important member of the health care team who has great influence on how efficiently the nursing unit functions.

Although the HUC position does not usually include direct management of people, how the HUC manages certain aspects of the job indirectly affects the other nursing unit personnel and the patients. Management can be divided into the following five areas:

1. Management of nursing unit supplies and equipment
2. Management of activities at the nurses' station
3. Management of patient medical records
4. Management related to the performance of tasks
5. Management of time
6. Management of stress

MANAGEMENT OF NURSING UNIT SUPPLIES

Responsibility for monitoring and maintaining supplies used on the nursing unit varies greatly among hospitals. However, this function definitely falls into the nonclinical category of tasks and is a part of the HUC job description in most hospitals with or without EMRs. Supplies stocked on a unit will vary depending on the unit specialty—for example, a pediatric unit will stock diapers, bottles, and similar items, and an orthopedic unit will stock slings, sandbags, and other orthopedic equipment and supplies.

Proper management of nursing unit supplies and equipment greatly enhances the delivery of patient care. Improper management can result in minor annoyances, such as the doctor's discovering that the batteries are burned out when attempting to use the unit's ophthalmoscope to examine a patient's eyes. Management of nursing unit supplies involves all areas of the nursing unit.

Common Areas Located on a Typical Nursing Unit

Nurses' station: Used as a reception desk and is the hub of activity. Contains the HUC workstation, and computers where doctors, nurses, and other health care professionals enter orders and other documentation into patients' electronic or paper records. Equipment located in the nurses' station includes computers, printers, scanner, telephones, and fax machine (see Fig. 1-1 on p. 3).

Patient rooms: Used to admit patients for treatment and care (medical, surgical, trauma, or obstetric patients).

Unit kitchen: Used to store food items and to prepare beverages and snacks for patients.

Linen room or cart: Used to store linens.

Employee lounge: Used by nursing unit personnel for conferences, breaks, and other activities.

Report room: Room used by nursing personnel who are going off duty to give a change-of-shift report to personnel who are coming on duty (report may be provided in person or may be tape-recorded).

Medication room or computerized medication cart: Used to store and to prepare medications for administration by nursing personnel.

Treatment room: Room used to perform invasive procedures such as lumbar puncture (spinal tap).

Central service closet or cart: Used to store items such as gauze pads, elastic bandages, adhesive tape, alcohol pads, masks, and protective gloves.

Utility room: Used for the storage and care of patient care equipment. Most hospitals have two utility rooms. One is referred to as a contaminated or "dirty" utility room, where used equipment such as intravenous pumps and air mattresses are stored until picked up by CSD personnel to be cleaned and sterilized for distribution as needed. The other is used as a storage room where frequently used equipment, such as intravenous poles, bedside commodes, and bedpans, is stored.

Visitor waiting room: Used as a visiting area for patients' relatives and friends

Conference room: Used for patient care conferences or as a place where a doctor or a pastor can speak to family members in private.

Departments that Provide Nursing Unit Supplies

The patient is charged for some items, such as catheter trays and medications, whereas other items, such as paper chart forms, hand soap, paperclips, and so forth, are charged to the nursing unit budget.

Purchasing Department

Purchasing department supplies consist of nonnursing items, such as paper chart and requisition forms, pencils, staples, flashlights, and numerous other items. Figure 7-1 illustrates an example of a purchasing department order form. Items received from the purchasing department are paid for from the nursing unit budget. A cost control center number for the nursing unit is placed on all requisitions issued by the unit. Restocking of purchasing department supplies is done

STANDARD REGISTER
STOCKLESS FORMS REQUISITION

NAME OF REQUESTOR	TELEPHONE NO.	AUTHORIZED SIGNATURE	DATE ORDERED
DEPARTMENT NAME	BUILDING/LOCATION	FLOOR	COST CENTER .460

NO. 01132

QTY	UNIT OF MEASURE	FORM NUMBER	DESCRIPTION
	500/BX	2044	ENV BLUE #9 SPEC WINDOW
	500/BX	2045	ENV INTER OFFICE BLUE #10
	1/EA	2046	ENV INTER OFFICE MAN/10x13
	500/BX	2051	ENV MANILLA PAYROLL WIND
	500/BX	2061	ENV WHITE ST JOSEPH #10
	1000/ROLL	2093	LABEL WHT 2-7/8 x 1-7/16
	500/PK	2177	ST JOSEPH LETTERHEAD
	500/BX	2881	ENV WHITE #9 OUTGOING
	1000/CTN	3224	PURCH 5 PT PAPER COLOR
	500/BX	3387	ENV WT WINDOW #10 PAT ACT
	2000/PK	3481	LABEL-ADDRESSOGRAPH-PACK
	25/PK	3623	HIV CONSENT FORM
	3000/CTN	61911G	WARD REPORT
	25/PD	ADM-1-4	CLASS ATTENDANCE SHEET
	25/PK	ADM-1104	ST JOE OCCURRENCE RPT
	10/PK	ADM-1196	ESP GRAM
	25/PK	ADM-1426	EMPL EXP REINBURSE
	50/PK	ADM-1775	PATIENT COMPLAINT SHEET
	100/PD	ADM-3-140	WHILE YOU WERE OUT PAD
	100/PD	ADM-503-127	REQ SPEC FOOD SERV
	100/PK	ADM-505	SPEED MEMO
	1930/CTN	ADMIT 1271	PATIENT INFO
	1000/CTN	ADMIT-1637	4 PT REQ INFO
	100/PD	BUS-1-222	OCCUPATIONAL THPY CHG
	100/PK	BUS-10	222 X-RAY CHGS
	100/PK	BUS-1000	GENERAL X-RAY
	200/PK	BUS-1001	RADIOLOGY CONSULT
	100/PK	BUS-1002	SP PROC X-RAY
	100/PK	BUS-1007	DEPT RAD CARDIO NUC MED
	100/PK	BUS-1008	GEN SERG DRUG CHGS
	50/PK	BUS-1016	CDV DIAG LAB
	10/PK	BUS-1040	CONTROLLED DRUGS ORAL A
	10/PK	BUS-1045	CONTROLLED DRUGS II
	10/PK	BUS-1055	CONTROLLED DRUGS-INJECT
	100/PD	BUS-1057	MEDICARE AS 2nd PAYOR
	100/PK	BUS-1057A	MEDICARE ADDENDUM A
	100/PK	BUS-1280	OP/PT CHRG-PROCEDURE
	100/PD	BUS-1476	BLOOD GAS LAB
	50/PK	BUS-15	EEG CHARGE SLIP
	100/PK	BUS-1597	PERINATAL AMNI BLOOD TEST
	100/PD	BUS-16-134	PHYS MED CHGE SLIP
	100/PD	BUS-178	CONDITIONS FOR TREATMENT
	100/PK	BUS-18	PHARMACY CHARGE SLIP
	100/PD	BUS-29-2	MISC CHARGE SLIP

QTY	UNIT OF MEASURE	FORM NUMBER	DESCRIPTION
	100/PD	BUS-30-135	CREDIT SLIP
	100/PK	BUS-33	SPEECH OTOLOGY CHARGE
	100/PD	BUS-35-295	MEMO PADS
	100/PD	BUS-35-295A	FULL SIZE MEMO PAD
	4950/CTN	BUS-42	BLOOD BANK CONTINUOUS
	100/PK	BUS-42B	OUTPT LAB REQUISITION
	100/PD	BUS-447	NEW INV CODING SHEET
	100/PD	BUS-448	PREPAID A/C CODE
	100/PK	BUS-50B	MICRO URNE FLDS LAB REQ
	100/PD	BUS-510-143	REQ FOR CK OR CASH
	100/PK	BUS-53B	CHEM, HEMA, SEROLO LAB REQ
	50/PK	BUS-60A	CYTOLOGY
	100/PK	BUS-61	TISSUES FORM
	100/PK	BUS-63	GENERAL SURGERY CHARGES
	250/PK	BUS-641	SPD CHARGE CARD
	100/PK	BUS-674	ER MEDICATION CHARGES
	100/PK	BUS-677	DELIVERY ROOM CHARGES
	100/PD	BUS-817	OCCUP THERAPY CHG SLIP
	100/PK	CRS-1421	GENERAL DIAGNOSTIC-CRS
	950/CTN	CRS-1483	CRS MTST PAPER
	100/PD	CS-3-291	NURSING CARE PLAN
	100/PK	DORM-508	DORM VISITATION SLIP
	100/PK	DORM-510	PRENATAL REC 2A MT ST
	250/PK	DP-2-163	BATCH HEADER/TRAILER
	250/PK	DP-2-163C	BATCH HEADER/TRAILER BLUE
	100/PD	DP-960	CREDIT/DEBIT RECORD
	100/PD	DP-962	BALANCE TRANSFER
	100/PD	DP-963	CREDIT/DEBIT SHEET
	250/PK	DP2-163B	BATCH HEADER/TRAILER PBS
	100/PD	EEG-609	PHYSICIAN TRANSCRIPTION
	100/PD	ENG-445	PLANT SERV SERVICE CALL
	100/PD	ER-508-172	PHONE REPORT OF LAB
	500/PK	ER-514	ER C/SERV ITEMS CHG SLIP
	5000/CTN	FS-1427	MENU LABEL
	100/PD	HB-17-96	WORK ORDERS
	1450/CTN	HB-1720	A/P BLUE
	200/PK	HB-54	RECEIPTS-PEGBOARD
	250/PK	HB-55	JOURNAL-PEGBOARD
	100/PK	HRS-2027	OPERATING ROOM PATH CONST
	2500/CTN	LAB-1684	1 PART LAB REPORT
	5000/CTN	LAB-1352	LAB LABEL-GREEN, MULTI-CUT
	5000/CTN	LAB-1353	LAB LABEL-WHT, SINGLE CUT
	2500/CTN	LAB-1354	LAB LABEL-RED
	1600/CTN	LAB-1428	12 PART CANARY-CONTINUOUS

QTY	UNIT OF MEASURE	FORM NUMBER	DESCRIPTION
	5700/CTN	LAB-1557	HEMO-CONTINUOUS
	1300/CTN	LAB-1621	3 PART LAB REPORT
	3000/CTN	LAB-1979	PATHOLOGY REPORT-LASER
	100/PD	LAB-501-79	PATHOLOGY CONSULTATION
	2500/CTN	LABEL 2-7/16 x 4	WHITE LABEL 2-7/16 x 4
	100/PK	MD-17	ADULT MCC ENCOUNTER
	100/PK	MD-300-01	MD PED HEME CHARGE
	100/PK	MR-1-302	SUMMARY SHEETS
	100/PD	MR-10-303	CONSENT TO OPERATION
	100/PK	MR-1012	ICU MEDICATION RECORD
	200/PK	MR-1016	MEDICATION REC UNIT DOSE
	100/PK	MR-1017	RESP THERAPY MOUNT SHEET
	100/PD	MR-1019-232	24-HR NWBRN NURSERY OBS
	100/PD	MR-1025-248	NB DEFIENCY SLIP
	100/PD	MR-1030-270	OB DEFIENCY SLIP
	100/PD	MR-11-41	GEN/BNI ANESTHESIA RECORD
	100/PK	MR-1117	MEDICATION ADMIN RECORD
	1350/CTN	MR-1134	MED ADMINISTRATION REC
	100/PK	MR-1142	MATERNITY PT CARE PLAN
	100/PD	MR-1156	PHYSICIAN IN CHARGE
	100/PK	MR-116	PED ADMISSION ASSESSMENT
	100/PK	MR-1262	MATERNITY PT CARE SUP
	100/PD	MR-1490	NURSES CARE PLAN
	100/PK	MR-1542	DISCHG PLAN WORKSHEET
	100/PD	MR-18-304	NURSES RECORD
	100/PD	MR-19-305	PROGRESS REPORT
	50/PK	MR-1904	BLANK FORM CARRIER
	25/PK	MR-1904A	ATRIAL LABEL
	25/PK	MR-1904ART	ARTERIAL LABEL
	25/PK	MR-1904CVP	CVP LABEL
	25/PK	MR-1904GP	GENERAL PURPOSE LABEL
	25/PK	MR-1904ICP	ICP LABEL
	50/PK	MR-1904IV	IV LABEL
	10/PK	MR-1904PA	PA LABEL
	250/PK	MR-20B-306	BLUE MD ORDERS
	200/PK	MR-20W-507	WHITE MD ORDERS
	100/PK	MR-210	ADMISS STATUS REC DORM
	100/PK	MR-245	PRE ADMIT PHYS ORDERS
	200/PK	MR-27	FOLLOW UP INSTRUCTIONS
	100/PK	MR-275	LABOR-DELIVERY FORM
	100/PD	MR-283	HEMODYNAMIC FLOWSHEET
	100/PK	MR-32	ER CLINICAL RECORD
	100/PK	MR-34-309	RECOVERY RM RECORD
	100/PK	MR-34A-318	RECOVERY RM REC CONT

QTY	UNIT OF MEASURE	FORM NUMBER	DESCRIPTION
	50/PD	MR-41-282	CONSENT PHOTOG-PUBLS
	100/PD	MR-417	REQ FOR PRIOR ORDERS
	100/PK	MR-43-216	MEDICATION RECORD
	100/PD	MR-46-158	DIABETIC CHART
	2850/CTN	MR-47	DISCHARGE FINAL REPORT
	2850/CTN	MR-48	WEEKLY LAB SUMMARY
	100/PK	MR-480	PHYS PARENTERAL NUT ORDER
	200/PK	MR-5	LAB REPORT
	100/PK	MR-509-98	ADMISSION ASSESSMENT
	500/CTN	MR-522	6-PLY MTST PAPER/CBNLESS
	650/CTN	MR-522	MTST 5-PT PAPER CBN
	50/PD	MR-533	MEDICAL RECORD OUT CARD
	100/PK	MR-571	VENTILATOR RESP THERAPY
	100/PK	MR-581	PATIENT RECORD
	100/PD	MR-583	CDV ICU FLOW SHEET
	100/PD	MR-593	DEFICIENCY RECORD
	100/PD	MR-595-179	PROBLEM SHEET
	100/PD	MR-600-643	PREOP CHECK LIST
	1100/CTN	MR-616	PULMONARY LAB REPORT
	2500/CTN	MR-616A	PULMONARY LAB REPORT 1-PT
	100/PD	MR-650	VITAL SIGNS
	100/PK	MR-671-730	PRE-ANESTHESIA QUES
	100/PK	MR-675	NEONATAL RECORD I
	100/PK	MR-676	NEONATAL II
	100/PK	MR-677	OB SUMMARY
	100/PK	MR-684	CONDITIONS OF ADMISSION
	100/PK	MR-685-755	NURSING DISCHARGE ASSESS
	100/PD	MR-692-783	X-RAY CASSETTES
	100/PK	MR-717	PERIOPERATIVE RECORD
	100/PD	MR-803	DIET SERVICE PROG NOTE
	100/PK	MR-895	CRITICAL CARE FLOWSHEET
	100/PK	MRS-1157	BACKING SHEET
	100/PK	NS-12-240	NOURISHMENT ORDER FORM
	100/PD	NS-507-114W	WEEKLY SCHEDULES
	100/PD	NS-510-215	REV TEAM ASSIGNMENT
	100/PD	NS-518-14	RN CLINICAL REPORT
	50/PK	NS-529-478	TREAT AND TEST PLAN
	100/PD	NS-530-115	FLUID FORMS
	100/PD	NS-7-100	TPR RECORD
	100/PD	NS-9-21	INTAKE/OUTPUT SHEETS
	1/EA	NSY-325	INFO ABOUT YOUR BABY
	50/PK	NSY-761	NURSERY ICU KARDEX
	200/PK	OPD-19	CLINICAL PRESCRIPTIONS
	100/PK	OPD-60-253	PED-PROGRESS NOTES

QTY	UNIT OF MEASURE	FORM NUMBER	DESCRIPTION
	100/PK	PER-1-196	EMPLOYMENT APPLICATION
	25/PD	PER-13-37	ACCIDENT EXPOSURE RC
	50/PK	PER-663-793	EMP/POS CHG REQUEST
	100/PD	PH-1-299	PRESCRIPTION BLANKS
	100/PD	PH-2-637	PHONE ORDER FOR MEDS
	4900/CTN	PRD-1923	NOTICE OF DEPOSIT
	100/PD	PULF-526	PULF TELEPHONE REPORTS
	100/PK	PUR-1	PURCHASE ORDERS
	25/PK	PUR-1622	OFFICE SUPPLY REQ
	25/PK	PUR-203	REQUISITION TO PURCHASE
	100/PD	PUR-4-53	GEN REQUISITION SM
	100/PK	PUR-IV	PURCHASE ORDER TOP COPY
	25/PK	PUR-9	FORMS REQUISITION
	2500/CTN	QA-1247	RSQUM WORKSHEET
	10/PK	QA-842	MONITORING SYSTEMS
	1/EA	RO-11-214	RADIATION ONCOLOGY BROCH
	25/PD	RAD-18	CAT HISTORY FORM
	100/PK	RAD-511-667	RADIOLOGY PRELIM REPT
	250/PK	RAD-516	DAYLIGHT FLASHER CARD
	250/PK	RAD-516A	BLANK DAYLIGHT FLASHER
	200/PK	RTD-504	RESP THERAPY CHG
	400/CTN	RTD-507	RESP THERAPY SCHEDULE
	100/PD	SSD-104-283	MED RECORD
	100/PD	TRAN-363	TUBE ROOM ROUTE SLIP
	100/PD	TRAN-564	TRAN CALL SLIP

PROCEDURE FOR COMPLETING FORM

1. FILL IN QUANTITY OF FORMS DESIRED. COMPLETE ALL BLANKS AT TOP OF FORM.
2. FOR ITEMS NOT APPEARING ON THIS REQUISITION, CONSULT FORMS CATALOG AND WRITE IN BELOW. (FOR NON-CATALOG FORMS, SPECIAL ORDERS OR NEW FORMS, CONTACT PURCHASING).
3. KEEP "REQUESTOR'S COPY" FOR YOUR RECORDS.
4. SEND ALL REMAINING COPIES TO PURCHASING.
5. FOR ASSISTANCE, CALL EXT. 3443.

QTY	UNIT OF MEASURE	FORM NUMBER	DESCRIPTION

Figure 7-1 Purchasing department order form.

weekly or bimonthly and is the most demanding of all supply tasks. It is important to order what is needed in a timely manner.

Central Service Department

Central service department (CSD) supplies used for nursing procedures that are stored in the CSD department need to be requisitioned and are charged to the patient. (See Fig. 11-2 for an example of a CSD computer screen.) Smaller items, such as adhesive bandages, tongue blades, alcohol, and sponges, are covered by the nursing unit's budget.

Pharmacy

The pharmacy issues supplies that include all medications administered to patients. Medications kept on the nursing unit include three classifications: (1) controlled substances, which are in a computerized dispensing cart or locked in the narcotics cupboard; (2) daily and as-needed (prn) medications that are currently being administered to patients according to doctors' orders; and (3) a unit stock supply of frequently used medications, such as Tylenol and aspirin. Restocking of medications is usually performed on a daily basis, and the stock supply is replenished as needed. Medications are charged to the patients who received them; therefore pharmacy supplies are not covered by the nursing unit's budget. Charges cover the cost of administration supplies, such as needles and syringes, and usually are determined on the basis of information found on the patient's medication record sheet.

Nutritional Care Department

Nutritional care department supplies include food items such as milk, juices, soft drinks, and crackers that are stored in the nursing unit kitchen and issued to patients as needed. These supplies are ordered and restocked daily and usually are charged to the nursing unit's budget.

Figure 7-2 illustrates an example of a nutritional care department stock supply order form.

Laundry or Linen Department

Laundry or linen department supplies include linens and bedding such as pillows, sheets, blankets, towels, washcloths, and patient gowns. The cost of linen supplies usually is absorbed into the charge for the patient's room. Most hospitals employ a laundry service to supply linen that is then delivered to each nursing unit by hospital personnel. If supplies run low during the day, the HUC may have to call the linen department or page personnel from the laundry department for additional items.

Systems Used in Determining Need and Restocking Unit Supplies

A busy nursing unit stocks a variety of supplies to keep the unit functioning smoothly. Two systems are used for restocking supplies. One system is used by the HUC and/or a unit aide, who determines the supplies needed and orders them from the supplying department. Supplies that the HUC is usually directly responsible for maintaining include consent forms or, if applicable, paper chart forms. In many hospitals, all patient chart forms are computerized and may be printed as needed. Other supplies include office supplies, batteries, nutritional care supplies, and other miscellaneous items. Only

```
NOURISHMENT ORDER FROM NUTRITIONAL CARE

UNIT_____ ORDERED BY_____

DATE_____ _____

======================================
  DESCRIPTION                | ORDER
--------------------------------------
Whole Milk                   |
Skim Milk                    |
Chocolate Milk               |
Orange Juice (unsw) (qts)    |
Apple Juice                  |
Cranberry Juice              |
Prune Juice                  |
Tomato Juice                 |
Nectar                       |
Decaffeinated Coffee (pkg of 20) |
Tea Bags (pkg of 30)         |
Graham Crackers (pkg of 12)  |
Saltines (pkg of 20)         |
Powdered non-dairy
Creamers (50 per box)        |
Sugar (per 100 ind.)         |
Ice Cream                    |
Sherbet                      |
Jello                        |
Custard                      |
Margarine (ind.)             |
Bouillon -Beef or Chicken(pkg/12) |
7-Up  (6 pk)                 |
Cola (6 pk)                  |
--------------------------------------
NOTE: BETWEEN MEAL FEEDINGS, TUBE FEEDINGS OR
LIQUID SUPPLEMENTS ARE TO BE ORDERED VIA
COMPUTER CARD.

NS-12-240    Received by_____
```

Figure 7-2 Nutritional care department stock supply order form.

the needed quantity of supplies should be maintained on the nursing unit. Overstocking may result in waste because some items become outdated and are no longer useful. Understocking may result in wasted time and a delay in a patient's treatment.

Most hospitals use a **standard supply list** (Fig. 7-3), a computerized or written record of the quantity of each item currently needed by the nursing unit to last until the next supply order date. Standard supply lists are sometimes located inside

Standard Supply List

Form	Amount
Doctors' order forms	10 pks
CABG orders	5 pks
Doctors' progress notes	10 pks
Nurses' admission notes	10 pks
Allergy adverse reaction documentations	10 pks
Patient valuables check list	10 pks
Patient care documentation records	10 pks
Kardexes	5 pks
Medication administration records	5 pks
Graphic records	5 pks
Surgical consents	8 pks
Blood transfusion consents	8 pks
Reviewer communication records	5 pks
IV therapy records	5 pks
Home instructions	10 pks
Coding summary forms	10 pks
Health information checklist	10 pks
Anticoagulant therapy records	8 pks
Diabetic records	5 pks

Figure 7-3 An example of a standard supply list. Patient chart forms would be included if not computerized.

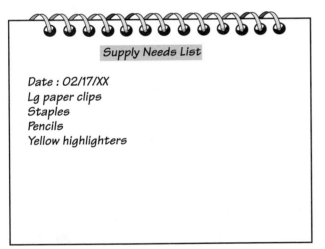

Figure 7-4 An example of a supply needs list.

cupboard doors or at the bottom of drawers where supplies are stored. To determine and order the number of supplies needed, simply compare the quantity on the standard supply list with the quantity of the item on the shelf, and requisition the difference. Keep in mind that the standard supply for many items may change and the standard supply list must be updated to reflect the changes. Another suggestion is to maintain on the nursing unit bulletin board a **supply needs list** for items (other than those maintained by the CSD) and ask all nursing unit personnel to record supplies that are running low (Fig. 7-4). This list may be used as a reference for items needed when you are ordering supplies for the nursing unit. The HUC may take inventory of nutritional care supplies such as crackers, juices, milk, coffee, and tea and order appropriate quantities for the nursing unit.

A second system, used by the supplying department such as the CSD, involves a computerized list of items used or a manual list made by a CSD technician making daily rounds throughout the hospital and restocking supplies as needed (similar to restocking of shelves in a grocery store). When electronic records are used, items taken from the supply closet are scanned into the patient's record, the patient is charged, and the CSD has a record of items used. A **central service discrepancy report** is a report that lists items that are missing from the supply closet or locker but were not charged to a patient. This discrepancy report and a list of items charged to patients from the previous day will be sent to the unit each afternoon from the CSD. The HUC compares the items on the discrepancy report with the list of items charged to patients to locate the missing items. Items are charged to the appropriate inpatients and a **central service department (CSD) charge slip** is used to charge items to a discharged patient's account when necessary to do so. A **central service (CSD) credit slip** is used to credit a patient for unused items left in the discharged patient's room or mistakenly charged to a patient. The cost of items that cannot be accounted for is charged to the nursing unit budget. Most hospitals have scanners located in the CSD closet or locker so items removed can be easily scanned and charged to the appropriate patient.

MANAGEMENT OF NURSING UNIT EQUIPMENT

Equipment Stored at the Nurses' Station

The HUC is responsible for monitoring all electronic equipment used on the nursing unit including computers, printers, copy machines, scanners, and phones and requesting repairs as needed. It is important to maintain the printer, copy machines, and fax machine by adding paper as needed and checking ink levels frequently. Flashlights, ophthalmoscopes, otoscopes, thermometers with disposable covers, blood glucose monitors, and other items used by doctors and nurses to examine patients are stored on the nursing unit. The HUC is responsible for checking this equipment frequently to make sure it is in working order and for ordering new light bulbs and/or batteries as needed. The HUC is the go-to person when the unit elevators, pneumatic tube system, patient call lights, or televisions are not functioning or there is a problem with plumbing or temperature. Burned-out electric light bulbs, an overflowing toilet, and other unpredictable problems need immediate attention. The HUC should know the appropriate person or department to call. The hospital information technology (IT) department would be responsible for the repair of communication equipment, such as computers and telephones; other repairs would be handled by the maintenance department. For immediate repair service, notify the maintenance department by telephone or pocket pager and, if necessary, complete the appropriate requisition.

Note: Larger hospitals may have divisions in the maintenance departments, such as "temperature control" and plumbing.

General Maintenance of Nursing Unit Equipment

General nursing unit equipment includes furniture, electrical fixtures, bathroom items, and other equipment. Equipment requires maintenance, and the old saying "An ounce of prevention is worth a pound of cure" applies here. Ideas for more efficient location of supplies offer an improvement opportunity and should be discussed with nursing management. Most hospital units have equipment lists that show when items are due for replacement.

Preventive management of nursing unit equipment may require that the HUC make rounds of the entire unit (i.e., kitchen, utility rooms, patient rooms, waiting rooms, linen room, and staff lounge) perhaps once a week or month to check on the functioning of equipment located in these areas. Leaky faucets, frayed electrical cords, and broken hinges are a few examples of the things to look for. Make a list of all items on the nursing unit that need to be checked. Then make rounds; check each item on the list for its working order. Make a note of the items that need repair. Request that nursing unit staff note needed repairs in the unit communication book.

Frequently, patients bring electrical devices such as electrical shavers, hair dryers, radios, and other items to the hospital for use during their stay. Before these items are used, they must be examined for electrical shorts by the hospital maintenance department. The HUC may place a call to initiate this process.

Patient Rental Equipment

Reusable equipment used by an individual patient, such as an intravenous infusion pump, is usually charged to the patient's bill on a daily basis. When the doctor discontinues a treatment that requires the rental equipment, nursing personnel usually place the equipment in the "dirty" utility room, where it is kept until it is returned to the proper department for cleaning. This equipment is picked up on a regular basis throughout the day. Personnel in the CSD will check the number printed on a label attached to the equipment to remove the daily charge to the patient. Often the HUC will receive a call from the central services department to check in the "dirty" utility room for intravenous pumps; shortages are frequent because so many are in use.

Nursing Unit Emergency Equipment

A *code* or *crash cart* (discussed in Chapter 21) is usually stored on each nursing unit or in an area between nursing units. The code or crash cart is a cart stocked by the CSD and pharmacy staff with advanced breathing supplies, intravenous solutions and appropriate tubing, needles, a heart monitor, a defibrillator, an oxygen tank, and emergency medication (used when a patient stops breathing or his or her heart stops beating, or both). The cart is kept locked with a plastic lock. It is a requirement of The Joint Commission (TJC) that the cart, according to a schedule set by hospital policy, be unlocked, the contents checked to ensure that all equipment and supplies are accounted for and are in working order, and that medications are not outdated. In some hospitals a registered nurse (RN) checks the cart and will request that the HUC order supplies or medication as needed. When the code or crash cart is completely checked and restocked, the nurse will again lock the cart after documenting the date and signing the form attached to the cart. In most hospitals the code or crash cart maintenance is the responsibility of the central supply and pharmacy departments. When the cart has been used for

⭐ **HIGH PRIORITY**

The health unit coordinator (HUC) must know the emergency procedures for the nursing unit; what emergency equipment and supplies are stored on the unit and where they are located; how to call a code; what the HUC's responsibilities are during a code; the signal codes and procedures for fire; behavioral alarms; disaster codes and evacuation procedures; and procedures for dealing with a hazardous materials spill. Although the HUC may not be directly responsible, knowing the procedures allows timely and safe removal of hazardous materials.

During a crisis, hospital personnel often approach the nurses' station and ask the HUC to locate emergency equipment and initiate emergency procedures. Frequent fire and disaster drills are conducted in hospitals to prepare personnel for disaster situations. The HUC and all hospital personnel must know what to do in the event of a fire or a disaster; these drills must be taken seriously.

Ignorance of code procedure or of the location of nursing unit emergency equipment may cause a delay in the delivery of emergency treatment, possibly resulting in serious consequences for patients.

Wireless mobile devices and mass communication capability have improved communication in emergency situations and disaster. (See Chapter 4 for more communication information. See Chapter 21 for emergency procedures and HUC responsibilities.)

a code, it is vital that the cart be restocked or replaced per hospital policy.

Other emergency equipment includes fire extinguishers and fire doors. Because of the importance of emergency equipment, it must be checked frequently and immediately after use and should be restored as soon as possible to be readied for future emergencies.

MANAGEMENT OF ACTIVITIES AT THE NURSES' STATION

As stated in Chapter 1, the HUC coordinates activities involving the doctor, the nursing staff, the other hospital departments, patients, and visitors to the nursing unit. Good management techniques are necessary to coordinate these activities effectively. The following guidelines may be of assistance in managing activities at the nurses' station.

Patient Activity and Information

A **change-of-shift report** is the statement by which an outgoing nurse informs the oncoming nurse about a patient's medical history and current condition. This information needs to be conveyed methodically, such as moving through each body system (cardiac, urinary, and so on) or going from head to toe. Other information includes pending diagnostic tests, transfers and discharges, and no codes. Patient safety hinges on a complete and correct exchange of information. The HUC may listen to the nurses' change-of-shift reports or will receive a report from the HUC going off duty.

Room #	Patient Name	Activities
301	Breath, Les	DC Today
302	Pickens, Slim	Surg 1100 x ray to be sent c̄ patient
303-1	Katt, Kitty	
303-2		
304	Bee, Mae	~~Call Dr. James c̄ ABG results~~ Called Sue 900
305	Honey, Mai	NPO for heart cath @ 900
306-1		
306-2		
307	Pack, Fanny	No calls to room
308	Bugg, June	DC today
309	~~Kynde, Bee~~	Trans to ICU 1130
310-1	Cider, Ida	DNR
310-2	Soo, Ah	~~Surg 800~~ Back @ 130
311-1	Bear, Harry	Resp isolation
311-2	Bread, Thad	
312-1	Kream, Kris	NINP
312-2	Pat, Peggy	~~Surg 930~~ Back @ 200

Figure 7-5 A census worksheet.

A **census sheet** is a printed copy of the *census screen* found on all nursing unit computers consisting of a list of the patients' names and ages with room and bed numbers, the patient's attending doctor, and the patient's acuity level.

A **census worksheet** may also be printed that consists of a list of just the patient's names with room and bed numbers, leaving a blank space next to each name for notations. A census worksheet may be printed at the beginning of each shift from a computer menu. Information from the change-of-shift report or from each patient's Kardex form (if used; see Chapter 9) can be recorded next to each patient's name. Record the patient activities including scheduled diagnostic procedures, surgeries, planned discharges, transfers, and other information that is pertinent to responsibilities of the HUC. Record the time that each activity will take place if known (Fig. 7-5).

Other data that are important to record so they can be referred to during the shift include (1) do not resuscitate (DNR) or no code, and similar information, (2) NINP (no information, no publication), (3) no visitors allowed,

SKILLS CHALLENGE

To practice preparing a unit census worksheet, complete Activity 7-1 in the *Skills Practice Manual*.

(4) no phone calls to the patient's room, (5) the patient is in respiratory isolation, (6) the patient is out on a temporary pass, (7) the nurse who is assigned to the patient, and (8) the resident or attending physician who is assigned to the patient.

Keep the census worksheet next to the telephone and near the computer for quick reference. During the shift, update the information as changes occur.

Patients and Patients' Charts that Leave the Unit

When EMRs or paper charts are used, record the time and destination next to the patient's name on the census worksheet when he or she leaves the nursing unit for surgery, for a diagnostic study, to visit the cafeteria with a relative, or for any other reason. When the patient returns to the nursing unit, draw a line through this recording. When paper charts are used, keeping track of and locating misplaced charts is essential for ensuring efficient use of time by doctors, nurses, and other professionals. Health care personnel, doctors, and visitors look to the HUC to know the whereabouts of patients and/or patients' charts. When the census worksheet is maintained, the answer can be found quickly.

Many hospitals have computerized systems such as the Hill-Rom NaviCare patient flow system to manage and improve the flow of patients, staff, and other resources. The NaviCare system uses colorful display monitors that depict a continuous, up-to-date picture of capacity and patient flow within the hospital, similar to information systems used in the air transportation industry. The NaviCare patient flow system features the Vocera communication system (discussed in Chapter 4), which allows caregivers in hospitals to communicate with the NaviCare system via wearable Vocera badges.

 HIGH PRIORITY

Many nursing units average 25 to 40 patients, so it would be impossible to mentally log the whereabouts of each patient.

Preparing Daily Forms

It may be the HUC's task to prepare forms for use by nursing team members, such as the patient assignment sheet (see Fig. 3-6), the admission, discharge, and transfer (ADT) sheet (may be prepared at the end of night shift or beginning of day shift), and work schedules. Because preparing these forms usually involves recording data pertinent to the individual nursing unit, this topic is not discussed further here. Daily tasks when paper charts are used may include preparing nurses' progress records by labeling with patient ID labels and filling in the headings, labeling CSD cards (not used when CSD items are scanned into patients' EMRs), and recopying medication administration records (MARs) if required. When preparing and filling out these forms is an HUC responsibility, plan to do this at the same time each day when possible.

Admission, Discharge, and Transfer Sheet

The HUC records all admissions, discharges, and transfers on the **admission, discharge, and transfer sheet (ADT sheet)** each day for quick reference regarding nursing unit activity for that day, and to determine the number of empty beds on the unit. The ADT sheet is usually used when EMRs or paper charts are used.

Admission, Discharge, and Transfer Log Book

When a patient is admitted to the nursing unit, the HUC places his or her label in the **admission, discharge, and transfer (ADT) log book** and writes the date and time of admission next to the label. If a patient is transferred to another unit within the hospital, the date and time of transfer and

the destination are written next to the patient's label in the ADT book. If the patient is discharged to another facility or to home, the date, time, and name of the facility to which he or she is going (if not to home) are written next to the patient label. The ADT log book is used when EMRs or paper charts are used.

Patient Label Book

Patient labels (at least five sheets) are stored in each patient's chart when paper charts are used, and newly discharged patient labels are often kept in a **patient label book** in case additional charges or credits have to be made to the discharged patient's account. When the EMR has been implemented, inpatient (at least five sheets) and newly discharged patient labels are stored in a patient label book.

The HUC is responsible for maintaining the unit census board (as discussed in Chapter 4), which may indicate patient names, initials, or an alias (if a patient is NINP); their room numbers; and the names of doctors and nurses assigned to each patient. This board may not be in plain sight to visitors, in order to protect patient confidentiality. The use of unit census boards varies from hospital to hospital.

Addressing Visitors' Requests, Questions, and Complaints

The HUC often has more contact with visitors than do most other nursing unit personnel, because visitors usually stop at the nurses' station for information or other types of communication regarding a patient's hospitalization. As a visitor approaches the nurses' station, the HUC should acknowledge his or her presence (if involved in a task that has to be finished or if on the telephone, smile and motion or advise the visitor that you will be with him or her shortly), and provide assistance as soon as possible. At that moment the HUC represents the entire hospital as well as the nursing unit. The manner in which visitors are responded to helps shape their attitudes about the care the patient is receiving and about the hospital as a whole. It is the responsibility of the HUC to (1) communicate appropriate and pertinent information to visitors, (2) respond to visitors' questions and requests, (3) initially handle visitors' complaints, and (4) locate the patient's nurse when necessary.

Pertinent information that is communicated to visitors includes the time for visiting hours, the number of visitors that may be in a patient's room at one time, isolation restrictions, and what items may or may not be taken into the patient's room. Examples of restricted items in the intensive care unit include flowers and plants. Latex balloons are banned in most hospitals because of latex allergies and the risk that children may aspirate broken pieces of the balloon. Refer to the hospital's policy manual for visitor regulations.

Visitors may ask the HUC such questions as, "May I take Mrs. Sanchez to the cafeteria?" or "Can Billy Mitchel have a milkshake?" or "When can Mr. Minard go home?" Many questions may be answered by checking information on the patient's computerized record or Kardex. However, if there is any doubt about the answer, check with the nurse.

Never discuss aspects of the patient's medical condition with the patient's visitors. Refer all of these questions to the patient's doctor or the nurse. If the answer to a question is not known or if the question should be referred to the nurse, respond to the visitor by saying, "I'll ask the nurse to come talk with you," or something similar, rather than saying, "I don't know" or "I'm not allowed to give out that information."

The HUC is often the first person to hear visitors' complaints, justified and unjustified. Visitors, especially the relatives of a critically ill patient, are under a great deal of **stress.** Their uncertainty of the course of the illness, unfamiliarity with the hospital routine, and many other factors contribute to their feelings of uneasiness and insecurity. Family members or friends may be dealing with emotions such as guilt and/or anger. Often these feelings are expressed in the form of complaints regarding the patient's care. The type of response that is given to the visitor's initial remarks may make the difference between whether the problem is solved at the nursing unit level or it escalates up through the nursing administration to the chief executive officer.

Guidelines for Dealing with Visitor Complaints

Follow these steps when dealing with visitor complaints:

1. Listen carefully and attentively to what the person is saying. If the person's voice is raised or is angry in tone, remember that this hostility is not being directed at you personally. It is important to understand that the person is upset and that listening carefully to what is being said is the first step toward dealing with a challenging situation.
2. Ask pertinent, objective questions, and gather as many facts as possible. Speak in a low tone of voice and demonstrate a caring attitude. Whether or not the complaint is justified is not important at this time.
3. Respond to the complaint appropriately. **Respond** verbally with a phrase such as "I understand what you're telling me" or "I understand how you feel." Do not **react** defensively with a statement such as "I wasn't here yesterday" or "That's not my job." If the complaint needs the attention of the nurse, say, "I'll ask the nurse to talk with you as soon as possible." If the person appears even the least bit anxious or angry, refer him or her to the nurse immediately, because time often causes a situation to be exaggerated. Anger may be acknowledged by saying, "I can see you're angry" or something similar before referring the person to the nurse. Doing this demonstrates a caring attitude.
4. Refrain from eating or chewing gum when communicating with visitors; it sends an "I don't care" message.
5. Try to avoid answering the phone, but if it must be answered, ask the person on the phone to hold; then return to handling the complaint.
6. Document the complaint and your responses after the conversation has ended, and relay the information to the patient's nurse as soon as possible.
7. Demonstrate empathy. Think about a loved one who is very close to you and imagine yourself in the family member's or friend's place facing the same situation involving your loved one.

★ HIGH PRIORITY

Check with the patient's nurse before giving permission for a patient to leave the nursing unit, to go outside, or to go to the cafeteria.

MANAGEMENT OF PATIENT MEDICAL RECORDS

Faxing and Receiving Faxed Medical Records

When an order is written to obtain a patient's medical records from another health care facility or doctor's office, the HUC prepares a medical record release form for the patient to sign. Usually it is the nurse or doctor who asks the patient to sign the release form. The HUC then notifies the facility or doctor's office of the request, obtains the appropriate fax number, and provides the return fax number as needed; the release form is then sent, and the requested records or reports are faxed to the nursing unit. When EMRs are in use, the signed release and faxed documents are scanned into the patient's EMR, and hard copies of the release and faxed documents are placed in a receptacle to be sent to the health information management department. If paper charts are in use, the HUC places the signed release form and the faxed documents into the patient's chart.

Scanning Records into the Patient's Electronic Medical Record

The HUC is responsible for scanning electrocardiogram reports, telemetry strips, medical records, reports from outside facilities (when requested), handwritten physician progress notes, and any other relevant documents related to the patient's medical record. After these documents have been scanned, they are certified by a health information specialist and are entered into the patient's EMR. Some hospitals may require the HUC to send the items to be scanned to the health information management system department (HIMS) to be scanned.

Guidelines for Scanning Records into the Patient's Electronic Medical Record

1. Label the document with the appropriate patient's ID label.
2. As required or requested, scan the records in a timely manner using the nursing unit scanner.
3. The records will then be certified by an HIMS specialist and will be entered into the patient's EMR.
4. Stamp the original documents as "scanned," and write the date, the time, and your initials.
5. Place the original documents in a box or bin to be delivered to HIMS.

Filing Medical Records in the Patient's Paper Chart

Each day, the nursing unit receives many typed and computer-generated records, such as diagnostic results, history and physical examination reports, pathology reports, and others, to be filed in the patient's chart. Efficient, timely filing of these records in the patient's chart is necessary for two reasons. First, during the patient's hospital stay, filed written records are readily available for viewing by the attending doctor and other hospital personnel. Diagnosis and/or treatment or therapy is often dependent on these records. Second, on the patient's discharge, HIMS personnel have the legal responsibility to assemble and store *all* records produced during the patient's hospital stay. Correct filing methods used during the patient's hospitalization assist HIMS personnel in completing this task.

Guidelines for Filing Medical Records in the Patient's Paper Chart

1. *When possible, file at the same time each day.* Filing near the end of the shift allows all records received during the shift to be filed at one time. It is important for the patients' nurses to have ready access to all laboratory results as soon as they arrive on the nursing unit.
2. *Separate the records according to patient name.* In this way, all records for a given patient are prepared at one time, so the chart holder must be accessed only once.
3. *Always check the patient's name within the chart with the name on the record before filing it.* Never select the patient's chart just by the room number on the record, because the room number on the record will be incorrect if the patient has been transferred to another bed on the nursing unit after the records were initiated. Often a doctor prescribes treatment according to test results, which may be delayed when records have been filed in the wrong patient's chart.
4. *Be especially alert when two patients on the unit have the same name.* When this happens, both patients' charts are flagged with a "name alert" sticker. File all medical records by their health record number. Many times, patients on the nursing unit will have the same or very similar names. The medical record number will never be duplicated.
5. *Place the record behind the correct chart divider.* Use consistent sequencing in filing the reports on the patient's chart to make it easier for the doctor and other health care personnel to locate them. Reports are usually filed with the latest report in front or on top of previously filed reports, right behind the divider.
6. *Initial each record before filing.* Follow the hospital's policy as to where to place initials if this practice is used.
7. *Never discard any patient's records.* Records that have not been filed for patients who have been discharged should be forwarded to HIMS. Records that have not been filed for patients who have been transferred within the hospital should be forwarded to the receiving unit.

⭐ **HIGH PRIORITY**

Additional health unit coordinator tasks regarding the health information management system (HIMS) and patient medical records are discussed in Chapter 18.

Locating Test Results When Using the Electronic Medical Record

The HUC can view diagnostic test results by choosing a patient and then choosing "Summary," which will display the patient's diagnostic test results as well as the code status, contact information, vital signs, task lists (icons for HUC tasks), and so on. There is no need for the HUC to print the results, as the patient's doctor(s) and nurse(s) have easy access to the test results.

Locating Test Results When Using Paper Charts

Most diagnostic test results may be retrieved from the computer by selecting "Laboratory results" or "Diagnostic imaging results" and then selecting the patient's name. The results will be displayed on the computer screen and may be printed. The HUC may print daily laboratory or diagnostic imaging results as requested. A summary of results may be printed daily for physicians to review on rounds or, if needed, to be sent to another facility if a patient is being transferred. In some hospitals recorded diagnostic test results may be obtained by telephone by calling a specified number.

MANAGING THE PERFORMANCE OF HEALTH UNIT COORDINATOR TASKS

Prioritizing Tasks

For an HUC, situations often occur in which several tasks have to be performed at the same time. Good management involves the ability to determine which task takes priority over another. Awareness and experience are necessary for one to develop skill in determining priorities. A task that is normally of lower priority sometimes becomes a high-priority task; for example, filing or scanning a report into a patient's chart may become a high priority if that patient is scheduled for surgery in a short time. Some of these tasks can be performed simultaneously, as when a HUC is ordering a stat laboratory test while conveying a message to the nurse regarding a patient's return from surgery.

The Usual Priority of Health Unit Coordinator Tasks

1. Orders involving a patient in a medical crisis; these always take precedence over all other tasks
2. Notifying the patient's nurse and doctor of stat laboratory results
3. Ordering and/or transcribing stat orders
4. Answering a nursing unit wireless device or nursing unit telephone (preferably before the third ring)
5. Communicating a telephoned message to the nurse that the surgery department is ready to pick up a patient for surgery or bring back a patient from surgery or that a patient is out of surgery and is in recovery
6. Monitoring or transcribing preoperative and postoperative orders
7. Monitoring or transcribing new admission orders and daily routine orders
8. Monitoring or transcribing discharge and transfer orders, so that clerical work can be processed by the time the patient is ready to leave or be transferred
9. Performing additional and routine tasks

⭐ **HIGH PRIORITY**

The health unit coordinator must have the ability to multitask—for example, ordering stat diagnostic tests for a patient in a medical crisis or notifying the nurse of stat lab results while answering the unit wireless device or telephone. Transcribing and/or calling in a doctor's order for a surgical or specialty consultation may be a high priority and is discussed in Chapter 18.

Not monitoring the patient's EMR or paper chart for orders could delay diagnostic tests and the patient's diagnosis, thereby delaying treatment. Delaying treatment could place the patient in danger.

The following time management and stress management techniques may assist the HUC in managing the workload.

Time Management

The ability to manage time may be the single most important factor in successful health unit coordinating. However, it is not easy to learn how to effectively use time. Experience, awareness, flexibility, and motivation are all necessary to achieve the goal of using time to its full potential.

There is a story that superbly demonstrates how the day tends to "go" when there is no plan for managing time:

A farmer told his wife, "I'll plow the south 40 tomorrow." The next morning, he went out to lubricate the tractor. But he needed oil; so he went to the shop to get it. On the way, he noticed that the pigs hadn't been fed. He started for the bin to get them some feed, but some sacks there reminded him that the potatoes needed sprouting. He walked over toward the potato bin. En route, he spotted the woodpile and remembered that he'd promised to carry some wood to the house. But he had to chop it first, and he'd left his ax behind the chicken coop. As he went for the ax, he met his wife, who was feeding the chickens. With surprise, she asked, "Have you finished the south 40 already?" "Finished!" the farmer bellowed. "I haven't even started."

Similar to the farmer, the HUC who is engaged in one part of the job is constantly seeing other tasks that need to be done. Knowing how to plan the day to make the best use of time helps avoid the pitfalls of the farmer. The following time management techniques may be of assistance to the HUC.

Time Management Techniques

1. *Ask for assistance when needed.* Most hospitals have a "SWAT HUC" who is available to assist on nursing units when additional help is needed. A HUC working on a neighboring unit may also be available to assist as needed.
2. *Monitor electronic medical records or paper charts for new orders frequently.* On returning from a break, check EMRs. When finding several charts lying about, check each chart for new orders, place those that do not have new orders in the chart rack, read all new orders, notify the patient's nurse of any stat orders and provide the nurse with a copy of the orders, and fax or send copies to the pharmacy. Then proceed to transcribe all other orders, one chart at a time. If CPOE has been implemented, check the computer for tasks. Delay in monitoring the patient's EMR or paper chart can result in delaying a diagnosis and effective treatment.
3. *Complete one task before beginning another.* This is not always possible because a stat order may take precedence over whatever else is being done. However, apply this principle as consistently as possible. Always finish transcribing a set of orders before you take a break.
4. *Follow the 10 steps of transcription (outlined in Chapter 9) if using paper charts.* Never sign off on orders before you ensure that each step has been completed.
5. *Plan for rush periods.* Take time at the beginning of each day to prepare for anticipated rush periods. For example, because it is always busy in the morning while the doctors are making rounds, allow time to assist the doctors in use

of the EMR if needed and for locating patient charts and for other assistance as needed. If several surgical patients are scheduled to be admitted, a rush can be anticipated in the afternoon, when they return to the unit from the post-anesthesia care unit (PACU). If there are several empty beds on the nursing unit in the morning, a rush during admitting time in the afternoon can be expected.

6. *Plan a daily schedule for routine HUC tasks.* Schedule routine tasks to be done at the time of day that produces the best outcome. Plan to perform regular tasks, such as monitoring the EMRs or transcribing doctors' orders and placing telephone calls, according to demand between the scheduled routine tasks. Verifying that the patient EMRs have current data and are within update guidelines may be the HUC's first task of the day. Follow the plan while making changes as required to improve use of time.
7. *Group activities.* Save time by grouping activities together, such as running necessary errands on the way to lunch, or if using paper charts checking to see if new forms are needed at the same time that reports are filed.
8. *Know the job and perform it well.* A nursing unit is made up of many people who work together to perform the overall function of caring for patients. For the nursing unit to function effectively, each person must know his or her job description and perform the tasks outlined in the job description. It is important to stay within the boundaries of the job and not drift over into performing tasks assigned to other health care personnel. For example, on a busy day it may seem appropriate to help out the nursing staff by assisting a patient to the restroom. This practice is not acceptable for two reasons: First, HUCs are not educationally prepared to perform clinical tasks; and second, when the HUC leaves the desk, health unit coordinating tasks are left unattended. An exception would be if a HUC is cross-trained as a certified nursing assistant (CNA) and is expected to do both jobs as necessary.
9. *Take breaks as assigned.* Often on a busy day, the immediate solution to getting the job done may appear to be to skip lunch and/or coffee breaks. Do not be tempted to do so. Often, spending a few minutes away from the pressure gives the HUC the opportunity to regroup and return to handle the situation with renewed vigor and speed.
10. *Delegate tasks to volunteers.* Determine which tasks hospital volunteers have been trained in and are allowed to do. Filing records in the chart and assembling patient information packets or admission packets are time-consuming tasks that can usually be performed by volunteer workers. Work out a plan to have volunteer assistance each day at the times that are most helpful. Remember that volunteer workers volunteer because they want to work. Verify that the volunteer has an ID badge if she or he has not been on the nursing unit before.
11. *Avoid unnecessary conversation.* Often, many other health care professionals gather at the nurses' station; thus it is very easy to be drawn into unnecessary conversation. Be aware of this, and avoid it when possible.
12. *Use a memory sheet.* Keep a notepad next to the telephone, to be used as a **memory sheet** to record names and the telephone line number when more than one caller is placed on hold.

Write down messages, and list tasks that cannot be completed at the moment (Fig. 7-6). To avoid delays in patient

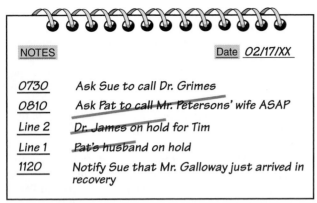

NOTES   Date _02/17/XX_

_0730_   Ask Sue to call Dr. Grimes

_0810_   ~~Ask Pat to call Mr. Petersons' wife ASAP~~

Line 2   ~~Dr. James on hold for Tim~~

Line 1   ~~Pat's husband on hold~~

_1120_   Notify Sue that Mr. Galloway just arrived in
            recovery

Figure 7-6 A notepad used as a memory sheet.

care and stress, write down all messages. Even a message that is urgent can be easily forgotten because of constant interruptions and activity on the nursing unit. Not relaying a message to a nurse that the surgery department needs to know if a patient is ready to be picked up will result in delays in the surgery schedule for the rest of the day. This will cause delays and stress to the surgeon, the surgery personnel, the nurse, and patients' families. Messages that are not urgent can be communicated to a member of the nursing team at a later time—for example, a message for Mary to call the pharmacy at her convenience. Rather than taking the time to find Mary, the information is recorded on the memory sheet, and when Mary returns to the nurses' station, the message can be given to her. A line is then drawn through the message on the memory sheet to indicate that the message has been communicated. Another use of the memory sheet would be to note that a call to a doctor's office that was not completed because the line was busy must be placed again. The doctor's telephone number and other pertinent data should be recorded, along with the time the first call was attempted. During an 8- or 12-hour shift, countless items will be recorded on the memory sheet. Near the end of the shift, all listed items should be checked to ensure that all have been completed, and any that remain should be completed.

> ⭐ **HIGH PRIORITY**
>
> The use of a memory sheet is an excellent method for remembering messages that need to be relayed and tasks that need to be completed. It also serves as a record of messages relayed and tasks completed.

Stress Management

Stress is a physical, chemical, or emotional factor that causes bodily or mental tension and may be a factor in disease causation. There are two types of stress: (l) **perennial stress**—the wear and tear of day-to-day living (e.g., traffic, school, work) with the feeling that one is a square peg trying to fit into a round hole—and (2) **crisis stress**, which results from common, uncontrollable, often unpredictable life experiences that have a profound effect on individuals (e.g., death, divorce, serious illness). Hospital units are often very stressful, and the personnel who deal with life-and-death situations often become extremely stressed. The HUC is at the center of all activity at the nursing station and is often said to be "in the

hot seat." The following stress management techniques may assist the HUC in dealing with stress.

Stress Management Techniques

1. Effective time management is the first step in managing stress.
2. Follow the time management techniques.
3. Realize that nurses, doctors, and other health care workers may be working under a lot of stress, so do not take their expressions of frustration personally.
4. Say "no" tactfully when asked to do additional work if there truly is not time.
5. Keep a sense of humor. Humor is a great stress reliever as long as it is timely and appropriate. Ethel Barrymore said, "You grow up the day you have your first real laugh at yourself."

Remember, 10% of stress is what actually happens, and 90% is the reaction to it.

Ergonomics for the Health Unit Coordinator

Ergonomics is the study of a workplace and equipment for the purpose of making the workplace more comfortable, improving comfort, efficiency, safety, and ease of use. Two types of common work-related injuries have been identified: (1) acute injuries, which consist of fractures, crushing, and low back strain injuries, and (2) cumulative injuries, which occur over time as a result of repetitive motion activity. Cumulative injuries include carpal tunnel syndrome, tendonitis, and low back pain. Discomfort and fatigue, whether personal or work related, can cause inefficiency, as well as workplace injuries. A comprehensive approach to ergonomics addresses three areas of work: physical, environmental, and emotional.

The following guidelines in each area may be of assistance in reducing injury risks for the HUC.

Guidelines for the Prevention of Workplace Injuries

- The computer monitor should be located where it will reduce awkward head and neck postures; position the monitor so that you must look slightly downward to look at the middle of the screen. The preferred viewing distance is 18 to 24 inches (Fig. 7-7).
- Chairs should be adjusted so that one can sit straight yet in a relaxed position, with a backrest supporting the small of the back and feet flat on the floor.
- Adjust the chair back to a slightly backward position and extend legs out slightly, so there are no sharp angles that result in pressure on hip or knee joints.
- Wrists should be straight while typing, with forearms level and elbows close to the body. Reduce bending of the wrists by moving the entire arm.
- Use a computer wrist pad.
- Eliminate situations that would require constant bending over to complete tasks.
- Shift weight in the chair frequently.
- Use proper body mechanics when lifting. Do not bend over with legs straight or twist while lifting, and avoid trying to lift above shoulder level.
- Take frequent mini-stretches of the neck (lower head in each direction for a 5-second count).

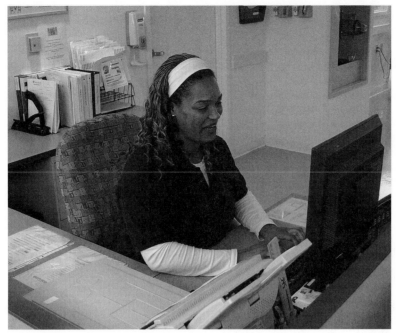

Figure 7-7 A health unit coordinator demonstrating proper body positioning when using a computer terminal.

BOX 7-1	ORGANIZING ITEMS WITHIN REACHING DISTANCE

- Counter space should be sufficient so people do not have to lean over others to obtain charts, office supplies, or other items.
- The label printer should be in close proximity to the work space.
- Frequently used forms should be stored within reaching distance.
- Charts (if paper charts are being used) should be located in an area where they can be easily reached.
- The telephone should be within easy reach.
- The fax machine should be in close proximity to the work space.
- The unit scanner should be in close proximity to the work space.
- The unit shredder or receptacle for paper to be shredded should be in close proximity.
- Any unit reference books and manuals should be kept within reaching distance.

- Stand, walk, and stretch back and legs at least every hour. These small breaks in position help avoid neuromuscular strain and alleviate the tension of job stress.

Organization of the Nurses' Station

A well organized and neat nurses' station gives the appearance of a well run nursing unit. First, use Box 7-1, *Organizing Items within Reaching Distance,* to check the work area at the nurses' station. Figure 7-8 shows the HUC with computer, telephone, scanner, label printer, and fax machine within close proximity. Before initiating a change in the work area, discuss these changes with all co-workers and the nurse manager. Take the time on occasion to stand back and observe the nurses' station area. Is it cluttered and disorganized in appearance? If so, take a moment to restore all items to their original places. Return charts to the chart rack (if paper charts are being used).

Nursing Unit Reference Materials

Most reference books and manuals are available on the nursing unit computers, and most doctors and nursing unit personnel have needed references books downloaded on their personal digital assistant (PDA) or smart phone. A small library of reference books and manuals may be kept on the nursing unit. These may include such sources as the following:

- *Physicians' Desk Reference* (PDR)
- The hospital formulary, which is used to define drugs and their uses and to check on dosages and on adverse effects
- The institutional policies and procedures manual, which is used to reference hospital policies and procedures
- A disaster manual, which is used to provide direction and to outline responsibilities in case of a disaster
- A laboratory manual, which is used to define laboratory tests, specimen amounts, and collections required to perform tests
- A diagnostic imaging manual, which is used to define diagnostic procedures and the preparations required to perform them

If not computerized, indexes of frequently used hospital extension numbers, in-hospital office numbers, and pager numbers are kept on the nursing unit and are kept up to date by the HUC. A communication book may be used to preserve organizational information between shifts (Fig. 7-9). Keeping co-workers informed helps the group work together as a team.

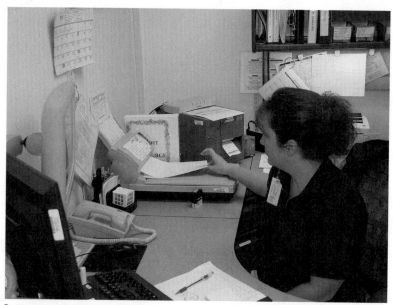

Figure 7-8 The health unit coordinator with the computer, telephone, scanner, label printer, and fax machine within close proximity.

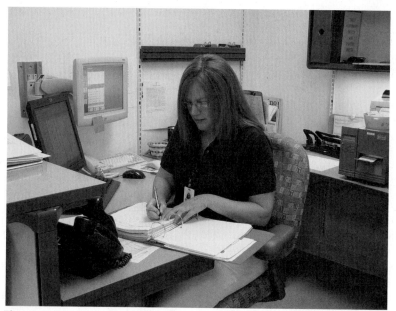

Figure 7-9 The health unit coordinator using a nursing unit communication book.

CONTINUOUS QUALITY IMPROVEMENT

Continuous quality improvement (CQI), a requirement of TJC, is the practice of continuously improving quality at every level of every department for every function of the health care organization. Most hospitals have CQI committees that oversee the assessment and improvement of work processes while focusing on what patients want and need.

How does this translate to the HUC? Quality improvement remains an important part of the job. Learn the language of quality. The quality movement is global because CQI results in products and services of better quality. Competition to provide the best product and service in the most efficient manner has increased worldwide. When completing HUC clinical hours or when newly hired as a HUC, one will likely have

more than one preceptor or trainer. It is beneficial to incorporate "best practices" from the efficient HUC and avoid the "inefficient practices" of the inefficient HUC. All experiences are learning opportunities. The HUC is often asked to serve on a committee to solve quality improvement problems involving nursing unit clerical processes. A committee that is focused on this process may use two techniques—application of the following five-step **problem-solving model,** and **brainstorming**.

The Five-Step Problem-Solving Model

1. Identify and analyze the problem.
2. Identify alternative plans for resolving the problem.
3. Choose the best plan.

4. Put the best plan into practice.
5. Evaluate the plan after it has been in place for a given time.

Application of the Five-Step Problem-Solving Model and Brainstorming

Example scenario: The admitting department reports to the nursing department that when patients are discharged, there is a long delay before the HUC provides this information to them. This causes inconvenience for patients who are going home and for those who are waiting for beds. The nurse manager asks Cynthia, a HUC, to join a committee (consisting of two admitting personnel, one nurse manager, and two HUCs) that has been assigned to find the cause and a solution to this problem. The committee meets several times and uses the five-step problem-solving model and brainstorming, as outlined below:

1. *Identify and analyze the problem:* The problem is discussed, and it is determined that discharged patients have to wait for their paperwork to be processed because the admitting department is not notified of the discharge in time, and new admissions have to wait for beds before they can be admitted—some lying on gurneys in the emergency room for hours or overnight. The group identifies possible causes of the problems and records them on slips of paper that Cynthia collects to share later with the entire group. It is determined that the probable cause of the problems is that nursing unit personnel want to get caught up with their work before receiving a new admission, so they ask the HUC to delay notifying the admitting department of discharges.
2. *Identify alternative plans for resolving the problem:* The brainstorming technique is used to identify alternative solutions to resolve the problem. Cynthia again collects the papers to share with the group as a whole. Some suggested solutions that are listed on a whiteboard are as follows: (a) ask the doctor to notify Admitting when discharging a patient, (b) hold a mandatory meeting for all HUCs to discuss the problem, and (c) create a policy requiring that a discharge order be sent to the Admitting department within 20 minutes after it has been written.
3. *Choose the best plan:* The committee members choose (c) as the best solution and plan the next meeting to create the policy.
4. *Put the best plan into practice:* The policy is created, approved, and implemented. The committee agrees to meet again in 6 weeks to evaluate the solution.
5. *Evaluate the plan after it has been in place for a given time:* The committee meets one last time to evaluate the plan and concludes that the discharge process has been greatly improved.

EXERCISE 3

Use the problem-solving model and the brainstorming technique to solve the following problem.

Hospital policy requires that a discharged patient be taken to his or her car via wheelchair. There is a long wait time after transport has been called until someone from transport arrives with a wheelchair. When asked why it takes so long to arrive, the transport personnel *blame the delay on "too many calls" or "a shortage of wheelchairs." The long waits causes anger and stress for the patients and their families and a delay in getting the room cleaned in preparation for a new patient. Because the HUC is stationary and the most visible, she or he is the person who hears the frustration and anger.*

1. Identify and analyze the problem.
2. Identify alternative plans for resolving the problem.
3. Choose the best plan.
4. Put the best plan into practice.
5. Evaluate the plan after it has been in place for a given time.

KEY CONCEPTS

To meet the challenge of management requires greater effort and motivation on the part of the HUC than just "getting the job done"; however, the effort and motivation are rewarding. Job success is self-made. To develop your career to its potential, take the step beyond "getting the job done," and employ essential management techniques. The use of the EMR and CPOE has increased management responsibilities and will require flexibility and additional education. Added responsibilities will vary greatly from hospital to hospital and will depend on the education, abilities, and motivation displayed by the HUC. Following ergonomic suggestions and adhering to time and stress management techniques will help make this job a more pleasurable experience.

Websites of Interest

"Time Management"—Improve time management skills: www.timethoughts.com/time-management.htm
Patient Room // 2020—Possibilities for future inpatients: www.nxthealth.org/51/patient-room-2020
Occupational Safety and Health Administration (OSHA): www.osha.gov/Safety and Health Topics / Ergonomics: www.osha.gov/SLTC/ergonomics/index.html
"The Basics of Stress": www.healthline.com/health/stress-information

REVIEW QUESTIONS

Visit the Evolve website to download and complete the following questions.

1. Define the following terms:
   a. ergonomics
   b. react
   c. respond

2. Describe the purpose and use of the following:
   a. census sheet
   b. memory sheet
   c. standard supply list
   d. supplies needs sheet
   e. census worksheet
   f. ADT sheet

3. List the five areas of management responsibilities as related to the HUC position.

4. List five departments that provide supplies to the nursing unit, and explain two systems used to restock supplies on the nursing unit.

5. Identify the department that would issue the following nursing unit supplies:
   a. pens and pencils
   b. patient snacks
   c. patient medications
   d. bed sheets and pillows
   e. elastic bandages and tongue blades

6. Identify the department that would be called to repair the following equipment or resolve the following problem:
   a. printer
   b. patient telephone
   c. nursing unit too hot
   d. scanner
   e. patient toilet backed up
   f. computer
   g. broken cupboard door

7. Discuss the emergency equipment that is located on a nursing unit.

8. Provide an example of patient equipment that would require a daily charge.

9. Explain the importance of the change-of-shift report, and list five items obtained from the change-of-shift report that would be recorded on the census worksheet for quick reference during a shift.

10. Discuss a method used to record the names of patients and patient charts that are temporarily away from the nursing unit, and explain the importance of recording this information.

11. Describe the process for sending and receiving medical records; list five guidelines for scanning medical records into the patient's EMR and seven guidelines for filing medical records in the patient's paper chart.

12. Explain the HUC responsibilities regarding the ADT sheet, ADT log book, and patient labels.

13. List nursing forms that the HUC may prepare on a daily basis.

14. List seven steps to follow when dealing with visitor complaints.

15. Explain the process of retrieving diagnostic test results with and without the EMR.

16. On arrival on the nursing unit, the following six tasks need be done:

   • There are two discharge orders to be processed.

   • A nurse comes out of a room and asks you to call a code arrest on a patient.

   • The unit telephone is ringing.

   • A doctor has entered an order for a surgery permit for a patient.

   • A doctor is waiting for medical records to be obtained from another hospital.

   • A tube has just arrived in the pneumatic tube system.

   a. Which task would take priority? (Write #1 next to that task.)

   b. Which task would be second in priority? (Write #2 next to that task.)

   c. Explain in what order you would handle the other tasks.

17. List 12 time management tips for the HUC.

18. List two types of stress, and provide an example of each.

19. List five techniques for dealing with stress on the job.

20. Identify two types of work-related injuries, and give an example of each.

21. List five guidelines that can be followed to avoid workplace injury.

22. List four items that should be within reaching distance of the HUC's desk area, and list at least six reference materials that would be located on the computers or stored in hard copy on the nursing unit.

23. Explain the possible consequences of not monitoring the patient's EMR or paper charts for HUC tasks or orders.

24. Explain the purpose of continuous quality improvement (CQI).

25. List the five steps that make up the problem-solving model.

26. Describe how you would respond to the following situations:
   a. Mrs. Robert Mendez, whose husband has been hospitalized for 3 weeks with a cerebral hemorrhage, walks up to the nurses' station and in a loud, angry voice states, "No one is taking care of my husband. When I came in today, his lunch tray was just sitting there, cold, no one was feeding him, and his bed was wet."
   b. Mr. Blair's doctor has written an order that only immediate family (his wife and son) may visit him. A female visitor with a small child asks what room Mr. Blair is in.
   c. A patient, Mrs. Lukas in room 365-1, complains that the other patient in her room has six people visiting her at this time, and she finds this very upsetting.

d. You have been employed for a month on a very busy surgical nursing unit. The scanner is located so far from the working area that each time you need to scan a document you must get up from your chair and walk to where it is located.

e. It is an especially hectic day, and one of the nurses is on a lunch break. You have completed all of the current tasks and are thinking of taking a break. A nurse approaches and asks, "Would you please help Mr. Tiesen to the restroom for me? His room is close to the nurses' station, so you'll be able to hear the telephone ring."

SURFING FOR ANSWERS

1. Go to www.mayoclinic.com/health/stress-assessment/ SR00029 and assess your stress level.
2. Locate two websites that provide tips for problem solving. List the two sites and discuss the tips provided.

CHAPTER **8**

The Patient's Electronic Medical Record or Chart

OUTLINE

CHAPTER OBJECTIVES

On completion of this chapter, you will be able to:

1. Define the terms in the vocabulary list.
2. Write the meaning of the abbreviations in the abbreviations list.
3. List six purposes for maintaining an electronic medical record (EMR) or paper chart for each patient.
4. Demonstrate knowledge of military time by converting military time to standard time and standard time to military time.
5. List five guidelines to be followed by all personnel when entering information into a patient's EMR.
6. Describe how the patient's medical records are organized and identified when paper charts are used, and list five guidelines to be followed by all personnel when writing on a patient's paper chart.

7. Identify four standard patient chart forms that are initiated in the admitting department.
8. State the purpose of seven standard chart forms included in a patient's electronic or paper admission packet, and list information that is included on the history and physical form.
9. Define what is meant by a *supplemental chart form*, and provide at least two examples of supplemental chart forms.
10. Explain the importance of accurately charting vital signs in a timely manner, and explain the correction of three types of errors on a graphic record.
11. Describe the purpose of a consent form, and list five guidelines to follow in the preparation of a consent form.
12. List four types of permits or release forms that patients may be required to sign during a hospital stay.
13. Describe the methods for correcting a labeling error and a written entry error on a patient's paper chart form.
14. List seven health unit coordinator (HUC) duties in monitoring and maintaining the patient's EMR.
15. List eight HUC duties in maintaining a patient's paper chart.
16. Explain the purposes and processes of splitting or thinning a patient's chart and reproducing chart forms.

VOCABULARY

Admission Packet A preassembled packet of standard chart forms to be used on admission of a patient to the nursing unit.

Allergy An acquired, abnormal immune response to a substance that does not normally cause a reaction; such substances may include medications, food, tape, and many other items.

Allergy Bracelet A plastic bracelet (usually red) that is worn by a patient that indicates allergies he or she may have.

Allergy Label A label affixed to the front cover of a patient's paper chart that indicates the patient's allergy/allergies.

Identification Labels Labels that contain individual patient information for identifying patient records or other personal items.

Name Alert A method of alerting staff when two or more patients with the same or similarly spelled last names are located on a nursing unit.

Old Record A patient's paper record from previous admissions, stored in the health information management department, that may be retrieved for review when a patient is admitted to the emergency room, nursing unit, or outpatient department; older microfilmed records also may be requested by the patient's doctor.

Split or Thin Chart Portions of the patient's current paper chart are removed when the chart becomes so full that it is unmanageable.

Standard Chart Forms Forms included in all inpatient paper charts that are used to regularly enter information about patients.

Stuffing Charts Placing extra chart forms in patients' paper charts so they will be available when needed.

Supplemental Chart Forms Patient chart forms used only when specific conditions or events dictate their use.

WALLaroo A locked workstation that is located on the wall outside a patient's room; it stores the patient's paper chart or a laptop computer, and when unlocked it forms a shelf to write on.

ABBREVIATIONS

Note: These abbreviations are listed as they are commonly written; however, they also may be seen in uppercase or lowercase letters and with or without periods.

Abbreviation	Meaning
H&P	history and physical
Hx	history
ID labels	identification labels
MAR	medication administration record
NKA	no known allergies
NKDA	no known drug allergies
NKFA	no known food allergies
NKMA	no known medication allergies

EXERCISE 1

Write the abbreviation for each term listed.

1. history
2. no known allergies
3. identification labels
4. history and physical
5. medication administration record
6. no known medication allergies
7. no known drug allergies
8. no known food allergies

EXERCISE 2

Write the meaning of each abbreviation listed.

1. ID labels	5. NKDA
2. NKFA	6. H&P
3. MAR	7. Hx
4. NKA	8. NKMA

PURPOSES AND USE OF A PATIENT'S ELECTRONIC MEDICAL RECORD OR PAPER CHART

The patient's electronic medical record (EMR) or paper chart serves many purposes, but for a health unit coordinator (HUC), the electronic record or chart is seen mainly as a means of communication between the doctor and the hospital staff.

The EMR or chart is also used for planning patient care, for research, and for educational purposes. As a legal electronic record or documentation, the medical record protects the patient, the doctor, the staff, and the hospital or health care facility. Careful entries and notations by doctors and other personnel provide an electronic or written record of the patient's illness, care, treatment, and outcomes of hospitalization. If the patient is readmitted to the hospital or health care facility, the paper chart may be retrieved from the health information management system (HIMS) department, also commonly called the *medical records department.* The advantage of the EMR is that all previous health information is immediately available on the computer.

HIGH PRIORITY

Purposes of a Patient's Electronic Medical Record or Paper Chart
- Means of communication
- Documentation and planning of patient care
- Research
- Education
- Legal record or documentation
- History of patient illnesses, care, treatment, and outcomes

The Patient Electronic Medical Record or Paper Chart as a Legal Document

When a patient is discharged, health information management personnel will analyze and check the EMR for completeness and will notify the appropriate nurses and/or doctors when they must go into the computer to complete the records. The patient's previous EMR will be available on computer to the patient's doctor, or if the patient is readmitted to the hospital. The Security Rule, a key part of the Health Insurance Portability and Accountability Act (HIPAA), protects a patient's electronically stored information (see Chapter 6).

The paper chart must be sent to HIMS as soon as possible. Health information management personnel will analyze and check the chart for completeness. When records are not complete or signatures are missing, those chart forms are flagged, and the appropriate nurses and/or doctors are notified that they must come to HIMS to complete or sign the chart forms.

Doctors and nurses must go to HIMS to see or complete old patient records if the patient has not been readmitted to the hospital. Completed paper charts are indexed and stored where they are available for retrieval as needed.

Older paper records are microfilmed (documents are placed on film in reduced scale) and stored. On request, health information management personnel may retrieve microfilmed records. The length of time that the record must be stored depends on the laws of the state. Unless a patient has been readmitted to the hospital, HIMS will not send an **old record** to nursing units.

The patient's electronic or paper medical record may be subpoenaed and may serve as evidence in a court of law. As a legal document, it must be maintained in an acceptable manner.

Military Time

Military time is a system that uses all 24 hours in a day (each hour has its own number) rather than repeating hours and using AM and PM. When military time is used, there are always four digits, the first two digits representing hours and the second two representing minutes. For example, 1:45 AM is recorded as 0145, and 1:45 PM is recorded as 1345; the colon is not needed when military time is used (Table 8-1). The hours after midnight are recorded as 0100, 0200, and so forth. Thirty minutes after midnight is written as 0030. Twelve noon is recorded as 1200, and the hours that follow are arrived at by adding the

TABLE 8-1 Standard and Military Time Comparisons

Standard Time	Military Time	Standard Time	Military Time
12:15 AM	0015	1:00 PM	1300
12:30 AM	0030	1:15 PM	1315
12:45 AM	0045	1:30 PM	1330
1:00 AM	0100	1:45 PM	1345
2:00 AM	0200	2:00 PM	1400
3:00 AM	0300	3:00 PM	1500
4:00 AM	0400	4:00 PM	1600
5:00 AM	0500	5:00 PM	1700
6:00 AM	0600	6:00 PM	1800
7:00 AM	0700	7:00 PM	1900
8:00 AM	0800	8:00 PM	2000
9:00 AM	0900	9:00 PM	2100
10:00 AM	1000	10:00 PM	2200
11:00 AM	1100	11:00 PM	2300
12:00 Noon	1200	12:00 Midnight	2400

hours after noon to 1200. Thus 1:00 PM is 1200 + 100 = 1300, 2 PM is 1200 + 200 = 1400, and so forth. See Figure 8-1 for a comparison of standard and military times. Military time is used with the EMR and paper chart systems and eliminates confusion because hours are not repeated, and AM or PM is unnecessary.

SKILLS CHALLENGE

To practice converting standard time to military time, complete Activity 8-1 in the *Skills Practice Manual.*

Confidentiality

As was discussed in Chapter 6, the EMR or paper chart is confidential, and the HUC is a custodian of all patient medical records (electronic or paper) on the unit. Any information provided by the patient to the health care facility and the medical staff is confidential. All health care personnel are required to have a code and a password to gain access to a patient's EMR. Portions of the patient's EMR may be available only to the patient's doctor and nurses.

HIGH PRIORITY

All access to a patient's electronic medical record (EMR) is monitored and recorded in the system. This serves to protect patient confidentiality and is a way to trace any errors or modifications made in the patient's EMR.

THE ELECTRONIC MEDICAL RECORD

The patient's EMR may be accessed by health care personnel after entering a user ID and a password. Once logged in, the health care personnel are able to access and should access only the EMR of the patients in their specific nursing unit. Health care personnel choose the patient's name from the nursing unit census displayed on the screen; this will allow them to view

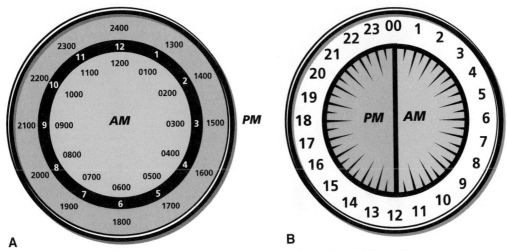

Figure 8-1 A, A 24-hour clock showing military time. **B,** Military time.

and enter information into the patient's EMR. An icon will be displayed next to a patient's name when there is a task or communication for the nurse or HUC written by the patient's doctor. A name alert flag may be placed on the patient's EMR when two or more patients with the same or similarly spelled names are located on the unit. If an order has been written stating that the patient's admission is not to be published, NINP (no information, no publication) is noted on the EMR or the patient may be listed as a "confidential patient."

Guidelines to Follow When Entering Information into the Patient's Electronic Medical Record

1. All entries into the EMR must be accurate.
2. Handwritten progress notes, electrocardiograms, consents, anesthesia records, and outside records and reports must be scanned into the EMR.
3. Errors made in care or treatment must be documented and cannot be falsified.
4. All entries into the EMR must include the date and time (military or standard) of the entry.
5. Abbreviations may be used in keeping with the health care facility's list of "approved abbreviations."

THE PAPER CHART

Guidelines to Follow When Writing in a Patient's Paper Chart

All persons who write in the paper chart follow standard guidelines. The HUC has minor charting tasks but is responsible for patient charts and so should be aware of the following basic rules:

1. All paper chart form entries must be made in ink. This is to ensure permanence of the record. Black ink is preferred by many health care facilities because it produces a clearer picture when the record is microfilmed, faxed, or reproduced on a copier.
2. Written entries on paper chart forms must be legible and accurate. Entries may be made in script or printed. Diagnostic reports, history and physical examination reports, and surgery reports are usually computer generated.

3. Recorded entries on the paper chart may not be obliterated or erased. The method for correcting errors is outlined later in this chapter.
4. All written entries on paper chart forms must include the date and time (military or standard) of the entry.
5. Abbreviations may be used in keeping with the health care facility's list of "approved abbreviations."

The Chart Binder

Forms that constitute the patient's paper chart are usually kept together in a three-ring binder. The binder may open from the bottom, or it may be a notebook that opens from the side, the top, or the bottom (Fig. 8-2).

The chart forms in the binder are sectioned off by dividers placed in the chart according to the sequence set forth by the health care facility (Fig. 8-3).

Paper charts are identified for each patient with a label that contains the patient's name and the doctor's name. The room and bed number may be written on the outside of the chart binder. Many health care facilities use colored tape on the outside of the chart to assist doctors in identifying their patients' charts. An **allergy label** is affixed to the chart binder if the patient has a medication, food, adhesive tape, or other type of allergy. Labels or tape affixed to chart binders are also used to alert the hospital staff of special situations. For example, a **name alert**, a piece of tape with *name alert* recorded on it, may be placed on the chart binder to remind staff that another patient with the same or a similarly spelled last name is housed on the unit. When an order indicates that a patient's admission is not to be published, *NINP* is often recorded on the chart binder to remind staff members that no information about a particular patient is to be issued.

The Chart Rack for Paper Charts

Many types of chart racks are available on the market. One type allows patient paper charts to be placed in a chart rack in which each slot on the rack holds one patient chart. Slots are labeled with the room and bed numbers; they usually are numbered in the same sequence as the rooms on the nursing unit (Fig. 8-4). Another type of chart storage is a **WALLaroo,** a locked

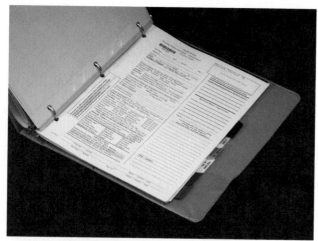

Figure 8-2 Patient's chart with dividers.

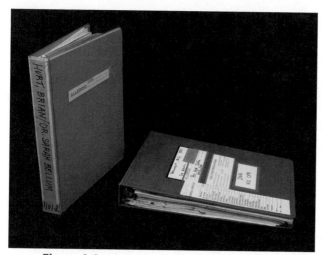

Figure 8-3 Patient chart binders properly labeled.

workstation that is located on the wall outside the patient's room. It stores a patient's paper chart or a laptop computer and when unlocked forms a shelf to write on (Fig. 8-5).

 HIGH PRIORITY

Health care facilities that have implemented the electronic medical record are utilizing the WALLaroo located just outside the patient's room as a computer workstation.

PATIENT IDENTIFICATION LABELS

A packet of patient **identification labels** is printed from the computer when the patient is admitted and as needed during the hospital stay. Information on the identification labels usually includes the following: the patient's name, age, sex, account number, health record number, admission date, and attending physician's name; a bar code may be included for identification purposes (Fig. 8-6). When the EMR is implemented, identification labels are kept in a "label book"; and when paper charts are used, they are kept in each patient's chart. The identification labels are used on consents, specimens, clothing, and

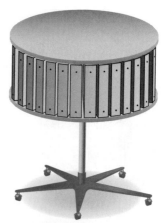

Figure 8-4 Chart rack.

other belongings. Labels may be generated from the computer and printed on a label printer.

STANDARD PATIENT CHART FORMS

Preparing the Patient's Paper Chart

Each health care facility has specific standard forms that are placed in all patients' paper charts. These forms are preassembled, clipped together (by the HUC or by volunteers), and filed in a drawer or on shelves near the HUC area. Some hospitals use computerized chart forms. These chart forms can be printed for individual patients with patient identification information printed on the forms. These assembled forms are often referred to as an **admission packet.**

On a patient admission, the HUC obtains an admission packet from the drawer or shelf and labels each form with the patient's identification (ID) label. If the forms are computerized, the HUC chooses the patient's name on the computer and prints the forms with the patient's identification information printed on them. Forms that need dates and days of the week are filled in and are then are placed behind the proper chart divider in a chart binder (Box 8-1, *Twelve Standard Chart Forms*).

 HIGH PRIORITY

When the electronic medical record (EMR) is implemented, information details are directly entered or scanned into the patient's EMR. Patient identification labels are placed in a binder that contains labels and face sheets for all patients on that nursing unit.

 SKILLS CHALLENGE

To practice preparing a patient's paper chart, complete Activity 8-2 in the *Skills Practice Manual.*

Standard patient chart forms are included in all inpatient paper charts and may vary in different hospitals. When the EMR is implemented, information is entered into the computer on similar electronic forms. The following **standard chart forms** are the most commonly used presently.

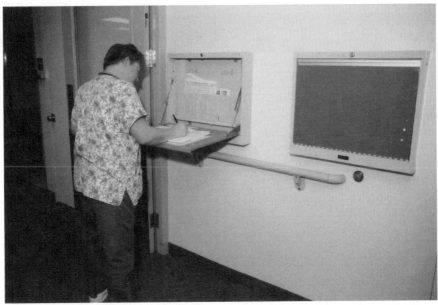

Figure 8-5 A workstation with storage for the patient's paper chart is called a WALLaroo.

Patient's name ——	Williams, John	175-09-02 —— Medical record #
Account number ——	0078376	Surg —— Type of service
Date of admission ——	DOA 01/14/20XX	DOB 05/07/39 —— Date of birth
Age - Sex ——	67Y M	Dr. Hy Hopes —— Attending doctor
Bar code ——	0‖‖‖‖‖‖‖‖	MC/BCBS —— Insurance

Figure 8-6 Patient identification label.

BOX 8-1	**TWELVE STANDARD CHART FORMS**

Initiated in the Admitting Department
1. Face sheet or information form
2. Admission and service agreement form
3. Patients' rights
4. Advance directive checklist

Initiated by the Physician
5. History and physical form (H&P)

Included in the Admission Packet
6. Physician's order form
7. Physician's progress record
8. Nurse's admission record
9. Nurse's progress notes or flow sheets
10. Medication administration record (MAR)
11. Nurse's discharge planning form
12. Physician's discharge summary

Standard Patient Chart Forms Initiated in the Admitting Department

1. Face Sheet or Information Form

The face sheet or information form (Fig. 8-7) contains information about the patient, such as name, address, telephone number, name of employer, admission diagnosis, health care insurance policy information, and next of kin. In most health care facilities, the form originates in the admitting department and is then sent to the unit to be placed in the patient's chart. When the EMR is implemented, the information is entered directly into the patient's EMR. Several face sheets (at least five) are kept in the binder containing patient labels when EMR is used and in each patient's chart when paper charts are used. Face sheets are taken by the attending physician and by consulting physicians to be used for billing purposes. The HUC can generate copies of the face sheet on the computer. The face sheet is also used on the nursing unit to locate information when staff must call the family or call consulting physicians.

2. Admission and Service Agreement Form (may also be called Conditions of Admission [COA])

The admission and service agreement form (Fig. 8-8) is signed by the patient in the admitting department and is then sent to the admitting unit to be scanned into the patient's EMR or placed in the patient's paper chart. The form provides legal permission to the hospital and doctor to treat the patient and also serves as a financial agreement.

3. Patients' Rights

The Joint Commission requires that all hospitals have a bill of rights and a notice of the facility's privacy practices. Copies must be given to each patient or legal guardian of the patient on admission. In addition, a copy of the bill of rights should be posted at entrances and other prominent places throughout the hospital. The patients' bill of rights varies in wording among hospitals, but all are based on the basic ethical principles outlined in Chapter 6.

Opportunity Medical Center

Account #	Admit Date	Admit Time	Reg Init	Brought By	Info Provided By	MR Number
01149408	01/14/XX	1430	EG	Wife	Patient	30897811

Admitting Physician	Primary Care Phys.	Room #	Type	Service	Discharge Date	Time
John Bauer	John Bauer	406		Surg		

Patient Last Name First Middle	Former Name	Race	Rel Pref	Social Security #
Williams, John		C	do not	111-11-1111

Patient Address	Apt. No.	City	State	Zip Code	Patient Phone #
294 W Filmore St		Sinclaire	NJ	90376-9009	222-222-2222

Driver's License #	Age	Birth Date	Birthplace	Gender	MS	Occupation	Accident? Date/Time
N/A	67	05/07/39	Ohio	M	M	Teacher	N/A

Patient Employer	Employer Address	Employer Phone
Retired May 2005		

Spouse Name	Spouse Address	City	State	Spouse Phone
Elaine Ann	9030 W. 3 Ave	Peoria	Ohio	200-330-3333

Emergency Contact	Relationship	Home Phone	Cell Phone	Work Phone
Jean Sounders	daughter	102-202-2002	N/A	102-101-1001

Admitting Diagnosis	Admit Type	ICD9	Admit Source
MVA - diabetes	Surg		Clinic

Primary Insurance Plan	Primary Policy #	Authorization #	Primary Policy Holder
Medicare	111-11-1111A		

Insurance Plan #2	Secondary Policy #	Authorization #	Secondary Policy Holder
Pacific Care	22020111		

Insurance Plan #3	Tertiary Policy #	Authorization #	Tertiary Policy Holder

Guarantor Name	Rel to Pt	Mailing Address	Guarantor Phone

Guarantor Occupation	Employer	Employer Address	Employer Phone

Billing Remarks: _____

Principal Diagnosis:	MVA	Code:	050
Secondary Diagnosis:	Diabetes	Code:	268

Operations and Procedures:	Physician	Date	Code

Consulting Physician: _____

Final Disposition: ◯ Discharged ◯ Transferred ◯ Left AMA ◯ Expired   ◯ Autopsy ◯ Yes ◯ No

I certify that my identification of the principal and secondary diagnosis and the procedures performed is accurate to the best of my knowledge.

Opportunity Medical Center

_____

Attending Physician   Date

Figure 8-7 Face sheet or information form. (Copyright 2004, Elsevier Inc. All Rights Reserved.)

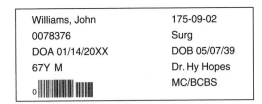

Williams, John	175-09-02
0078376	Surg
DOA 01/14/20XX	DOB 05/07/39
67Y M	Dr. Hy Hopes
	MC/BCBS

MEDICAL TREATMENT AGREEMENT
(Conditions of Admission)

Patient or the patient's legal representative agrees to the following terms of hospital admission:

1. **MEDICAL TREATMENT :**
    The patient consents to the treatment, services and procedures which may be performed during this hospitalization or on an outpatient basis, which may include but are not limited to laboratory procedures, X-ray examinations, medical and surgical treatments or procedures, anesthesia, or hospital services rendered under the general or specific instructions of the responsible physicians or other health care providers. The hospital may establish certain criteria which will automatically trigger the performance of specific tests which the patient agrees may be performed without any further separate consent. This Medical Treatment Agreement covers E-ICU services and outpatient services provided by the hospital's extended treatment facilities, including services at other Banner facilities. Where the hospital routinely provides services for inpatients at an outpatient facility in close proximity to the hospital, the patient consents to transport to the outpatient facility for the requested services. This Medical Treatment Agreement is effective for this inpatient admission/outpatient visit and/or for recurring outpatient services of the same type for a period of one year following its execution. For obstetrical patients this Medical Treatment Agreement covers both outpatient and inpatient services and also covers and applies to both the obstetrical patient and the newborn(s). Photographs or videotapes may be made of diagnostic and surgical procedures for treatment and/or training purposes.

2. **LEGAL RELATIONSHIP BETWEEN HOSPITAL AND HEALTH CARE PROVIDERS:**
    The patients will be treated by his/her attending physician or health care providers and be under his/her care and supervision. Physicians and other health care providers furnishing services to the patient, including but not limited to the emergency room physician, hospitalist, radiologist, pathologist, and anesthesiologist, are generally not employees or agents of the hospital. These providers may bill separately for their services. Questions about whether a health care provider is an agent or employee of the hospital should be directed to Administration during normal business hours, and the Administrator On Call or the Chief Nursing Officer/Designee after hours, weekends, and holidays.

3. **MONEY AND VALUABLES:**
    VALUABLES AND MONEY SHOULD BE RETURNED TO YOUR RESIDENCE. The hospital has a safe in which to keep money or valuables. The hospital will not be responsible for loss of or damage to items not deposited in the safe (such as glasses, dentures, hearing aids, contact lenses, jewelry or money).

4. **TEACHING PROGRAM:**
    The hospital participates in training programs for physicians and heath care personnel. Some patient services may be provided by persons in training under the supervision and instruction of physicians or hospital employees. These persons in training may also observe care given to the patient by physicians and hospital employees.

5. **RELEASE OF INFORMATION:**
    The patient acknowledges and agrees that medical and/or financial records (INCLUDING INFORMATION REGARDING ALCOHOL OR DRUG ABUSE, HIV RELATED OR OTHER COMMUNICABLE DISEASE RELATED INFORMATION) may be released to the following.
    A. Health care providers who are providing or have provided health care to the patient or their agents; any individual or entity responsible for the payment of hospital's or other provider's charges; to health care providers or organizations accrediting the facility or conducting utilization reveiw, quality assurance, or peer review; and to the hospital's and provider's legal representatives and professional liability carriers.
    B. Individuals and organizations engaged in medical education and research, provided that information may only be released for use in medical studies and research without patient identifying information.
    C. Individuals and entities as specified by federal and state law and/or in the hospital's Notice of Privacy Practices.
    D. Patient records of services provided at any Banner facility or Banner Surgicenter may be exchanged among these facilities where necessary to provide appropriate patient care. This Release shall continue for so long as the medical and/or financial records are needed for any of the above-stated purposes.

6. **CONTRABAND:**
    Drugs, alcochol, weapons and other articles specified as contraband by the hospital may not be brought onto hospital premises. Any illegal substance will be confiscated and turned over to law enforcement authorities. If the presence of contraband is suspected, the patient's room and belongings may be searched, and visitors may be searched before visitation.

ACKNOWLEDGEMENTS
☐   I acknowledge receipt of the hospital's "Patient Rights and Responsibilities" brochure.
☐   I acknowledge receipt of the hospital's "Notice of Privacy Practices".
☐   I acknowledge receipt of either the "Important Message from Medicare" or the "Important from Tricare" (if applicable).
I have read and understand this Medical Treatment Agreement, have received a copy of this agreement, the hospital's "Notice of Privacy Practices," the hospital's "Patient Rights and Responsibilities" brochure, and where applicable the "Important Message from Medicare/Tricare." I am the patient, the parent of a minor child, or the legal representative of the patient and am authorized to act on the patient's behalf to sign this agreement.

_____   _____
Patient/Parent of Minor Child/Court-Appointed Guardian   Witness
Patient-Appointed Agent/Statutory Surrogate
Please circle the correct title   _____
                                                                Date: Time:

WHITE - Chart Copy, **CANARY** - Patient Services Copy, **PINK** - Patient Copy

Figure 8-8 Admission and service agreement.

Continued

Williams, John	175-09-02
0078376	Surg
DOA 01/14/20XX	DOB 05/07/39
67Y M	Dr. Hy Hopes
	MC/BCBS

MEDICAL TREATMENT AGREEMENT
(Conditions of Admission)

HEALTH CARE DIRECTIVES

If you have a Health Care Power of Attorney and/or Living Will you should provide it to the hospital to best assure that the hospital is aware of your wishes and that they are followed if you become unable to make or communicate your own health care decisions. If you do not have a Living Will or Health Care Power of Attorney and wish to have one, we can provide information and assistance.

I have completed a Health Care Power of Attorney

<u>If Yes:</u>
- ☐ Power of Attorney presented to hospital
- ☐ Power of Attorney requested from family

<u>If No:</u>
- ☐ "Making Decisions About Your Health Care" brochure provided
- ☐ Power of Attorney form provided
- ☐ Information declined

I have completed a Living Will

<u>If Yes:</u>
- ☐ Living Will presented to hospital
- ☐ Living Will requested from family

<u>If No:</u>
- ☐ "Making Decisions About Your Health Care" brochure provided
- ☐ Living Will form provided
- ☐ Information declined

Health Care Power of Attorney

To be completed by the **patient** only when a Health Care Power of Attorney has not been provided to the hospital.

Health Care Power of Attorney A.R.S. § 36-3224: I, as principal, designate:

_____

Name

_____

Address

_____

Phone

as my agent to act in all matters relating to my health care, including, without limitation, full power to give or refuse consent to all medical, surgical, hospital and related health care. This Health Care Power of Attorney is effective upon my inability to make or communicate health care decisions. All of my agent's actions under this power during any period when I am unable to make or communicate health care decisions, or when there is uncertainty whether I am dead or alive have the same effect on my heirs, devisees and personal representatives as if I were alive, competent, and acting for myself. This health care directive is authorized under A.R.S. § 36-3221 and continues in effect including for subsequent admissions, for all who may rely upon it except to those to whom I have given notice of its revocation.

_____   _____   _____

Patient   Date   Time

I was present when the patient signed and dated this Health Care Power of Attorney. The Patient appears to be of sound mind and free from duress at the time he/she executed this Power of Attorney.

_____

*Witness

(*The witness may **not** be related to the patient by blood, marriage, or adoption; may **not** be the agent appointed as the Health Care Power of Attorney; may **not** be entitled to any portion of the patient's estate; and may **not** be directly involved in the patient's care.)

☐ **Unable to complete due to the need for immediate medical attention**

Additional attempts to complete

Date: _____ Time: _____ Initials: _____ Reasons: _____

Date: _____ Time: _____ Initials: _____ Reasons: _____

Date: _____ Time: _____ Initials: _____ Reasons: _____

WHITE - Chart Copy, **CANARY** - Patient Services Copy, **PINK** - Patient Copy

Figure 8-8, cont'd

Williams, John	175-09-02
0078376	Surg
DOA 01/14/20XX	DOB 05/07/39
67Y M	Dr. Hy Hopes
	MC/BCBS

FINANCIAL AGREEMENT

I agree that, in return for the services provided to the patient by the hospital or other health care providers, I will pay the account of the patient or make financial arrangements for payment prior to discharge satisfactory to the hospital and all other providers. I will pay the hospital's charges as set out in the hospital's chargemaster, which are the rates currently on file with the Arizona Department of Health Services. I understand that the chargemaster is available for inspection upon request. I understand that the rates charged for services rendered to the patient may differ from the amounts other patients are obligated to pay based upon each patient's private insurance coverage, Medicare/AHCCCS coverage, or lack of any such coverage. A delinquent account will be subject to interest at the legal rate of 10% per annum.

I request that payment of any authorized Medicare benefits be made on my behalf. I assign the benefits payable for physician services to the physician or organization furnishing the services or authorize such physician or organization to submit a claim to Medicare for payment.

If any signer (or the patient) is entitled to benefits of any type whatsoever, under any policy of health of liability insurance insuring patient, or any other party liable to patient, that benefit is hereby assigned to hospital and/or to the provider group rendering service, for application on patient's bill. HOWEVER, IT IS UNDERSTOOD THAT THE UNDERSIGNED AND PATIENT ARE PRIMARILY RESPONSIBLE FOR PAYMENT OF PATIENT'S BILL.

IN GRANTING ADMISSION OR RENDERING TREATMENT, THE HOSPITAL AND OTHER PROVIDERS ARE RELYING ON MY AGREEMENT TO PAY THE ACCOUNT. EMERGENCY CARE WILL BE PROVIDED WITHOUT REGARD TO THE ABILITY TO PAY.

X _____   _____
Patient or Other Party Agreeing to Pay   Relationship to Patient

_____   _____
Witness   Date & Time

WHITE-Medical Record Copy • **CANARY**-Patient Services Copy • **PINK**-Patient Copy

Figure 8-8, cont'd

4. Advance Directive Checklist Form

An advance directive checklist form (Fig. 8-9) documents that a patient has been informed of his or her choice to declare health care decisions. Advance directives are discussed in Chapter 19. The Patient Self Determination Act of 1990 mandates that all patients admitted to a health care facility must be asked whether they have or wish to have an advance directive. The patient or guardian signs the advance directive checklist, then it is sent to the admitting unit to be scanned into the patient's EMR or placed in the patient's paper chart to document that the patient was advised of his or her choices. When the EMR is being used, the advance directive form may be converted into an electronic version.

Standard Patient Chart Forms Included in the Admission Packet

1. Physician's Order Form

The physician's order form or doctor's order sheet is the form on which the doctor requests care and treatment procedures for the patient (see Chapter 9, the *Skills Practice Manual*, and the Evolve website for examples of orders). All orders must be dated and signed by the physician writing the order. When the EMR is implemented, the physician enters orders directly into the computer, and the orders are routed to the appropriate departments, including the pharmacy. When paper charts are used, the physician's order form may be available in a single-page format (in which case the HUC will fax or scan and send a copy to the pharmacy) or in duplicate format (in which case the HUC will send the copy of the original physician's order [commonly called the *pharmacy copy*] to order the patient's medications). It is essential that the pharmacist see the original physician's orders to eliminate errors in the transcription process. A copy may also be created on a fax machine and given to the appropriate nursing personnel.

2. Physician's Progress Record

The progress record is a form on which the physician records the patient's progress during the patient's hospitalization. Medical staff rules and regulations and the patient's condition

ADVANCE DIRECTIVE CHECKLIST

Patient Name: _____

❏ Advance Directives Brochure Provided   ❏ Advance Directives Brochure Refused

The Following Information Was Obtained From: ❏ Patient   ❏ Other: _____

❏ **Patient HAS executed the following Advance Directive(s):**	COPY RECEIVED		COPY REQUESTED
	THIS ADMIT	**PRIOR ADMIT**	
❏ Declaration for Health Care Decisions (Living Will)	❏	❏	❏
❏ Medical Power of Attorney (MPOA)	❏	❏	❏
Name: _____			
Relationship: _____			
❏ Mental Healthcare Power of Attorney (MHPOA)	❏	❏	❏
Name: _____			
Relationship: _____			
❏ Combination Power of Attorney (that includes MPOA language)	❏	❏	❏
❏ Other: (specify)	❏	❏	❏

❏ Patient **HAS NOT** executed Advance Directive(s). (Check items below **ONLY** when talking with patient.)	**PATIENT Was Advised On** _____ . (date)
❏ **PATIENT** requests more information.	❏ of the *right to accept or refuse medical treatment.*
❏ Social Services notified.	❏ of the *right to formulate Advance Directives.*
❏ **PATIENT** chooses not to execute Advance Directives at this time.	❏ of the *right to receive medical treatment whether or not there is an Advance Directive.*

For Home Health/Hospice Use Only:

❏ Patient **HAS** EXECUTED Prehospital Medical Care (Arizona's Orange Card).

❏ Patient was advised of the *right to have Advance Directives followed by the health care facility and caregivers to the extent permitted by law.*

Signature of Facility Representative:	Department:	Date:

IF ADVANCED DIRECTIVE IS UNAVAILABLE, the patient indicates that the substance of the directive is as follows: *(see reverse for script)*

Living Will: _____

Medical Power of Attorney: _____

❏ Patient signature (legal representative if applicable): _____

❏ Witness signature (if patient physically unable to sign): _____ Reason: _____

Verification Upon Admit/Re-Admit or Transfer:

Verified with patient/legal representative that Advance Directives in medical record are current.	Verified with patient/legal representative that Advance Directives in medical record are current.	Verified with patient/legal representative that Advance Directives in medical record are current.
Signature:	Signature:	Signature:
Date:	Date:	Date:

PATIENT IDENTIFICATION

Williams, John	175-09-02
0078376	Surg
DOA 01/14/20XX	DOB 05/07/39
67Y M	Dr. Hy Hopes
‖‖‖‖‖‖	MC/BCBS

Figure 8-9 Advance directive checklist.

Directions for Completing the Advance Directive Checklist

A. Complete the first section as follows:

1. Write patient's name in the designated area and place patient label in lower right corner.
2. Offer a brochure. Check the appropriate box.
3. Indicate from whom the information was obtained: Patient or Other.
   If "Other", indicate the relationship to the patient.

B. Information for the second section may come from someone other than the patient.

1. Ask which (if any) advance directives the patient has executed and verify currency. Check all boxes that apply.
2. If a copy is provided check the box in the "Copy Received, This Admit" column across from the specific advance directive. If a copy was provided prior to this visit, check the appropriate box in the "Copy Received, Prior Admit" column. If neither, ask for a copy and check the "Copy Requested" column.

C. Information for the third section must be obtained from the patient.

1. If the patient has not executed advance directives, ask if the patient would like more information (in which case, Social Services should be notified) or if the patient chooses not to execute advance directives at this time. Check the corresponding box.
2. Advise the patient of his/her rights as listed on the form, check each box as you read each right, and list the date in the space provided.

D. Fourth section to be completed by Home Health/Hospice admitting RN.

E. Sign the form, indicate your department and date of signing. <u>The patient, or if applicable, the patient's legal representative must sign the form. In the event the patient is mentally competent and able to communicate but physically unable to sign the form, a witness may sign the form. A reason must be indicated describing the physical ailment preventing the patient from signing.</u> The original form is kept in the medical record.

To determine substance of the document, it is best to query the patient in this way:

"Mr./Mrs. _____ , I understand you have a Living Will/MPOA.......Can you tell me what it says?" (If the patient is unable to indicate this, offer to have them execute new documents and refer to Social Services.)

F. The final section should be completed by any PHCT member receiving the patient upon admit/re-admit or transfer. Verify with patient/legal representative that Advance Directives in medical record are current. Signature and date required.

*   **Refer to Advance Directives Policy, in the Patient Rights section of the Clinical Policy & Procedure Manual.**

Figure 8-9, cont'd

dictate the interval allowed between notations (usually daily). The attending physician, residents, hospitalist, and consultants may write on this form. When the EMR is implemented, the physician may enter progress notes directly into the computer or may handwrite them and request that the HUC scan them into the patient's EMR. When paper charts are used the progress notes are kept in the patient binders.

3. Nurse's Admission Record

The nurse's admission record (Fig. 8-10) usually precedes or leads into the nurse's notes. On admission to the nursing unit, the patient answers printed questions on the form. A member of the nursing care team also compiles a short nursing history (Hx) from the patient or family member regarding the patient's daily living activities, present illness, and medications the patient is taking. Also recorded on the nurse's admission history form are the patient's vital signs, height, weight, and any allergies to food or medications. When the EMR is implemented, the nurse enters the admission information, including patient allergies, height, and weight, directly into the patient's EMR. The clinical decision support system then provides an allergy alert on the ordering screen if the doctor orders a medication for which a patient allergy has been documented. When paper charts are used, the HUC enters this vital information, including height, weight, and allergies, into a patient profile screen on the computer. It is a responsibility of the HUC to label the front of the patient's chart with an **allergy** sticker. It is standard practice in some facilities to use red ink to note patients' allergies on chart forms including the patient's medication administration record (MAR) and Kardex (discussed in Chapter 9). If the patient has reported having no known allergies **(NKA),** that is also noted. **NKDA or NKMA** may be used to indicate no known drug or medication allergies on the MAR. A patient's food allergy or no known food allergies **(NKFA)** would also be noted on chart forms including the patient's Kardex and MAR and the nutritional care department would be informed. Some facilities provide a separate allergy form that is included under the hard cover of the chart binder. When using the EMR or paper chart, the HUC places an insert into a plastic **allergy bracelet** for the patient to wear.

4. Nurse's Progress Notes or Flow Sheet

The nurse's progress notes are a standard chart form that is used to outline the patient's care and treatment and to record the treatment, progress, and activities of the patient. The nurse's observations of the patient are recorded on the nurse's progress notes. Entries must be dated, timed, and signed by the nurse who is making the entry; the signature usually includes the nurse's first name, last name, and professional status (RN, LPN). These notes relate to the patient's behavior and reaction to treatment and other care ordered by the physician. The form serves as the written communication between the doctor and the nursing staff. When the EMR is implemented, the nurse's progress notes are entered directly into the patient's EMR. The nurse may use portable computers (discussed in Chapter 4) to enter information into the EMR at the patient's bedside. The form is used during patient care conferences to evaluate patient progress and to plan discharge and future care.

When paper charts are used the form is often located on a nurse's clipboard, outside the room in a chart rack or the WALLaroo. Nursing students, registered nurses (RNs), licensed practical nurses (LPNs), and, in some facilities, certified nursing assistants (CNAs) may record on this form. Black ink is preferred for all shifts because colored ink, especially red and green, does not photocopy or microfilm well.

5. Medication Administration Record

When the EMR is implemented, medications are entered directly into the patient's computerized medication record when the doctor orders them. The nurse enters documentation regarding administration of those medications on the patient's computerized medication record.

When paper charts are used, all medications given by nursing personnel are recorded on a medication administration record (MAR). As the doctor orders new medications, the date, drug, dosage, administration route, and time and frequency of administration of the medication are written on this form. This may still be a part of the transcription procedure and is sometimes a task for the HUC in some health care facilities. Some hospital pharmacies provide a computerized medication record for every patient each day. When a new medication is ordered, the nurse or HUC handwrites the name of the medication with administration instructions on the computerized form. Pharmacy personnel will add the new medications to the following day's printed MAR from the copy of the doctors' orders sent by the HUC.

6. Nurse's Discharge Planning Form

The nurse's discharge planning form is used to prepare the patient for discharge from the health care facility (see the Evolve website). The nurse usually records information about the patient's health status at the time of discharge and provides instructions for the patient to follow after discharge from the health care facility. When the EMR is implemented, the nurse enters information and instructions directly into the patient's EMR. When paper charts are used, the form is kept in the patient's chart. When the patient is discharged, the HUC or nurse prints the discharge instructions from the computer or photocopies the handwritten form to give to the patient.

7. Physician's Discharge Summary

The physician's discharge summary is used by the physician to summarize the treatment and diagnosis the patient received while hospitalized, and it includes discharge information. A coding summary or diagnosis-related group (DRG) sheet may be part of the physician's discharge summary, or it may be a separate chart form.

When the EMR is implemented, the physician enters the discharge summary directly into the patient's EMR; and when paper charts are used, the form is kept in the patient's chart.

Standard Patient Chart Form Initiated by the Physician
History and Physical Form

The history and physical (H&P) form is used to record the medical history and the present symptomatic history of the patient. A review of all body systems or physical assessment of the patient is also recorded. When the EMR is implemented, the doctor, hospitalist, or resident may enter information directly into the patient's EMR; alternatively, the health care provider may dictate the information so the medical transcriptionist can enter it into the patient's EMR. When paper charts are used, the H&P form is usually dictated by the patient's doctor, hospitalist, or resident.

Williams, John	175-09-02
0078376	Surg
DOA 01/14/20XX	DOB 05/07/39
67Y M	Dr. Hy Hopes
0	MC/BCBS

Nursing Admit Data Form - Adult Patient

PATIENT STORY

Pain /Comfort Evaluation: Check all that apply

Frequency: ☐ None ☒ Currently have ☐ Acute ☐ Chronic
Onset / Duration
Type: ☐ Constant ☒ Intermittent ☐ Sharp ☐ Dull ☐ Burning
☐ Crushing ☐ Stabbing ☒ Radiating ☐ Other _____
Pain Severity _3_ Location: _LOWER LEGS - RIBS_
Pain Scale: ☒ Numeric ☐ Wong-Baker ☐ Objective Sign/Symptom
If using OS/S, document values: _____
What makes it better? _MEDICATION_
What makes it worse? _MOVING_

Substance Use (per patient)   Info is Unknown or UTA ☐
Tobacco: ☒ No ☐ Yes (answer the following) ☐ Smoke ☐ Chew
   Amt per day: _____ # of years _____ If quit, when _____
Alcohol: ☒ No ☐ Yes (answer the following) Last drink _____
   What kind: _____ Amt: _____ Frequency _____
Drugs: ☒ No ☐ Yes (answer the following) Last used _____
   What kind: _____ Frequency _____

Emotional / Spiritual / Religious   Info is Unknown or UTA ☐
Religion / faith _DO NOT PUBLISH_ ☐ None
Requesting Chaplain visit ☐ No ☐ Yes ☐ Chaplain notified (ext5437)
What spiritual /cultural practices/beliefs would you like supported while
being hospitalized _____ ☐ None
How can we support these _____ ☐ N/A

Are there any concerns that are troubling you while being hospitalized?
☐ Finances ☐ Job ☒ Insurance ☐ Housing ☐ Child care ☐ Pay for meds
☐ Homeless ☐ None ☐ Other _____

Educational   Info is Unknown or UTA ☐
Does the patient indicate he/she is motivated to learn? Yes ☒ No ☐
How does the patient best learn? ☐ Video ☐ Discussion ☒ Reading
☐ Audio tapes ☐ Pictures ☐ Demonstration ☐ Other _____
Based on the above, are there any barriers to learning ☒ No ☐ Yes
Describe _____
If yes, what alternatives to barriers are being suggested _____

Communication   Info is Unknown or UTA ☐
Language at home: ☒ English ☐ Spanish ☐ Other (identify below)
                              (don't forget sign language)
Able to speak: ☒ Y N   Write: ☒ Y N   Read ☒ Y N
Visual Impairment? ☒ No ☐ Yes ( ) R ( ) L ( ) UTA
Hearing Impairment? ☒ No ☐ Yes ( ) R ( ) L ( ) UTA
Was an interpreter used ☒ N/A ☐ Yes Name _____
Language spoken _ENGLISH_
Outcomes Management   Info is Unknown or UTA ☐
Anticipate D/C to ☒ Home ☐ Nursing Home ☐ Rehab Facility ☐ Hospice
☐ Correctional Facility ☐ Foster Care ☐ Other _____
Who will care for patient at D/C ☒ Self ☐ Spouse /SO ☒ Family
☐ Attendant ☐ Other _____
May need: HomeHealth ☒ No ☐ Yes Community Resources ☐ No ☐ Yes

NOTIFICATIONS
Social Service Notified via STAR ☒ N/A ☐ Yes Date/ time _____
Rehab Services notified (0945) ☒ N/A ☐ Yes Date/time _____
Form faxed (5453) to Pharmacy ☐ Yes ☒ No, why? _____

Prior Level of Function Info is Unknown or UTA ☐
In the last 3 months pt was ☒ Independent
☐ Partial Care ☐ Total Care
In the last 3 months pt has needed help with
☒ NA ☐ Ambulation ☐ Bathing ☐ Eating ☐ Dressing
☐ Transferring ☐ Toileting ☐ Other _____
If any green area has been checked order a Rehab referral

**Circle if a concern or deficit in an area seems to be
present Info is Unknown or UTA ☐**
Mobility   Balance   Ambulation
Upper Extremity   Lower Extremity   ADLs
Self Care   Cognition   Swallow
If any green area has been checked order a Rehab referral
Circle what medical equipment is used at home
Wheelchair   Ostomy   Walker
Cane   Crutches   Oxygen
Venous access device Glucose Meter Feeding tube
Foley   Suprapubic   Ostomy
Other _____

Immunizations – Info is Unknown or UTA ☐
If any pink highlighted area has been checked, the patient
should be offered pnuemo / flu vaccine. See Pneumococcal
and influenza pre-printed order form for details
Patient 65 or older? ☒ Yes ☐ No
Pnuemovac: ☐ Yes When? _____ ☒ No
Current diagnosis of Pneumonia ☐ Yes ☒ No
Influenza: ☐ Yes When? _____ ☒ No
Tetanus: ☒ Yes When? _2005_ ☐ No
Medical History: Info is Unknown or UTA ☐
Per: ☒ Patient   ☐ Family   ☐ Chart
Frequent admissions due to inability to meet the expense
of medication: ☐ Yes ☒ No
Dates of previous hospitalizations/surgeries: _____
2005 - PNEUMONITIS

# of ED visits or clinic visits in the last 6 months: ☒
*Circle all that apply. If circled, you may provide additional
detail in narrative area below*
Alzheimer's/Dementia: Psychiatric   Depression
GI Bleeds/Ulcer: Heart Disease   Hepatitis
Arthritis/Osteoporosis Asthma/COPD   HIV / AIDs
Blood Disorders   Emphysema   Diabetes
Sickle Cell   Chronic Alcohol Cancer
Hepatitis / Cirrhosis Spleenectomy   Stroke
Blood Transfusions   Kidney Problems Thyroid
Current Pregnancy   Substance abuse Rehab TB
Chronic Immunosuppresion   Other _____

Is there anything else the patient or family thinks would be
helpful for us to know in order to plan the care for this patient?
☒ No ☐ Yes _____

Printed Name / Credentials	Signature / Credentials / Initials
printed Name / Credentials	Signature / Credentials / Initials

Page 2 of 2

Figure 8-10 Nurse's admission record.

Continued

Nursing Admit Data Form - Adult Patient
PATIENT STORY

Williams, John	175-09-02
0078376	Surg
DOA 01/14/20XX	DOB 05/07/39
67Y M	Dr. Hy Hopes
	MC/BCBS

DT102

Date/Time **6/10 1810** Unit **3C** Room # **306** Age **67**

Admit Dx: **MVA - DIABETES**

Addl Dx: **HYPERTENSION**

Height **182** cm (1 in /2.54 cm) Weight **89** kg. (2.2lb/kg.)
☐ Stated ☐ Bed scale ☐ Standing scale ☐ Other

Emergency Contact: Name / Phone / Relationship to patient
1. **JEAN SOUNDERS - DAUGHTER**
2. **102-202-2082**

Personal Property ☒ Taken by family ☐ In safe ☐ None
Property at bedside: ☐ Cane ☐ Walker ☐ WC ☒ Glasses /Contacts
☐ Hearing Aids ☒ Dentures: Upper / Lower / Partial
☐ Clothes_____ ☐ Prosthesis_____

Advance ☐ None ☒ In Chart ☐ Has Directive but not available
Directives: ☐ Refused info ☐ Info given to _____
Type: ☐ Advance directive ☐ Living will ☐ POA (medical)
What is the patient/family's intent if Advance Directive not available?

A Social Service referral may be needed to help pt / family (ext. 5321)
Social Services notified ☐ Yes Date/ time_____ ☒ N/A
Allergies: ☒ No known   **Info is Unknown or UTA** ☐
☐ Iodine (reaction_____) ☐ Tape (reaction_____)
☐ Latex (reaction_____)
☐ Meds (List/reaction)_____
☐ Food (List/reaction) **N/A**
☐ Other (List/reaction)_____
Allergy Band applied? ☐ Yes   ☐ No, why?

Safety Alerts: ☐ Fall ☐ Skin ☐ Seizure ☐ Aspiration ☐ Flight ☐ None
☐ Harm to self ☐ Harm to others ☐ Isolation (type)

Nutrition: Diet at home: **DIABETIC** Last ate at **1200**
Poor oral health ☐ Yes ☒ No Tube Feeding/TPN ☐ Yes ☐ No
Vomiting, nausea, clear liquids or NPO > 3 days ☐ Yes ☐ No
Modified Diet (such as Low Sodium, Diabetic, Renal) ☐ Yes ☐ No
New Diabetic ☐ Yes ☒ No Breastfeeding ☐ Yes ☐ No
Pregnant ☐ Yes ☐ No Decubitis III / IV ☐ Yes ☐ No
Surgical patient and over 70 years ☐ Yes ☐ No
Difficulty with chewing or swallowing ☐ No ☐ Yes, why_____
Unplanned weight loss within last 3 months of 10+ lbs. ☐ Yes ☐ No
If any yellow area has been checked order a Nutrition referral

Domestic Violence Do you feel safe in your home? ☒ Yes ☐ No ☐ None
Do you feel safe in your current relationship? ☒ Yes ☐ No ☐ None
Do your children feel safe in your current relationship ☒ Yes ☐ No ☐ None
If any blue area has been checked order a Social Service referral
Oriented to unit: ☒ Call light ☒ Bed Controls
☒ Phone/TV ☒ Mealtimes ☒ ID bands
☐ Smoking Policy ☒ Visiting Hours ☒ Side rails
☒ Pain Assessment Chart ☐ Isolation rules ☐ Hand washing
Info given to: ☐ Patient ☒ Family ☐ Unable to

NOTIFICATIONS
Nutrition Services faxed (1203) ☒ N/A ☐ Yes Date/time_____
Social Service Notified via STAR ☒ N/A ☐ Yes Date/time_____
Form faxed (5453) to Pharmacy ☒ Yes ☐ No, Why? _____
Infection Control Called (5276) ☒ N/A ☐ Yes Date/time_____

(sidebar, left margin:) If an area in yellow has been checked, order a Nutrition referral / If an area in blue has been checked, order a Social Service referral / Do not forget to fax this page to the pharmacy / If an area in pink has been checked notify Infection Control

Briefly describe the events that led to the admit
(Include where patient arrived from, ie: ED, PACU, home)
ADMITTED FROM ER STATUS POST MVA

Brief Social History / Support System
SEPARATED FROM WIFE FOR 5 YRS. HAS ADULT CHILDREN LIVES WITH DAUGHTER

Referred to Social Services ☒ N/A ☐ Yes Date/ time_____
Reason_____

**List the medications the patient is taking
including dose and frequency
Remember OTCs & Herbal supplements**

AVALIDE 300/12.5 mg ī PO SD.
LIPITOR 40mg ī PO QD
GLYBURIDE 5mg ī QAM

Other / Updates:

Printed Name / Credentials _____
Signature / Credentials / Initials _____

2155 (07/04)

Figure 8-10, cont'd

A medical transcriptionist in HIMS types the dictated report and sends it to the nursing unit to be placed in the patient's chart. The H&P form may be completed after the patient has been admitted to the hospital. Some doctors send a completed copy of the patient's H&P form with the patient, or they may send it to the hospital before the time of the patient's admission to be scanned into the patient's EMR or to be placed in the paper chart.

⭐ HIGH PRIORITY

In some health care facilities using electronic medical records (EMRs), the health information management services department (HIMS) is responsible for scanning paper forms to the patient's EMR.

SUPPLEMENTAL PATIENT CHART FORMS

Supplemental patient chart forms are additional to the standard chart forms according to specific care and treatment provided. For example, if the patient has diabetes, is receiving medication, and is being monitored, the supplemental form called the *diabetic record* is added. When the EMR is implemented, information is entered into the patient's EMR on electronic forms; and when paper charts are used, the forms are inserted into the patient's paper chart. This allows information to be recorded separately from other data, making interpretation easier. It is the responsibility of the HUC to obtain and label (with the patient's ID label) the needed paper supplemental forms and place them behind the appropriate chart divider in the patient's chart binder. If the hospital uses computerized **supplemental chart forms,** the HUC chooses the appropriate patient's name, prints the form with that patient's identification information on the form, and places the forms behind the proper chart divider in the chart binder. Other examples of supplemental patient chart forms include the following:

Clinical Pathway Record Form

Most hospitals use clinical pathway record forms for particular diagnoses or conditions, such as coronary artery bypass graft or total hip or knee replacement. The clinical pathway record form is placed in the chart for those particular patients. The clinical pathway record form includes the surgeon's orders, a plan of care with treatment, and predicted outcomes (Fig. 8-11).

Anticoagulant Therapy Record

The anticoagulant record is used to document blood test results and the anticoagulant medication received by the patient who is undergoing anticoagulant therapy. A flow sheet allows the doctor to make a comparison of the patient's blood test results and the medications prescribed over time.

Diabetic Record

The diabetic record is placed in the charts of patients who are receiving medication for diabetes (see Evolve). Results of the blood tests performed to monitor the effects of diabetic medications are also documented on the diabetic record.

Consultation Form

The patient's attending physician may wish to obtain the opinion of another doctor. In this event, the physician requests a consultation by writing it on the doctor's order sheet. Most doctors dictate their report on completion of the consultation. The hospital medical transcription department types the dictated report and sends it to the nursing unit to be filed in the patient's paper chart. Some doctors may prefer to write their findings on a consultation form. Additional information regarding consultations is presented in Chapter 18.

Operating Room Records

The number of forms required for maintaining a record of a patient's operation varies; these forms are usually assembled into a surgery packet. Such records are used by the preoperative department, anesthesiologist, operating room staff, and recovery room personnel). Additional responsibilities regarding the surgery chart are discussed in Chapter 19.

Therapy Records

Health care facilities use individual record sheets for recording treatments. It is possible to have record sheets for physical therapy, occupational therapy, respiratory care, diet therapy, radiation therapy, and others. These departments are discussed in Section Three of this text.

Parenteral Fluid or Infusion Record

A parenteral fluid record is placed in the chart of a patient who receives an intravenous infusion. This form, when completed, is a written record of types and amounts of intravenous fluids administered to the patient. If bedside charting is in use, the parenteral fluid record or vital signs record may be initiated when the information is entered into the computer.

Graphic Record Form

The graphic record form is usually included in the nurse's notes and completed by the patient's nurse, but it may be a separate form in some hospitals and completed by the HUC. The graphic record form is a form used to graph patient vital signs including temperature (Fahrenheit or Celsius), pulse, and respiration (TPR) (discussed in Chapter 10). TPRs are usually taken three times each day or according to specific hospital policy, to monitor the patient's condition. Intake and output and daily weights are also recorded on the graphic record form (Box 8-2, *Recording Vital Signs;* Box 8-3, *Method for Correcting Errors on the Graphic Record in Paper Charts;* Figs. 8-12 and 8-13).

SKILLS CHALLENGE

To practice recording the vital signs and other data on the graphic record, complete Activities 8-3 and 8-4 in the *Skills Practice Manual.* (See Chapter 10 for information regarding vital signs and other data to record on graphic record.)

History: _____
IV: _____

Procedures: _____

Date _____   A = achieved - N = not achieved

	Pre-hospital	Day of Surgery	Post-op day 1	PO day 2	PO day 3	PO day 4 Discharge
Consult	Medical Clearance if necessary	PT consult in PM	PT therapy BID	PT BID Home Care and SS as appr	PT BID	PT ☐
Tests	CXR, CBC, UA, PT, SMA20, EKG, Labs appropriate for age & health 72 hrs before	T & C 2 units (pre-op) (autologous when able) X-ray (in PACU)	H & H ☐ PT (if on coumadin) ☐	H & H ☐ PT ☐	H & H ☐ PT ☐	PT ☐
Mobility		dangle - stand prn	Knee exercises Chair BID (30 min) - up for dinner Stand/Amb	Cont exercises - Amb BID Chair BID (45 min) - up for lunch and dinner BRP	Continue mobility Chair (60 min) - up for all meals	Continue mobility Chair (60 min) - up for all meals
Treatments		Trapeze Drain IV therapy, incentive spir q2° DVT prophylaxes : (TED, foot compression device, coumadin , Lovenox) CPM 0 - 50°	Trapeze Drain Cap IV, incentive spir q2° DVT prophylaxes CPM 0 - 50°	Trapeze DC drain Cap IV, incentive spir q2° DC IV DVT proph Dressing change by physician CPM 0 - 60°	Trapeze Incentive spirometer DC IV DVT proph CPM 0 - 70°	CPM 0 - 80°
Meds		Pain Med (IV, IM) Pt states pain relief: A N Antibiotics DAT ____	Pain Med (IV, IM) Pt states pain relief: A N DC Antibiotics DAT ____	PO pain meds Pt states pain relief: A N DAT ____	PO pain meds prn Pt states pain relief: A N DAT ____	PO pain meds prn Pt states pain relief: A N DAT ____
Nutrition Metabolic						
Elimination		Catheter of choice prn st cath foley after 3rd time	DC foley	Eval. bowel function (BCOC)	Bowel movement: A N	Bowel movement: A N
Health /Home Management			Screen for Home Care & Social Service needs	Prescription for home equipment identified by PT Order equipment	Complete transfer form	☐ Home ☐ ECF
Health Perception	TKA pre-op teaching by Interdisciplinary Team	Review: ☐ TCDB, ☐ incentive spirometry, ☐ ankle pumps, ☐ ROM to arms, ☐ CPM, ☐ pain management	Instruct on: ☐ knee precautions	Instruct on: ☐ incisional care ☐ pain management	Discharge teaching: ☐ Medication ☐ review knee book	☐ Written discharge instructions to patient and family
Signature						
Signature						
Signature						

Outcomes	Date met/initials	Outcomes	Date met/initials
1. In-out of bed ☐ indep or with min assist ☐ mod - max assist		5. Evidence of wound healing, no drainage	
2. On-off commode or chair ☐ indep or with min assist ☐ mod - max assist		6. Performs total knee exercises without assistance	
3. Ambulates with assistive devices. ☐ 75 feet indep or with min asst ☐ 50 feet		7. Re-establish elimination pattern.	
4. AROM ☐ 0 - 70 - 90° ☐ 0 - 60°		8. Utilizes oral analgesics for pain control.	

Figure 8-11 Clinical pathway (care plan with treatment and predicted outcomes) for total knee arthroscopy.

| BOX 8-2 | **RECORDING VITAL SIGNS** |

The graphing of vital signs is usually completed by the patient's nurse. In some hospitals using paper charts, the nursing personnel record patient vital signs on a temperature, pulse, and respiration (TPR) sheet. It then may be the health unit coordinator's (HUC's) task to record data from the TPR sheet onto each patient's graphic record. The HUC should record vital signs and other data as soon as they are recorded on the TPR sheet, so the information is readily available to doctors when they make rounds to see their patients. Accuracy and timeliness in the recording of vital signs information is a must, because the doctor may use this information to prescribe treatment for the patient. Most often the temperature is taken and recorded using the Fahrenheit scale, but it is sometimes taken and recorded on the Celsius scale, also known as the *Centigrade* scale.

Frequent Vital Signs Record

The frequent vital signs record is used when vital signs are taken more often than every 4 hours.

CONSENT FORMS

Surgery or Procedure Consent Form

A number of conditions require the patient or a responsible party to sign a special form granting permission for surgery or other invasive procedures to be performed on the patient (Fig. 8-14).

Patients who are hospitalized for surgery are required to sign a consent form permitting their doctor to perform the surgery named on the form. This form should not be signed until the physician has explained the surgery or invasive medical procedure and its risks, alternatives, and likely outcomes (informed consent). After having received an explanation, a competent patient can give informed consent.

Other invasive procedures that require the signing of consent forms by the patient or a responsible party are covered in chapters related to those specific procedures.

The HUC usually prepares the consent form for the physician or nurse to take to the patient for signature. If the surgery should be cancelled, the surgery permit is still valid unless the doctor or the surgical procedure has been changed.

Consent forms for surgery and other invasive medical procedures are legal agreements between the patient and the physician. In some health care facilities it may be the physician's responsibility to write the name of the doctor who is to perform the surgery or invasive medical procedure and to write the name of the procedure to be done.

Procedure for Preparing Consent Forms

In most facilities the HUC prepares the consent form for the nurse or doctor to present to the patient for signature. The following steps assist the HUC in preparing the consent form:

1. Affix the patient's ID label to the consent form.

| BOX 8-3 | **METHOD FOR CORRECTING ERRORS ON THE GRAPHIC RECORD IN PAPER CHARTS** |

Minor graphic errors may be corrected on the original graphic record. However, correction of major errors may require that the original graphic record be recopied. The following procedure for correcting errors should be followed.

1. To correct a *minor error on the graphic portion* of the record, write "mistaken entry" or "error" in ink on the incorrect connecting line, and record your first initial, your last name, and your status above the error; then graph the correct value (see Fig. 8-12).
2. To correct a *numbered entry*, such as the respiration value, draw a line through the entry in ink, and write in ink "mistaken entry" or "error," your first initial, your last name, and your status near it. As close as possible, insert the correct numbers (see Fig. 8-12).
3. To correct a *series of errors* on the graphic record, the entire record must be recopied to show the correct data (see Fig. 8-13, *A*).
   a. Prepare a new graphic record and label with the patient's ID label (see Fig. 8-13, *B*).
   b. Transfer in ink *all* the information onto the new graphic record, including the correction of errors (see Fig. 8-13, *B*).
   c. Draw a diagonal line through the old graphic record in ink, and record in ink on the line "mistaken entry" or "error" (see Fig. 8-13, *A*).
   d. Place the old record behind the recopied record because it must remain as a permanent part of the chart.
   e. In ink, write "recopied," followed by your name, your status, and the date on the new graphic record (see Fig. 8-13, *B*); place the new record behind the correct divider in the patient's chart.

2. Write in black ink the first and last names of the doctor who is to perform the surgery or invasive medical procedure.
3. Write in black ink the surgery or invasive medical procedure to be performed exactly as the physician wrote it on the physician's order sheet, except that abbreviations must be spelled out. For instance, if the doctor's order reads "amp of rt index finger," the consent form should read "amputation of the right index finger."
4. Spell correctly, and write all information legibly
5. Do not record the date and time. The person who obtains the patient's signature will enter the date and time.

The patient may be required to sign other permit or release forms during hospitalization. Following are examples of situations that usually require a signature by the patient or by the patient's representative:

1. Release of side rails
2. Consent to receive blood transfusion (Fig. 8-15)

3. Refusal to permit blood transfusion (Fig. 8-16)
4. Consent form for human immunodeficiency virus (HIV) testing (Fig. 8-17)

When paper charts are used, signed consent forms are filed in the patient's chart. When the EMR is implemented, all printed or handwritten signed consent forms are scanned into the patient's EMR by the HUC.

Most health care facilities require that only licensed personnel witness the signing of consent forms. Personnel must follow these general rules when asking patients to sign consent forms.

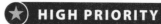

★ HIGH PRIORITY

When paper charts are used, signed consent forms are filed in the patient's chart. When the electronic medical record (EMR) is implemented, all printed or handwritten signed consent forms are scanned into the patient's EMR by the health unit coordinator.

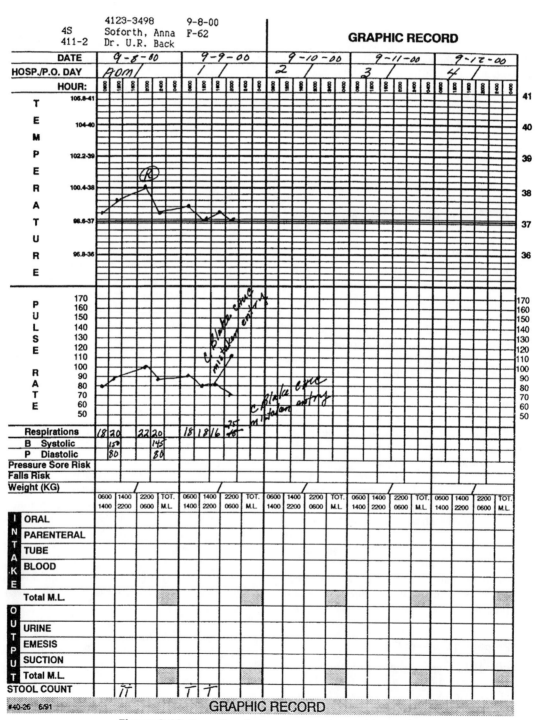

Figure 8-12 Correction of minor errors on the graphic record.

1. The patient must not be under the influence of any "mind-clouding" medications.
2. The patient must be of legal age (18 years in most states).
3. The patient must be mentally competent.

METHODS OF ERROR CORRECTION ON PAPER CHART FORMS

Because the patient's chart is considered a legal document, information recorded on a chart form must not be erased or obliterated by pen, by covering with a label, or by using liquid correction fluid. Only certain methods of correcting errors recorded on a patient's chart form are permitted.

Patient chart forms that are affixed with the wrong or incorrect ID label may be shredded if no notations have been made

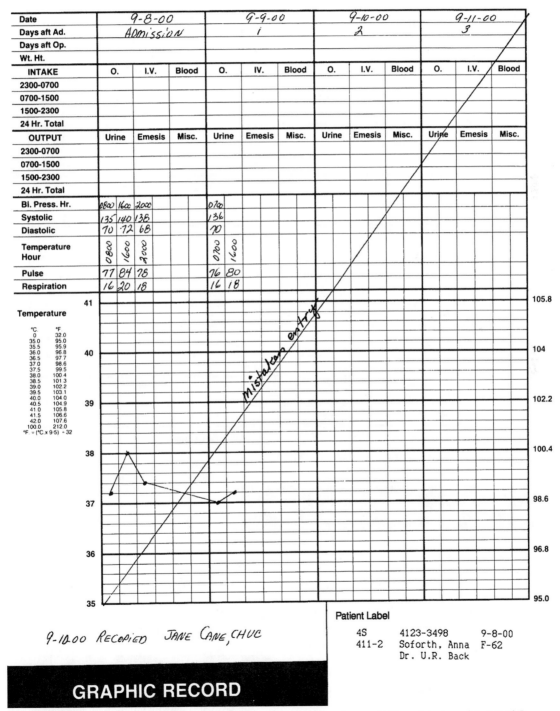

GRAPHIC RECORD

Figure 8-13 Recopied graphic record used to correct a series of errors. **A,** The original graphic record. **B,** A copied graphic record.

Continued

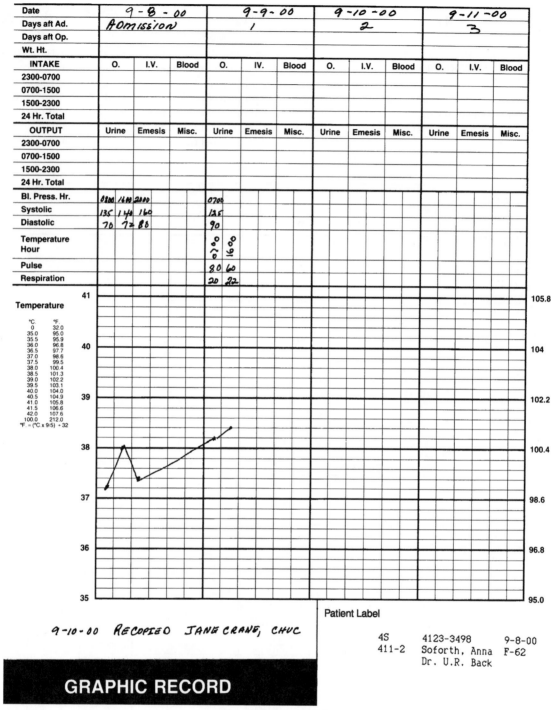

Date	9-8-00			9-9-00			9-10-00			9-11-00		
Days aft Ad.	Admission			1			2			3		
Days aft Op.												
Wt. Ht.												
INTAKE	O.	I.V.	Blood	O.	IV.	Blood	O.	I.V.	Blood	O.	I.V.	Blood
2300-0700												
0700-1500												
1500-2300												
24 Hr. Total												
OUTPUT	Urine	Emesis	Misc.	Urine	Emesis	Misc.	Urine	Emesis	Misc.	Urine	Emesis	Misc.
2300-0700												
0700-1500												
1500-2300												
24 Hr. Total												
Bl. Press. Hr.	0800 1600 2000			0700								
Systolic	135 140 160			125								
Diastolic	70 72 80			90								
Temperature Hour	0700 1600											
Pulse	80 60											
Respiration	20 22											

Temperature

°C.	°F.
0	32.0
35.0	95.0
35.5	95.9
36.0	96.8
36.5	97.7
37.0	98.6
37.5	99.5
38.0	100.4
38.5	101.3
39.0	102.2
39.5	103.1
40.0	104.0
40.5	104.9
41.0	105.8
41.5	106.6
42.0	107.6
100.0	212.0

°F. = (°C x 9/5) + 32

9-10-00   RECOPIED   JANE CRANE, CHUC

Patient Label

4S   4123-3498   9-8-00
411-2   Soforth, Anna   F-62
          Dr. U.R. Back

GRAPHIC RECORD

Figure 8-13, cont'd

on them. If a chart form has notations on it, the chart form cannot be shredded. Draw an X with a black ink pen through the incorrect label and write "mistaken entry" with the date, time, and first initial, last name, and status (of the person correcting labeling error) above the incorrect label. Affix the correct patient ID label on the form next to the incorrect label (do not place the correct label over the incorrect label). It is also permissible to hand print the patient information in black ink next to the incorrect label that has an X drawn through it (Fig. 8-18).

To correct an error in a written entry made on a paper chart form, draw (in black ink) one single line through the error. Record

the words "mistaken entry" or "error," along with the date, the time, and your first initial, your last name, and your status in a blank area near (directly above or next to the error) (Fig. 8-19). Follow the facility policy for correction of erroneous computer entries.

⭐ **HIGH PRIORITY**

Errors in care or treatment must be documented on both the EMR and paper chart, and an incident report must be completed, as discussed in Chapter 21.

Williams, John	175-09-02
0078376	Surg
DOA 01/14/20XX	DOB 05/07/39
67Y M	Dr. Hy Hopes
0‖‖‖‖‖‖‖ ‖‖‖	MC/BCBS

CONSENT FOR
SURGERY/PROCEDURES/SEDATION/ANESTHESIA

1.　　I authorize the following operation(s) or procedure(s) **(No Abbreviations)** _____

_____

to be performed by Dr. _____ and/or the associates or assistants of his/
her choice, which may include medical or surgical residents. I understand a representative from a medical company, such as
a sales representative, may be present during the surgical procedure to provide verbal technical advice to the surgeon,
anesthesiologist, and/or staff.

2.　　During the course of the operation(s)/procedure(s), unforeseen conditions may arise, which may necessitate additional
surgery or other therapeutic procedures to promote my well-being. I consent to other surgery / procedures as may be
considered necessary or advisable by my physician(s) under the circumstances.

3.　　I consent to the use of sedation/anesthetics, as may be necessary and advisable,except _____
I understand that sedation/anesthesia may involve serious risk, even though administered in a careful manner. I further
understand that a patient should not drive, operate equipment, or drink alcoholic beverages for at least 24 hours after
sedation/anesthesia.

4.　　To further medical and scientific learning, I consent to the photographing and/or video taping of the operation(s)/ procedure(s)
that may reveal portions of my body, with the understanding that my identity is not to be revealed. To advance medical
education, I give my permission for physicians, nurses, medical students, interns, residents, and other individuals who are
participating in an educational process approved by the hospital to be present during the operation(s)/procedure(s).

5.　　I consent to the examination for anatomical purposes and disposal by the hospital of any tissue or body parts that may be
removed during the operation(s)/procedure(s).

6.　　I understand that some physician(s) performing the operation(s)/procedure(s), administering sedation/anesthesia and
those physicians providing services involving pathology and radiology, may not be the agents, servants, or employees of the
hospital nor of one another and may be independent contractors.

7.　　I have been advised that prosthetic devices including, but not limited to, dentures, bridges, caps, crowns, fillings, dental
implants, etc. are more easily damaged than normal teeth. I have been advised to remove all removable prosthetic devices
prior to surgery, and I agree that responsibility for loss or damage will be mine if I fail to remove such dental or other
prosthetic devices.

8.　　My physician has explained to me the nature, purpose, and possible consequences of the operation(s)/procedure(s) as
well as significant risks involved, possible complications, expected postoperative functional level, expected alterations in
lifestyle/health status and alternative methods of treatment. I further understand that the explanation I have received is not
exhaustive and that there may be other, more remote risks and consequences. I have been advised that a more detailed
explanation will be given to me if I so desire. I have received no guarantee or warranty concerning the results/outcome and
cure and have been given an opportunity to ask questions, and have my questions answered to my satisfaction.

9.　　In the event a device is implanted during the operation(s)/procedure(s) and federal law requires the tracking of the device, I
consent to the release of my social security number to the manufacturer of the device.

10.　　The patient is unable to sign for the following reason:

　　　　☐　　The patient is a minor.

　　　　☐　　The patient lacks the ability to make or communicate medical treatment decisions because of:

_____

_____	_____	_____
Patient or Legally Authorized Representative	Date	Time

_____
Relationship to Patient

_____	_____	_____
Witness	Date	Time

Figure 8-14 Surgery consent form.

CONSENT FOR TRANSFUSION OF BLOOD OR BLOOD PRODUCTS

1.   I HAVE BEEN INFORMED that I need or may need, during treatment, a transfusion of blood and/or one of its products in the interest of my health and proper medical care.

2.   I HAVE BEEN INFORMED of the risks and benefits of receiving transfusion(s). These risks exist despite the fact that the blood has been carefully tested.

3.   I HAVE BEEN INFORMED that the blood has been tested using all FDA-required, routine tests and that new, unlicensed, and experimental testing may or may not have been performed.

4.   The alternatives to transfusion, including the risks and consequences of not receiving this therapy, have been explained to me.

5.   I have read, or have had read to me, the Blood Transfusion Information regarding blood transfusions and have had the opportunity to ask questions.

6.   I have been given the Paul Gann Safety Act Booklet (CA only).

7.   I hereby consent to the transfusion(s).

This consent is valid for the following period of time(check one):

☐ One specific date only: _____

☐ Start Date: _____   End Date: _____

☐ This hospital admission

_____   _____   _____
Patient's Signature   Date   Time

_____
Signature of parent, legally appointed guardian or responsible person *(for patients who cannot sign)*

_____   _____   _____
Witness   Date   Time

Consent obtained under the direction of Dr. _____

_____   _____   _____
Physician Signature *(if required by local policy)*   Date   Time

NOTE:
Refusal form on reverse side
Chart Consent or Refusal Form
Separate "Blood Transfusion Information" sheet and give to patient, parent, or legal guardian.

Williams, John	175-09-02
0078376	Surg
DOA 01/14/20XX	DOB 05/07/39
67Y M	Dr. Hy Hopes
0 ‖‖‖‖‖ ‖‖‖	MC/BCBS

Figure 8-15 Consent form for receiving blood transfusion.

SKILLS CHALLENGE

To practice correcting labeling and written errors on a chart form, complete Activities 8-6 and 8-7 in the *Skills Practice Manual.*

MONITORING AND MAINTAINING THE PATIENT'S ELECTRONIC MEDICAL RECORD

The HUC position has changed with the implementation of the EMR, but monitoring and maintaining patients' records is still the responsibility of the HUC.

Health Unit Coordinator Duties for Monitoring and Maintaining the Patient's Electronic Medical Record

1. Monitor the patient's EMR consistently, and complete HUC tasks as required and in a timely manner.
2. Assist nurses, doctors, and ancillary personnel as necessary in entering information and orders into the computer.
3. Report any necessary repairs regarding nursing unit computers and/or printers to the hospital information systems department.
4. Scan documents as required, such as handwritten progress notes, electrocardiograms, outside medical records,

REFUSAL TO PERMIT TRANSFUSION OF BLOOD OR BLOOD PRODUCTS

1. I request that no blood components be administered to _____
    during this hospitalization.   (patient name)

2. I hereby release the hospital, its personnel, and the attending physician from any responsibility whatsoever for unfavorable reactions
    or any untoward results due to my refusal to permit the use of blood or its components.

3. I fully understand the possible consequences of such refusal on my part.

    ☐ Physician aware of patient's refusal.   Physician notified: _____

Physician notified by:

_____	_____	_____
Signature	Date	Time
_____	_____	_____
Patient's Signature	Date	Time

Signature of parent, legally appointed guardian or responsible person *(for patients who cannot sign)*

_____	_____	_____
Witness	Date	Time
_____	_____	_____
Witness	Date	Time

REFUSAL

Williams, John	175-09-02
0078376	Surg
DOA 01/14/20XX	DOB 05/07/39
67Y M	Dr. Hy Hopes
0 ‖‖‖‖‖‖‖‖	MC/BCBS

Figure 8-16 Form for refusal to permit blood transfusion.

consent forms, operating room records, and reports, in a timely manner.

5. Place and maintain patient ID labels in a patient label book.
6. Place patient face sheets into the face sheet binder, which may be the same as the label book, to provide to physicians as requested.
7. Always log out of the EMR when not in use to protect patient confidentiality.

MAINTAINING THE PATIENT'S PAPER CHART

As the person in charge of the clerical duties on the nursing unit, the HUC is responsible for maintaining the patient's chart.

Health Unit Coordinator Duties for Effective Maintenance of the Patient's Paper Chart

1. Place all charts in proper sequence (usually according to room number) in the chart rack when they are not in use.

2. Place new chart forms in each patient's chart before the immediate need arises. In many health care facilities, this is referred to as **stuffing charts.** Label each chart form with the patient's ID label before placing it in the chart. New chart forms are placed on top of old chart forms for easy access. The new forms may be folded in half to show that the old form has not been completely used.
3. Place diagnostic reports in the correct patient's chart behind the correct divider. Match the patient's name on the report with the patient's name within the chart (do not depend on room numbers because patients are often transferred to another room).
4. Review the patient's charts frequently for new orders (always check each chart for new orders before returning the chart to the chart rack).
5. Properly label the patient's chart so it can easily be located at all times.
6. Check each chart to be sure that all forms are labeled with the correct patient's name. Chart forms should be filed in the proper sequence.

CONSENT FOR HIV TESTING

1. My physician, _____, has recommended that I (my child) receive a blood test to detect the presence of antibodies to Human Immunodeficiency Virus (HIV), the virus that causes Acquired Immune Deficiency Syndrome (AIDS). I consent to this testing.

    It has been explained to me that in some cases the tests may be positive when I have (my child has) not been infected with HIV. This is a false positive.

    If the screening is positive, a second confirming test is done.

    I understand that a negative result usually means that I have (my child has) not been exposed to HIV. However, there is a possibility of a false-negative result, especially in the time period immediately after exposure to the virus.

2. I have been advised by my physician and I understand the following:

    ● Positive test results could mean that I have (my child has) been exposed to the HIV; this would not necesarily mean that I have (my child has) AIDS, or will develop AIDS.

    ● That if I am (my child is) HIV positive, I (my child) can transmit the virus to other individuals by sexual contact, by sharing needles, or by the donation of organs, blood, and blood products.

    ● That if I am (my child is) HIV positive, I (my child) should not donate blood or blood products, or body organs because the virus can be transmitted to the recipient.

3. I understand that Arizona State Law and Regulations require the reporting of HIV cases to the Department of Health Services and that if my (my child's) test results are positive, they will be submitted to the Arizona Department of Health Services, and others whose authority is established by law, regulation, or court order.

4. I also understand that my request for the test and the test results will be part of my (my child's) hospital medical record and may therefore be requested by others, including insurers, third party payors or other individuals as outlined in the Conditions of Admission.

I have been given the opportunity to ask quesitons, I understand what is involved in HIV testing, and I freely consent to it.

_____   _____
DATE   SIGNATURE

_____   _____
LEGAL GUARDIAN   WITNESS SIGNATURE
(If patient cannot sign or under age)

Figure 8-17 Consent form for human immunodeficiency virus (HIV) testing.

7. Check the chart frequently for patient information forms or face sheets. Usually five copies are maintained in the chart. Physicians may remove copies for billing purposes. The HUC may print additional copies of the face sheet from the computer or may order them from admitting.
8. Assist physicians or other professionals in locating the patient's chart.

Splitting or Thinning the Chart

The paper chart of a patient who remains in the health care facility for a long time becomes very full and eventually becomes unmanageable. When this occurs, the HUC may **split** or thin the chart. A doctor's order is not required to thin a patient's chart. In thinning the chart, some categories of chart forms may be removed and placed in an envelope for safekeeping on the unit.

The following guidelines will assist the HUC in thinning a patient's chart:

1. Remove older nurse's notes, medication forms, and other forms that are no longer needed in the chart binder. (Check the hospital policy and procedures manual to verify forms that may and may not be removed.)
2. Place the removed forms in an envelope.
3. Place the patient's ID label on the outside of the envelope.
4. Write "thinned chart" and record the date with your first initial and your last name (if you are the person thinning the chart) on the outside of the envelope.
5. Place a label on the front of the patient's chart stating that the chart was thinned, along with the date and the first initial and last name of the person thinning the chart.

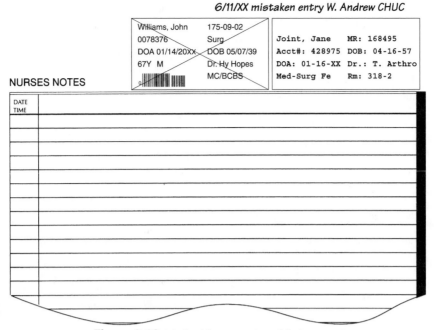

Figure 8-18 Method for correcting a labeling error.

MEDICATION RECORD

Routine Medications

○ **- CIRCLE ALL DOSES NOT GIVEN - STATE REASON IN NURSES NOTES**

DATE			6/10/XX	6/11/XX	6/12/XX	6/13/XX	6/14/XX
DAY OF WEEK			Sun.	Mon.	Tues.	Wed.	Thurs.
MEDICATION *11/6/XX mistaken entry* *prednisalone* *A. Hay, Chuc*			11-7				
			7-3				
DOSE *5 mg*	ROUTE	FREQUENCY	3-11				
MEDICATION *Prednisone*			11-7				
			7-3				
DOSE *5 mg*	ROUTE *p.o.*	FREQUENCY *Bid.*	3-11				
MEDICATION			11-7				
			7-3				
DOSE	ROUTE	FREQUENCY	3-11				
MEDICATION			11-7				
			7-3				
DOSE	ROUTE	FREQUENCY	3-11				
MEDICATION			11-7				
			7-3				
DOSE	ROUTE	FREQUENCY	3-11				
ICATION			11-7				
	ROUTE	FREQUENCY					

Figure 8-19 Method for correcting a written error on the chart.

6. If the patient is transferred to another unit, transfer the thinned-out forms with the patient's chart.
7. When the patient is discharged, send all thinned-out forms with the patient's paper chart to the health information management department.

Reproduction of Chart Forms that Contain Patient Information

Availability of patient medical records is necessary to ensure continuity of care when a patient is discharged to another facility. When the EMR is used, the patient's EMR is available on computer to other health care facilities, or the records may be printed from the computer. The patient will be required to sign a release form for the records to be available or copied in this situation. When paper charts are used, the records will need to be reproduced using a copy machine. The patient's doctor must write an order specifying the specific chart forms to be copied, and the patient will be required to sign a release form. Depending on hospital policy, the HUC may have the responsibility of copying the paper chart forms, or the patient's chart may be sent to HIMS to be copied. After the forms have been reproduced on the copier, the original forms are replaced in the patient's chart and the copied records are sent to the receiving facility.

★ HIGH PRIORITY

After reproducing records, be certain that original records are returned to the patient's binder and the copies are placed in a labeled envelope to be sent to the receiving facility.

KEY CONCEPTS

The patient's chart (electronic or paper) is a record of care rendered and the patient's response to care during hospitalization. When the EMR is implemented, all health care information is entered into or scanned into the patient's electronic chart. When paper charts are in use, the nursing unit to which the patient is assigned adds forms to the patient's chart. The patient's medical information (electronic or paper) is a legal record and should be maintained as such.

Standard chart forms are included in the patient's EMR or placed in all patients' paper charts; supplemental forms may be added according to the need dictated by each patient's treatment and care. The purpose of the forms is the same for each hospital, but the sequence of forms in the chart and the placement of blank forms that are added may differ from hospital to hospital. Information contained in the patient's EMR or paper chart must always be regarded as confidential.

Websites of Interest

Military time conversion and time table: www.247clocks.com/Military_Time.htm
"Dos and Don'ts of Nursing Documentation": www.medismart.com/nursing-resources/documentation
U.S. Department of Health and Human Services—"Effective Communication in Hospitals": www.hhs.gov/ocr/civilrights/resources/specialtopics/hospitalcommunication
American Management Association official website www.amanet.org/

REVIEW QUESTIONS

Visit the Evolve website to download and complete the following questions.

 1. Define the following terms:
    a. stuffing charts
    b. split or thin chart
    c. identification labels
    d. name alert
    e. allergy labels
    f. old record
    g. WALLaroo
    h. admission packet

 2. List six purposes for maintaining an EMR or paper chart for each patient.

 3. List five guidelines for entering information into a patient's EMR.

 4. List five guidelines for writing on a patient's paper chart.

 5. List four standard patient electronic or paper chart forms that are initiated in the admitting department, and describe the purpose of each.

 6. State the purpose of the following standard forms contained in a patient's electronic or paper admission packet:
    a. physician's order form
    b. nurse's admission record
    c. physician's progress record
    d. nurse's progress notes or flow sheet
    e. medication administration record (MAR)
    f. physician's discharge summary
    g. nurse's discharge planning form

 7. List the information that is included in a patient's history and physical form.

 8. Define what is meant by a *supplemental patient chart form*, and list at least two examples of a supplemental form.

 9. Explain the importance of charting vital signs accurately and in a timely manner.

10. Describe how the following errors on a patient's graphic record would be corrected:
    a. a minor error on the graphic portion of the record
    b. a numbered entry, such as the respiration value
    c. a series of errors on the graphic record

11. Discuss the purpose of a consent form, and list five guidelines for preparing consent forms.

12. Describe how patients' medical records are organized and identified when paper charts are used.

13. Convert the following standard times to military times:
    a. 3:00 PM
    b. 7:15 AM
    c. 12:30 PM
    d. 1:15 AM

14. Convert the following military times to standard times:
    a. 1020
    b. 1940
    c. 1119
    d. 2130

15. List four types of permit or release forms that a patient may be required to sign during a hospital stay.

16. List seven duties that will assist the HUC in properly maintaining and monitoring a patient's EMR.

17. List eight duties that will assist the HUC in properly maintaining a patient's paper chart.

18. Explain the purpose and process for each of the following:
   a. splitting or thinning a patient's paper chart
   b. stuffing a patient's paper chart
   c. reproducing a patient's paper chart

19. Describe how to correct the following errors on a paper chart form.
   a. written entry error
   b. labeling error

SURFING FOR ANSWERS

1. Research "Guidelines for retention of patient medical records." List at least three factors to be considered regarding length of time for which patient records should be retained. Provide two websites used.
2. Search the Internet for benefits of using EMRs over paper charts. List at least five and document two websites used.

Health Unit Coordinator Role in Processing of Electronic, Preprinted, and Handwritten Doctors' Orders

OUTLINE

CHAPTER OBJECTIVES

On completion of this chapter, you will be able to:

1. Define the terms in the vocabulary list.
2. Identify four methods that may be used by a doctor to provide orders for a hospitalized patient.
3. Name two criteria the health unit coordinator can use to recognize a new set of handwritten doctors' orders that need transcription.
4. List the four categories of doctors' orders, and explain the characteristics of each.
5. Describe the health unit coordinator's role in processing doctors' orders when computer physician order entry (CPOE) is used and in transcribing doctors' orders when paper charts are used (handwritten or preprinted orders).
6. Identify five common areas found on the Kardex form and describe the purpose of Kardexing.
7. Describe the process of ordering diagnostic procedures, treatment, medication, or supplies via computer.
8. Name and describe the purpose of the symbols used in transcribing doctors' orders, and describe the purpose and process of signing off on a set of doctor's orders.
9. List in order the 10 steps of transcribing handwritten doctors' orders.
10. Discuss why accuracy is important in the transcription procedure, the types of errors that may occur during the transcription procedure, and the methods of avoidance that may be used.

VOCABULARY

Flagging A method used by the doctor to notify the nursing staff that a new set of orders has been written.

Kardex File A portable file that contains and organizes the Kardex forms for each patient on the nursing unit.

Kardex Form A form on which the health unit coordinator records doctors' orders; it is used by the nursing staff for a quick reference to the patient's current orders.

Kardexing The process of recording and updating doctors' orders on the Kardex form (many hospitals have eliminated the paper Kardex form in favor of entering all patient orders into the computer).

One-Time or Short-Series Orders Doctors' orders that are executed according to the qualifying phrase and then automatically discontinued.

Ordering The process of requesting diagnostic procedures, treatments, or supplies from hospital departments other than nursing.

Preprinted Orders A typed set of orders for a specific diagnosis or procedure that has been approved for use in the hospital.

prn Orders Similar to standing orders, except that orders of this type are executed according to the patient's needs.

Requisition A paper form used to order diagnostic procedures, treatments, or supplies from hospital departments other than nursing when the computer is down (also called a *downtime requisition*).

Set of Doctor's Orders An entry of doctor's orders written on the doctor's order sheet, dated, notated for time, and signed by the doctor.

Signing Off A process by which the health unit coordinator records data (date, time, name, and status) on the doctor's order sheet to indicate the completion of transcription of a handwritten set of doctor's orders.

Standing Orders Doctors' orders that remain in effect and are executed as ordered until the doctor discontinues or changes them.

Stat Orders Doctors' orders that are to be executed immediately then automatically discontinued.

Symbols Notations which consist of words or letters written in black or red ink on the doctor's order sheet to document completion of a step of the transcription procedure.

Telephoned Orders Orders for a patient called into a health care facility (usually to the patient's nurse) by the doctor.

DOCTORS' ORDERS

Hospitals across the nation are in the process of implementing electronic medical records (EMRs) and computer physician order entry (CPOE). When the EMR with CPOE is used, the doctor enters orders for a patient's care and diagnostic studies directly into the computer on a physician's order form and the appropriate departments automatically receive the computerized orders. The doctor records the date and time and electronically signs each entry. The doctor may write one order or a collection of orders; this is referred to as a **set of doctor's orders.** The doctor may also enter orders from a remote location such as from his or her office computer.

When paper charts are being used, the doctors' orders are handwritten or preprinted on a paper doctors' order sheet located in the patient's chart binder. **Preprinted orders** are a typed set of orders for a specific diagnosis or procedure that has been approved for use in the hospital. The physician will have options for diagnostic and treatment orders that may be selected by marking the appropriate box or by placing a checkmark next to the order. Preprinted orders greatly reduce the potential for errors resulting from the inability of the health unit coordinator (HUC) to read the physician's handwriting. Physician's orders include such items as diagnostic procedures; medications; nursing, surgical, and other treatments; diet, patient activities; and discharge. As stated in Chapter 8, handwritten and preprinted doctors' orders are legal documents that become a permanent record of the patient's chart.

The doctor writes all orders in ink, records the date and time, and signs each entry. Again, the doctor may write one order or a collection of orders that is referred to as a set of doctor's orders. The doctor indicates to the nursing staff that a new set of orders is included by **flagging** the chart. Flagging techniques vary among health care facilities (e.g., they may involve dog-earing the order sheet or using a slide indicator on the side or top of the chart binder). New orders can be identified by the absence of symbols and by the absence of sign-off information. See Figure 9-1 for an example of a set of written doctor's orders. Sometimes, the doctor may write new orders and forget to flag the chart. Always check for new orders before returning a chart to the area where it is stored.

If the new orders are recorded at the top of the doctor's order sheet, check to see if the orders are a continuation from the previous sheet. When orders are recorded near the bottom of the doctor's order sheet instead of at the top, make diagonal lines

Physicians' Order Sheet

		Joint, Jane MR: 168495
		Acct#: 428975 DOB: 04-16-57
		DOA: 01-16-XX Dr.: T. Arthro
		Med-Surg Fe Rm: 318-2

Date	Symbol	Physicians' Orders
01/16/XX		Admit to med-surg
		CBR
		STAT CBC
		consultation with Dr. T.L. Payne
		HOB ↑ 30°
		Wt daily
		Rectal temp q 4°
		Intake and output
		Compazine 10 mg IM for nausea ana vomiting
		Dr. Thomas Arthro, M.D.

Figure 9-1 Example of a set of written doctor's orders. Interpretation of the abbreviations used in this figure and in subsequent figures in this chapter may be found in the Glossary and is explained in future chapters.

across the remaining space so new orders will not be recorded there, and then continue to the following page (Figure 9-2).

Doctors may also call the nursing unit and give **telephone orders** to the patient's nurse. The nurse would then write the order(s) on the patient's doctor's order sheet and sign the order with the physician's name along with his or her name (e.g., *Dr. John Tabler MD/Julie Brown RN*). The doctor is required to sign the orders at a later time.

Categories of Doctors' Orders

Doctors' orders may be categorized according to when they are carried out and the length of time for which they are in effect. The transcription procedure varies according to the category of the order; therefore it is necessary to recognize each category. The four categories include (1) **standing (continuing) orders**, (2) **prn orders**, (3) **one-time or short-series orders**, and (4) **stat orders**.

Standing (Continuing) Orders

Most doctors' orders fall into the group called *standing* or *continuing orders*. **Standing orders** are in effect and are executed routinely as ordered until they are discontinued or changed by a new doctor's order. For example, in following order:

- BP lying, sitting, and standing tid

the doctor has ordered that the patient's blood pressure (BP) be taken with the patient lying, sitting, and standing and that it be recorded three times a day (tid). A time sequence such as 0800, 1400, and 2000 is set up by the nursing personnel for the BP to be taken daily. This routine continues until it is changed or discontinued by the doctor.

Another example of a standing order includes the following:

- Regular diet

This order means that the patient receives a regular diet on each day of the hospital stay unless the order is changed or discontinued by the doctor.

prn Orders

The Latin words *pro re nata*, meaning "as circumstances may require," are abbreviated as *prn* and are used by the doctor in a written order to indicate that the order is to be executed as needed. Similar to standing orders, prn orders are in effect

until they are changed or discontinued by the doctor. They differ from standing orders in that they are executed according to the patient's needs. For example, in the following order:

- Acetaminophen 325 mg i or ii PO q4h prn H/A

the nurse may give 325 mg i or ii capsules as often as every 4 hours (q4h) as needed by the patient to relieve a headache. This does not mean that the medication is administered every 4 hours, because the patient may not have a headache at those times; therefore it is impossible to set up a time sequence as discussed for the standing order.

In the following order:

- Compazine 10 mg IM q6h for nausea or vomiting

the doctor uses a qualifying phrase—*for nausea or vomiting*—to indicate that it is a prn order.

Remember: A prn order may be recognized by the abbreviation *prn* or by the content of a qualifying phrase and is in effect until it is changed or discontinued by the doctor.

One-Time or Short-Series Order

The doctor may want a treatment or medication carried out once only or for a short period of time. A one-time or short-series order is indicated by a qualifying phrase, such as "give at 2:00 PM," or "give tonight and in AM." On completion of the one-time or short-series order, the order is automatically discontinued. For example, in the following orders:

- Give patient Fleets enema this PM

the phrase "this PM" makes it a one-time order—thus the order is discontinued after the enema has been given.

In the following order:

- Blood pressure q2h until awake

the phrase "until awake" makes it a short-series order.

> ★ **HIGH PRIORITY**
>
> A one-time or short-series order may be recognized by the content of the qualifying phrase and is automatically discontinued after completion.

Physicians' Order Sheet

```
Joint, Jane    MR: 168495
Acct#: 428975  DOB: 04-16-57
DOA: 01-16-XX  Dr.: T. Arthro
Med-Surg Fe    Rm: 318-2
```

Date	Symbol	Physicians' Orders
01/16/XX	Ord K	May have reg diet
		Dr. Thomas Arthro, M.D.
01/16/XX	1000	Ellen Green CHUC

Figure 9-2 Diagonal lines drawn at the bottom of a nearly filled doctors' order sheet.

Stat Orders

Stat is the abbreviation for the Latin word *statim*, which means "at once." When included in a doctor's order, it indicates that the order is to be carried out immediately. Stat orders are usually written during an emergency or for patients who are critically ill. Because of the urgency of stat orders, they are communicated immediately to the nurse and/or department personnel responsible for carrying out the order. Stat orders are transcribed first when included in a set of orders. Stat orders are recognized by the word *stat* (meaning "now") included in the order, as in the following examples:

- CBC stat
- CBC now (or CBC immediately)

The words *now* and *immediately* are usually considered to indicate stat orders that should receive urgent attention.

★ HIGH PRIORITY

Categories of Doctors' Orders

Standing: In effect and given routinely until discontinued or changed by the doctor

prn: In effect and given as needed by the patient until automatically discontinued or changed by the doctor

One-time or short-series: In effect for one time or a short period; automatically discontinued when the order has been completed

Stat: Given immediately, then automatically discontinued

Processing of Doctors' Orders with Computer Physician Order Entry

When CPOE has been implemented, the role of the HUC remains acting as the primary communicator in helping to coordinate patient care activities on the nursing unit. When orders have been entered into the computer directly by the physician, there are many tasks that must still be performed by the HUC. Orders for consultations are usually denoted by a telephone icon that appears next to the patient's name on the computer screen. Documentation of the consultation phone calls in detail is important and is discussed in more detail in Chapter 18 (Miscellaneous Orders). Additional phone call requests include requests by the nursing staff for the HUC to page or place calls to physicians. Another responsibility of the HUC that results directly from a physician's order is the coordination of patient discharge or transfer (which may be denoted by a "bed icon"). A physician may input an order that requires an outside appointment that must be scheduled and documented by the HUC.

The tasks related to patient discharges, transfers, and scheduling of appointments are also discussed in Chapters 18 and 20. The physician may input a request for patient medical records from a different facility; this may require HUC follow-up. One icon that may appear next to a patient's name in the computer as a direct result of CPOE is an order for the patient to be "NPO" (nothing to eat or drink). This is informational and can be an important icon for the HUC to verify in case the patient requests food or other hospital personnel need to verify the nutritional status. The HUC is responsible for many tasks that facilitate workflow related to doctor's orders and patient care. These tasks include communicating with the bed placement or admitting department; requesting outside health records; coordinating and printing discharge paperwork; printing and labeling consent forms; updating unit forms such as admission, discharge, and transfer sheets as well as face sheets and labels; managing equipment and delivering equipment in the pneumatic tube system; and checking utility and supply rooms.

Chart management includes scanning documents, reports and other items, such as telemetry strips or electrocardiogram (ECG) tracings, signed consent forms, discharge paperwork, and blood transfusion records, into the EMR. Unit management tasks may include assisting the clinical manager with staffing and bed and nurse assignments and allocating wireless communication devices and other technology such as workstations on wheels (WOWs) or Howard carts (combined computer and computerized medication drawer). As the EMR facility must ensure that the patient's medical record is up to date, it may be the HUC's responsibility to poll several EMRs at the beginning of the shift and verify that the information (such as lab results) is current (i.e., no more than 2 hours old). When the EMR system is to undergo a planned "downtime" session, it is the HUC's responsibility to print copies of part of the EMR (such as the last medication administration record [MAR] and set of lab results) and create temporary paper charts for all patients.

TRANSCRIPTION OF PREPRINTED AND HANDWRITTEN DOCTORS' ORDERS

Transcription of doctors' handwritten or preprinted orders is a process that is used to communicate doctors' orders to the nursing staff and other hospital departments. The transcription procedure includes Kardexing, ordering, using symbols, the signing-off process, and sometimes other steps. How the HUC goes about performing this procedure varies among health care facilities and from individual to individual

The Kardex File and the Kardex Form

Each nursing unit may use a portable file that is referred to as the *Kardex*. This file contains one **Kardex form** for each patient on the nursing unit. Approximately 15 to 20 individual patient Kardex forms can be included in one **Kardex file;** larger nursing units of 30 or more patients may need to use two Kardex files. Patient information such as room number, name, doctor's name, and diagnosis are recorded at the bottom of the Kardex form, so when filed in the Kardex file, the information remains visible (Figure 9-3).

Five main areas common to most Kardex forms are as follows:

1. Activity
2. Diet
3. Vital sign frequency
4. Treatment
5. Diagnostic studies

Other areas, such as intravenous therapy, intake and output, and weight, are usually included on the form.

The Kardex form also may include an area for a patient care plan, which is completed by the nursing staff. The purpose

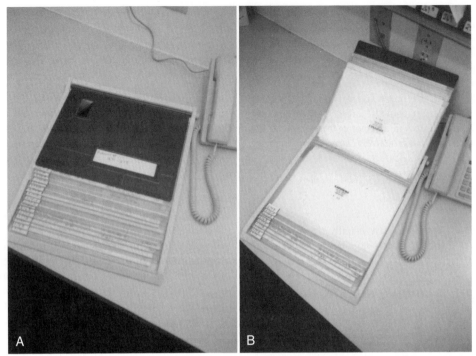

Figure 9-3 A portable file (a Kardex) as it appears closed **(A)** and open **(B).**

of the Kardex is to maintain a current profile of a patient's information, current doctors' orders, and the patient's nursing needs. It provides a quick reference for the nursing staff, is used for planning and designating patient care, and is used for reporting patient information to the oncoming shift. The design of the Kardex form varies according to hospital and nursing unit needs, but the basic concept remains the same.

Kardexing

Kardexing is the process of recording all new doctors' orders onto each patient's Kardex form. The purpose of Kardexing all the doctors' orders is to communicate new orders to the nursing staff and to update the patient's profile on the Kardex form. Kardexing is usually done in pencil because new doctors' orders may involve changing or discontinuing an existing order. However, information not subject to change, such as the patient's name, is usually recorded in black ink, and allergies are always recorded in red ink.

Accuracy in Kardexing is absolutely essential. An error could result in the patient's receiving the wrong, and perhaps harmful, treatment. The patient's Kardex form is usually not considered a legal document, and in the past, it was usually discarded when the patient was discharged from the hospital. However, the present trend is toward filing the nursing care plan portion of the Kardex form with the patient's chart in the health information management department.

★ HIGH PRIORITY

Many hospitals that have not completely implemented the electronic medical record (EMR) are using a computerized Kardexing system, eliminating the need for the form and the Kardex file. When the EMR is fully implemented, the Kardex is not used.

Ordering

Ordering is the process of inputting the handwritten doctors' orders into the computer or onto a paper or downtime **requisition.** Paper requisitions are seldom necessary, even when paper charts are used, because computer maintenance downtime is usually scheduled at night when few orders are written. The procedure for using paper requisitions is included in this chapter to assist one in learning the tests and procedures performed in each of the various departments of the hospital. The purpose of the ordering step is to communicate the doctors' orders to the hospital departments that will execute the orders. It is often the method by which the patient is charged for tests, treatments, and supplies.

Doctors' orders that involve diagnostic procedures, treatment, or supplies from hospital departments usually require the ordering step. Ordering by computer requires the HUC to select the patient's name from a computer screen and follow the steps to input the ordering information (according to the hospital computer program used). Ordering by downtime requisition requires the HUC to affix that patient's ID label on the requisition and to fill in all pertinent data from the doctors' orders.

★ HIGH PRIORITY

The completion of additional forms may be included in step 6 of transcription—for example, the preparation of surgical or invasive procedure consent forms, consultation forms, and blood transfusion consents. Documentation of these activities on the chart is important.

Symbols

As the HUC completes a part of the transcription procedure, a **symbol that consists of words or a letter** is recorded on the

Patient Label Information

Physicians' Order Sheet

Pharm Copy Sent @1445 EG

Date	Symbol	Physician's Orders
01/16/XX	K	Admit to med-surg
	K	CBR
	Ord, K	STAT CBC *called Pat @1450*
	K	Consultation with Dr. T. L. Payne *called Michele 1455*
	K	HOB ↑ 30°
	K	Wt daily
	K	Rectal temp q 4°
	K	Intake and output *I&O form prep*
	M	Compazine 10 mg IM for nausea and vomiting
		Dr. Thomas Arthro, M.D.
01/16/XX	1505	*Ellen Green, CHUC*

Figure 9-4 Example of a transcribed set of doctor's orders, showing use of the symbols to indicate that the pharmacy copy has been faxed (step 2), the telephone call has been placed and documented (step 4), the test has been ordered (step 6), the orders have been Kardexed (step 7), and the medication has been written on the medication administration record (MAR) (step 8). The set of orders has been signed off by the health unit coordinator, indicating completion of transcription (step 10).

doctors' order sheet to indicate completion of the task. The symbol may be written in black or red ink, depending on hospital policy, in front of the doctor's order (see Figure 9- 44).

By using symbols, the HUC provides a written record of the steps completed, which reduces the possibility of omitting or forgetting to complete a part of the transcription procedure. There are constant interruptions, and this could make it easy to forget where one left off when returning to transcribing a set of orders. Lack of order completion can cause delays in treatment, which may cause delays in or be harmful to the patient's recovery.

The following list of symbols is used in this textbook; however, symbols vary among hospitals. The instructor, therefore, may prefer that HUC students become familiar with symbols commonly used in hospitals in their area.

PC sent, faxed, or scanned: Indicates that the pharmacy copy of the doctors' order sheet was forwarded to the pharmacy. Initial and record the time it was sent on the copy or original if faxed. *Note:* Some hospitals have a "faxed" or "scanned" stamp with an area in which to fill in initials and the time sent.

Ord: Indicates that diagnostic tests, treatments, or supplies have been ordered by computer or by requisition. When using the computer method, record the computer order number above each ordered item.

K: Indicates that the order has been transcribed on the patient's Kardex form. It is also used to indicate that a discontinued order has been erased from the Kardex. Each order Kardexed requires the date and its own line on the Kardex.

M: Indicates transcription of a medication order on the MAR form.

Called (name and time): Indicates completion of a telephone call necessary to complete the doctor's order. Document the time of the call and the name of the person contacted above the order on the doctor's order sheet, and initial it.

Notified (name and time): Indicates that the appropriate health care team member has been notified of a stat order. Document above the order on the doctor's order sheet the time of notification and the name of the person contacted, and initial it.

Signing Off on a Set of Doctors' Orders

Signing off is the process that is used to indicate completion of the transcription procedure of a set of doctors' orders. To sign off, the HUC records the date, time, full name, and status (may use the abbreviation *SHUC* if a student HUC, or *CHUC* if certified) on the line directly below the doctor's signature (see Figure 9-4). Once again, this is done in black or red ink because the doctors' order sheet is a legal document. In many hospitals, a registered nurse is required to cosign the

⭐ **HIGH PRIORITY**

A panel of experienced nurses and health unit coordinators (HUCs) developed 10 steps of transcription to reduce the risk of errors. There will always be differences among what is done in the classroom, what is done in different hospitals, and even what is done in different nursing units within hospitals. Hospital or unit policy may dictate the process and may include the following variations: Symbols may be different or not be used at all, red ink or black ink only may be used to note orders, patient identification (ID) cards with imprinter machines may be used in place of labels, and different forms may be used. This and other chapters will assist the reader in coping with these variances. If the electronic medical record (EMR) with computer physician order entry (CPOE) is used, the HUC will not have the responsibility of transcribing written or preprinted doctors' orders but may still have to perform and document many of the tasks included in transcription, such as making telephone calls.

Flexibility is the key!

Doctor Ordering __Hy Hopes__   ☒ Stat   Joint, Jane   MR: 168495
Today's Date _____01/16/XX_____   ☐ Routine   Acct#: 428975   DOB: 04-16-57
Collection Date _01/16/XX_____ Time _____   DOA: 01-16-XX   Dr.: T. Arthro
Collected by _____   Med-Surg Fe   Rm: 318-2
Requested by ___J. Phoebe_____

Hematology	**Serology**	**Urinalysis/Urine Chemistry**
☐ Bleeding Time, Ivy	☐ ANA	☐ Routine UA
☒ CBC c̄ Diff	☐ ASO Titer	☐ Reflex UA
☐ CBC c̄ Manual Diff	☐ CEA	☐ Amylase (2 hr)
☐ Factor VIII	☐ CMV	☐ Bilirubin
☐ Fibrinogen	☐ IgG	☐ Calcium
☐ HCT	☐ IgM	☐ Chloride
☐ HGB	☐ Cocci Screen	☐ Creatinine Clearance
☐ H & H	☐ EBV Panel	☐ Glucose Tolerance
☐ Eosinophil Ct Absolute	☐ Enterovirus Ab Panel 1	☐ Nitrogen
☐ Eosinophil Smear	☐ Enterovirus Ab Panel 2	☐ Occult Blood
☐ ESR	☐ FTA	☐ Osmolality
☐ LE Cell Prep	☐ HbsAb	☐ Phosphorus
☐ Platelet Ct	☐ HbsAg	☐ Potassium
☐ PT	☐ Hepatitis Screen	☐ Pregnancy
☐ PTT (APTT)	☐ HIV	☐ Protein
☐ RBC	☐ Monospot	☐ Sodium
☐ RBC Indices	☐ PSA Screen	☐ Sp Gravity
☐ Reticulocyte Ct	☐ RA Factor	☐ Uric Acid
☐ Sickle Cell Prep	☐ RPR	
☐ WBC	☐ RSV	
☐ WBC c̄ Diff	☐ Rubella Screen	
☐ WBC c̄ Manual Diff	☐ Streptozyme	
☐ Other	☐ Other	

Write in Orders: _____

_____

Revised 3/12/XX

Figure 9-5 Completed downtime laboratory requisition.

transcribed orders. All hospitals require that registered nurses perform 24-hour chart checks, during which they will sign off on their assigned patients.

The sign-off procedure varies among health care facilities. For example, some health care facilities use black ink for the sign-off procedure. Some hospitals use red ink to distinguish the sign-off information from the written doctors' orders, and some require that the HUC draw a line to box off the orders when signing off.

Ten Steps for Transcription of Doctors' Handwritten or Preprinted Orders

In the following list are the 10 steps that make up the transcription procedure. It is important to note that each type of doctors' orders may require some or all of the steps to complete the transcription procedure. Always compare each order with the 10 steps of transcription when choosing the steps that are required for complete transcription of each order. This procedure is the simplest, yet most efficient, method used for transcribing doctors' orders. See Figure 9-4 for a transcribed set of doctors' orders.

The following 10 steps of transcription will assist the HUC in transcribing doctors' handwritten orders efficiently and accurately:

1. Read the complete set of doctor's orders.
2. Order medications by sending or faxing the pharmacy copy of the doctors' order sheet to the pharmacy department.

3. Complete all stat orders.
4. Place telephone calls as necessary to complete the doctor's orders.
5. Select the patient's identifying information (e.g., name, account number) from the census on the computer screen, or collect all necessary forms.
6. Order diagnostic tests, treatments, and supplies (see Figure 9-5 for a completed downtime laboratory requisition).
7. Kardex all the doctor's orders except medication orders (see Figure 9-6 for a completed Kardex).
8. Complete medication orders by writing them on the MAR.
9. Recheck each step for accuracy and thoroughness.
10. Sign off the completed set of the doctor's orders.

Procedure 9-1 describes a method of carrying out the 10 steps of transcription.

Avoiding Transcription Errors

Throughout this chapter, the importance of accuracy during the transcription procedure has been emphasized. Errors may cause serious harm or delay in treatment for the patient. Consider, for example, the consequences for the HUC who, during the transcription procedure, overlooks a doctor's order for the patient to have a stat medication, or orders a diet for a patient who has been ordered by the doctor to have nothing by mouth for a pending surgery or invasive medical procedure.

Table 9-1 outlines the types of errors that may occur during the transcription procedure and methods that may be used to avoid making these errors.

Kardex Form

Activity *1/16 C*Ⓑ*R* *HOB* ↑*30°*	Date Ord	Treatments	Date Ord	Laboratory	Date Ord	Allergies	
	1/16	*Consult Dr. T.L. Payne*	1/16	*stat CBC*			
						Diagnostic Imaging	Date to
Diet							be Done
Vital signs *1/16 Rtemp q 4 h*							
Weight *1/16 Daily*							
IV		Respiratory Care		Pre OP Orders		Diagnostic Studies	
				Daily Lab			
I & O *1/16*							
Retention Cath (Foley) ☐ Health Records _____		Physical Medicine					
Adm. Date *1/16*		Consultations:		Surgery: Date:			
Name *Joint, Jane*	Doctor *T.Arthro*		Age *51*	Diagnosis *Osteoarthritis*		Date of admission *1/16/xx*	

Figure 9-6 Completed Kardex.

PROCEDURE 9-1
TRANSCRIPTION OF DOCTORS' ORDERS

TASK	NOTES
1. Read the complete set of doctor's orders.	Reading the complete set of orders gives an overview of the task at hand. Accurate reading and interpretation of each word of a doctor's handwritten orders are vital because each word and/or abbreviation carries a specific meaning.

2. Order medications.
  a. Remove and send the pharmacy copy of the doctors' order sheet, or fax original copy of doctors' order sheet to the pharmacy.
  b. Write "PC sent" (or "faxed"), time, and initials on the doctors' order sheet (see Figure 9- 4).
	Sending a copy or faxing the original doctor's order to the pharmacy helps avoid medication errors because no rewriting is involved. Completing this step first allows the patient to receive the medication as soon as possible.

3. Complete all stat orders.	Stat orders are always transcribed first.
4. Place telephone calls as necessary to complete the doctor's orders. On completing this task, insert the symbol *called* and the time *called* (be sure to include AM or PM, or use military time) and the name of the person receiving the call in ink in front of the doctor's order on the doctors' order sheet (see Figure 9- 4).	Doctors' orders may require a telephone call to be placed to another department or health agency to schedule appointments, procedures, and so on. Recording the time of the call and the name of the person who is receiving the call is helpful if follow-up is necessary.
5. Select the correct patient's name on the computer screen, and/or collect all necessary forms.	This varies according to the type of doctors' orders included in the set. Collecting necessary forms at once saves time.

6. Order all diagnostic tests, treatments, and supplies.
Using a computer with CD-ROM, which simulates a hospital computer system, do the following:
  a. Select the correct patient's name on the viewing screen.
  b. Select the department from the department menu on the viewing screen.
  c. Select the test, treatment, or supply from the menu on the viewing screen.
  d. Fill in required information.
  e. Order test, treatments, or supplies.
  f. Insert the symbol *ord* or computer number in ink in front of the doctor's order on the doctors' order sheet (see Figure 9- 4).
	This step includes ordering diagnostic procedures, treatments, and supplies from appropriate hospital departments.
	Check both the patient's name and the hospital number with the same information in the chart.

Using handwritten requisitions: Although handwritten requisitions are seldom used, this process will assist the student in learning which departments would perform tests and procedures ordered.
  a. Affix the patient's identification (ID) label to the requisition (or imprint).
  b. Place a checkmark on the requisition to indicate the test, treatment, or supply that is being requisitioned.
  c. Fill in today's date and the date the test or treatment is to be done in the appropriate spaces.
  d. Write in pertinent data, such as "patient blind" or "isolation."
  e. Sign name and status in the appropriate space on the requisition form.
  f. Write the symbol *ord* in ink in front of the doctor's order on the doctors' order sheet (see Figure 9-4).
	Selection of the correct patient when one is filling out requisitions is absolutely essential. The wrong selection could easily cause a patient to receive a diagnostic test or treatment intended for another patient. Always compare the name and hospital number on the requisition form with the same information in the chart. Remember: There may be more than one patient on the unit with the same last name. Label all requisitions for the patient whose orders are being processed at the same time.

7. Kardex all the doctor's orders. Begin with the first order, then proceed to the next until all the orders have been completed (see Figure 9-6). Complete Kardexing by doing the following: a. Write the date followed by the order in pencil under the correct column of the Kardex form. Carefully read what is already written in the column to evaluate whether the new order cancels an existing order. If this occurs, erase the existing order. If an order is discontinued, erase it from the Kardex.	Nursing orders that need to be implemented during the shift are often recorded on a clipboard in order to bring them to the immediate attention of the nurse. *All doctors' orders are Kardexed. Make sure the right patient's Kardex form is selected; many patients' Kardex forms are filed in a single Kardex file. To ensure accurate selection, check the name of the patient and the doctor on the Kardex form with the patient information in the chart.

PROCEDURE 9-1—cont'd

TRANSCRIPTION OF DOCTORS' ORDERS

TASK	NOTES
b. Write the symbol *K* in ink in front of the doctors' order on the doctors' order sheet (see Figure 9-4).	*There may be more than one patient on the unit with the same last name. Note: Many hospitals are using a computerized Kardexing system.
8. Complete medication orders by doing the following: a. Write the medication order on the medication administration record (MAR). b. Place the symbol *M* in ink in front of the doctor's order on the doctors' order sheet (see Figure 9-4).	This procedure is covered in greater detail in Chapter 13.
9. Recheck the performance of each task for accuracy and thoroughness.	This is an important step because it is easy to miss an order or a detail of an order.
10. Sign off the completed set of orders by writing the following in ink on the line directly below the doctor's signature: a. Date b. Time c. Full signature d. Status Figure 9-4 provides an example of this step.	It is important to have completed all the tasks of transcription before signing off. *Signing off on a set of doctors' orders is an indication that all the transcription steps necessary for the orders to be carried out as written have been performed.

TABLE 9-1 Avoiding Transcription Errors

Types of Errors	Method of Avoidance
Errors of omission	Read and understand each word of the doctor's orders. If in doubt, check with the patient's nurse or the doctor. Use symbols. It is especially important to write the symbol after each step of transcription has been completed. When new orders are recorded at the top of the doctors' order sheet, check the previous order sheet to see whether these orders are continued from the previous page. If the set of orders finishes near the bottom of the doctors' order sheet, cross through the remaining space with diagonal lines. This is done so that newly written orders will begin at the top of the new doctors' order form. When orders are recorded at the bottom of one page and are continued onto the next, it is easy to miss transcribing those recorded on the first page. Record the signing-off information on the line directly below the doctor's signature to avoid leaving space in which future orders could be written and missed. Check for new orders before returning a chart from the counter or elsewhere to the chart rack.
Errors of interpretation	When in doubt about the correct interpretation of doctors' orders, always check with the registered nurse or the doctor.
Errors in the selection of the patient's identification (ID) label or errors in selection of the patient's name on the computer screen	Compare the patient's name and the hospital number on the order requisition form or on the computer screen with the same information in the patient's chart. Never select computer labels by the patient's room number only. *Note:* Other staff members frequently use the computer to retrieve information and may change screens while orders are being transcribed. Always double-check the patient information when entering orders into the computer.
Errors in selection of the patient's Kardex form	Compare the patient's name and the doctor's name on the Kardex form with the same information in the patient's chart. Never select by using room number alone. If the patient has been transferred, the room number imprinted on chart forms may no longer be correct. *Note:* Many nursing staff members use the Kardex for a quick reference and may flip to another patient's Kardex form while orders are being transcribed. Remove the Kardex form from the holder when transcribing orders and return it to its proper place in the Kardex holder when order transcription has been completed.
Errors in reading a doctor's poor handwriting	When an order cannot be read because of the doctor's handwriting, refer to the progress record form in the patient's chart. The orders are often recorded on this form also, and using this information may assist in interpreting the orders on the physician's order form. If the order remains unclear, ask the doctor who wrote it or ask the patient's nurse for clarification. If a doctor has a reputation for poor handwriting, ask to go over the orders for clarification before the doctor leaves the nursing unit.

HIGH PRIORITY

How to Avoid Errors of Transcription
- Ask the doctor or nurse for assistance if a doctor's order cannot be read or understood.
- Use information from the chart to correctly select the patient from the computer screen or to correctly label requisitions.
- Record the sign-off information on the line directly below the doctor's signature.
- Check the previous page for orders when the orders begin at the top of the page.

KEY CONCEPTS

Unless the EMR with CPOE is implemented, the transcription of doctors' orders is the single most important task that a HUC performs. An error may result in harm to a patient or in his or her recovery time being extended. Completing the transcription procedure promptly, accurately, and thoroughly is always the best practice in providing high-quality care for patients. When CPOE is being used, the HUC continues to communicate and coordinate many activities that affect patient care and the workflow on the hospital unit.

Websites of Interest

Centers for Medicare and Medicaid Services overview of e-prescribing: www.cms.gov/eprescribing

U.S. Department of Health and Human Services—"Health Information Privacy": www.hhs.gov/ocr/privacy/hipaa/faq/right_to_access_medical_records

Medline Plus—"Personal Health Records": www.nlm.nih.gov/medlineplus/personalhealthrecords.html

REVIEW QUESTIONS

Visit the Evolve website to download and complete the following questions.

1. Define the following terms:
   a. ordering
   b. Kardexing
   c. requisition
   d. flagging
   e. preprinted orders
   f. set of doctor's orders

2. Identify four methods that may be used by a doctor to provide orders for a hospitalized patient.

3. List two ways that the HUC would recognize newly written doctors' orders that need transcription.

4. Describe the health unit coordinator's role in the processing of physician orders when CPOE is used and in transcription of physician orders when paper charts are used.

5. Provide examples used to indicate completion of the following:
   a. ordering
   b. writing of a medication order on the MAR
   c. Kardexing
   d. telephone call
   e. pharmacy copy sent or faxed
   f. notification to appropriate person of a stat order

6. Symbols are recorded on the doctors' order sheet (circle the letter of the correct answer):
   a. after the step of transcription is completed
   b. before the step of transcription is completed
   c. at any time, as long as they are recorded accurately
   d. after the patient's nurse has verified that the step of transcription is complete

7. Explain the purpose of the HUC "signing off" on a set of doctors' orders and demonstrate how the HUC would sign off.

8. List *in order* the 10 steps of transcribing handwritten doctors' orders.

9. Describe the purpose of Kardexing, and list five common areas found on a Kardex

10. Why are doctors' orders written on the Kardex form in pencil?

11. Describe the process of ordering diagnostic procedures, treatment, or supplies via computer.

12. Explain why accuracy is essential when transcribing doctors' orders.

13. Identify six types of errors and precautions that can be taken to avoid them.

14. Identify each type (category) of order written:
   a. blood pressure q3h until alert
   b. morphine 8 to 12 mg IM q3-4h prn pain
   c. diazepam 10 mg PO now
   d. Premarin 1.25 mg PO daily
   e. regular diet
   f. Fleet enema this pm and repeat in am
   g. TWE this a.m.

15. How would a stat order be identified?

SURFING FOR ANSWERS

1. Research patient medication safety tips. List three, and document at least two websites used.
2. Research and document the federal agency that tracks medication errors.

CHAPTER 10

Patient Activity, Patient Positioning, and Nursing Observation Orders

CHAPTER OBJECTIVES

On completion of this chapter, you will be able to:

1. Define the terms in the vocabulary list.
2. Write the meaning of the abbreviations in the abbreviation list.
3. Explain how and why The Joint Commission's "Do Not Use" list was developed and identify abbreviations that are on the "Do Not Use" list.
4. Identify patient activity and patient positioning orders.
5. List the four measurements included in a patient's daily vital signs.
6. Describe five methods of taking a patient's temperature.
7. Explain how orthostatic vital signs are measured.
8. Identify at least three tests that may be performed at the point of care or bedside (POCT).
9. Explain what type of patient would require blood glucose monitoring, and identify two types of blood glucose monitors that are commonly used.
10. Identify the hospital areas in which pulse oximetry would be used and the reason for it.
11. Identify the nursing unit that would employ a cardiac monitor technician.
12. Explain the function of nursing observation orders, and list at least four examples of nursing observation orders.

13. Explain the reason for a doctor ordering intake and output (I&O), and list the items that would be included in "intake" and "output."

VOCABULARY

Activity Order A doctor's order that defines the type and amount of activity a hospitalized patient may have.

Afebrile Without fever.

Apical Rate Heart rate obtained from the apex of the heart.

Axillary Temperature The temperature reading obtained by placing the thermometer in the patient's axilla (armpit).

Bedside Commode A chair or wheelchair with an open seat, used at the bedside by the patient for the passage of urine and stool.

Blood Pressure The measurement of the pressure of blood against the artery walls.

Cardiac Monitor Device that shows the electrical and pressure waveforms of the cardiovascular system for measurement and treatment. Monitors heart function, providing visual and audible record of heartbeat.

Cardiac Monitor Technician A person who observes the cardiac monitors; health unit coordinators may be cross-trained to this position.

Celsius (C) A scale used to measure temperature in which the freezing point of water is 0° and the boiling point is 100° (formerly called *Centigrade*).

Daily TPRs A patient's temperature, pulse, and respiration, taken at certain times each day.

Dangle the patient sits and hangs their feet over the edge of the bed.

Diastolic Blood Pressure The minimum level of blood pressure measured between contractions of the heart; in blood pressure readings, it is the lower number of the two measurements.

Emesis Vomit.

Fahrenheit (F) A scale used to measure temperature, in which 32° is the freezing point of water and 212° is the boiling point.

Febrile Having an elevated body temperature (a fever).

Fowler's Position A semi-sitting position.

Intake and Output The measurement of the patient's fluid intake and output.

Neurologic Vital Signs (neuro checks) Measurable indicators of the function of the body's neurologic system; includes checking pupils of the eyes, verbal response, and so forth.

Nursing Observation Order A doctor's order that requests the nursing staff to observe and record certain patient signs and symptoms.

Oral Temperature The temperature reading obtained by placing the thermometer in the patient's mouth under the tongue.

Orthostatic Hypotension A temporary lowering of blood pressure (hypotension) usually resulting from suddenly standing up; also called *postural hypotension*.

Orthostatic Vital Signs Measurement (Orthostatics) Recording the patient's blood pressure and pulse rate while the patient is supine (lying) and again while he or she is erect (sitting and/or standing).

Oxygen Saturation A noninvasive measurement of gas exchange and red blood cell oxygen-carrying capacity.

Pedal Pulse The pulse rate obtained on the top of the foot.

Point-of-Care Testing (POCT) Medical testing at or near the site of patient care.

Positioning Orders Doctors' orders that request that the patient be placed in a specified body position.

Pulse Deficit The discrepancy between the ventricular rate detected at the apex of the heart and the arterial rate at the radial pulse.

Pulse Oximeter A device that measures gas exchange and red blood cell oxygen-carrying capacity by attaching a probe to either the ear or the finger (also called an *oxygen saturation monitor*).

Pulse Oximetry A noninvasive method of measuring gas exchange and red blood cell oxygen-carrying capacity (considered to be the fifth vital sign).

Pulse Rate The number of times per minute the heartbeat is felt through the walls of the artery.

Radial Pulse Pulse rate obtained on the wrist.

Rectal Temperature The temperature reading obtained by placing the thermometer in the patient's rectum.

Respiration Rate The number of times a patient breathes per minute.

Systolic Blood Pressure The blood pressure measured during the period of ventricular contraction; in blood pressure readings, it is the higher, upper number of the two measurements.

Temperature The quantity of body heat, measured in degrees—Fahrenheit or Celsius.

Trendelenburg Position A position in which the head is low and the body and legs are on an inclined plane (sometimes used in pelvic surgery to displace the abdominal organs upward, out of the pelvis, or to increase the blood flow to the brain in hypotension and shock).

Tympanic (aural) Temperature The temperature reading obtained by placing an aural (ear) thermometer in the patient's ear.

Vital Signs Measurements of body functions, including temperature, pulse, respiration, and blood pressure.

ABBREVIATIONS

Abbreviation	Meaning	Example of Usage on a Doctor's Order Sheet
A&O	alert and oriented	D/C to home when A&O
ABR	absolute bed rest	ABR × 12 hr
ac	before meals	accu ✓ ac
ad lib	as desired	up ad lib
amb	ambulate	amb c̄ help
asst	assistance	Up c̄ asst
as tol	as tolerated	up as tol
ax	axilla or axillary	ax temp tid
bid	two times per day	up in chair 20 min bid
BP	blood pressure	BP tid, call if systolic ↑ 150
BR	bed rest	BR until A&O
BRP	bathroom privileges	BRP only
BSC	bedside commode	may use BSC
c̄	with	up c̄ help
CBR	complete bed rest	CBR today
CMS	circulation, motion, sensation	check CMS fingers rt hand
CMT	cardiac monitor technician	HUC may be cross-trained as a CMT
C/O	complains of	Call me if pt c/o SOB
CVP	central venous pressure	measure CVP q4h
DBP	diastolic blood pressure	Call me if DBP ↑ 90
D/C *or* DC	discontinue *or* discharge	D/C BSC *or* DC to home today
HOB	head of bed	↑ HOB
h, hr, hrs	hour, hours	flat in bed for 8 h
hs	hour of sleep	accu ✓ ac & hs
I&O	intake and output	Strict I&O
lt, Ⓛ	left	↑ lt arm on pillow
min	minutes	up in chair for 5 min today
NVS or neuro ✓s	neurologic vital signs or checks	NVS q4h & record
°	degree or hour	elevate head of bed 30 degrees
OOB	out of bed	OOB ad lib
P	pulse	BP&P q4h
pc	after meals	up in chair for 1 hr pc
prn	as necessary	up prn

q	every	wt q day
qd	every day or daily	wt q day
qh *or* q-h	every hour *or* every (fill in number) hour	check VS q2h
qid	four times a day	VS qid
qod	every other day	wt q other day
R	rectal	R temp
RR	respiratory rate	monitor RR q1h
rt, ®	right	↑ rt arm on pillow
rout	routine	rout VS
s̄	without	
SBP	systolic blood pressure	call me if SBP ↑ 160
SOB	shortness of breath	evaluate for SOB & notify physician
temp or T	temperature	rectal temp
tid	three times a day	up in chair tid
TPR	tempera-ture, pulse, respiration	TPR & BP q4h
U/O	urine output	✓ cath U/O q2hr
VS	vital signs	VS q4h
w̄	with	
wt	weight	wt daily
×	times	position on lt side × 2 hr

↑ or >	increase, above, elevate, or greater than	↑ arm on 2 pillows call me if P > 110
↓ or <	decrease, below, lower, or less than	call me if BP ↓ 100/60 call me if BP < 100/60

THE JOINT COMMISSION

The Joint Commission (TJC), founded in 1951, has been acknowledged as the leader in developing the highest standards for quality and safety in the delivery of health care. Today more than 19,000 health care providers use TJC standards to guide how they administer care and continuously improve performance. In 2001 TJC issued a Sentinel Event Alert on the subject of medical abbreviations, and 1 year later a National Patient Safety Goal (NPSG) requiring accredited organizations to develop and implement a list of abbreviations not to use. In 2002 TJC established its NPSG program to help accredited organizations address specific areas of concern regarding patient safety. A panel called the Patient Safety Advisory Group composed of nurses, physicians, pharmacists, risk managers, clinical engineers, and other professionals works with and advises TJC staff to identify and address emerging patient safety issues. In 2004 TJC created its "do not use" list of abbreviations as part of the requirements for meeting that goal (Table 10-1).

TABLE 10-1 The Joint Commission's Official "Do Not Use" List*

Do Not Use	Potential Problem	Use Instead
U, u (unit)	Mistaken for "0" (zero), the number "4" (four) or "cc"	Write "unit"
IU (International Unit)	Mistaken for IV (intravenous) or the number 10 (ten)	Write "International Unit"
Q.D., QD, q.d., qd (daily)	Mistaken for each other	Write "daily"
Q.O.D., QOD, q.o.d, qod (every other day)	Period after the Q mistaken for "I" and the "O" mistaken for "I"	Write "every other day"
Trailing zero (X.0 mg)†	Decimal point is missed	Write X mg
Lack of leading zero (.X mg)		Write 0.X mg
MS	Can mean morphine sulfate or magnesium sulfate	Write "morphine sulfate"
MSO4 and MgSO4	Confused for each other	Write "morphine sulfate" or "magnesium sulfate"

Additional Abbreviations, Acronyms, and Symbols for Possible Future Inclusion in the Official "Do Not Use" List

> (greater than)	Misinterpreted as the number "7" (seven) or the letter "L"	Write "greater than"
< (less than)	Confused for each other	Write "less than"
Abbreviations for drug names	Misinterpreted due to similar abbreviations for multiple drugs	Write drug names in full
Apothecary units	Unfamiliar to many practitioners Confused with metric units	Use metric units
@	Mistaken for the number "2" (two)	Write "at"
cc	Mistaken for U (units) when poorly written	Write "mL" or "ml" or "milliliters" ("mL" is preferred)
μg	Mistaken for mg (milligrams), resulting in one thousand–fold overdose	Write "mcg" or "micrograms"

Courtesy The Joint Commission, 2011.

*Applies to all orders and all medication-related documentation that is handwritten (including free-text computer entry) or on preprinted forms.

†*Exception:* A trailing zero may be used only where required to demonstrate the level of precision of the value being reported, such as for laboratory results, imaging studies that report size of lesions, or catheter or tube sizes. It may not be used in medication orders or other medication-related documentation.

⊖ EXERCISE 1

Write the abbreviations for each term listed.

1. complete bed rest
2. with
3. alert and oriented
4. four times a day
5. degree or hour
6. blood pressure
7. every
8. ambulatory
9. absolute bed rest
10. increase, above, or elevate
11. bathroom privileges
12. respiratory rate
13. as desired
14. every other day
15. two times a day
16. every day
17. three times a day
18. every hour
19. temperature
20. as tolerated
21. right
22. left
23. discontinue or discharge
24. vital signs
25. intake and output
26. out of bed
27. minutes
28. weight
29. bed rest
30. rectal
31. axilla or axillary
32. temperature, pulse, respiration
33. pulse
34. hour or hours
35. as necessary
36. neurologic vital signs or neuro checks
37. decrease, below, or lower
38. head of bed
39. bedside commode
40. every 4 hours
41. circulation, motion, and sensation
42. shortness of breath
43. central venous pressure
44. routine
45. cardiac monitor technician
46. times
47. assistance
48. diastolic blood pressure
49. systolic blood pressure
50. urine output
51. before meals
52. hour of sleep
53. complains of
54. after meals

⊖ EXERCISE 2

Write the meaning of each abbreviation listed.

1. lt or Ⓛ
2. rt or Ⓡ
3. D/C or DC
4. VS
5. BP
6. tid
7. CBR
8. c̄
9. TPR
10. BR
11. min
12. BRP
13. ad lib
14. ↑ or >
15. OOB
16. A&O
17. wt
18. amb
19. q other day
20. q day
21. bid
22. qid
23. qh
24. ABR
25. temp or T
26. as tol
27. I&O
28. q
29. P
30. ax
31. R
32. prn
33. RR
34. q4h
35. h, hr, or hrs
36. NVS or neuro ✓s
37. ↓ or <
38. rt
39. SOB
40. HOB
41. BSC
42. CMS
43. CVP
44. rout
45. CMT
46. ×
47. asst
48. DBP
49. SBP
50. U/O
51. ac
52. hs
53. C/O
54. pc

PATIENT ACTIVITY ORDERS

Background Information

Patient activity refers to the amount of walking, sitting, and other motions that the patient may do in a given period during a hospital stay. The prescribed activity changes to coincide with the patient's stage of recovery. For example, after some major surgical procedures, the doctor may prefer that the patient remain in bed; as the patient recovers, the doctor increases the level of activity accordingly. The doctor indicates the degree of activity the patient should have by writing an **activity order** on the doctors' order sheet or by entering the order directly into the patient's electronic record when the electronic medical record (EMR) has been implemented. Common activity orders are listed here with interpretations.

 Doctors' Orders for Patient Activities

CBR

The patient is to remain in bed at all times.

BR c̄ BRP

The patient may use the bathroom for the elimination of urine and stool but otherwise must remain in bed.

Dangle Tonight

The patient may sit and **dangle** his or her legs and feet over the edge of the bed. The doctor may specify the number of times per day the patient should dangle, such as *Dangle bid*, or may specify a period of time, such as *Dangle 5 min tid*.

Use Bedside Commode or Use BSC
The patient may use a portable commode at the bedside.

Note: The health unit coordinator (HUC) may need to order a **bedside commode** from the central service department (depending on the type of nursing unit; a geriatrics or rehabilitation unit may have them available on the unit).

Up c̄ Help
The patient may be out of bed when assisted by a member of the nursing staff.

Up in Chair
The patient may sit in a chair. The doctor may specify the length of time and/or the number of times per day, especially if this activity is ordered after complete bed rest (CBR). Example: *Up in chair 20 min tid*.

BRP When A&O
The patient may use the bathroom as desired when alert and oriented.

Up in Hall
The patient may walk in the hall.

Up as Tol
The patient may be out of bed as much as can be physically tolerated.

Up ad Lib
The patient has no restriction on activity.

OOB
The patient may be out of bed. The doctor may qualify this order with another statement, such as *OOB bid. c̄ asst*.

Amb
This is another way of saying that the patient may be up as desired.

May Shower
The patient may have a shower. A doctor's order is necessary for a hospitalized patient to have a shower or tub bath.

These orders are written in abbreviated form as the doctor would write them on the doctor's order sheet, *with one exception:* They are not written in a doctor's handwriting. Reading doctors' handwriting can be a difficult task. However, the repetitive reading of doctors' handwritten orders helps the HUC become more adept in this area. For assistance with abbreviations, refer to the Abbreviations list at the beginning of the chapter. ■

SKILLS CHALLENGE

To practice transcribing an activity order, complete Activity 10-1 in the *Skills Practice Manual*.

PATIENT POSITIONING ORDERS

Background Information

Patient positioning is often determined by the nursing staff; however, the doctor may want the patient to remain in a special body position to maintain body alignment, promote comfort, and facilitate body functions. For example, the doctor may order the head of the bed to be elevated to ease the patient's breathing or may want the nurse to turn the patient to the unaffected side to promote healing. The doctor indicates a special position by writing the order on the doctor's order sheet. Because it would be impossible to discuss all patient **positioning orders,** only those that are most typical are described here. The following positioning orders are written in the same terms as are found on a doctor's handwritten order sheet. Refer to the Abbreviations list at the beginning of the chapter for assistance.

Doctors' Orders for Patient Positioning

↑ HOB 30° or Elevate Head of Bed 30 Degrees
The head of the bed is to be elevated 30 degrees. (The degree of elevation may vary according to the purpose of the order; for example, the doctor may write ↑ *head of bed 20 degrees*.)

↑ Lt Arm on 2 Pillows or Elevate Lt Arm on Two Pillows
The left arm is to be elevated on two pillows. Variations on this order include the degree of elevation and may involve other limbs; for example, *Elevate rt foot on pillow*.

Fowler's Position
The patient is placed in a semi-sitting position by elevating the head of the bed approximately 18 to 20 inches, or 45 degrees, with a slight elevation of the knees. The semi-**Fowler's position** is the same as the Fowler's position, but with the head of the bed elevated 30 degrees (Fig. 10-1).

Trendelenburg Position
The patient is placed in a position in which the head is low and the body and legs are on an inclined plane (sometimes used in pelvic surgery to displace the abdominal organs upward out of the pelvis, or to increase the blood flow to the brain in hypotension and shock.)

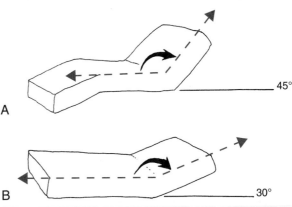

Figure 10-1 A, Fowler's position. **B,** Semi-Fowler's position.

Log Roll

The patient is turned from side to side or from side to back while keeping the back straight like a log, with a pillow between the knees.

Turn to Unaffected Side

The doctor wishes the patient to lie on the side that is free of injury.

Flat in Bed × 8 hr—No Pillow

The patient is to remain flat in bed for 8 hours, after which the standing activity order is resumed.

Turn q2h

The patient's position is changed every 2 hours to prevent skin breakdown (bedsores). ∎

SKILLS CHALLENGE

To practice transcribing a patient positioning order, complete Activity 10-2 in the *Skills Practice Manual*.

NURSING OBSERVATION ORDERS

Background Information

The doctor will often write a **nursing observation order** for periodic observation of the patient's condition, referred to as *signs and symptoms*. Some doctors may write "call" orders, if they want to be called in the event of certain circumstances. An example would be, *Call if P > 110, R <10, T > 101°, B/P systolic ↑ 160, diastolic ↑ 90.* The doctor may need this information to assist in diagnosing the patient's illness or interpreting the patient's progress. The doctor writes or electronically enters an order to request the information wanted. It is difficult to include all doctors' orders that may be encountered in this area. Outlined in the following sections are some of the more common ones as they might be written. For assistance with the interpretation of these abbreviations, refer to the Abbreviations list at the beginning of the chapter.

Vital Sign References

Vital Sign	Age	Normal	Average
Body temperature	Adult	Oral: 98.6° F (37° C)	Rectal: 99.6° (F) 37.6° (C)
	1 yr old	Oral: 99.7° (F) 37.6° (C)	
Pulse	Adult	60-80	80
	1 yr old	80-170	120
Respiration	Adult	12-20	18
	1 yr old	20-40	30
Blood Pressure	Adult	Systolic 100-140	120
		Diastolic 60-90	80*
	Infant	Systolic 65-115	90
		Diastolic 42-80	61

*Recommendation for normal blood pressure is ↓ 120/80 mm Hg.

Vital signs consist of the following:
- Temperature—Oral, tympanic (aural), axillary, rectal
- Pulse—Apical, radial, pedal, femoral, carotid, popliteal, brachial
- Respiration rate
- Blood pressure

Vital Signs Measurement

Vital signs include **temperature, pulse rate, respiration rate**, and blood pressure reading. Each hospitalized patient's vital signs are taken on a daily basis and are called **daily TPRs**. A patient's **tympanic (aural) temperature** is taken using a tympanic thermometer (Fig. 10-2, *A*), **oral temperature** and **axillary temperature** using an oral thermometer, or **rectal temperature** using a rectal thermometer. Oral and rectal thermometers may be glass or electric (see Fig. 10-2, *B* and *C*). Results of the temperature may be recorded using the **Celsius (C)** or **Fahrenheit (F)** scale and will indicate whether the patient is **febrile** or **afebrile** (Table 10-2). The pulse is obtained from the radial artery in the wrist, unless otherwise indicated (see Fig. 10-3 for locations of pulse points on the body). A **pulse deficit** is the difference between the patient's **radial pulse** (arterial rate) and the **apical rate** (ventricular rate) taken at the apex of the heart. **Blood pressure** is the measurement of the pressure of blood against the artery walls. The higher upper number measured during the period of ventricular contraction is called the **systolic blood pressure,** and the lower number, the minimum level of blood pressure measured between contractions of the heart, is called the **diastolic blood pressure.**

Orthostatic Vital Signs Measurement (Orthostatics)

When a doctor writes an order for orthostatic vital signs measurement (**orthostatics**), the nurse will record the patient's blood pressure and pulse rate while the patient is supine (lying) and again while he or she is erect (sitting and/or standing). A significant change in vital signs may signify dehydration or **orthostatic hypotension**, which is a temporary lowering of blood pressure *(hypotension)* owing usually to sudden standing up *(orthostatic)*. Hypotension is more common in older people when they rise quickly from a chair, especially after a meal, and may be accompanied by a few seconds of disorientation. The change in position causes a temporary reduction in blood flow and therefore a shortage of oxygen to the brain. This leads to light-headedness and sometimes to a loss of consciousness. A positive test result occurs if the patient becomes dizzy or has a pulse increase of 20 or more beats per minute or a systolic blood pressure decrease of 20 or more mm Hg (millimeters of mercury).

Point-of-Care Testing

Point-of-care testing (POCT) bring tests conveniently and immediately to the patient. The patient, physician, and care team will receive the results more quickly, which allows for quicker treatment decisions to be made. Blood glucose testing, blood gases, pulse oximetry, and electrolyte analysis are just a few tests that can be performed at the bedside; others will be discussed in Chapter 14.

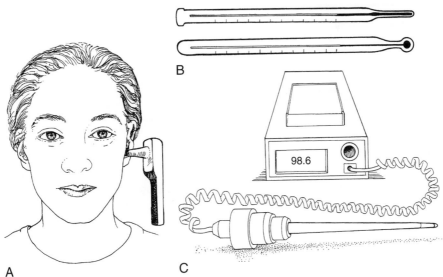

Figure 10-2 Types of thermometers. **A,** Aural—used to take tympanic membrane temperature in the ear. **B,** Glass—used to take oral, rectal, and axillary temperatures. **C,** Electric—used to take oral and rectal temperatures. A temporal thermometer (not pictured) is a totally non-invasive system that involves a gentle forehead scan with advanced infrared technology. It is the ideal thermometer for use with newborns, infants, children, or adults.

TABLE 10-2 Celsius-Fahrenheit Conversion

Conversion from Fahrenheit to Celsius	Conversion from Celsius to Fahrenheit
Subtract 32	Multiply by 9
Multiply by 5	Divide by 5
Divide by 9	Add 32

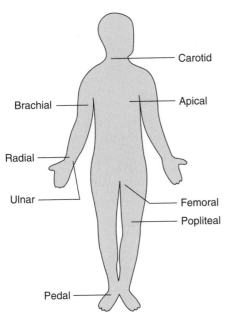

Figure 10-3 Location of the pulse points on the body.

Blood Glucose Monitoring Orders

Blood glucose monitoring is a point-of-care test routinely performed by the nursing staff for diabetic patients or patients who are receiving nutritional support (total parenteral nutrition). Different types of blood glucose monitoring devices are used to obtain capillary blood, usually from the patient's finger. One type of monitor is the ACCU-CHEK Advantage (referred to as *ACCU-CHEK*), in which a drop of blood is placed on a chemically treated strip. The strip is placed in a blood glucose monitor, and the patient's blood glucose results are displayed in numbers. The monitor is turned off by pressing the "O" button. Another type of blood glucose monitor is the OneTouch, which can be used on the patient's arm rather than on the finger. The nurse uses the results of the blood glucose level test to administer or adjust insulin dosage according to the doctor's orders (see Chapter 13). The order for blood glucose monitoring is usually written on the Kardex form during the transcription procedures. The doctor may use the trade name of the device, such as ACCU-CHEK (Roche Diagnostics, Basel, Switzerland) or OneTouch (LifeScan, Milpitas, California, United States), or may write "fingersticks" when ordering blood glucose monitoring (Fig. 10-4).

Note: Other types of POCT will be discussed in Chapter 14.

Oxygen Saturation (Pulse Oximetry) Orders

Pulse oximetry is a noninvasive measurement of gas exchange and red blood cell oxygen-carrying capacity. Oximetry is often referred to as the fifth vital sign. A probe is usually attached to the ear or the finger or, in the case of an infant, across a foot. A **pulse oximeter** (Fig. 10-5) is often ordered to be applied continuously in the recovery room, an intensive care unit, a pediatric unit, or any setting in which a patient's oxygenation is considered unstable. An alarm will sound when the **oxygen saturation** is too low. An order for pulse oximetry would be sent to the respiratory department and will be discussed in Chapter 16. The nurse observes and documents the oximeter results as ordered.

Cardiac Monitors and Cardiac Monitor Technicians

A **cardiac monitor** is a device that shows the electrical and pressure waveforms of the cardiovascular system for measurement and treatment. HUCs may be cross-trained to be a **cardiac monitoring technician (CMT)** who would work on a telemetry unit

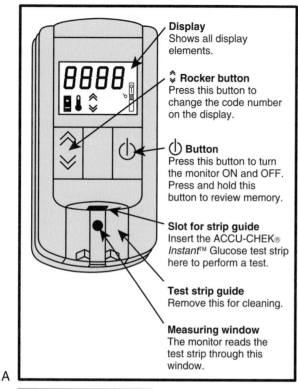

Display
Shows all display elements.

≋ Rocker button
Press this button to change the code number on the display.

⏻ Button
Press this button to turn the monitor ON and OFF. Press and hold this button to review memory.

Slot for strip guide
Insert the ACCU-CHEK® Instant™ Glucose test strip here to perform a test.

Test strip guide
Remove this for cleaning.

Measuring window
The monitor reads the test strip through this window.

A

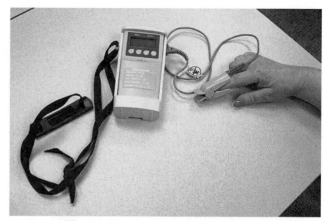

Figure 10-5 A handheld pulse oximeter.

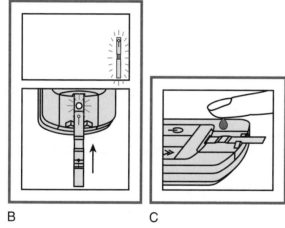

B
C

Figure 10-4 A, Example of a blood glucose monitor. **B,** The strip is placed on the monitor. **C,** Blood glucose results are displayed in numbers; the monitor is turned off by pressing the "O" button. (From Stepp CA, Woods MA: *Laboratory procedures for medical office personnel,* Philadelphia, 1998, Saunders.)

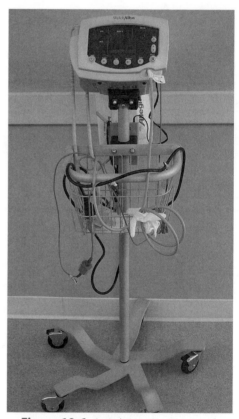

Figure 10-6 A vital signs monitor stand.

(see Fig. 3-2). Cardiac monitoring technicians monitor patients' heart rhythms and inform nurses of important physiologic changes. They monitor up to 32 patients at a time and have direct and instant audio and visual contact with patients and nurses.

Doctors' Orders for Nursing Observation

VS q4h
The patient's vital signs are to be taken and recorded every 4 hours. Variations on this type of order may include other time sequences and can read, for example, *VS q1h* or *VS q2h,* or the order may include a qualifying phrase, such as *VS q1h until stable then q4h.*

BP q h × 4
The blood pressure is to be taken and recorded every hour for 4 hours. Variations on this order may involve other time sequences, such as *BP q4h, BP tid,* and so forth, or a qualifying phrase, such as *BP q3h while awake* or *BP q4h if ↓ 100/60, call me.* Figure 10-6 shows a vital sign monitor stand with a screen that will register the vital signs.

Observe for SOB and Notify Physician
The patient will be observed for shortness of breath (SOB) and, if severe, the nurse will notify the physician of the patient's condition.

24-Hour Intake and Output	Name _Mary Ryan_						
	Room _403A_						
	Date _9/10/XX_						

Shift	Fluid Intake			Fluid Output		Other	Stools
	Oral	I.V.	Piggy Back	Urine	Emesis	Suction ☐	
0700-1500	08³⁰ 100 cc 10⁰⁰ 30 cc 12⁰⁰ 320 cc 15⁰⁰ 500 cc 210	Credit _300_ Add _1000_ Add ____	50	07³⁰ 200 cc 11⁰⁰ 300 cc 13⁰⁰ 175 cc	200 cc		x1 lg amt
8 hr.	1160		50	675			
1500-2300		Credit _500_ Add ____ Add ____					
8 hr.							
2300-0700		Credit ____ Add ____ Add ____					
8 hr.							
24 hr.							

Iced Tea - 6 oz. (180 cc)	Cup of Coffee or Tea - 7 oz. (210 cc)
Water Glass - 6 oz. (180 cc)	Styrofoam Cup - 150 cc
Milk (carton) - 8 oz. (240 cc)	Paper Cup - 150 cc
Fruit Juice - 4 oz. (120 cc)	Coffee Creamer - 0.5 oz. (15 cc)
Soup - 4 oz. (120 cc)	Cereal Creamer - 2 oz. (60 cc)
Ice Cream - 3 oz. (90 cc)	Coca Cola and Sprite - 12 oz. (360 cc)
Jello - 3.5 oz. (105 cc)	H_2O Pitcher - 30 oz. (900 cc)

Figure 10-7 An intake and output form.

Orthostatics q Shift

The nurse will take the patient's blood pressure and pulse rate while the patient is supine (lying) and again while he or she is erect (sitting and/or standing).

Apical Rate

The patient's heart rate is to be taken at the apex of the heart with a stethoscope.

Check Pedal Pulse Rt Foot q2h

Pulses are obtained from an artery (dorsalis pedis) on top of the foot.

Neuro ✓s q2h

The patient's **neurologic vital signs (neuro checks)** are taken and recorded every 2 hours.

NVS q 4 hrs until stable

The patient's neurologic vital signs are taken and recorded every 4 hours until stable.

I&O

The patient's fluid **intake and output** are measured and recorded at the completion of each shift to monitor the patient's fluid balance. The I & O is then calculated for 24-hour periods. Intake includes any oral liquid consumed and intravenous fluids infused; output consists of urine, **emesis,** wound drainage, and liquid stools. Figure 10-7 shows a typical intake and output form used by the nursing staff to calculate the patient's intake and output for an 8-hour shift.

U/O q 2 hr

The patient's catheter bag contents would be emptied and measured every 2 hours.

Wt Daily

The patient is to be weighed daily and the weight recorded. A variation of this order may be *daily wt.*

Tympanic Temp q4h

The temperature is to be measured every 4 hours with the tympanic (aural) thermometer (see Fig. 10-2, *A*) as opposed to the oral method. A third method of measuring the body temperature is the axillary method. The doctor's order for this method may read *axillary temp q4h*. A fourth method is the rectal method. The doctor's order will read *rectal temp q4h.*

CVP q2h

A catheter is inserted, usually through the right or left subclavian vein, and is threaded through the vein until the tip reaches the right atrium of the heart (see Fig. 11-11). The catheter is inserted by the doctor, and pressure readings are taken by the nurse.

Pulse Oximetry q4h

Oxygen saturation is to be measured every 4 hours. A portable pulse oximeter with a special sensor is used. The sensor is often left in place for continuous monitoring (see Fig. 10-5).

Check CMS Fingers Rt Hand

The circulation, motion, and sensation (CMS) of the patient's right-hand fingers are to be checked as often as the nurse determines necessary. This type of order specifies observation of the patient's signs and symptoms relative to the patient's diagnosis and treatment. For example, this order was written after a cast had been applied to the patient's right arm and hand.

ACCU-CHEK qid ac and hs

ACCU-CHEK is a type of commercial blood glucose monitor that is used to check the glucose level of blood. The doctor has ordered the test to be done four times a day before meals and at hour of sleep. (The order may also be written *fingersticks ac and hs*.)

Move Patient to Telemetry Unit, Place on Telemetry, and Notify Hospitalist of any Arrhythmias

The patient would be moved to the telemetry unit and placed on telemetry, and the CMT would monitor the patient's telemetry; if any abnormal heart rhythms are seen, the CMT would run a strip, notify the patient's nurse, and call the hospitalist if requested to do so.

VS q shift

Vital signs are measured to detect changes in the patient's condition, assess response to treatment, and recognize life-threatening situations. Accurate recording of vital signs is essential.

★ HIGH PRIORITY

An order for pulse oximetry would be sent to the respiratory department. This will be discussed in greater detail in Chapter 16.

SKILLS CHALLENGE

To practice transcribing a nursing observation order, complete Activity 10-3 in the *Skills Practice Manual*.

To practice transcribing a blood glucose monitor order, complete Activity 10-4 in the *Skills Practice Manual*.

To practice transcribing, automatically canceling, and discontinuing doctors' orders, complete Activity 10-5 in the *Skills Practice Manual*.

To practice transcribing a review set of doctor's orders, complete Activity 10-6 in the *Skills Practice Manual*.

To practice recording telephoned messages, complete Activity 10-7 in the *Skills Practice Manual*.

KEY CONCEPTS

When paper charts are used, transcription of doctors' orders is a major responsibility of the HUC. This chapter has introduced doctors' orders for patient activity, patient positioning, and nursing observation. Refer back to this chapter as needed.

Websites of Interest

The Joint Commission—Patient safety: www.jointcommission.org/topics/patient_safety.aspx

Point of Care Testing: www.pointofcare.net

Nursing Times—Nursing research, jobs, careers, articles and news: www.nursingtimes.net

Use of the Trendelenburg Position by Critical Care Nurses: ajcc.aacnjournals.org/content/6/3/172.short

REVIEW QUESTIONS

Visit the Evolve website to download and complete the following questions.

1. Define the following terms.
   a. dangle
   b. febrile
   c. afebrile
   d. emesis
   e. Celsius
   f. Fahrenheit
   g. pulse deficit

2. Write out each doctor's order:
   a. CBR
   b. BR c̄ BRP when A&O
   c. wt q other day
   d. VS q shift
   e. TPR&BP tid
   f. ↑HOB 20°
   g. ✓ dressing for drainage q2h
   h. temp R or ax only
   i. neuro ✓s q4h
   j. I&O q shift
   k. OOB ad lib
   l. up as tol
   m. T q4h
   n. amb today
   o. DC VS
   p. ↑HOB 30 degrees
   q. may use BSC
   r. CVP q hr
   s. check CMS toes lt foot qid
   t. ACCU-CHEK qid ac and hs
   u. call me if pt c/o SOB
   v. call me if DBP > 90
   w. call me if U/O < 1000 mL

3. Explain how and why TJC's "do not use" list was developed.

4. Identify the following doctors' orders as nursing observation, activity, or positioning orders.
   a. BRP
   b. log roll on lt side
   c. pulse oximetry
   d. TPR q4h
   e. CMS q2h
   f. wt 0700 q AM
   g. BSC prn
   h. HOB↑30°
   i. Up ad lib
   j. May dangle 20 min bid
   k. NVS q4h
   l. Fowler position
   m. up in chair
   n. call if T > 101°

5. List four measurements included in daily vital signs.

6. List five methods of taking a patient's temperature.

7. Explain how orthostatic vital signs are measured.

8. Identify at least four tests that may be performed at the patient's bedside (POCT).

9. Explain what type of patient would require blood glucose monitoring, and identify two types of blood glucose monitors that are currently used.

10. Identify the hospital areas and the reason that pulse oximetry would be used.

11. Identify the measurement that is often considered the "fifth vital sign."

12. Identify the nursing unit that would employ a CMT.

13. Explain the function of nursing observation orders, and list at least four examples of nursing observation orders.

14. Explain the reason for a doctor to order intake and output (I&O), and list the items included in the measurement of a patient's I&O.

SURFING FOR ANSWERS

1. Research medical errors caused by use of dangerous abbreviations. Discuss errors and risks of using certain abbreviations, and document websites used.
2. Find the recommended systolic and diastolic blood pressure levels for adults, and document two websites used.

CHAPTER 11

Nursing Intervention or Treatment Orders

CHAPTER OBJECTIVES

On completion of this chapter, you will be able to:

1. Define the terms in the vocabulary list.
2. Write the meaning of the abbreviations in the abbreviations list.
3. Describe what is included in holistic care, and provide an example of a nursing intervention.
4. Describe the function of the central service department with regard to nursing treatment orders.
5. List the types of items stored in the central service stock supply closet (C-locker or cart) on the nursing units and the types of items stored in the central service department.
6. Explain why discontinued reusable equipment should be returned to the central service department as quickly as possible.
7. List four types of enemas.

8. Explain the procedure and purpose of a urine flow test.
9. Explain two types of urinary catheterization procedures and two methods of measuring postvoid residual urine volume.
10. Describe two methods and four purposes of administering intravenous therapy.
11. Explain the major difference between peripheral intravenous therapy and a central line.
12. List four types of central venous catheters.
13. Explain the purpose of a heparin lock, and describe how a heparin lock is kept patent.
14. List three parts of a physician's order for intravenous therapy.
15. Identify three commercially prepared intravenous solutions, and explain how the health unit coordinator (HUC) would determine how long a bag of intravenous solution would take to empty.

16. List the four blood types and explain the importance of correct labeling of a blood specimen that is being sent for a type and crossmatch.
17. Explain the HUC's role in obtaining blood from the blood bank and the correct storage of blood.
18. Discuss the purposes of an arterial line and a Swan-Ganz catheter.
19. Identify three types of suction devices inserted during surgery.
20. List at least two heat applications and at least two applications used for cold therapy.
21. Explain why most comfort, safety, and healing orders require a doctor's order, and identify at least five items or types of equipment these orders may include.
22. List at least four complementary or alternative approaches or therapies that may be recommended or provided to hospitalized patients.

VOCABULARY

Ace Wraps Elastic gauze used for temporary compression to various parts of the body to decrease swelling and reduce skin breakdown.

Adult Disposable Diapers An absorbent garment worn by patients who are incontinent.

Aquathermia Pad A waterproof plastic or rubber pad used to apply heat or cold that is connected by hoses to a bedside control unit that contains a temperature regulator, a motor for circulating the water, and a reservoir of distilled water (also called a *K-pad* or a *water flow pad*).

Arterial Line (art-line or a-line) A catheter placed in an artery that is used to measure the patient's blood pressure continuously and/or to obtain samples for arterial blood gas measurements.

Autologous Blood The patient's own blood donated previously for transfusion to be used as needed by the patient (also called *autotransfusion*).

Binder A cloth or elastic bandage that is usually used for abdominal or chest support.

Bladder Ultrasound (BUS) A noninvasive method of assessing bladder volume and other bladder conditions using ultrasonography to determine the amount of urine retention or postvoid residual urine. A portable, ultrasound device called a *bladder scanner* is used.

Catheterization Insertion of a catheter into a body cavity or organ to inject or remove fluid.

Central Line A catheter inserted into the jugular or subclavian vein or a large vein in the arm and threaded to the superior vena cava or the right atrium of the heart.

Chux A disposable pad placed in areas where patients either lie or sit.

Compression Garments Tight-fitting, custom-made garments that are used to put constant pressure on healed wounds to reduce scarring.

Donor-Specific or Donor-Directed Blood Blood donated by relatives or friends of the patient to be used for transfusion as needed.

Egg-Crate Mattress A foam rubber mattress.

Elevated Toilet Seat (ETS) An elevated seat that fits over a toilet and has handrails; used for patients who have difficulty sitting on a lower seat.

Enema The introduction of fluid and/or medication into the rectum and sigmoid colon.

Extravasation The accidental administration of intravenously infused medicinal drugs into the surrounding tissue, by leakage (as with the brittle veins of elderly patients) or directly (by means of a puncture of the vein).

Foley Catheter A type of indwelling catheter (tube) that is inserted into the bladder for urine collection and measurement.

Gastric Suction Used to remove gastric contents.

Harris Flush or Return-Flow Enema A mild colonic irrigation that helps expel flatus.

Hemovac A disposable suction device (evacuator unit) connected to a drain that is inserted into or close to a surgical wound.

Heparin Lock A vascular access device (also called *intermittent infusion device, heplock,* or *saline lock*) that is placed on a peripheral intravenous catheter when used intermittently.

Incontinence Inability of the body to control the elimination of urine and/or feces.

Indwelling or Retention Catheter A catheter that remains in the bladder for a longer period until a patient is able to void completely and voluntarily, or as long as hourly accurate measurements are needed.

Infiltration Process by which the tip of an intravenous (IV) catheter comes out of the vein or pokes through the vein and IV solution is released into surrounding tissue. This also can occur if the wall of the vein becomes permeable and leaks fluid.

Intermittent (Straight) Catheter A single-use catheter that is introduced long enough to drain the bladder (5 to 10 minutes) and is then removed.

Intravenous Infusion The administration of fluid through a vein.

Irrigation Washing or flushing out of a body cavity, organ, or wound.

Intravenous (IV) Infusion Pump A device used to regulate the flow or rate of intravenous fluid; more commonly called an *IV pump*.

Jackson-Pratt (JP) A disposable suction device (evacuator unit) that is connected to a drain that is inserted into or close to a surgical wound.

Nasogastric (NG) Tube A tube that is inserted through the mouth or nose into the stomach and is used to feed the patient, or to drain stomach contents to prevent vomiting.

Needleless Heplock or Saline Lock A safe, sharp device that is placed on a peripheral intravenous catheter when used intermittently.

Patent (Patency) A term that indicates that there are no clots at the tip of the needle or catheter and that the needle tip or catheter is not against the vein wall (open).

Penrose Drain A drain that is inserted into or close to a surgical wound; it may lie under a dressing, extend through a dressing, or be connected to a drainage bag or suction device.

Peripheral IV Therapy An infusion of a liquid prepared solution directly into a vein intermittently or continuously.

Peripherally Inserted Central Catheters (PICC or PICs) Catheters inserted into the arm and advanced until the tip lies in the superior vena cava; placement is checked with an x-ray examination.

Pneumatic Hose Stockings that promote circulation by sequentially compressing the legs from ankle upward, promoting venous return (also called *sequential compression devices or pneumo boots*).

Postvoid Residual Urine Volume The measurement of urine left in the bladder after urination.

Rectal Tube A plastic or rubber tube designed for insertion into the rectum; when written as a doctor's order, *rectal tube* means the insertion of a rectal tube into the rectum to remove gas and relieve distention.

Restraints Devices used to control patients who exhibit dangerous behavior or to protect the patient.

Sheepskin A pad made out of lamb's wool or synthetic material; used to prevent pressure sores (used frequently in long-term care).

Sitz Bath Application of warm water to the pelvic area.

Splinting Holding the incision area to provide support, promote a feeling of security, and reduce pain during coughing after surgery; a folded blanket or pillow is helpful for use as a splint.

Straight Catheter See *Intermittent (Straight) Catheter.*

Swan-Ganz Catheterization Placement in the neck or the chest of a catheter that measures pressures in the patient's heart and pulmonary artery.

T.E.D. Hose (Thrombo-embolic-deterrent) A brand name for antiembolism (AE) hose.

Urinary Catheterization A tube is placed in the body to drain and collect urine from the bladder.

Urine Flow Test A test that evaluates the speed of urination, or amount voided per second, and the total time of urination.

Urine Residual Urine that remains in the bladder after urination.

Uroflowmeter a funnel-shaped device that reads, measures, and computes the rate and amount of urine flow.

Venipuncture Needle puncture of a vein.

Void (micturate or urinate) To empty, especially the urinary bladder.

ABBREVIATIONS

Abbreviation	Meaning	Example of Usage on a Doctor's Order Sheet
$\bar{a}$	before	Start IV of 1000cc D_5LR $\bar{a}$ surg
@	at	Run @ 100 mL/hr
abd	abdominal	Up $\bar{c}$ abd binder
ASAP	as soon as possible	Start IV ASAP
B/L	bilateral (both sides)	B/L TEDs
cath	catheterize	Cath q 8 hr prn
CBI	continuous bladder irrigation	CBI $\bar{c}$ NS 50 mL/hr
cm	centimeter	Chest tube 20 cm neg pressure
con't	continue, continuous	Foley cath to con't drainage
CVC	central venous catheter	Blood draws through CVC
drsg	dressing	Change drsg q shift & PRN
D/LR	dextrose in lactated Ringer's	IV 1000 mL 5% D/LR at 125 mL/hr
D_5W	5% dextrose in water	1000 mL D_5W @ 125 mL/hr
$D_{10}W$	10% dextrose in water	1000 mL $D_{10}W$ @ 100 mL/hr
DW or D/W	distilled water	Irrig cath prn $\bar{c}$ DW
ETS	elevated toilet seat	Order ETS for home use
gtt(s)	drop(s)	IV @ 60 gtts/min
HL or heplock	heparin lock Also called a *saline lock*	Convert IV to heplock
H_2O_2	hydrogen peroxide	Irrigate wound $\bar{c}$ H_2O_2 & NS equal strength
irrig	irrigate	Irrig cath $\bar{c}$ NS prn
IV	intravenous	Con't IVs as ordered
IVF	intravenous fluids	DC IVF at 1000 mL today
KCl	potassium chloride	Add 20 mEq KCl to IV
KO	keep open	KO IV $\bar{c}$ 1000 mL 5% D/W
LIS	Low intermittent suction	Connect NG to LIS
LR	lactated Ringer's	1000 mL LR 125 mL/hr
min, m	minute	Run @ 30 gtts/min
mL	milliliter Same as *cc*, which may not be allowed in some institutions, may be confused with "U" or "u" if poorly written	1000 D_5W @ 100 mL/hr
MR	may repeat	SSE now MR × 1
nec	necessary	SSE now MR if nec
NG	nasogastric	Insert NG tube
NS	normal saline	Give NS enema now
N/V	nausea and vomiting	Notify HO of any N/V
ORE	oil-retention enema	ORE today
$\bar{p}$	after	Up $\bar{p}$ breakfast
PICC	peripherally inserted central catheter	Insert PICC, follow protocol
PVR or RV	postvoid residual urine volume residual volume	Obtain PVR this a.m. Obtain RV this am
SCD	sequential compression device	Apply SCD when in bed

sol'n	solution	Irrig cath c̄ NS sol'n
SSE	soap suds enema	SSE now
st	straight retention	Cath to st drain
stat	urgent—*rush*	Prepare for stat
(from Latin	may be written	surgery
word *statim*,	in uppercase	
meaning	or lowercase	
"immediately"		
TCDB	turn, cough, and	TCDB q2h
	deep breathe	
TKO	to keep open	1000 mL D₅W TKO
TWE	tap water enema	Give TWE
VAD	vascular access	Use VAD for blood
	device	draws
WA or W/A	while awake	BP q 4 hr W/A
Δ	change	Δ catheter daily
/	per, by	IV @ 150 mL/hr

EXERCISE 1

Write the abbreviation for each term listed.

1. soap suds enema
2. keep open
3. may repeat
4. solution
5. necessary
6. centimeter
7. tap water enema
8. nasogastric
9. normal saline
10. nausea and vomiting
11. dextrose in lactated Ringer's
12. distilled water
13. at
14. oil-retention enema
15. irrigate
16. intravenous
17. catheterize
18. lactated Ringer's
19. straight
20. sequential compression device
21. immediately
22. after
23. abdominal
24. turn, cough, and deep breathe
25. minute
26. drops
27. change
28. as soon as possible
29. per
30. hydrogen peroxide
31. continue
32. continuous bladder irrigation
33. to keep open
34. milliliter
35. intravenous fluids
36. postvoid residual urine volume or residual volume
37. elevated toilet seat
38. while awake
39. peripherally inserted central catheter
40. vascular access device
41. central venous catheter
42. 5% dextrose in water
43. 10% dextrose in water
44. bilateral
45. heparin lock
46. before
47. dressing
48. low intermittent suction
49. potassium chloride

EXERCISE 2

Write out each doctor's order.

1. 1000 mL LR @ 125mL/hr, then DC
2. SSE HS MR ×1
3. Give ORE follow c̄ TWE if nec

4. Irrig cath tid c̄ NS sol'n
5. 1000 mL D₅W 0.9 NS TKO
6. Insert NG tube
7. TCDB q2h
8. Δ IV tubing ASAP
9. Please obtain ETS for patient
10. Start IVF of D₁₀W @ 120 mL/hr
11. Insert HL
12. Shave B/L inguinal groin area
13. Apply SCD when in bed
14. Obtain PVR today
15. Insert HL stat

NURSING INTERVENTION OR TREATMENT ORDERS

Background Information

A nursing intervention is any act performed by a nurse that implements the nursing care plan or any specific objective of the clinical plan or pathway, such as turning a comatose patient to avoid the development of decubitus ulcers (bedsores), or teaching insulin injection technique to a diabetic patient before the time of discharge. Interventions may include support measures, activity limitations, administration of medications, or treatments given to relieve the current condition or to prevent the development of further stress. The emphasis is on a holistic approach in nursing care. Holistic nursing or comprehensive care consists of total patient care that considers the physical, emotional, social, economic, and spiritual needs of the patient; the patient's response to illness; and the effects of the illness on the ability to meet self-care needs. Nursing interventions and treatment orders are discussed in this chapter.

★ HIGH PRIORITY

The Evolve website associated with the *Health Unit Coordinator Skills Manual* includes a simulated hospital electronic medical record program that may be used for practice.

Instruction and paper requisitions (which are seldom used) are also provided for learning purposes and for health unit coordinators who are working in settings without a computerized requisition process or implementation of the electronic medical record.

COMMUNICATION WITH THE CENTRAL SERVICE DEPARTMENT

The central service department (CSD) distributes the supplies that are used for nursing procedures. The supply purchasing department (SPD) is another name for the CSD. Although CSD supplies are frequently used (even when they are not mentioned in a doctor's orders), obtaining these supplies for the nursing staff may require a separate step in the transcription procedure for nursing treatment orders. For example, for the order *footboard to bed*, the health unit coordinator (HUC) would order the footboard from the CSD. Other items may include **adult disposable diapers** or **chux** for a patient with leakage or **incontinence.** It is therefore necessary for the HUC to be familiar with frequently used CSD items and to learn the hospital's system for obtaining them.

The process for obtaining central service supplies may vary among hospitals; thus it is impossible to outline one procedure that would cover all hospital systems. Disposable or frequently used items are stored on each nursing unit (items will vary depending on the specialty of the nursing unit). That storage space is often referred to as the *CSD closet, CSD room,* or *C-locker.* When paper charts are used, the charging process is done by removing a bar code label from the item and placing it on the patient's CSD charge card. Figure 11-1, *A,* shows a CSD card. The person who removes the supplies is responsible for placing the bar code label on the patient's CSD card. In hospitals using an electronic medical record (EMR) system, a computer with a scanner is located in the storage area and nurses may scan items with bar code labels directly into the appropriate patient's EMR. Figure 11-1, *B,* shows a computer used for this purpose located in a CSD closet.

When paper charts are used, a central service technician usually takes a daily inventory of the items stored in the closet or C-locker. Used items are replaced, and the patient's CSD current charge cards are collected. Some hospitals use a system with an exchange cart that is supplied with frequently used items and is exchanged every 24 hours. The unit receives another completely supplied cart while the CSD replenishes the used cart.

Reusable or infrequently used items are stored in the CSD. Refer to Table 11-1 for a comparison of items commonly stored on nursing units and items often stored in the CSD (items in each category may vary among hospitals).

The HUC, when transcribing an order for treatment, orders only those items stored in the CSD because the nursing staff can quickly obtain needed items from the CSD stock supply. The nurse may ask the HUC to order items as needed. Items from the CSD are usually ordered by computer or with the use of a downtime requisition (if the computer is down). Figure 11-2 shows a CSD downtime requisition.

Many items used for nursing treatments, such as enema bags or urinary catheterization trays, are disposable. This means that once the item has been used for the patient, it is discarded or is given to the patient for future use. The patient is charged for the disposable equipment. Other items charged to the patient, such as **compression garments, T.E.D. hose,** and **Ace wraps,** are sent home with the patient when he or she is discharged.

Other items are reusable, such as an **intravenous (IV) infusion pump, pneumatic hose,** or an **elevated toilet seat (ETS),** and are cleaned or sterilized, if necessary, after use by a patient. The patient usually is charged a rental fee for the use of these items. Reusable items are numbered and tracked for charging or discontinuing the charge. When a reusable item, such as an IV infusion pump, is discontinued, it is placed in the dirty utility room. A central service technician picks up the item and returns it to the CSD. It is important for these items to be returned as quickly as possible so that if a rental charge has been assessed, it will be terminated, and the equipment will be readied for use by other patients.

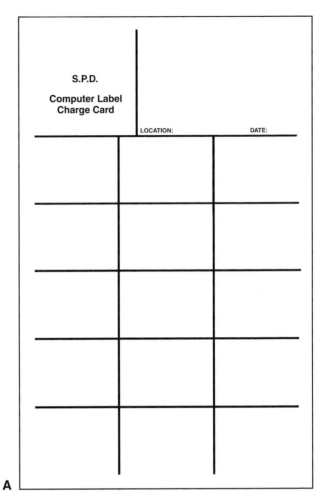

A

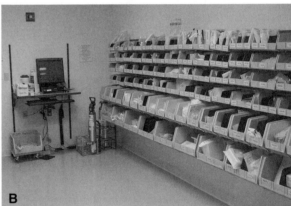

B

Figure 11-1   A, Central service department (CSD) patient charge card. **B,** Bar code labels are scanned into the patient's electronic medical record via a computer located in the CSD closet.

Equipment is discussed and illustrated throughout this chapter as it relates to nursing treatment orders. It is important that the HUC recognize the frequently used items that are required and must be requested during the ordering step of the transcription procedure. It is also important for the HUC to learn which items are stored on the unit and which are stored in the CSD. If information on size and/or weight is required for the ordering of an item (e.g., T.E.D. hose), the HUC needs to check with the patient's nurse and enter this information when ordering the item.

TABLE 11-1 Items Obtained from the Central Service Department (CSD)

Items that May Be Stored in the Nursing Unit CSD Closet or the C-Locker	Items that May Be Stored in the CSD
Abdominal pads	Adult disposable diapers
Alcohol pads	Alternating pressure pad
Chux	Bedside commode
Disposable suture removal kits	Bone marrow
Dressings	Central line
Examination gloves	Colostomy kit
Fleet enema	Egg-crate mattress
Gauze pads in various sizes	Elastic abdominal binder
Glycerin swabs	Feeding pump and tubing
Irrigation kits	Footboard
Irrigation solutions	Foot cradle
Irrigation trays	Hypothermia machine
IV catheters and needles	IV infusion pump
IV solutions*	K-pad
IV tubing	Lumbar puncture (spinal tap)
Kling	Paracentesis
Masks	Pneumatic hose
Rectal tube	Restraints
Sterile gloves	Sitz bath, disposable
Suction catheters and tubing	Sterile trays
Syringes and needles	Stomal bags
Tape (various types)	T.E.D. (thrombo-embolic-deterrent) hose
Telfa pads	Thoracentesis
Urinary catheter trays	Tracheostomy
Vaseline gauze	

IV, Intravenous

*Certain IV solutions are obtained from the pharmacy in some hospitals.

★ HIGH PRIORITY

The health unit coordinator (HUC) can best assist the nursing staff when transcribing nursing treatment orders by learning about equipment and supplies used on the nursing unit and ordering needed items.

INTESTINAL ELIMINATION ORDERS

Background Information

Enemas, rectal tubes, and colostomy irrigations are treatments used to remove stool and/or flatus (gas) from the large intestine.

An **enema** is the introduction of fluid into the rectum and sigmoid colon for the purpose of relieving distention (trapped gas) or constipation, or to prepare the patient for surgery and/or diagnostic tests. A doctor may order a "high" or a "low" cleansing enema. The terms *high* and *low* refer to the height from which the enema container is held; this determines the pressure with which the fluid is delivered. High enemas are

given to cleanse the entire colon; low enemas cleanse only the rectum and the sigmoid colon. Common types of enemas include the following:

1. Oil-retention
2. Soap suds
3. Tap water
4. Normal saline

Figure 11-3 is an example of a disposable enema bag used to administer these types of enemas.

A Fleet enema is a disposable, commercially prepackaged sodium phosphate enema that is frequently used (Fig. 11-4).

The order for a **rectal tube** refers to the insertion of a disposable plastic, latex-free, or rubber tube into the rectum for the purpose of relieving distention or draining feces. The rectal tube may be attached to a bag that captures the flatus and/or feces (Fig. 11-5).

A **Harris flush** is a **return-flow enema** that is used to relieve distention. A disposable enema bag is used to inject fluid into the rectum. This fluid is allowed to return into the bag. The process is repeated several times.

Colostomy (an artificial opening in the colon for passage of stool) **irrigation** (the flushing of fluid resembling an enema) is used to regulate the discharge of stool. Figure 11-6 shows a disposable colostomy irrigation bag used for this treatment.

A doctor's order is required for the administration of an enema, rectal tube, or Harris flush. The order contains the name of the treatment, the type (when pertinent), and the frequency. If the frequency is not indicated (as in the order *tap water enema*), it is considered a one-time order.

Examples of intestinal elimination orders are listed in the accompanying box as they are usually written on the doctors' order sheet. Refer to the abbreviations list at the beginning of this chapter for assistance in interpreting the abbreviations.

Doctors' Orders for Intestinal Elimination

TWE now MR ×1 prn
Give ORE followed by NS enemas this A.M.
Harris flush for abdominal distention
NS enemas until clear
Give Fleet enema daily prn constipation
Rectal tube prn for distention ■

BLADDER AND URINARY CATHETERIZATION ORDERS

Urine Flow Test
Background Information

During a **urine flow test,** the patient is asked to **void** into a **uroflowmeter** that reads, measures, and computes the rate and amount of urine flow. The patient cannot urinate for at least 2 hours before the test. The test takes approximately 10 minutes to perform. A urine flow test is performed to evaluate the speed of urination, or amount voided per second, and the total time of urination. The test can indicate a problem in bladder function, such as an obstruction, that will need further tests to diagnose. An average urine flow rate varies depending on age and gender.

Doctor ordering _____ ☐ Stat
Today's date _____ ☐ Routine
Requested by _____

| Patient Label |

CENTRAL SERVICES DEPARTMENT (CSD) REQUISITION

☐ Adult disposable diapers
☐ Alternating pressure pad
☐ Colostomy kit
☐ Colostomy irrigation bag
☐ Egg-crate mattress
☐ Elastic abdominal binder   size _____
☐ Feeding pump with bag and tubing
☐ Feeding bag and tubing
☐ Footboard
☐ Foot cradle
☐ Hypothermia machine
☐ Isolation pack
☐ IV infusion pump with tubing
☐ K-pad with motor
☐ Nasal gastric tube   type _____   size _____
☐ Pleur-evac
☐ Pneumatic hose
☐ Restraints   type _____
☐ Sitz bath, disposable
☐ Stomal bags   type _____   size _____
☐ Suction canister and tubing
☐ Suction catheter   type _____   size _____
☐ TED hose   size _____
☐ Vaginal irrigation kit

Sterile Trays:
☐ Bone marrow
☐ Central line
☐ Lumbar puncture (spinal tap)
☐ Paracentesis
☐ Thoracentesis
☐ Tracheostomy

☐ Write in item _____

Figure 11-2 An example of a central service department (CSD) downtime requisition.

Urinary Catheterization

Background Information

Urinary catheterization is the insertion of a latex-free tube called a *catheter* through the urethral meatus into the bladder for the purpose of removing urine. The tube is usually made of silicone or natural rubber, and varies in size. The doctor may order one of two types of catheterization procedures: retention or nonretention. Disposable sterile catheterization trays are used for both types, and each tray is marked with the size and type of catheter it contains.

An intermittent nonretention catheter, sometimes referred to as a **straight catheter**, is used to empty the bladder, to collect a sterile urine specimen, or to check the **urine residual**. The **intermittent (straight) catheter** is removed from the bladder after completion of the procedure (5 to 10 minutes) (Fig. 11-7). The **postvoid residual (PVR) urine volume** may be measured by two methods: a portable bedside **bladder ultrasound**, called a *bladder scanner*, and by **catheterization** using a straight catheter. Both methods are effective in measuring the urine remaining after voiding (urine residual), but the convenience, efficiency, and safety of bladder ultrasound makes its use preferable.

An **indwelling or retention catheter** (also called a **Foley catheter**) remains in the bladder and is usually connected to a

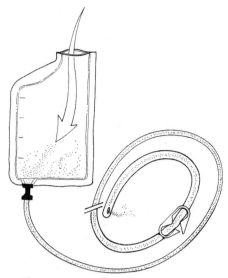

Figure 11-3 A disposable enema bag.

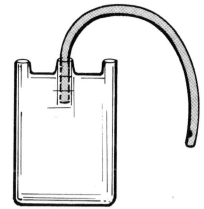

Figure 11-5 A disposable rectal tube in a flatus bag.

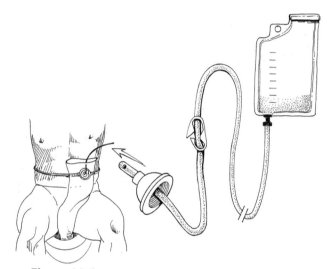

Figure 11-6 A disposable colostomy irrigation apparatus.

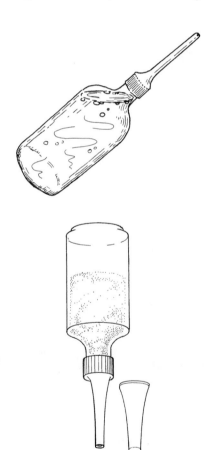

Figure 11-4 Commercially prepackaged enema.

drainage system that allows continuous flow of urine from the bladder to the container. Doctors refer to this type of drainage system as a *straight drain* (Fig. 11-8).

The doctor may order the indwelling catheter to be irrigated on an intermittent or continuous basis to maintain patency (to keep the catheter open). This is referred to as a *closed system,* and it is usually used for those who have had surgery involving the urinary or reproductive system. The open irrigation system

is used for irrigating the catheter at specific intervals. The open system requires the nurse to open a closed drainage system and insert an irrigation solution. A disposable irrigation tray is used for this procedure. The doctor indicates the solution to be used (normal saline, acetic acid, distilled water). For continuous and intermittent irrigation, special setups are used (Fig. 11-9).

Several types of typical doctors' orders related to urinary catheterizations are listed in the text that follows, recorded in abbreviated form as they would appear on the doctors' order sheet. Refer to the abbreviations list at the beginning of the chapter for assistance with these abbreviations.

Doctors' Orders for Catheterization

Intermittent (Straight) Catheter
May cath q8h prn
Straight cath prn
Cath in 8 hr if unable to void

Postvoid Residual Urine Volume
Bladder US for PVR
Cath for PVR

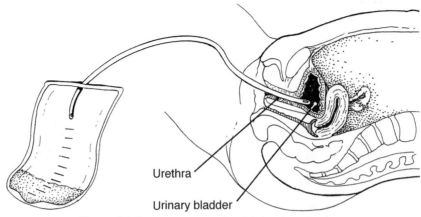

Figure 11-7 An intermittent (straight) catheter in place.

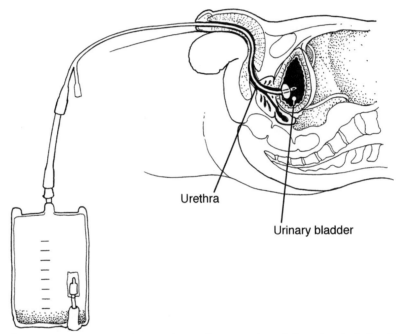

Figure 11-8 An indwelling (Foley) catheter in place and connected to a drainage bag (called *straight drainage*).

Indwelling (Retention) Catheter

Insert Foley
Indwelling cath to st drain
Cath for residual; if more than 200 mL, leave in
DC cath in A.M.; if unable to void in 6 hr, reinsert
DC cath this A.M.
Clamp cath x 4 hr, then drain
Catheter Irrigation
CBI; use NS @ 50 mL/hr
Irrig Foley NS bid
Irrig cath prn patency
Intermittent CBI q4h × 6 ■

 SKILLS CHALLENGE

To practice transcribing intestinal elimination and urinary catheterization orders, complete Activity 11-1 in the *Skills Practice Manual.*

INTRAVENOUS THERAPY ORDERS

Background Information

Until 1949, IV therapy consisted of the administration of simple solutions, such as water and normal saline, through peripheral veins. Equipment consisted of a glass bottle, a rubber tube, and a needle. Today, IV therapy may be used to correct electrolyte imbalances, to deliver medications, to transfuse blood, or to correct dehydration with fluid replacement. IV fluids may be administered through peripheral veins and through central veins. The IV route is the fastest way to deliver fluids and medications throughout the body. Some medications, as well as blood transfusions and lethal injections, can be given only intravenously. The availability of sophisticated equipment allows IV therapy to be administered to the patient at home, as well as in the hospital. Fluids can be administered by two methods—continuously or intermittently—and IV administration is done by the nurse, by the

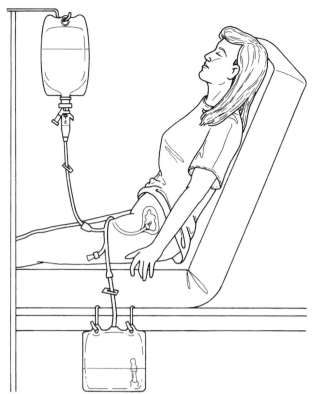

Figure 11-9 A setup used for intermittent or continuous bladder irrigation.

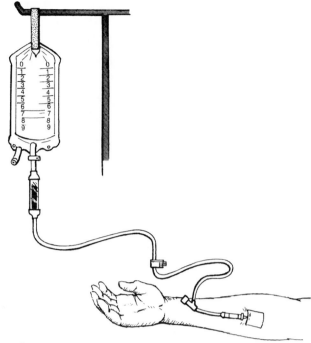

Figure 11-10 Peripheral intravenous therapy (venipuncture).

patient, or by the patient's family. IV therapy is given to do the following:

- Administer nutritional support such as total parenteral nutrition (TPN) (covered in Chapters 12 and 13)
- Provide for intermittent or continuous administration of medication
- Transfuse blood or blood products
- Maintain or replace fluids and electrolytes

> ⭐ **HIGH PRIORITY**
>
> **Infiltration** is the process by which the tip of an intravenous (IV) catheter comes out of the vein or pokes through the vein and IV solution is released into surrounding tissue.
>
> **Extravasation** is the accidental administration of intravenously infused medicinal drugs into the surrounding tissue, by leakage (as with the brittle veins of elderly patients) or directly (by means of a puncture of the vein).

Peripheral Intravenous Therapy

Peripheral IV therapy (*peripheral* refers to blood flow in the extremities of the body) has the following characteristics:
- It is usually initiated by the nurse at the bedside.
- Usually the needle is inserted into a vein **(venipuncture)** in the arm or hand or, on rare occasions, in the foot (adult); a vein in the scalp or foot is often used when peripheral IV therapy is administered to infants.
- Peripheral IV therapy is used for short-term treatment (i.e., a week or less).

- It is basic and easiest to initiate and is commonly used in hospitals.
- Sometimes, peripheral IV therapy is administered through a vascular access device (VAD). The cannula is short (less than 2 inches), so it ends in the extremity. It is not threaded to the larger veins or to the heart as in central venous therapy (Fig. 11-10).

Central Line Intravenous Therapy

With a **central line** (*central* refers to the blood flow in the center of the body), a catheter is inserted into the jugular or subclavian vein or a large vein in the arm and is threaded to the superior vena cava or the right atrium of the heart. A central venous catheter (CVC) is used. The central line is commonly referred to as a *central venous line* or a *subclavian line* (Figure 11-11 shows various types of CVCs.) The HUC orders a *central line tray or a triple lumen tray* and an IV infusion pump from the CSD and prepares a consent form.

Types of Central Venous Catheters

Peripherally inserted central catheters (PICCs or PICs) generally have the following characteristics:

- Catheterization is initiated by the doctor or by a nurse who is certified in the procedure, usually at the bedside but sometimes in the special procedures department or surgery.
- The procedure requires a consent form.
- The catheter is inserted into the arm and advanced until the tip lies in the superior vena cava.
- Placement is verified with a radiograph.
- This type of catheter is used when therapy is needed for longer than 7 days.

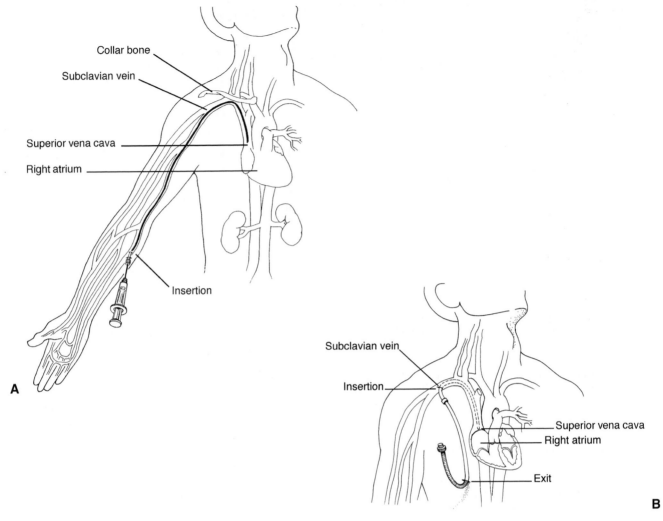

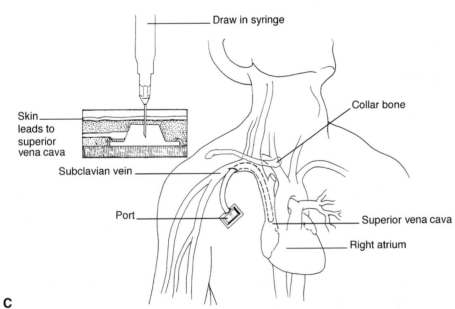

Figure 11-11 Types of central venous catheters (CVCs). **A,** Peripherally inserted central catheter (PICC). **B,** Percutaneous CVC. **C,** Implanted port.

- PICCs are used for antibiotic therapy, TPN, chemotherapy, cardiac drugs, or other drugs that are potentially harmful to peripheral veins.
- Sometimes PICCs are used for blood draws.

Percutaneous central venous catheterization has the following characteristics:

- A percutaneous CVC is sometimes referred to as a *subclavian line.*
- It is usually initiated by the doctor at the bedside but sometimes in the special procedures department or surgery.
- It requires a consent form.
- The catheter is inserted through the skin directly into the subclavian (most common) or jugular vein.
- The catheter is then advanced until the tip lies in the superior vena cava or the right atrium of the heart.
- Placement is verified with a radiograph.
- This type of catheterization is used for short-term therapy (i.e., 7 days to several weeks).
- The percutaneous CVC is used for antibiotic therapy, TPN, or chemotherapy.
- It is sometimes used for blood draws.

Tunneled catheters have the following characteristics:

- They are initiated by the doctor and are considered a surgical procedure.
- They require a consent form.
- They are inserted through a small incision made near the subclavian vein.
- They are inserted and advanced to the superior vena cava.
- They are used with a device called a *tunneler,* which exits the catheter low in the patient's chest.
- They are designed to allow the patient to administer his own therapy; the tips can be placed under clothing.
- They are available in various types, including Hickman, Raaf, Groshong, and Broviac.
- They are inserted for long-term IV therapy (i.e., longer than a month).
- They are used for home care, in long-term care facilities, and for self-administration.
- Sometimes they are used for blood draws (usually requires a doctor's order).

An *implanted port* has the following characteristics:

- The implantation is a surgical procedure that is performed by the doctor in a surgical setting.
- The procedure requires a consent form.
- The port is inserted into the subclavian or jugular vein.
- A container is implanted under the skin in the chest wall.
- The port is inserted with the use of an incision; after insertion, the incision is closed, and the device cannot be seen but can be identified by a bulge.
- The port is different from other long-term catheters in that it has no external parts, is located under the skin, and does not require daily care.
- It is used with a special needle that is inserted into the port to administer therapy.

- The port is available in different types, including Port-A-Cath, MediPort, and Infuse-a-Port.
- The port is used for long-term and or intermittent treatment; often it is used for chemotherapy administration.

Heparin Lock (Heplock) or Saline Lock

A **heparin lock** *(heplock),* or *saline lock,* is a venous access device (also called an *intermittent infusion device)* that is placed on a peripheral IV catheter when used intermittently. The heplock or saline lock is used to maintain an intermittent line when IV fluids are no longer needed but IV entry is still required. It is commonly used for the administration of medication. It consists of a plastic needle with an attached injection cap. A **needleless heplock or saline lock** is also available. The device is kept **patent** with heparin or saline flushes ordered by the doctor to be administered at specific intervals (Fig. 11-12).

Intravenous (IV) Infusion Pump

An intravenous (IV) **infusion pump** is an electrical device that is used for **intravenous infusion** (the administration of IV fluid). It is used to measure a precise amount of fluid (regulates drips per hour) to be infused for a stated amount of time. The pump is ordered from the CSD and is manufactured under several brand names (Fig. 11-13).

Intravenous Fluids

The doctor orders the type, the amount, and the flow rate of solutions to be given. For example, in the following IV order:

1000 mL D_5 W @ 125 mL/hr

D_5W is the type of solution. A large variety of solutions are available on the market, and the doctor must select the one that best meets the patient's needs.

In this example, 1000 mL is the amount of solution the doctor wants the patient to have. Solutions are most commonly packaged in amounts of 1000 mL; however, 250 mL or 500 mL also may be ordered.

The notation "125 mL/hr" indicates the rate of flow per hour of the solution into the vein. Other examples of phrases used in stating the rate of flow are "60 gtts per min, to run for 8 hr" and "to keep open (usually 50 to 60 mL/hr)."

If the HUC is required to order IV solutions at specific intervals, it would be necessary to know the length of time it takes

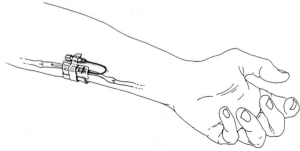

Figure 11-12 Intermittent infusion device (heparin or saline lock).

the IV solution to infuse. An IV injection of 1000 mL running at 125 mL/hr runs for 8 hours (1000 mL/125 mL = 8 hours). How many hours will an IV injection running at 100 mL/hr take to infuse?

★ HIGH PRIORITY

To determine the amount of time it will take for an intravenous (IV) infusion to be completed, divide the number of milliliters in the IV bag by the rate of flow. In the doctor's order *1000 mL 5% D/W @ 125 mL/hr*, divide 1000 by 125. The answer is 8. The IV will run for 8 hours. Use this information to order the number of 1000-mL IV bags needed for a given amount of time.

Several one-time, continuous, and discontinuation IV orders, written in abbreviated form as commonly seen on the doctor's order sheet, follow. Use the abbreviations list at the beginning of this chapter for assistance in interpreting these, if necessary. Box 11-1 provides a list of commercially prepared IV solutions that are commonly used.

Doctors' Orders for Intravenous Therapy

1000 mL LR @ 125 mL/hr then DC
Con't IVs alternate 1000 mL/RL 1000 mL D₅W, each to run for 8 hr via CVC
1000 mL NS TKO
DC IV when present bottle is finished
D₅LR 100 mL/hr follow c̄ 1000 mL 5% Isolyte M at same rate
Alternate the following IVs:
    1000 mL D₁₀LR via Groshong cath
    1000 mL 5% D/W 20 mEq KCl to run at 125 mL/hr
    1000 mL D₅W 0.9 NS @ 100 mL/hr if pt not tol fluids
DC IV fluids, convert to heplock c̄ rout saline flushes
Have IV team insert PICC
Use Port-a-Cath for blood draws ∎

SKILLS CHALLENGE

To practice transcribing intravenous therapy orders, complete Activity 11-2 in the *Skills Practice Manual*.

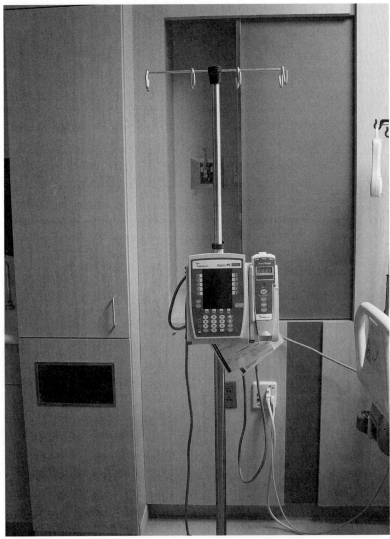

Figure 11-13 Infusion pump on intravenous pole.

TRANSFUSION OF BLOOD, BLOOD COMPONENTS, AND PLASMA SUBSTITUTES

Background Information

An IV infusion of blood is called a *blood transfusion*. It is a safe procedure and is done after a loss of blood from surgery or injury or when the body cannot properly make blood because of an underlying illness. There are four blood types: A, B, AB, and O, and either Rh positive or Rh negative. A person undergoing a blood transfusion must receive blood that matches his or her type or she or he can become extremely ill. In the U.S., about 44% of the population has type O blood; 42% has type A; 10% has type B; and 4% has type AB. O negative may be given to most people in an emergency, so it is called the universal donor blood type. A person with AB blood is said to be a universal receiver. Before the administration of blood and blood products, the patient must sign a specific consent form. A refusal form must be signed if the patient refuses to have a blood transfusion. Refer to Chapter 8 to see a blood transfusion refusal form.

There are very few indications for the use of whole blood transfusions. The major indication for whole blood transfusion would be in some cases of cardiac surgery or situations of massive hemorrhage when more than 10 units of red blood cells are required in any 24-hour period. Parts or components of blood are often used. The following are commonly seen transfusion orders:

1. Packed cells (red blood cells) (frequently used)
2. Plasma
3. Platelet concentrate
4. Washed cells
5. Fresh frozen plasma (FFP)
6. Cryoprecipitates
7. Gamma globulins
8. Albumin
9. Factor VIII

BOX 11-1	**COMMERCIALLY PREPARED INTRAVENOUS (IV) SOLUTIONS THAT ARE COMMONLY USED**

- Sodium chloride 0.45% (NaCl 0.45%, or half-strength NaCl)
- Sodium chloride 0.9% (NaCl 0.9%, or normal saline)
- 5% Dextrose in water (5% D/W, or D_5W)
- 10% Dextrose in water (10% D/W, or $D_{10}W$)
- 5% Dextrose in 0.2% sodium chloride (5% D/0.2% NaCl)
- 5% Dextrose in 0.45% sodium chloride (5% D/0.45% NaCl)
- 5% Dextrose in 0.9% sodium chloride (5% D/0.9% NaCl)
- Lactated Ringer's solution with 5% dextrose (LR/5%D)
- 5% Dextrose in 0.2% normal saline
- 5% Dextrose in 0.45% normal saline
- Lactated Ringer's solution

Other IV solutions that contain essential body elements are sold under various trade names. For example, McGaw, a manufacturer of parenteral fluids, markets an IV solution with electrolytes under the trade name Isolyte M. The same formula is sold by Abbott Laboratories as Ionosol T.

Transcribing Doctors' Orders for Blood Transfusions

A type and crossmatch is a laboratory study that is performed to determine the type and compatibility of blood; it must be done before the patient receives blood or certain blood components. A type and crossmatch is performed in the blood bank division of the hospital laboratory. It is essential that the HUC match the patient's name and information on the patient ID label affixed to the blood specimen with the patient name and information on the doctors' order sheet and with the name and information on the computer order screen. The specimen will be discarded if the specimen patient ID label and the patient name on the requisition are not the same. The patient then will need to have blood redrawn, causing additional discomfort, a delay in treatment, and additional charges.

The equipment used for infusion of blood is similar to that used for infusion of IV solutions. Blood is packaged in plastic containers and is ordered by the unit. The IV tubing used for blood contains a filter. Normal saline solution generally is used, along with blood administered via IV infusion pump. All containers and tubing must be disposed of after the blood is transfused.

The transfusion of blood is a potentially dangerous procedure. Special precautions are taken by the nursing staff to ensure the correct administration of blood. Proper storage of blood is essential to ensure safe administration. Blood is stored in the blood bank, in a special refrigerator designed to maintain a constant temperature for safe storage of blood. It is often the HUC's responsibility to pick up the blood from the blood bank and bring it to the nursing unit. If blood for two different patients is to be obtained from the blood bank at the same time, two different health care personnel should pick up the blood. It is important for the HUC to know that if the blood is not used immediately, it must be returned to the blood bank for storage. Blood should be stored only in refrigerators designated for blood storage.

Planning for blood transfusions is becoming common practice because it greatly reduces the risk that a blood-borne pathogen or infection such as human immunodeficiency virus (HIV) or hepatitis B will be acquired. Patients, family members, or friends may donate blood for a patient in advance. Transfusion with the patient's own blood is called *autologous transfusion* or an *autotransfusion;* the blood of relatives or friends is called **donor-specific or donor-directed blood.** Blood may also be collected from the patient at the surgery site during surgery. This blood is then transfused back to the patient. The blood is collected in a device called a *Cell Saver* or *autotransfusion* system.

Plasma extenders or plasma substitutes are ordered by the doctor to increase the level of circulating fluid in the body. These may be obtained from the pharmacy.

Doctors' Orders for Transfusion of Blood, Blood Components, and Plasma Substitutes

The nurse carries out the following orders for administration of blood, blood components, and plasma substitutes; however, the transcription procedure requires the ordering step of transcription. Blood bank ordering and the definition of the following abbreviations may be found in Chapter 14, "Laboratory Orders."

Give 2 units of whole blood now

T & X-match 2 units PC & hold for surgery

Give 1 unit of packed cells tonight and one in the a.m.

Give 2 units of FFP stat

Give 1 unit PC now, draw stat H & H $\overline{p}$ completion of transfusion

Give 2 units PCs $\overline{c}$ 20 mg Lasix $\overline{p}$ 1st unit

Transfuse 1 unit of **autologous blood** today

Autotransfusion per protocol ■

Doctors' orders for total parenteral nutrition and for intravenous medication are covered in Chapter 13.

HIGH PRIORITY

Ordering and Obtaining Blood

A mistake in labeling of a blood specimen sent to the laboratory for a type and crossmatch will result in the specimen being discarded and the patient having to have blood drawn again.

To avoid an error in labeling, which will cause the patient additional discomfort and a delay in treatment, match the patient's name and information on the ID label affixed to the blood specimen to the patient name and information on the computer order screen and if applicable, the name and information on the doctors' order sheet.

If two units of blood need to be picked up from the blood bank for two different patients on the nursing unit:

- Have another person go to the blood bank to pick up the second unit *or*
- Make two trips to pick up one unit at a time

When blood is brought to the nursing unit and cannot be given within a reasonable time, the blood is to be returned to the blood bank for storage; the proper storage temperature will ensure the safety of the blood.

MONITORING LINES AND CATHETERS

Arterial Line

An **arterial line (art-line or a-line)** is a thin catheter inserted into an artery. It is most commonly used in intensive care and anesthesia to monitor the blood pressure in real time (rather than by intermittent measurement) and to obtain samples for arterial blood gas measurements.

Swan-Ganz Catheterization

Swan-Ganz catheterization is the passing of a thin tube (catheter) into the right side of the heart and the arteries leading to the lungs to monitor the heart's function and blood flow, usually in persons who are very ill.

SUCTION ORDERS

Background Information

Suction may be ordered by the doctor to remove fluid or air from body cavities and surgical wounds. Suction may be ordered intermittently or continuously and may be accomplished manually or mechanically. The doctor may set up some types of suction apparatus during surgery, and the nursing staff may initiate some other types, such as **gastric suction.** The doctor may write orders for the establishment, maintenance, or discontinuance of suction. Wall suction usually is installed at each patient's bedside. Usually the canisters, tubing, and suction catheters used with wall suction are stored in the nursing unit supply closet or C-locker. The HUC may be asked by the nurse to order additional tubing or a specific type and/or size of catheter for a patient.

Following are doctors' orders related to suctioning, along with a brief interpretation. Refer to the abbreviations list at the beginning of the chapter for assistance, if necessary.

Doctors' Orders for Suctioning

Suction Throat prn to Clear Airway

When a patient is unable to clear respiratory tract secretions by coughing, the doctor may order manual (bulb suction device) or mechanical (wall suction) suctioning to clear the airways (Fig. 11-14). Three pathways for suctioning respiratory tract secretions are through the nose, through the mouth, and through an artificial airway, all with the use of tubing connected to the wall suction.

The health unit coordinator (HUC) may be asked by the nurse to order additional tubing or a specific type and/or size of catheter for a patient.

Suction Tracheostomy prn

A tracheostomy is an artificial opening into the trachea (windpipe) that is performed to facilitate breathing. When the patient is unable to cough, suctioning is necessary to remove secretions. Usually, small catheters and tubing connected to wall suction are used to remove secretions (Fig. 11-15). The HUC may be asked by the nurse to order additional tubing or a specific type and/or size of catheter for a patient.

Assess Character of Penrose Drainage

Patients often return from surgery with a drain inserted into or close to the surgical wound if a large amount of drainage is expected. A drain such as a **Penrose drain** may lie under a dressing, extend through a dressing, or be connected to a drainage bag or a disposable wound suction device (also called *evacuator units*).

Keep Hemovac Compressed
Empty and Record JP Drainage q Shift

Hemovac and **Jackson-Pratt (JP)** are names of disposable wound suction devices (evacuator units) that are attached to an incisional drain during surgery. These devices exert a constant low pressure as long as the suction device is fully compressed. Figure 11-16 shows various surgical suction devices.

Insert NG Tube, Connect to LIS (low intermittent suction)

The nurse or doctor inserts a **nasogastric (NG) tube** through the nose or mouth into the stomach. Correct placement of the NG tube is usually checked by inserting air into

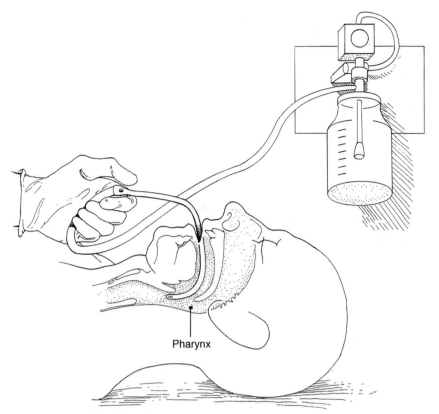

Figure 11-14 Throat-suctioning apparatus.

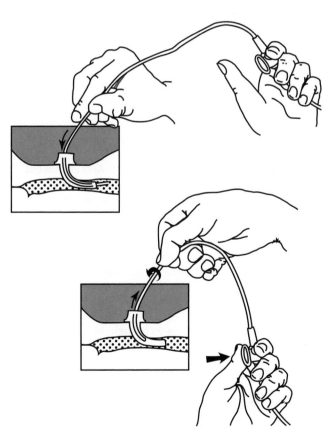

Figure 11-15 Suctioning of a tracheostomy with the use of a small catheter and tubing attached to wall suction.

the tubing and listening to the stomach with a stethoscope. The tube then is connected to a wall-mounted suction unit, which provides intermittent removal of gastric contents and is usually set on low. (A high-pressure setting is never used without specific orders to do so.) Gastric suction often is ordered after gastrointestinal or other abdominal surgery, to prevent vomiting or for various other reasons.

Irrig NG per Rout

The nurse irrigates the nasogastric tube per facility policy. An irrigation tray, usually disposable, is used for this procedure.

Clamp NG Tube Intermittently q1h

A clamp is applied to the NG tube or a plug is inserted into the distal end of the tube at 1-hour intervals and then is reconnected to the suction machine for 1-hour intervals.

Remove NG Tube and Gastric Suction

This is a typical example of an order to discontinue gastric suction.

Chest Tube 20 cm Neg Pressure

A chest tube is a catheter that is inserted through the thorax (chest) to reexpand the lungs by removing air or fluids that collect in the pleural cavity. Chest tubes are used after chest surgery and chest trauma. The chest tube is connected to a closed chest drainage system, such as Pleur-evac (Fig. 11-17). The drainage system and chest tubes are disposable items. ■

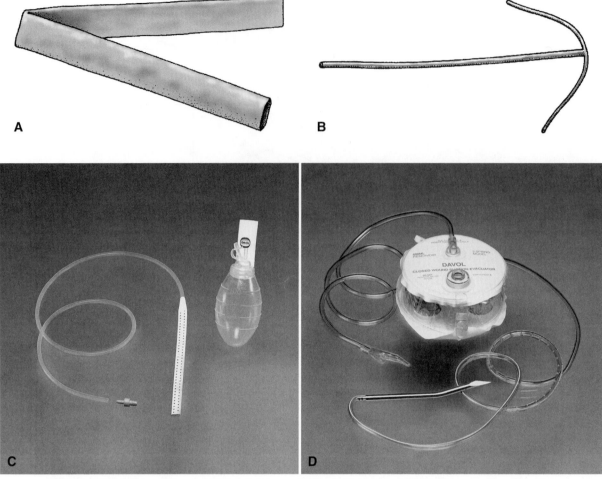

Figure 11-16 Types of surgical drains. **A,** Penrose. **B,** T tube. **C,** Jackson-Pratt. **D,** Hemovac. (From Ignatavicius D, Workman L: *Medical-surgical nursing,* ed 5, Philadelphia, 2006, Saunders. **C** and **D** courtesy C.R. Bard, Inc., Covington, Georgia.)

SKILLS CHALLENGE

To practice transcribing suction orders, complete Activity 11-3 in the *Skills Practice Manual.*

HEAT AND COLD APPLICATION ORDERS

Background Information

Heat and cold treatments are ordered for the patient by the doctor. Heat treatment is used to promote comfort, relaxation, and healing; to reduce pain and swelling; and to promote circulation. Cold treatment may be used to relieve pain, reduce inflammation, control hemorrhage, and decrease circulation.

Various methods for application of heat and cold are used; thus a variety of doctors' orders are used to prescribe the methods intended. Typical doctors' orders for commonly used procedures for heat and cold applications follow, along with explanations.

Doctors' Orders for Heat Applications

Aquathermia Pad with Heat to Lower lt Arm 20 min qid
An **aquathermia pad** (also called a *K-pad* or a *water flow pad*) is a device with a waterproof plastic or rubber pad that can be applied to various parts of the body. The pad contains channels through which heated or cooled water flows. The device includes hoses that are connected to a bedside control unit that consists of a temperature regulator, a motor for circulating the water, and a reservoir of distilled water. The pad and the patient's skin should be checked periodically to prevent accidental burns (Fig. 11-18).

Hot Compresses to Abscess on lt Ankle 10 min qh
Hot compresses are warm, wet gauze applied to a body part. They are used to treat small areas of the body. Usually, disposable items are used for this procedure.

Soak rt Hand 20 min in Warm NS Solution q4h while Awake
A soak is usually ordered to facilitate healing. For this order, the right hand is placed in a container of the prescribed

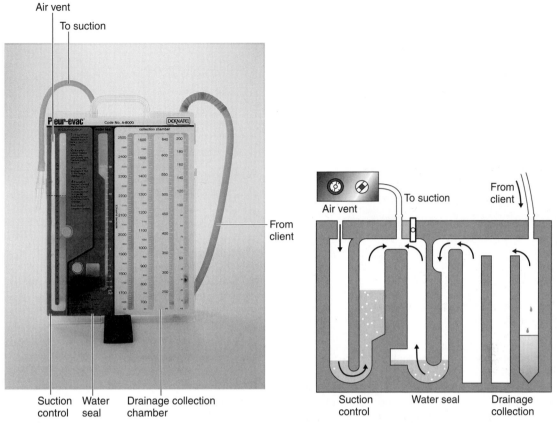

Air vent
To suction
From client
Suction control
Water seal
Drainage collection chamber
Air vent
To suction
From client
Suction control
Water seal
Drainage collection

Figure 11-17 Pleur-evac—one of many available brands of chest draining systems. (From Ignatavicius D, Workman L: *Medical-surgical nursing,* ed 5, Philadelphia, 2006, Saunders.)

solution to soak for 20 minutes every 4 hours while the patient is awake.

Sitz Bath 30 min tid
A **sitz bath** is used for the application of warm water to the pelvic area. Special tubs may be used for this procedure, or a disposable sitz bath that fits under a toilet seat may be ordered from the central service department (Fig. 11-19). Obstetric units may include sitz baths in patient bathrooms. ■

Doctors' Orders for Cold Applications

Alcohol Sponge for Temp over 102°
An alcohol sponge is the bathing of a patient with a solution of alcohol and water for the purpose of reducing the patient's temperature.

Ice Bag to Scrotum as Tolerated × 24 hr
An ice bag may be a reusable plastic container, a commercially prepared disposable ice bag, or sometimes a disposable rubber glove filled with ice.

Hypothermia Machine prn if Temp > 104°
The hypothermia machine or cooling blanket circulates fluid through a network of tubing in a mattress-sized pad. It is used for prolonged cooling and to reduce body surface temperature. This is a reusable item that is returned to the central service department when discontinued by the doctor. ■

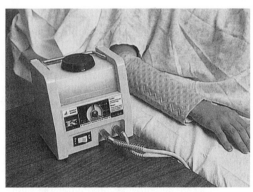

Figure 11-18 Aquathermia pad. (From Potter PA, Perry AG: *Fundamentals of nursing,* ed 6, St Louis, 2005, Mosby.)

COMFORT, SAFETY, AND HEALING ORDERS

Background Information

The nursing staff selects and performs many tasks to promote the comfort, safety, and healing of the patient. However, doctors' orders are also written to address these needs. Most comfort, safety, and healing orders do require a doctor's order for the patient's insurance to pay for items or equipment used. Because such orders are varied, only typical examples with the interpretation of each are listed.

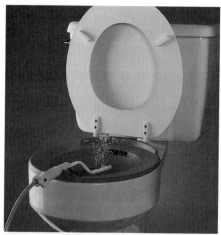

Figure 11-19 A disposable sitz bath. (Courtesy Andermac, Inc. From *Mosby's medical dictionary*, ed 7, St Louis, 2006, Mosby.)

 Doctors' Orders for Patient Comfort, Safety, and Healing

Specialty Beds

Many types of specialty beds are available to reduce the hazards of immobility to the skin and the musculoskeletal system; just a few are discussed here.

The *Hill-Rom air fluidized bed* provides body support through the use of thousands of tiny soda-lime glass beads suspended by pressurized temperature-controlled air. The beads are covered with a polyester filter sheet. The bed is used to relieve pressure and to treat burn patients (Fig. 11-20). KinAir III beds provide controlled air suspension to redistribute body weight away from bony prominences (see Evolve site), and FluidAir Elite beds use airflow and bead fluidization to achieve this. The Clinitron bed is filled with tiny sandlike pieces that are moving gently all the time. The RotoRest bed is specifically designed to support the trauma patient who is at risk for pulmonary complications. A circo-electric bed rotates inside circular bars that look like a giant hamster treadmill. These beds are used for patients in traction, with severe skin conditions, with severe burns, or with spinal injuries who cannot be moved but must be turned every 2 hours according to standard hospital policy.

The critical care bed provides programmable kinetic therapy that administers lateral rotation to a range of 62 degrees in both directions. The health unit coordinator (HUC) must include the patient's height and weight when ordering these beds from the central service department (CSD).

Egg-Crate Mattress

The **egg-crate mattress** is a foam rubber pad that resembles an egg crate or carton; it is used to distribute body weight evenly (Fig. 11-21). This is a disposable item that is used frequently in long-term care.

Other mattresses used to reduce the hazards of immobility to the skin and the musculoskeletal system include the Lotus Water Flotation Mattress, Bio Flote (an alternating air mattress), a static air mattress, and a foam mattress.

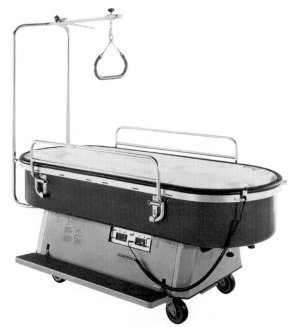

Figure 11-20 A Hill-Rom air fluidized bed. (Copyright © Hill-Rom Services, Inc. Used with permission. From *Mosby's medical dictionary*, ed 7, St Louis, 2006, Mosby.)

Sheepskin on Bed

A **sheepskin** is made of lamb's wool or of a synthetic material and usually measures about the same length and width as the patient's bed. The sheepskin is placed directly below the patient and is used to relieve pressure and prevent bedsores (decubitus ulcers). A sheepskin is usually considered a disposable item and is used frequently in long-term care.

Footboard on Bed

A footboard is placed at or near the foot of the bed so that the patient's feet, when placed against it, are at a right angle to the bed. It is used to prevent footdrop of patients who are in bed for long periods (Fig. 11-22). A footboard is a reusable item that would be ordered from the CSD.

Foot Cradle to Bed

A foot cradle is a metal frame that is placed on the bed to prevent the top sheet from touching a specified part of the body. It is a reusable item that would be ordered from the CSD.

ETS for Patient

An extended toilet seat (ETS) is ordered from the CSD and is placed over the patient's toilet to make lowering and rising from a sitting position easier (Fig. 11-23).

Immobilizer to lt Knee 20 Degrees Flexion

Immobilizers are used to keep a limb or body part in alignment (Fig. 11-24). They are reusable and are usually stored in the CSD closet or the C-locker on an ortho unit, but they are ordered from the CSD if they are needed for a patient on another unit. In some hospitals, they may be ordered through the Physical Therapy Department.

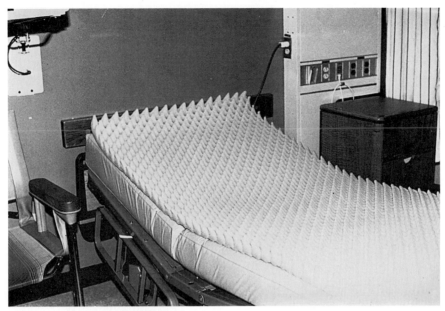

Figure 11-21   An egg-crate mattress.

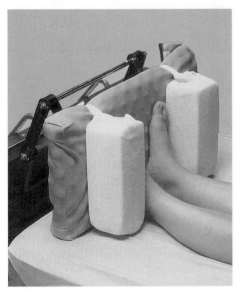

Figure 11-22   A footboard. (Courtesy JT Posey Co. From *Mosby's medical dictionary*, ed 7, St Louis, 2006, Mosby.)

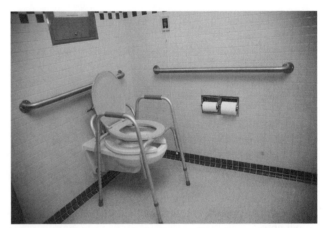

Figure 11-23   An extended toilet seat. (From Ignatavicius D, Workman L: *Medical-surgical nursing*, ed 5, Philadelphia, 2006, Saunders.)

Sandbags to Immobilize lt Leg

Sandbags are placed on both sides of the leg to immobilize it. Sandbags are stored in the CSD closet or the C-locker on ortho units, but they would need to be ordered from the CSD for other units.

Out of Bed with Elastic Abd Binder

An elastic abdominal **binder** is a disposable item that is often ordered after surgery to provide patient support (Fig. 11-25). Measurements of the patient's waist and hips are usually required on the requisition to obtain the correctly sized binder. The doctor may also order an elastic binder for the chest after chest surgery.

Sling to rt Arm when Up

A sling is a disposable bandage that is used to support an arm. Slings may be stored in the CSD closet or the C-locker on an ortho unit, but they would need to be ordered from the CSD if they are needed for a patient on another unit.

Thigh-High T.E.D. Hose to Both Legs

T.E.D. is a brand name for antiembolism (AE) hose, which are ordered to promote circulation to the lower extremities to help prevent blood clots. They are made in various sizes and may be ordered as thigh high or knee high, so the correct size and style information must be obtained from the patient's nurse. The patient takes the stockings home when discharged.

Jacket Restraint for Agitation and Patient Safety

When restraint is absolutely necessary for patient safety, it requires a doctor's order. Various methods of restraint, including soft wrist, jacket **restraints**, and several types of commercial equipment, are available. The patient's mental and physical status must be assessed at close and regular intervals as prescribed by law and the agency's policies. Careful nursing documentation is essential when any type of restraint is applied. The HUC may have to place a

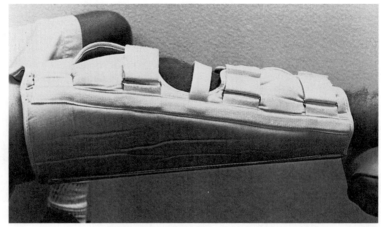

Figure 11-24 A knee immobilizer.

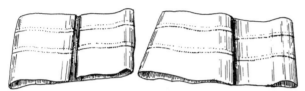

Figure 11-25 An elastic binder.

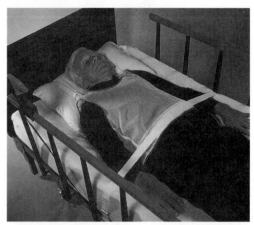

Figure 11-26 A jacket restraint. (Courtesy Medline Industries. From *Mosby's medical dictionary*, ed 7, St Louis, 2006, Mosby.)

restraint documentation form in the patient's chart. Figure 11-26 shows a patient in a jacket restraint.

May Shampoo Hair
Depending on the patient's condition, a doctor's order may be necessary for the hospitalized patient to have a shampoo. Appropriate equipment needed to do this for a bedridden patient usually is requisitioned from the CSD and is reusable. Some hospitals may have a beauty shop located on the campus for the use of ambulatory patients.

Change Surgical Drsg bid
A bandage or other application over an external wound is called a *dressing*. Items used for this treatment are disposable and usually are stored in the nursing unit supply closet or the C-locker.

Pneumatic Compression to Left Calf
Pneumatic compression devices (also called *sequential compression devices [SCDs]*) or pneumo boots are used to enhance venous blood flow by providing periods of compression. These devices prevent deep vein thrombosis (DVT) from forming in the legs as the result of inactivity. Different types of pneumatic compression devices may include boots, sleeves, or wraps to be placed on the patient's legs. T.E.D. hose may be worn, in addition to the boots, to reduce some of the uncomfortable sensations produced by the boots, such as itching, sweating, and heat. Figure 11-27 shows various types of pneumatic compression devices.

TCDB q2h Splinting
The doctor may write an order for a postsurgical patient to turn, cough, and deep breathe every 2 hours after surgery to expel secretions, keep the lungs clear, and prevent

pneumonia. **Splinting** or holding the incision area provides support and security and reduces pain during coughing. The doctor may also write an order for "do not cough" for patients who should avoid coughing.

Ostomy Nurse Referral
An ostomy nurse or wound care nurse is trained to care for ostomy patients. The ostomy nurse is notified and will perform the care needed or will provide ostomy training to the patient. During the patient's stay in the hospital, the HUC will order supplies for ostomy care. Figure 11-28 displays stoma supplies used in the care of a colostomy.

Note: A colostomy is the creation of an artificial opening into a patient's colon. The patient then wears a bag over the opening (called a *stoma*) to catch stool.

**Ask ostomy nurse to do ostomy teaching
Irrigate colostomy q A.M.** ■

SKILLS CHALLENGE

To practice transcribing heat and cold applications and performing tasks related to comfort, safety, and healing orders, complete Activity 11-4 in the *Skills Practice Manual*.

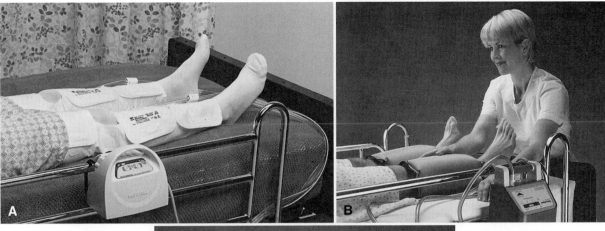

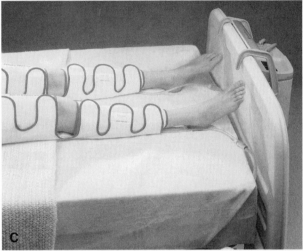

Figure 11-27 Types of pneumatic compression devices. **A,** Kendall SCD Compression System Controller, SCD Sleeves, and T.E.D. Anti-Embolism Stockings. **B,** Venodyne pneumatic compression system. **C,** Flowtron DVT calf garments. (**A** courtesy Kendall Healthcare Company, Mansfield, Massachusetts; **B** courtesy Venodyne, Norwood, Massachusetts; **C** courtesy Huntleigh Healthcare, Eatontown, New Jersey. From Ignatavicius D, Workman L: *Medical-surgical nursing,* ed 5, Philadelphia, 2006, Saunders.)

TYPES OF NURSING TREATMENT ORDERS

- Intestinal elimination orders
- Urinary catheterization orders
- Intravenous therapy orders
- Blood transfusion orders
- Suction orders
- Heat and cold application orders
- Comfort, safety, and healing orders

COMPLEMENTARY AND ALTERNATIVE APPROACHES AND THERAPIES

Complementary and alternative medicine is defined and discussed in Chapter 3. Many Americans are using complementary therapies (additional treatment) and/or alternative therapies (substitutions for traditional treatment) because they want to be treated in a holistic fashion. Nurses believe in a holistic, caring philosophy; therefore, complementary and alternative therapies are consistent with nursing practice. It would not be common to see complementary or alternative therapies ordered in the hospital setting, but reference may be made to them, so a few are listed here, along with a brief description of each.

- *Acupressure* is a Chinese ancient healing art in which the fingers are used to gradually press key healing points, which stimulate the body's natural self-curative abilities.
- *Aromatherapy* involves the use of essential oils obtained from the flowers, leaves, bark, wood, roots, seeds, and peels of plants, which are applied in compresses, in baths, or topically on the skin.
- *Imagery* is used during painful procedures or treatments; the nurse may ask a patient to think about a pleasant event or a beautiful scene to ease anxiety.
- *Journaling* is a reflective therapy in which the processes of one's life are recorded. Writing provides a vehicle by which a person can express feelings, gain new perspectives, and pay attention to what is in the unconscious. The writing is done for oneself and need not be shared.
- *Magnets* are applied via wide belts and orthotics or in mattresses and pillows and are used for a particular type

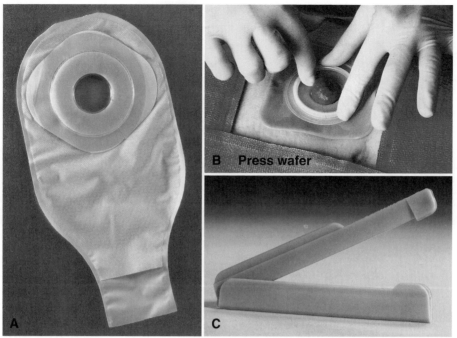

Figure 11-28 A, Stoma wafer that fits around a stoma on a patient with a colostomy. A drainable pouch is applied over the wafer and clamped **(B)** until the pouch is to be emptied **(C).** (Courtesy ConvaTec, Bristol-Myers Squibb, Princeton, New Jersey. From *Mosby's medical dictionary*, ed 7, St Louis, 2006, Mosby; and Ignatavicius D, Workman L: *Medical-surgical nursing*, ed 5, Philadelphia, 2006, Saunders.)

of energy therapy. One of the primary reasons for using magnets is to relieve chronic pain, particularly back and joint pain.

- *Massage* has a long history in nursing practice. Until recently, daily backrubs were a standard nursing procedure administered to all hospitalized patients. Hand massage can be used with persons with dementia to provide relaxation and to lessen aggressive behaviors. Patient permission must be obtained before massage is performed.

- *Music therapy* is an established health care profession in which music is used to address physical, emotional, cognitive, and social needs of patients of all ages. Music therapy interventions are used to elevate patients' moods and to counteract depression; in conjunction with anesthesia or medication to alleviate pain; to promote movement for physical rehabilitation; to calm, sedate, or induce sleep; to help counteract apprehension or fear; and to lessen muscle tension in areas such as the autonomic nervous system for the purpose of achieving relaxation.

- *Tai chi* is a traditional Chinese martial art that has been adapted to become a mind-body exercise. The goal of tai chi is to integrate body movements, mind concentration, muscle relaxation, and breathing to promote a flow of energy throughout the body.

- *Therapeutic touch* is the use of hands on or near the body with the intention to heal. The practitioner directs his or her own interpersonal energy to help or heal another. Therapeutic touch has been used to reduce anxiety and pain, improve the immune system, and improve functional ability.

SKILLS CHALLENGE

To practice transcribing a review set of doctor's orders, complete Activity 11-5 in the *Skills Practice Manual*.

To practice recording telephone messages, complete Activity 11-6 in the *Skills Practice Manual*.

KEY CONCEPTS

The procedure for nursing treatment orders is fairly simple after one has become familiar with the supplies and equipment necessary to implement each order. Ordering the wrong supplies and/or equipment may delay treatment. When in doubt about the supplies or equipment needed, check with the nurse or with the CSD. Whether an EMR or paper charts are used, the HUC who is able to recognize supplies and equipment and their uses and to effectively use the CSD plays an invaluable role in helping the nursing staff to provide high-quality patient care.

Websites of Interest

Strategic Health Care Communications: www.strategichealthcare.com

American Hospital Association—"Strategies for Leadership: Patient- and Family-Centered Care": www.aha.org/advocacy-issues/communicatingpts/pt-family-centered-care.shtml

What is Bladder ultrasound? www.wisegeek.com/what-is-bladder-ultrasound.htm

National Heart, Lung, and Blood Institute—"What Is a Blood Transfusion?": www.nhlbi.nih.gov/health/health-topics/topics/bt

⊖ REVIEW QUESTIONS

Visit the Evolve website to download and complete the following questions.

1. Define the following terms.
   a. splinting
   b. patent (patency)
   c. autologous blood
   d. donor-specific blood
   e. catheterization
   f. central venous catheter
   g. Ace wraps
   h. compression garment
   i. infiltration
   j. chux
   k. elevated toilet seat
   l. extravasation
   m. irrigation

2. Describe what holistic care includes, and provide an example of a nursing intervention.

3. Briefly describe the function of the CSD as it relates to nursing treatment orders.

4. List five nursing treatment items that would be located in the nursing unit supply closet or C-locker and five that would need to be ordered from the CSD.

5. Explain why discontinued reusable equipment should be returned to the CSD as quickly as possible.

6. List four types of enemas that a doctor may order.

7. Explain the procedure and purpose of a urine flow test.

8. List two types of urinary catheters, and describe the function of each.

9. List two methods of measuring postvoid residual urine volume (PVR)

10. Describe two methods and four purposes of administering intravenous therapy.

11. List three parts of an IV order.

12. Explain the major difference between "peripheral intravenous therapy" and a "central line."

13. List four types of central venous catheters.

14. Label the following statements as true or false:
    a. Consent is required for insertion of a PICC.
    b. Consent is required to follow this order: *start IV of 1000cc D₅LR*
    c. Consent is required for insertion of a heplock.
    d. A Hemovac is connected to a drain in or near the surgical site and is inserted during surgery.
    e. A central line tray would have to be ordered for insertion of a PICC.

15. List three types of commonly used prepared intravenous solutions, and explain how the HUC would determine how long a bag of IV solution would take to empty.

16. Explain the purpose of a heparin lock (heplock or saline lock), and describe how a heplock is kept patent.

17. List the four blood types.

18. Explain what would happen if a patient's blood specimen sent for a type and crossmatch was labeled incorrectly (the patient's name on the ID label does not match the patient's name on the order requisition).

19. A patient's nurse asks the HUC to pick up a unit of packed cells from the blood bank. When the HUC returns to the nursing unit with the packed cells, the nurse states that the transfusion will not be started for hours. Explain what the HUC should do with the packed cells until the nurse can start the transfusion.

20. The HUC is asked to pick up 2 units of packed cells from the blood bank for two separate patients on the nursing unit. Explain what the HUC should do.

21. Explain the purpose of a Swan-Ganz catheter and an arterial line (a-line or art-line).

22. Identify three suction or drainage devices that are inserted during surgery.

23. List items that the HUC may be asked to order for a patient requiring gastric, throat, or tracheostomy suctioning.

24. List two devices used for heat application.

25. List two devices used for cold application.

26. Explain why most comfort, safety, and healing orders require a doctor's order, and identify at least five items or equipment these orders may include.

27. List at least four complementary or alternative approaches or therapies that may be recommended or provided to hospitalized patients.

SURFING FOR ANSWERS

1. Research and document five risks of intravenous therapy, and document the website used.

2. Research ways in which hospitals are trying to improve patient satisfaction. Document at least three ways patient satisfaction is being improved, and list two websites used.

CHAPTER 12

Nutritional Care Orders

OUTLINE

CHAPTER OBJECTIVES

On completion of this chapter, you will be able to:

1. Define the terms listed in the vocabulary list.
2. Write the meaning of the abbreviations in the abbreviations list.
3. Explain the importance of communicating diet changes and patient food allergies to the nutritional care department.
4. Discuss the methods that may be used by the health unit coordinator (HUC) to order a late tray for a patient.
5. Discuss two eating disorders and other factors that a doctor would need to consider when ordering a hospitalized patient's diet.
6. List three groups of diets that may be ordered for the hospitalized patient.
7. List five consistency changes that can be made to a standard diet, and explain what is included in each.
8. List four diet options that may be selected for the patient who has started on clear liquids and has an order for *diet as tolerated,* and explain how the selection would be made.
9. Identify two diets that may be requested by patients.
10. Identify at least five therapeutic diets that the patient's doctor may order.
11. Discuss the reasons a patient would require a tube feeding, and list three methods of administering tube feedings.
12. List three items a HUC may need to order when transcribing an order for tube feeding.
13. Explain the purpose of the doctors' orders *force fluids, limit fluids,* and *calorie count,* and discuss the importance of sending all doctors' orders regarding a patient's diet or modifications to a patient's diet to the nutritional care department.
14. Discuss the importance of sending total parenteral nutrition (TPN) orders to the pharmacy in a timely manner.

VOCABULARY

Anorexia Nervosa Condition characterized by intense fear of gaining weight or becoming fat, although underweight.

Body Mass Index Body weight in kilograms divided by height in square meters; this is the usual measurement to define overweight and obesity.

Bolus Rounded mass of food formed in the mouth and ready to be swallowed; also defined as a concentrated dose of medication or fluid, frequently given intravenously (discussed in Chapter 13).

Bulimia Nervosa Recurrent episodes of binge eating (rapid consumption of a large amount of food in a discrete period of time) and self-induced vomiting, often along with use of laxatives or diuretics.

Calorie A measurement of energy generated in the body by the heat produced after food is eaten.

Dehydration Excessive loss of body water. Causes may include diseases of the gastrointestinal tract that cause vomiting or diarrhea, heat exposure, prolonged vigorous exercise (e.g., in a marathon), kidney disease, and medications (diuretics).

Diet Manual Hospitals are required to have available in the dietary office and on all nursing units an up-to-date diet manual that has been jointly approved by the medical and nutritional care staffs. May also be called the *diet formulary* (may be available on computer).

Diet Order A doctor's order that states the type and quantity of food and liquids the patient may receive.

Dietary Reference Intake (DRI) The framework of nutrient standards now in place in the United States; this provides reference values for use in planning and evaluating diets for healthy people.

Dietary Supplements A product (other than tobacco) taken by mouth that contains a "dietary ingredient" intended to supplement the diet; dietary supplements come in many forms, including extracts, concentrates, tablets, capsules, gel caps, liquids, and powders.

Duodenostomy Surgical formation of a permanent opening into the duodenum. May be performed for the purpose of introducing a tube for postpyloric feeding.

Dysphagia Difficulty eating and swallowing.

Enteral Feeding Set Equipment needed to infuse tube feeding; includes plastic bag for feeding solution and may be ordered with or without pump.

Enteral Nutrition The provision of liquid formulas into the gastrointestinal tract by tube or by mouth.

Feeding Tube A small flexible plastic tube that is usually placed in the patient's nose and that goes down to the stomach or small intestine to provide and/or increase nutritional intake.

Food Allergy A negative physical reaction to a particular food that involves the immune system (people with food allergies must avoid offending foods).

Food Intolerance Nonallergic food hypersensitivity—a more common problem than food allergies, involving digestion (people with food intolerance can eat some of the offending foods without developing symptoms).

Gastritis Inflammation of the stomach.

Gastroenteritis Inflammation of the stomach and intestines.

Gastrostomy A surgical procedure for inserting a tube through the abdominal wall and into the stomach. The tube may be used for feeding or drainage.

Gavage Feeding by means of a tube inserted into the stomach, duodenum, or jejunum through the nose or an opening in the abdominal wall; also called *tube feeding*.

Hydration Adequate water in the intracellular and extracellular compartments of the body.

Ingest To take in food by mouth.

Ingestion The act of taking in food by mouth.

Intravenous Hyperalimentation The administration of nutrients by intravenous feeding, especially to individuals unable to take in food through the alimentary tract.

Jejunostomy A creation of an artificial opening into the jejunum that may be used for enteral feeding when it is necessary to bypass the upper gastrointestinal tract.

Kangaroo Pump A brand name of a feeding pump used to administer tube feeding.

Kosher Adhering to the dietary laws of Judaism; the conventional meaning in Hebrew is "acceptable" or "approved."

Morbid Obesity An excess of body fat that threatens necessary body functions such as respiration.

Nutrients Substances derived from food that are used by body cells, for example, carbohydrates, fats, proteins, vitamins, minerals, and water.

Obese Having an excess amount of body fat, usually defined by body mass index.

Obesity Condition characterized by an excess amount of body fat, usually defined by body mass index.

Parenteral Nutrition A mode of feeding that does not use the gastrointestinal tract, instead providing nutrition by intravenous delivery of nutrient solutions.

Partial Parenteral Nutrition (PPN) A solution containing some essential nutrients injected into a vein to supplement other means of nutrition, usually a partially normal diet of food.

Percutaneous Endoscopic Gastrostomy Insertion of a tube through the abdominal wall into the stomach under endoscopic guidance.

Recommended Dietary Allowance (RDA) The average daily intake of a nutrient that meets the requirements of nearly all (97% to 98%) healthy people of a given age and sex. Also commonly known as *recommended daily allowance*.

Registered Dietitian One who has completed an educational program, served an internship, and passed an examination sponsored by the American Dietetic Association.

Regular Diet A diet that consists of all foods and is designed to provide good nutrition.

Rehydration Restoration of normal water balance in a patient through the administration of fluids orally or intravenously.

Therapeutic Diet A diet with modifications or restrictions (also called a *special diet*) that must be ordered by the doctor.

Total Parenteral Nutrition (TPN) The provision of all necessary nutrients via veins (discussed in detail in Chapter 13).

Tube Feeding Administration of liquids into the stomach, duodenum, or jejunum through a tube.

ABBREVIATIONS

Abbreviation	Meaning	Example of Usage on a Doctor's Order Sheet
ADA	American Diabetes Association	1200 cal ADA diet
ADD	attention-deficit disorder	ADD diet
AHA	American Heart Association	Follow AHA diet
BMI	body mass index	Calculate BMI
cal	calorie	1800 cal diet
CHO	carbohydrate	High-protein, low-CHO diet
chol	cholesterol	Low-chol diet

Abbreviation	Meaning	Example of Usage on a Doctor's Order Sheet
cl	clear	Cl liq diet
DAT	diet as tolerated	Advance DAT
FF	force fluids	Soft diet FF
FS	full strength	Jevity FS @ 50 mL/hr
K or K+	potassium	Low K+ diet
Liq	liquid	Full liq diet
MN	midnight	NPO MN
Na or Na+	sodium	2000 mg Na diet (2000 mg/2 g)
NAS	no added salt	Reg diet, NAS
NPO	nothing by mouth	NPO after midnight
NSA	no salt added (same as NAS)	
PEG	percutaneous endoscopic gastrostomy	PEG in A.M.
RD	registered dietitian	RD consult requested
reg	regular	Reg diet

⊜ EXERCISE 1

Write the abbreviation for each term listed.

1. sodium
2. midnight
3. nothing by mouth
4. regular
5. clear
6. calorie
7. American Diabetes Association
8. liquid
9. cholesterol
10. diet as tolerated
11. force fluids
12. carbohydrate
13. no salt added
14. full strength
15. percutaneous endoscopic gastrostomy
16. no added salt
17. registered dietitian
18. potassium
19. body mass index
20. American Heart Association
21. attention-deficit disorder

⊜ EXERCISE 2

Write the meaning of each abbreviation listed.

1. Na or Na+
2. NPO
3. reg
4. MN
5. liq
6. cal
7. NSA
8. ADA
9. DAT
10. cl
11. chol
12. CHO
13. FF
14. FS
15. PEG
16. NAS
17. RD
18. K or K+
19. BMI
20. AHA
21. ADD

COMMUNICATION WITH THE NUTRITIONAL CARE DEPARTMENT

When the electronic medical record (EMR) with computer physician order entry (CPOE) is implemented, the physician orders are entered directly into the patient's electronic record, and the dietary order is automatically sent to the nutritional care department. The health unit coordinator (HUC) may have tasks to perform, such as ordering equipment from the central service department (CSD). A computer icon may indicate a HUC task, may indicate important information such as "nothing by mouth" (NPO), or may indicate a nurse request. There will still be late patient trays to order after completion of tests or procedures for which it was necessary for the patient to be NPO or after a patient has undergone minor surgery.

The procedure for ordering a new diet or a change or modification to an existing diet when paper charts are used requires the HUC to communicate the order by computer to the nutritional care department. The HUC chooses the correct patient from the unit census screen on the computer, selects the nutritional care department from the department ordering screen, then checks the box to order the specific diet from the options on the dietary screen, along with other items that apply (e.g., dietitian consultation). The HUC must communicate with the nutritional care department (by computer or telephone) when ordering a diet for a patient who has completed a procedure or test that requires him or her to be NPO. The patient's food allergies and intolerances must be communicated to the nutritional care department (usually on admission). Some food allergies or intolerances cause minor discomforts such as hives or an upset stomach. True food allergies such as allergies to tree nuts, fish, shellfish, and peanuts can produce life-threatening changes in circulation and bronchioles called *anaphylactic shock*. The notation *NKFA* indicates that the patient has no known food allergies.

A "write-in" option is provided for additional comments. The **diet order** would be sent to the nutritional care department by pressing "enter" on the computer keyboard.

If the computer system is unavailable, the diet is ordered from the nutritional care department via a written downtime requisition. The diet order is later entered into the computer to maintain a record (Fig. 12-1).

Most health care facilities provide each patient with the next day's menu of items that are allowed for the particular diet the doctor has ordered for the patient. The patient checks what foods he or she would like from the menu. The menu is then sent to the nutritional care department. Many facilities have initiated a system to better serve patients and save the cost of printing menus. This requires the diet aide or technician to interview each patient on admission to obtain and record food preferences and allergies. The diet aide may use a laptop computer to record the information. With the increase in computerization, many patients are encouraged to submit their preferences online. The doctor, nurse, diet aide, or diet technician may ask the **registered dietitian** to consult with the patient.

★ HIGH PRIORITY

The health unit coordinator must communicate with the nutritional care department (by e-mail or telephone) when requesting a diet tray for a patient who has completed a procedure or test that requires him or her to be NPO.

Note: Some hospital nutritional care departments require that *all* diet orders be submitted in writing via computer.

Doctor ordering ______________________

Today's date ______________________

Requested by ______________________

Patient Label

NUTRITIONAL CARE DEPARTMENT REQUISITION

☐ Bland	☐ Mechanical soft	☐ Soft
☐ ________ Calorie ADA	☐ Modified fat ________	☐ Tube Feeding ________
☐ Clear liquid	☐ Pediatric	________
☐ Dysphagia ________	☐ Protein modified ________ g	________
☐ Finger food	☐ Prudent cardiac	☐ Vegetarian
☐ Force fluids	☐ Pureed	☐ Calorie count
☐ Full liquid	☐ Regular	☐ Dietitian consult
☐ Gluten free	☐ Renal	☐ Early tray
☐ Kosher	☐ Restrict Fluids to ________	☐ Guest tray
☐ Low cholesterol	☐ Snacks / supplements	☐ Hold tray
☐ Low sodium	☐ ________ Sodium	☐ NPO ________
		☐ Release from hold

☐ Other ______________________

Food Allergies ______________________

Preferences ______________________

Comments ______________________

Figure 12-1 A nutritional care department requisition.

All dietary information, including orders for NPO, tube feedings, allergies, limit fluids, force fluids, and **calorie** count, must be sent to the nutritional care department, so necessary adjustments will be made when the patient's trays are prepared. The dietitian also maintains a record (usually on computer) on each patient, which is updated with each order received.

> **HIGH PRIORITY**
>
> A patients' **food allergy** and/or **food intolerance** must be communicated to the nutritional care department (usually on admission). Some food allergies and intolerances cause minor discomforts such as hives or an upset stomach. True food allergies such as allergies to tree nuts, fish, shellfish, and peanuts can produce life-threatening changes in circulation and bronchioles called *anaphylactic shock.* "NKFA" indicates that the patient has no known food allergies.

> **HIGH PRIORITY**
>
> Downtime requisitions are included in this chapter for learning purposes. The Evolve website associated with the *Health Unit Coordinator Skills Manual* includes a simulated hospital computer program that may be used as well.

Background Information

During hospitalization, the doctor will order the type of diet the patient is to receive depending on the patient's diagnosis. There are many factors the doctor must consider when ordering diets for a hospitalized patient, including whether the patient has an eating disorder such as **anorexia nervosa** or **bulimia nervosa,** is **obese** (20% over recommended weight and having a **body mass index** (BMI) of 30 or over), has **dehydration,** or has inability to swallow, chew, and/or **ingest** food. The doctor may also order between-meal **dietary supplements** or *snacks* for patients as needed. The food is prepared by the nutritional care department and is designed to attain or maintain the health of the patient. Hospitals are required to have an up-to-date **diet manual** or diet formulary (may be available on computer) with the **dietary reference intake (DRI)** values and **recommended dietary allowance (RDA)** (or *recommended daily allowance*) values available in the dietary office and on all nursing units for use by the hospital staff for reference.

Diets for the hospitalized patient can be divided into three groups: standard diets, therapeutic diets, and tube feedings (Table 12-1).

> **HIGH PRIORITY**
>
> It is essential that all dietary information, including orders for nothing by mouth, tube feedings, allergies, limit fluids, force fluids, and calorie count, be sent to the nutritional care department, so necessary adjustments will be made when the patient's tray is prepared. All admitted patients require a diet order.

STANDARD DIETS

Standard hospital diets consist of a **regular diet** and diets that vary in consistency or texture of foods (from clear liquid to solid). A regular diet, also called *general, house, routine,* and *full* diet, is planned to provide good nutrition and consists of all items in the four basic food groups. This diet is ordered for hospitalized

TABLE 12-1 Description and Purpose of Common Hospital Diets

Type	Description	Purpose	Tray Condiments
Bland diet	May be used for patients who experience stomach irritation. Spicy foods containing black or red pepper and chili powder are omitted. Beverages that contain caffeine, cola, coffee, cocoa, and tea are omitted. Chocolate is also omitted. Any foods known to cause discomfort are omitted.	For patients with ulcers and other problems.	Salt, sugar
Prudent cardiac—low cholesterol, reduced sodium	Controls the type of fat in the diet. Limits saturated fat and cholesterol found in foods from animal sources such as eggs, dairy products, meat, and fish. Limits salt added to foods and on tray.	For patients who have high levels of blood cholesterol.	Pepper, sugar, salt substitute, or herbal seasoning mix
Sodium-controlled diet	Controls the amount of sodium in the diet. Salt and foods that contain salt are high in sodium and are limited. The sodium-controlled diet will vary according to the amount of sodium allowed.	For patients with heart disease, high blood pressure, or kidney disease or who are using certain drugs.	Sugar, pepper, salt substitute, if ordered
Diabetic diet	Total amount of food (calories) is carefully planned. Diabetic individuals cannot receive too much or too little food; therefore portion sizes must be followed. Concentrated sweets such as syrup, jelly, sweet desserts, and sugar are omitted. Snacks may be planned between meals to keep blood sugar levels balanced.	For patients who cannot produce enough insulin. Insulin is a substance that is important for helping sugar enter body cells. When insufficient insulin is made, sugar builds up in the blood.	Salt, pepper, sugar substitute
Renal diet	On the basis of individual needs, diet is controlled in terms of one or more of the following: protein, sodium, potassium, total fluid, and phosphorus.	For patients with renal disease.	Sugar, pepper, no salt substitutes
Neutropenic diet—no fresh fruits or vegetables, low bacteria	No fresh fruits or vegetables allowed.	Reduce the number of bacteria entering the stomach for patients on chemotherapy or those with immune deficiency diseases.	Sugar, no pepper or salt
Lactose-controlled diet	Limits intake of milk and milk products.	For patients who experience stomach disturbances after drinking or eating milk-containing foods.	Salt, pepper, sugar
NPO—nothing by mouth	Patient cannot receive fluids or solid foods.	Presurgery or as indicated for procedure or test.	None
Clear liquid	Foods that are liquid or that become liquid at room or body temperature. Includes foods such as tea, coffee, clear broth, gelatin, and carbonated beverages, as well as foods that can be seen through (e.g., apple, cranberry, grape juice).	For patients who are very sick and cannot eat anything else. For patients before or after surgery.	Sugar
Full liquid diet	This diet includes food from the clear liquid diet, with the addition of juices with pulp, such as orange. It also includes milk, ice cream, puddings, refined cooked cereals, strained cream soups, and eggnog.	For patients who cannot eat solid foods. For patients after surgery and after the clear liquid diet.	Salt, pepper, sugar
Regular diet/DAT	All foods and beverages are allowed.	For patients who have no dietary restrictions.	Salt, pepper, sugar
Gastrointestinal soft diet	Limits raw, highly seasoned, and fried foods.	For patients with nausea and for distention in the postsurgical patient.	Salt, pepper, sugar
Mechanical soft diet	Any diet made soft, with ground meats, soft canned fruits, and well cooked vegetables.	For patients who have trouble chewing or swallowing.	Salt, pepper, sugar

TABLE 12-1 Description and Purpose of Common Hospital Diets—cont'd

Type	Description	Purpose	Tray Condiments
Purée	Mechanically altered foods and full liquids allowed.	For patients with problems in chewing and swallowing.	Salt, pepper, sugar
No thin liquids/thick liquids only	No milk (except milkshakes), juice (except nectars), broth soups (only cream soups), coffee, tea, or soda pop.	To prevent choking.	Salt, pepper, sugar
DAT, diet as tolerated	Usually ordered as a consistency variation on a regular diet, although may be seen combined with some therapeutic diets.	To allow a consistency best tolerated by the patient	Salt, pepper, sugar

patients who do not require restrictions or modifications of their diets. Clear liquid, full liquid, soft, mechanical soft, and puréed are types of diets that vary in food texture or consistency.

 Doctors' Orders for Standard Progression Diets

Clear Liquid

This diet is used for patients who cannot tolerate solid foods, including those in whom an acute illness has been diagnosed and patients who have just had surgery. It includes clear liquids only, such as broth, bouillon, coffee, tea, carbonated beverages, clear fruit juices, gelatin, and popsicles.

Full Liquid

Clear liquids with the addition of smooth-textured dairy products, custards, refined cooked cereals, vegetables, and all fruit juices. This diet is often ordered as a transitional step between a clear liquid diet and a soft diet.

Puréed

Most foods including meats, vegetables, and fruits can be processed (cooked and blended) to a puréed (smooth) consistency. No lumps or chunks, coarse textures, dried fruits, nuts, seeds, or raw vegetables or fruits. Foods that require chewing are excluded from this diet. Some commercially prepared products are acceptable, including applesauce, pudding without rice, smooth custard, farina cereal, and stage 1 baby food.

Mechanical Soft

Includes the addition of ground or finely diced meats, flaked fish, cottage cheese, cheese, rice, potatoes, pancakes, light breads, cooked vegetables, cooked or canned fruits, bananas, soups, or peanut butter. This diet is prepared to meet the needs of patients who have difficulty chewing. Some variations of the mechanical soft diet are the *minced diet* and the *dental soft diet*.

Soft

This diet is often used in the progression from a full liquid diet to a regular diet. It combines foods considered nonirritating, easily digestible foods and with modified fiber content, such as broiled chicken and boiled vegetables. It may be ordered postoperatively, for patients with acute infections, or for those with gastrointestinal (GI) disorders.

Regular

No restrictions unless specified.

Diet as Tolerated (DAT)

Frequently the doctor will order an initial diet such as clear liquid and then request that the diet progress as the patient's condition improves. The nurse can determine and select the consistency of the patient's diet. This means that the nurse can select a full liquid, soft, mechanical soft, or regular diet for the patient, according to the patient's tolerance of food. For example, after the patient has tolerated clear liquids following a morning surgery, the nurse may order a full liquid diet for the evening meal. Usually the patient is advanced from clear liquid to full liquid, to soft, and then to a regular diet, according to the current stage of recovery. Because DAT is nonspecific, some hospitals may not allow this as a dietary order and require that the physician write or enter a specific consistency. ■

 HIGH PRIORITY

An order sent to nutritional care for a liquid diet must indicate *clear* or *full*, or nutritional care personnel will not know what to send to the patient.

HIGH PRIORITY

When the doctor writes an order to *advance diet as tolerated* (DAT), the order usually includes the initial diet. The nurse may then select from standard (consistency) diets such as full liquid, soft, or regular to advance the diet. Variations may include mechanical soft or puréed, depending on the patient's ability to chew.

Note: The health unit coordinator must ask the patient's nurse for the diet selection, then send this information to the nutritional care department. The order for "DAT" should not be sent as a diet, as the nutritional care department cannot determine what the patient can tolerate.

Patient-Requested Diets

Many patients have food preferences or restrictions that are based on their culture, religion, religious holidays, or personal preference. This information is used in conjunction with any therapeutic or consistency requirements to prepare food

BOX 12-1	OTHER RELIGIOUS DIETARY RESTRICTIONS

Islam
- Pork
- Alcohol
- Caffeine
- Ramadan: fasting (actually NPO—no food or drink) sunrise to sunset for a month
- Ritualized methods of animal slaughter required for meat ingestion

Christianity
- Minimal or no alcohol (for some religions)
- Holy day observances may restrict meat

Hinduism
- All meats

Church of Jesus Christ of Latter-Day Saints (Mormons)
- Alcohol
- Tobacco
- Caffeine

Seventh-Day Adventists
- Pork
- Shellfish
- Alcohol
- Vegetarian diet encouraged

for those patients. Two examples of patient-requested diets include vegetarian diets and kosher diets.

Vegetarian diets are those in which the patient follows a plant-based diet and limits or excludes animal foods. Several types of vegetarian diets are available, such as the following:

- Ovolactovegetarian—includes all plant foods, dairy, and eggs
- Lactovegetarian—includes all plant foods and dairy
- Vegan—includes plant foods only
- Flexitarian—includes predominantly plant foods with nonvegetarian foods, such as fish or poultry, on occasion

Kosher diets are those that adhere to the dietary laws of Judaism. A kosher diet involves the following:

- Certain categories of animals—only healthy animals that have split hooves and chew their cud (hogs and pigs do not chew their cud) and only fish with scales and fins.
- Manner in which food is processed—animals properly slaughtered and no mixing of milk and meat.
- Time—leavened product properly disposed of before Passover and no food cooked on Sabbath.
- All fresh fruits and vegetables are kosher.
- Unprocessed grains and cereals are kosher.
- Chicken eggs are kosher.

See Box 12-1, *Other Religious Dietary Restrictions*, for additional examples of dietary restrictions.

SKILLS CHALLENGE

To practice transcribing a standard hospital diet order, complete Activity 12-1 in the *Skills Practice Manual.*

THERAPEUTIC DIETS

A therapeutic diet, which must be ordered by a doctor, differs from the regular diet in that the foods served are modified to vary in caloric content, level of one or more **nutrients**, bulk, or

flavor. The following list contains some common therapeutic diets and diets for specific conditions.

- ADD diet—The attention-deficit disorder (ADD) diet is designed to provide adequate nutrition while avoiding certain foods or food ingredients that may exacerbate ADD. May also include ADHD (attention-deficit/hyperactivity disorder). Was originally developed as the Feingold Diet.
- Bland diet—This diet is designed to provide adequate nutrition during treatment of patients with inflammatory or ulcerative conditions of the esophagus, stomach, and intestines. It is mechanically, chemically, physiologically, and sometimes thermally nonirritating to the gastrointestinal (GI) tract. A bland diet disallows caffeine, alcohol, black pepper, spices, or any other food that could be considered irritating.
- BRAT diet—This diet is commonly used as short-term dietary treatment for diarrhea, **gastritis, gastroenteritis,** and some incidences of food poisoning. The name *BRAT* is an acronym for bananas, rice, applesauce, and toast. Oral **rehydration** solution or other liquids are usually given to the patient immediately. A BRAT diet is usually administered to prevent dehydration about 24 hours after the diarrhea or gastroenteritis has started, once vomiting has stopped and the patient is able to eat.
- Soft or low-residue diet—Addition of low-fiber, easily digested foods, such as pastas, casseroles, moist tender meats, and canned cooked fruits and vegetables. Desserts, cakes, and cookies without nuts or coconut are included. A variation is the GI soft diet.
- Low-cholesterol diet—A diet including 300 mg of cholesterol per day is in keeping with American Heart Association (AHA) guidelines for serum lipid reduction.
- Low-sodium diet—A diet including 4 g (no added salt), 2 g, 1 g, or 500 mg of sodium. These diets vary from no added salt to severe sodium restriction (500-mg sodium diet) that requires selective food purchases. Sodium intake is often restricted for patients with cardiovascular disease, hypertension, and kidney disease.
- Low-protein diet—Protein intake may be controlled in Parkinson disease and in chronic kidney disease.

- High-fiber diet—Fresh uncooked fruits, steamed vegetables, bran, oatmeal, and dried fruits are added.
- Diabetic (American Diabetes Association [ADA]) diet—Included food exchanges are recommended by the ADA. Usually, caloric recommendations are made for around 1800 calories. The exchange diet results in a balanced intake of carbohydrates, fats, and proteins. Total calories may vary to accommodate the client's metabolic demands, which may be affected by an exercise program, pregnancy, or, in some situations, another illness. Variations include the gestational diabetic diet and the consistent carbohydrate diet.
- Calorie-restricted diet—Diet may be limited to 1200 calories or 1400 calories.
- Renal diet—This diet is ordered for patients with renal disease. On the basis of individual needs, diet is controlled in terms of one or more of the following: protein, sodium, potassium, total fluid, and phosphorus. The many variations of the renal diet include prerenal, chronic kidney disease, hemodialysis, peritoneal dialysis, acute renal failure, and acute post–renal transplant diets.
- Prudent cardiac diet—This diet is based on variations of diet recommendations of the AHA for low cholesterol and low sodium.
- Low-fat diet—Diets high in fat, especially saturated fat, are linked to high blood cholesterol levels and heart disease. High-fat diets can also increase risk of **obesity** and cancer. This is a diet low in fat, saturated fat, and cholesterol.
- High-potassium diet—A shortage of potassium in body fluids may cause a potentially fatal condition known as *hypokalemia*, which typically results from diarrhea, increased diuresis, and vomiting. Eating a variety of foods that contain potassium is the best way to get an adequate amount. Foods with high sources of potassium include orange juice, potatoes, bananas, avocados, apricots, parsnips, and turnips, although many other fruits, vegetables, and meats contain potassium. Diets high in potassium can reduce the risk of hypertension.
- Potassium-restricted diet—Some people with kidney disease are advised to avoid large quantities of dietary potassium. Patients with end-stage renal failure who are undergoing therapy by renal dialysis must observe strict dietary limits on potassium intake because the kidneys control potassium excretion, and buildup of blood concentrations of potassium may trigger fatal heart dysrhythmias.
- Hypoglycemic diet—The purpose of the hypoglycemic diet is to normalize blood sugar levels, thereby normalizing levels of stress hormones such as adrenaline and cortisol, which are thought to be responsible for the symptoms of mood swings, depression, anxiety, phobias, alcoholism, and drug addiction. This diet limits sugar, coffee, strong tea, nicotine if possible, refined carbohydrates, sugary drinks, candy bars, colas, cookies, and so forth. The diet consists of high levels of protein plus complex carbohydrate snacks every 3 hours or less, to provide a slow release of glucose and to prevent the hypoglycemic dip. A high-protein breakfast must be considered the most important meal of the day. Good sources of protein include eggs and white meat (e.g., chicken, fish). Plenty of green vegetables and fruits are eaten. The more varied the diet, the better it is.
- Low-carbohydrate diet—This diet involves restricted carbohydrate consumption, based on research that ties consumption of certain carbohydrates with increased blood insulin levels, and overexposure to insulin with metabolic syndrome (the most recognized symptom of which is obesity). Foods high in digestible carbohydrates (sugars and starches) are limited or are replaced by foods that contain a higher percentage of proteins, fats, and/or fiber.

Dysphagia diets include the following:

- Level I (most restricted): Severe dysphagia—Patients are just beginning to eat by mouth (unable to safely swallow chewable foods and unable to safely drink thin liquids). The diet consists of foods with thick homogenous semiliquid textures and decreased fiber; no coarse textures, nuts, or raw fruits or vegetables are included. May also be called a *dysphagia purée diet.*
- Level II: Moderate dysphagia—Patients can tolerate a minimal amount of easily chewed foods and cannot swallow thin liquids safely. The diet consists of liquids thickened with commercial thickener as needed, very thick juices and milk products, and decreased fiber; no coarse textures, nuts, or raw fruits or vegetables are included.
- Level III: Patients have difficulty chewing, manipulating, or swallowing foods. Patients are beginning to chew, and the diet is mechanically soft or suitable for edentulous (absence of teeth) patients. No tough skins, nuts, or dry, crispy, raw, or stringy foods are included. Meats have to be minced or cut into small pieces; liquids are taken as tolerated. May also be called a dysphagia altered diet.
- Level IV (least restricted): Persons can chew soft textures and swallow liquids safely. The diet includes foods with soft textures that do not require grinding or chopping; no nuts or raw, crisp, or deep fried foods are included; liquids are taken as tolerated. May also be called a dysphagia advanced diet.

The postoperative diet for the gastric bypass procedure consists of the following:

- Stage 1: Clear liquids—1 ounce allowed at the beginning; continued for two to three meals
- Stage 2: Gastric bypass liquids—begun after clear liquids are tolerated; continued for 3 to 4 weeks
- Stage 3: Puréed—begun after postoperative week 4 (4-ounce meals, six to eight times a day); continued for 1 to 2 weeks
- Stage 4: Soft, solids—begun after postoperative week 6; continued indefinitely

Patients who have had gastric bypass surgery owing to **morbid obesity** will be placed on a gastric bypass diet. Gastric bypass liquids include nonfat milk, blenderized soups, 100% fruit juice (diluted ½ water, ½ juice), vegetable juice (e.g., V8, tomato), sugar-free Carnation Instant Breakfast powder mixed with nonfat milk, grits, oatmeal, cream of wheat, mashed potatoes (thinned down enough that the mixture could go through a straw), nonfat sugar-free milkshakes, thinned baby food, and sugar-free drinks (e.g., sodas, tea).

As there are many different hospital manuals, there are a wide variety of additional therapeutic diets. The HUC should become familiar with the approved diets at his or her facility. Additional diets include the following:

- Caffeine-free diet
- Dumping syndrome diet
- Encephalopathy diet
- Esophagogastrectomy diet
- Finger-foods diet (for cath lab patients who must lie flat)
- Hyperemesis diet (may be called *wet and dry diet*)
- Ketogenic diet
- Low-bacteria or neutropenic diet
- Low-oxalate diet
- MAOI diet (monoamine oxidase inhibitor diet)
- Pediatric diet (specific for age)
- Postgastrectomy diet
- Six small meals diet
- T&A (tonsillectomy and adenoidectomy) diet

★ HIGH PRIORITY

An order modifying a nutrient or number of calories would not change the consistency of a patient's diet.
Example 1: If a patient is on a soft diet and the doctor writes an order for *low fat,* the patient's diet would be "soft, low fat."
Example 2: If a patient is on a mechanical soft diet and the doctor writes an order for *2 g Na,* the patent's diet would be "mechanical soft, 2 g Na."

SKILLS CHALLENGE

To practice transcribing a therapeutic diet order, complete Activity 12-2 in the *Skills Practice Manual.*

TUBE FEEDING

Tube feeding, also called **gavage,** is the administration of **enteral nutrition** or liquefied nutrients into the stomach, duodenum, or jejunum through a tube inserted through the nose (a nasogastric or nasoenteral tube; Fig. 12-2) or through an opening in the abdominal wall (**gastrostomy, duodenostomy,** or **jejunostomy;** Fig. 12-3). **Percutaneous endoscopic gastrostomy** is a procedure performed to insert a tube through the abdominal wall into the stomach under endoscopic guidance. Tube feedings are ordered for patients who have **ingestion** problems owing to difficulty swallowing, who are unable to eat sufficient nutrients, or who cannot absorb nutrients from the foods they eat.

Tube feedings may be administered in a bolus, continuous, or cyclic manner:

- Administration of a **bolus** (intermittent feeding) involves infusing 300 to 400 mL of formula over a short time (10 minutes) with a syringe (Fig. 12-4), or 300 to 400 mL every 3 to 6 hours over a 30- to 60-minute period with the use of an enteral feeding bag (Fig. 12-5).
- Continuous administration requires the use of a mechanical feeding infusion pump (called an *enteral feeding pump* or a **Kangaroo pump**) to control the rate of infusion (Fig. 12-6).

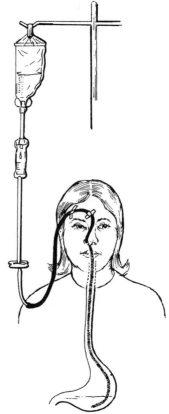

Figure 12-2 A nasogastric **feeding tube.** (Courtesy Baxter Travenol Laboratories.)

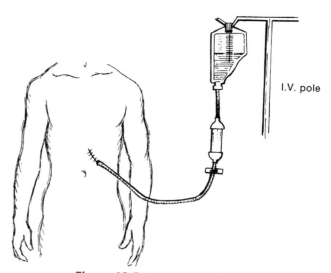

Figure 12-3 A gastrostomy feeding.

- With cyclic administration, feedings are infused over 8 to 16 hours during the day or night. Nighttime feedings allow greater freedom during the day. Daytime feedings are recommended for patients who have a greater chance of aspiration or tube dislodgment.

Types of nasogastric or nasoenteral tubes used for feedings include Entron, Dobbhoff, and Levin. Some of the commercially prepared formulas, including Isocal HN, Deliver 2.0,

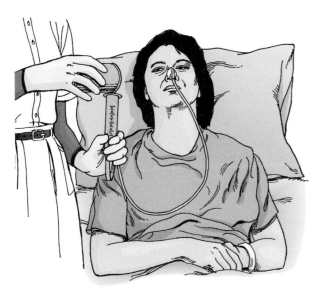

Figure 12-4 Administration of a bolus or intermittent feeding through a syringe. (From Potter PA, Perry AG: *Fundamentals of nursing*, ed 6, St Louis, 2005, Mosby.)

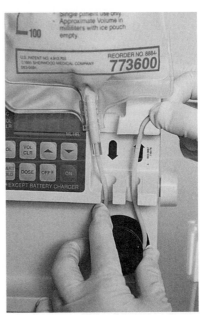

Figure 12-6 Connecting tubing through an enteral feeding pump to administer a continuous feeding by monitored drip. (From Potter PA, Perry AG: *Fundamentals of nursing*, ed 6, St Louis, 2005, Mosby.)

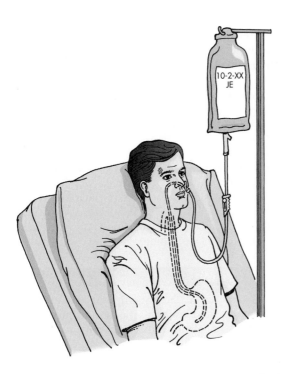

Figure 12-5 Administration of a bolus or intermittent feeding via an enteral feeding bag. (From Potter PA, Perry AG: *Fundamentals of nursing*, ed 6, St Louis, 2005, Mosby.)

Ultracal HN Plus, Pulmocare, Jevity, Boost High Nitrogen, Boost Plus, Respalor, and Magnacal, may be ordered for tube feedings.

To transcribe a tube feeding order, the HUC may have to order an **enteral feeding set,** which includes bags and tubing and/or a specific-sized nasogastric tube, formula, and a feeding infusion pump and if necessary an x-ray examination to verify placement.

Doctors' Orders for Tube Feeding

Several types of formulas and other preparations are available to meet nutritional needs for different disease states. More than 50 medical food products are available, and changes are constantly made as new knowledge is acquired. Examples of a typical doctor's order for tube feeding are provided here.

Insert nasogastric (NG) feeding tube, verify placement, and begin feeding of Isocal HN (1 cal/mL) FS @ 40 mL/hr. Progress by 10 mL/hr q2h as tolerated to final rate of 90 mL/hr
The nurse may verify tube placement by withdrawing a small amount of stomach contents or by injecting air with a syringe through the tube and listening with a stethoscope as air enters the stomach. The doctor has ordered that the prepared formula be started at full strength and the amount increased every 2 hours as tolerated to a final rate.

Tube feeding of Boost Plus (1.5 cal/mL) FS bolus by syringe 45 mL q6h given over 20 min. Flush tube c̄ 5 mL H₂O q2h
The doctor is ordering the formula to be given full strength by bolus with the use of a syringe every 6 hours and to be given over 20 minutes. The nurse will flush the tube with water as ordered.

Magnacal FS @ 40 mL/hr through gastrostomy tube. Insert jejunostomy tube. Chest x-ray for placement. When in proper position, begin via pump to deliver 2 cal/mL @ 30 mL/hr for 8 hr, then 40 mL/hr for 8 hr, then increase to final rate of 50 mL/hr
In this order for tube feedings, the doctor is requesting a chest x-ray examination to determine correct placement of the tube before formula is administered. ■

Doctors' Orders: Other Dietary Orders

The following orders pertain to the patient's intake of foods and liquids but are not orders for a specific type of diet.

Force Fluids

This order is probably written in addition to the patient's dietary order. The doctor wants to encourage the patient to drink more fluids for **hydration** or rehydration purposes. The health unit coordinator would send this order to the nutritional care department so that more fluids would be included on the patient's trays.

Limit Fluids to 1000 mL per Day

This order is also written in addition to the diet order. The patient's fluid intake is to be restricted to 1000 mL per day. Restriction of fluids is usually ordered for patients who are retaining fluids (a condition known as *edema*) because of a disease process. The nutritional care department should be notified of this order, so fluids would be limited on the patient's trays; the dietitian would also become involved.

NPO

This order means the patient is to have nothing by mouth. This is usually ordered after major surgery or during a critical illness. This information is sent to the nutritional care department to update the patient's dietary record, so a tray would not be prepared for the patient.

NPO Midnight

The patient is to have nothing by mouth after midnight. This is ordered to prepare a patient for surgery, treatment, or a diagnostic procedure. The nutritional care department is notified, so a breakfast tray would not be sent to the patient in the morning. In some facilities, an order to "resume previous diet" may not be acceptable, and the physician must write or enter the complete diet order.

Sips and Chips

The patient may have only sips of water and ice chips. This order would also be sent to the nutritional care department to update the patient's dietary record.

Have Dietitian See Patient

The doctor is requesting that the registered dietitian discuss the diet with the patient or teach the patient about the diet. This order may require a phone call, in addition to sending a requisition to the nutritional care department.

Calorie Count Today and Tomorrow

This is usually ordered to document the quantities and types of food consumed by the patient for further nutritional evaluation by the dietitian. Send this information to the nutritional care department and notify the nurse who is caring for the patient. It may be required to prepare a form on which the patient's caloric intake will be recorded. ■

PARENTERAL NUTRITION

Parenteral nutrition provides nutrients to patients who are unable to receive food via the digestive tract. Nutrients, including carbohydrates, proteins, fats, water, electrolytes, vitamins, and minerals, are prepared by the pharmacist under sterile conditions, and not by the dietary department. **Total parenteral nutrition (TPN)** is the provision of all necessary nutrients via veins (discussed in detail in Chapter 13). **Partial parenteral nutrition (PPN)** contains some essential nutrients injected into a vein to supplement other means of nutrition, usually a partially normal diet of food. **Intravenous hyperalimentation** is the administration of nutrients by intravenous feeding, especially to individuals unable to take in food through the alimentary tract. Changes in TPN orders need to be sent to the pharmacy as soon as possible, as TPN is very expensive and is customized for each patient; if a formula is prepared before the changes are received, the already prepared formula must be discarded. TPN is administered through *central* or *peripheral venous catheters* depending on the type of solution.

The complex composition of a TPN solution requires a written doctor's order (usually preprinted with details that are filled in by the physician). Printed or written orders are still required in many facilities even if CPOE is used for the majority of other orders. Parenteral nutrition is discussed in more detail in Chapter 13 (Medications).

KEY CONCEPTS

Accuracy is essential in the transcription of dietary orders because an error could result in serious consequences. Imagine, for example, a patient who is NPO for surgery receiving breakfast, or a severely diabetic patient receiving a regular diet.

Hospitalized patients are dependent on hospital personnel to meet their dietary preferences and needs. The diet ordered by the doctor for the patient may be an integral part of the treatment plan, or it may be ordered to maintain health. In either case, mealtime is an important time for many patients, and for some it may be the most positive experience of the day. The HUC is responsible for ordering late trays when a patient has missed a meal because of a test or procedure. It is important that the tray be ordered and delivered to the patient promptly. The nutritional care and nursing departments must work closely together to provide the patient with proper and pleasant meals. Thorough and prompt communication by the HUC facilitates this tremendously.

Websites of Interest

Health-Diets.net—Health and nutrition advice and resources:
   www.health-diets.net
WebMD—"Vegetarian and Vegan Diet": www.webmd.com/diet/
   guide/vegetarian-and-vegan-diet
Judaism 101—Kosher dietary laws:
   www.jewfaq.org/kashrut.htm
The Food Allergy and Anaphylaxis Network:
   www.foodallergy.org

 REVIEW QUESTIONS

*Visit the Evolve website to download and complete the following
questions.*

1. Define the following terms:
   a. calorie
   b. dehydration
   c. gastritis
   d. hydration
   e. gastrostomy
   f. Kosher
   g. ingest or ingestion
   h. dysphagia
   i. morbid obesity
   j. jejunostomy
   k. duodenostomy
   l. obese or obesity
   m. gavage

2. Rewrite the following doctors' orders using symbols and/
   or abbreviations. Or, to practice writing doctors' orders,
   have someone read the orders while you record them.
   Practice using symbols and abbreviations.
   a. nothing by mouth after midnight
   b. clear liquid breakfast, then nothing by mouth
   c. 1000-calorie American Diabetes Association diet
   d. low-cholesterol diet
   e. diet as tolerated
   f. regular diet
   g. low-sodium diet
   h. no salt added

3. Discuss the methods that may be used to order a late tray
   for a patient.

4. List two eating disorders and other factors that a doctor
   would need to consider when ordering a hospitalized
   patient's diet.

5. Explain the importance of communicating diet changes and
   patient food allergies to the nutritional care department.

6. Explain the possible consequences of a true food allergy.

7. List three groups of diets that may be ordered for a hospitalized patient.

8. List five consistency changes that can be made to a standard diet, and explain what is included in each.

9. List four diet options that may be selected for a patient
   who has started on a clear liquid diet and has an order
   for "diet as tolerated," and explain how the selection
   would be made.

10. Explain why a doctor's order for DAT requires the HUC
    to ask the nurse what diet to order from the nutritional
    care department.

11. List two diets that may be requested by patients.

12. List four therapeutic diets that the doctor may order.

13. Discuss the reasons a patient would require a tube
    feeding, and list three methods of administering tube
    feedings.

14. List three items that the HUC may have to order for a
    tube feeding.

15. Explain why a doctor would write the following orders:
    a. force fluids
    b. calorie count

16. List two reasons why a doctor would order the patient
    NPO MN.

17. Would a doctor's order *2.5 g Na* change a patient's previ-
    ous order for a soft diet?

18. Would a doctor's order *limit fluids to 1200 mL/day* change
    a patient's previous order for a regular diet?

19. Would an order for a patient to have sips and chips need
    to be sent to dietary?

20. Discuss the importance of sending all doctors' orders
    regarding a patient's diet or modifications to a diet to the
    nutritional care department.

21. Explain the importance of sending TPN orders to the
    pharmacy in a timely manner.

SURFING FOR ANSWERS

1. Research the eight most common food allergies. List them,
   and identify the website used.
2. Research and document the number of deaths caused by
   anaphylactic reactions to foods annually, and identify the
   website used.
3. Locate and document the importance of diet in diabetes,
   and identify the website used.

Medication Orders

CHAPTER OBJECTIVES

On completion of this chapter, you will be able to:

1. Define the terms in the vocabulary list.
2. Write the meaning of the abbreviations in the abbreviations list.
3. Identify at least four causes of medication errors, and explain how the use of computer physician order entry (CPOE) with clinical decision support systems (CDSS) decreases the risk of errors.
4. Compare the health unit coordinator (HUC) roles regarding medication orders with and without electronic medical records (EMRs) with CPOE.
5. Discuss two types of medicine carts and their use, and identify two medications that would be found in the medication stock supply.

6. Discuss the use of the medication administration record (MAR) when EMRs are used and when paper charts are used.
7. List the five components of a medication order.
8. List at least four routes by which medications may be administered.
9. Describe the general purpose for provided drug groups.
10. Identify four categories of medications that are controlled substances.
11. Explain the importance of notifying the pharmacy of changes or pending changes to a patient's total parenteral nutrition (TPN) orders.
12. Define standing, prn, one-time, short-series, and stat medication orders.
13. Name three common skin tests performed, and explain the purpose of each.

14. Discuss how medications are renewed, discontinued, and changed when the EMR is used and when paper charts are used.

VOCABULARY

Admixture The result of adding a medication to a bag of intravenous solution.

Adverse Drug Events (ADEs) Injuries or harmful reactions that result from the use of a drug.

Bolus Concentrated dose of medication or fluid, frequently given intravenously (may also be referred to as a loading dose).

Computerized Medication Cart Storage cart that requires confidential user ID and a password to gain access to medications (e.g., Pyxis MedStation).

Drug Enforcement Administration (DEA) A U.S. Department of Justice law enforcement agency tasked with suppressing the sale of recreational drugs by enforcing the Controlled Substances Act of 1970. It shares concurrent jurisdiction with the Federal Bureau of Investigation (FBI) in narcotics enforcement matters.

Food and Drug Administration (FDA) U.S. government agency whose purpose is to ensure that foods, drugs, cosmetics, and medical devices are safe and properly labeled.

Hypnotics Drugs that induce sleep.

Inhalation The act of breathing in; liquid medications are most commonly administered by the respiratory care department as part of its treatment procedures.

Injectable Medication that is given by forcing a liquid into the body by means of a needle and syringe (intraarterial, intradermal, intramuscular, intravenous, and subcutaneous).

Instillation To slowly introduce fluid into a cavity or a passage of the body to remain for a specific length of time before it is drained or withdrawn. (The purpose is to expose tissues of the area to the solution, to hot or cold, or to a drug or substance in the solution.)

Intradermal Injection Injection of a substance between the layers of the skin (used for skin tests).

Intramuscular (IM) Injection Injection of medication directly into the muscle.

Intravenous Infusion Administration of a substance directly into a vein.

Intravenous or IV Piggyback (IVPB) A method of administering a medication in 50 to 100 mL of solution through an intravenous line that is inserted into a patient's vein and given by hanging it above the level of the primary fluid bag.

Intravenous or IV Push (IVP) Method of giving concentrated doses of medication directly into the vein.

Medication Administration Record (MAR) Computerized list of medications that each individual patient is currently taking; it is used by the nurse to administer and document medications.

Narcotic Controlled drug that relieves pain or produces sleep.

Oral (PO) By mouth.

Over-the-Counter (OTC) Drugs Drugs for which a prescription is not needed. The FDA defines OTC drugs as safe and effective for use by the general public without a doctor's prescription.

Parenteral Routes Pertaining to a medication administered by a route that bypasses the gastrointestinal (GI) tract, such as a drug given by injection, or intravenously.

Patient-Controlled Analgesia (PCA) Medications administered intravenously by means of a special infusion pump controlled by the patient within order ranges written by the physician.

Rectal Instillation Medications prepared specifically for insertion into the rectum. Enemas are also instilled into the rectum.

Sedatives Agents given to reduce or relive anxiety, stress, or excitement.

Sedative-Hypnotics Agents given to induce sleep and to relieve anxiety.

Skin Tests Tests given to determine the reaction of the body to a substance injected intradermally or applied topically to the skin. Skin tests are used to detect allergens, to determine immunity, and to diagnose disease.

Subcutaneous Injection (sq or sub-q) Injection of a small amount of a medication under the skin into fatty or connective tissue.

Sublingual (subling) Under the tongue.

Suppository Medicated substance mixed in a solid base that melts when placed in a body opening; suppositories are commonly used in the rectum, vagina, or urethra.

Topical Direct application of medication to the skin, eye, ear, or other parts of the body.

Unit Dose Medicine Cart Cart that contains "unit doses" in separate drawers or bins specifically labeled for each patient as ordered by the doctor(s).

ABBREVIATIONS

Abbreviation	Meaning	Example of Usage on a Doctor's Order Sheet
ADE	adverse drug event	[ADEs are common and costly]
ASA	acetylsalicylic acid or aspirin	ASA 81 mg PO q day
BCOC or LOC	bowel care of choice or laxative of choice	BCOC as per patient request LOC as per patient request
BS	bedside	NTG 0.4 mg subling prn, keep @ BS
cc (same as "mL" and may not be allowed in some facilities, as it may be confused with "U" or "u" if poorly written)	cubic centimeters	MOM 30cc po prn
G, gm, or g	gram	cefadroxil 1 g IVPB q6h
gr	grain	chloral hydrate gr XV PO hs prn
HA or H/A	headache	Tylenol 650 mg prn H/A
IM	intramuscular	vitamin B_{12} 1000 mcg deep IM tomorrow
IV	intravenous	D/C IV if infiltrates

Abbreviation	Meaning	Example of Usage on a Doctor's Order Sheet
IVP	intravenous push	theophylline 5 mg/kg IVP now
IVPB	intravenous or IV piggyback	cephalothin 0.5 g IVPB q8h
KCl	potassium chloride	Add 40 mEq KCl to each IV
L	liter	1 L 5% D/W to run @ 125 mL/hr
mcg	microgram	vitamin B$_{12}$ 1000 mcg IM
mEq	milliequivalent	Give 20 mEq KCl per open heart protocol
mg	milligram	ciprofloxacin 250 mg PO q12°
mL or ml	milliliter (same as cubic centimeter)	1000 mL 5% D/W @ KO rate
noc	night	Ambien 10 mg po q noc
NTG	nitroglycerin	NTG 0.4 mg subling for heart pain prn
OTC	over-the-counter	The patient was not taking any OTC medications
oz	ounce	Add 8 oz of juice to Metamucil packet
PCA	patient-controlled analgesia	PCA morphine sulfate 2 mg q15 min
PCN	penicillin	PCN 250 mg PO q 6 hr
PO or po	*per os* (by mouth)	lorazepam 2 mg PO tid
Pr or R	*per rectum*	bisacodyl supp 10 mg pr now
prn	*pro re nata* (as needed)	Maalox 30 mL prn GI discomfort
sq, or sub-q	subcutaneous	heparin 5000 unit sub-q daily
subling, sl	sublingual (under tongue)	nitroglycerin tab sl prn anginal pain

Abbreviation	Meaning	Example of Usage on a Doctor's Order Sheet
supp	suppository	acetaminophen supp prn for temp ↑ 100°(R)
syr	syrup	ipecac syr 15 mL now
tinct or tr	tincture	Apply tinct of benzoin around operative site before applying tape

See Table 10-1 for a list of incorrect and correct abbreviations, as approved by The Joint Commission (TJC). Some hospitals have additional abbreviations to avoid using, such as those listed in Table 13-1.

⭐ **HIGH PRIORITY**

The use of electronic medical records (EMRs) and e-prescribing greatly reduces confusion and medication errors involving medical abbreviations.

⊜ EXERCISE 1

Write the abbreviation for each term listed.

1. aspirin
2. liter
3. adverse drug event
4. milligram
5. potassium chloride
6. penicillin
7. gram
8. milliliter
9. milliequivalent
10. grain
11. sublingual
12. tincture
13. by mouth
14. ounce
15. ampoule
16. suppository
17. subcutaneous
18. microgram
19. night
20. syrup
21. intravenous piggyback
22. per rectum
23. patient-controlled analgesia
24. intravenous push
25. laxative of choice
26. pro re nata (*as needed*)
27. over-the-counter
28. intravenous
29. bowel care of choice
30. nitroglycerin
31. bedside
32. cubic centimeters
33. headache

TABLE 13-1 A Hospital's List of Additional Abbreviations to Avoid

Abbreviation	Potential Problem	Preferred Term
IM	Because of poor writing, often misinterpreted as "IV," causing the medication to be given via the wrong route	Write out "intramuscular"
D/C	Patient's medications may be prematurely discontinued when D/C means "discharge" and is followed by a list of medications	Write out "discontinue"
HS	May be misinterpreted as "hour of sleep" when written as meaning "half-strength"	Write out "half-strength"
IVP	When written to mean "intravenous push," may be mistaken for "intravenous piggyback" (IVPB)	Write out "intravenous push"
S/C or S/Q	When poorly written, often mistaken for "SL" (sublingual)	Write out "subcutaneous"
Slash mark: /	Misunderstood as the number "1" rather than the intended meaning "per"	Write out "per"

⊜ E X E R C I S E 2

Write the meaning of each abbreviation listed.

1. KCl
2. ADE
3. amp
4. syr
5. noc
6. ASA
7. mcg
8. oz
9. sq, or sub-q
10. mEq
11. PCN
12. mL
13. PO
14. tinct
15. gr
16. mg
17. supp
18. G, gm, or g
19. L
20. subling, sl
21. IVPB
22. PCA
23. pr, p
24. prn
25. LOC
26. IVP
27. OTC
28. IV
29. BCOC
30. NTG
31. BS
32. cc
33. HA, H/A

COMPUTER PHYSICIAN ORDER ENTRY AND CLINICAL DECISION SUPPORT SYSTEM

Adverse drug events (ADEs) result in more than 770,000 injuries and deaths each year and cost up to $5.6 million per hospital, depending on size. Illegible doctors' handwriting and transcription errors are responsible for as much as 61% of the medication errors. Medication errors may involve the wrong drug or the incorrect dose. Errors can go undetected unless there is an adverse event. A simple mistake such as putting the decimal point in the wrong place can have serious consequences because a patient's dose could be 10 times the recommended amount. Drugs with similar names are also a common cause of error, such as *quinine* (used to treat malaria) and *quinidine* (used to normalize the heartbeat in people with certain heart rhythm disorders) or *Zyrtec* (used to treat allergies) and *Zyprexa* (used to treat schizophrenia and bipolar disorder). Other ADEs occur as a result of administration mistakes, including the wrong frequency or time, or the incorrect route, or medication not administered at all.

U.S. hospitals that have switched to computer physician order entry (CPOE) systems have experienced a 66% drop in prescription errors according to a new review of studies. When CPOE is used, the doctor enters orders directly into the patient's electronic medical record (EMR) via computer, and the orders are automatically sent to the pharmacy, reducing the risk of errors in interpreting doctors' handwriting. E-prescribing is the process of sending a medication order or prescription from the prescriber's computer to the pharmacy computer. The clinical decision support system (CDSS) provides the doctor with prompts that warn against the possibility of drug interaction, allergy, or overdose at the point of order entry.

Health Unit Coordinator Role Regarding Medication Orders with and without an Electronic Medical Record with Computer Physician Order Entry

Health unit coordinators (HUCs) working in hospitals that have implemented an EMR system with CPOE no longer have the responsibility of interpreting doctors' handwritten medication orders. It is, however, beneficial that the HUC recognize medication orders. The HUC will still have some responsibilities involving medications, such as ordering stock medications for the nursing unit and printing required computerized medication pamphlets prior to a patient's discharge. The HUC may also be required to include some types of medications on requisitions (such as anticonvulsants for a neurodiagnostics test). The goal is for all hospitals to have EMR with CPOE in 2014, but as of 2012 most hospitals do not have electronic prescription systems (stand-alone or as part of an EMR program) in use. Electronic prescription systems are costly and difficult to integrate into the sometimes chaotic hospital structure. The HUC is still transcribing medication orders in many hospitals. Transcription of medication orders will vary among hospitals and may involve writing ordered medications on the patient's paper medication administration record (MAR) or entering medications into the patient's computerized MAR. (Review transcription of medication orders in Chapter 9.)

★ HIGH PRIORITY

Until all hospitals have implemented the electronic medical record (EMR) with computer physician order entry (CPOE), medication orders will be included in this text.

ADMINISTRATION OF MEDICATION

Medication Carts

Medications are usually stored in a medicine cart that is prepared by the pharmacy and sent to the units daily. Use of medication carts reduces the risk of mislabeled medications, ensuring that regulations of the **Food and Drug Administration (FDA)** are met. Two types of medication carts are used. One is a **unit dose medicine cart** that contains "unit doses" in separate drawers or bins specifically labeled for each patient as ordered by the doctor(s). The pharmacist fills these orders by reading the computerized orders written by the physician, or by reading a hard or faxed copy of the physician's orders. The unit dose medication cart can be wheeled to the patient's bedside for administration of the medication (Fig. 13-1). The second type is a **computerized medication cart** such as a Pyxis that requires the nurse to enter a confidential user identification (ID) and password to unlock the cart. The nurse always verifies the name of the medication, the dose, and the patient's name before removing the medication. The computerized medication carts remain in the medication room and are not taken from room to room. Some hospitals lock intravenous (IV) solutions in a storage cabinet that is located next to the computerized medication cart, and both can be opened only when a nurse enters an assigned code (Fig. 13-2). All medications and/or IV solutions that are removed can be tracked on the computer by the code entered at the time of removal. When a computerized medication cart is used, the pharmacist enters the instructions for each patient's medications into the cart (usually for a 24-hour period).

A registered nurse or a licensed practical nurse who is caring for a number of specific patients will administer medications to those patients. Alternatively, a registered nurse or a licensed practical nurse may be assigned to serve as the "med

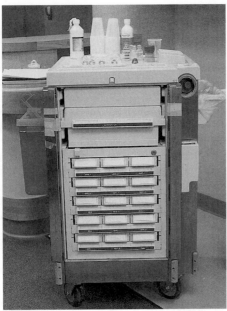

Figure 13-1 Medication cart. (From Lilley LL, Aucker RS: *Pharmacology and the nursing process*, ed 3, St Louis, 2001, Mosby.)

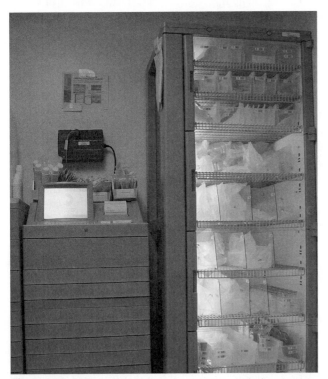

Figure 13-2 Computerized medication cart, including intravenous solutions.

nurse" and will administer medications to all patients on the nursing unit.

Medication Stock Supply

Hospitals store a supply of medications on nursing units, often in the computerized medication cart. This supply is often called the *medication stock supply*, and it includes many over-the-counter (OTC) drugs such as aspirin, acetaminophen, mineral oil, and milk of magnesia. When floor stock medicines are ordered from the pharmacy, they are charged to the unit budget.

The Medication Administration Record

The **medication administration record (MAR)**, as described in Chapter 8, is a form on which nursing personnel record all medications given to the patient; it is a permanent part of the patient's chart (electronic or paper). Nurses use the MAR as a reference while preparing medications for administration (if medication carts are not used) and while administering medications. The nurse signs the MAR electronically (when the EMR is used) or manually (when paper charts are used) at the bottom of the form at the end of each shift to indicate that the patient received the medications as charted or did not receive any medications if none were ordered. Currently, three methods of completing MARs are used.

If the EMR is implemented in the facility, the medications are entered on the MAR when the doctor writes the order, and the registered or licensed practical nurse enters the time at which the medications are administered into each patient's computerized MAR. The electronic MAR is a permanent part of the patient's EMR.

If the EMR is not being used, the pharmacy prepares a printed medication record for each patient, which is sent to the nursing unit each morning. The registered nurse or the HUC adds to the MAR any new medications ordered, along with any changes to medication orders made during the day. The pharmacist, after having received the faxed physician orders, makes those changes, and the printed MAR sent the next morning reflects those changes. When the patient is discharged, the printed MARs become a permanent part of the patient's chart.

A handwritten MAR is used when CPOE or the printed MAR initiated by the pharmacy has not been implemented. Transcribing of medication orders may require the HUC to write the order on the MAR. In some hospitals, nurses are responsible for writing their assigned patients' medication orders on the MAR. Accuracy in copying the medication order from the physician's order sheet onto the MAR is absolutely essential. The HUC initiates the record on the patient's admission. The record varies in the number of days (3 to 10 days) that medications may be entered. When the last date of the dated period on the MAR has been reached, a new record with new dates is prepared, and all medications still in use are copied onto the new form. Handwritten MARs are also a permanent part of the patient's chart. The MAR is a legal document, so entries are required to be written in ink (usually black) (Fig. 13-3). To discontinue medications on the MAR, indicate "DC" on the correct day and time, and draw a line through the days the medication will not be given. A yellow or pink highlight is usually drawn over the medication entry that is discontinued (see Fig. 13-3, *A*).

RECOGNIZING MEDICATION ORDERS

Five Components of a Medication Order

Each medication order is written with specific components that include directions for the person who is giving the drug.

Part A

Date / Exp.	MEDICATION ADMINISTRATION RECORD SCHEDULED: A	24 01 02 03	04 05 06 07	08 09 10 11	12 13 14 15	16 17 18 19	20 21 22 23	RN ✓	Date 6/10/XX 23	07	15	Date 6/11 23	07	15	Date 6/12 23	07	15	Injection Code
6/10	atorvastatin 40 mg P.O. qd						zz				NN			NN				**RU:** RUQ
6/10	ezetimibe 10 mg P.O. qd						zz				NN							**LU:** LUQ
6/10 / 6/13	zolpidem 30 mg P.O. qH.S						zz				NN	DC						**LA:** Left Arm
6/10	Coreg 25 mg P.O. qd		09						NN			NN						**RA:** Right Arm

RT: Right Thigh
OU: Both Eyes
ABD: Abdomen
OD: Right Eye
OS: Left Eye

LT: Left Thigh

IV MEDS

Allergies **PCN - ALL DAIRY PRODUCTS**
Diagnosis _MVA- Diabetes - CAD_ Age _67_
Name _Williams, John_ MD _Hy Hopes_

Recopy Check

A

Part B

PATIENT _Williams, John_ ALLERGIES **PCN- DAIRY PRODUCTS**

Date / Exp.	MEDICATION ADMINISTRATION RECORD PRN-ONE TIME & STAT: B	RN ✓	Date 6/10/XX 23	07	15	Date 6/11 23	07	15	Date 6/12 23	07	15
	temezepam; P.O. HS PRN										

PRN

ONE-TIME

B

Figure 13-3 A, Medication administration record (side A) shows a method of discontinuing a standing medication. **B,** Medication administration record (side B).

These may be written in slightly different order, but the components remain the same.

For example:

Tylenol   325 mg   PO   q4h   prn for pain
1   2   3   4   5

The numbered portions of this drug order are as follows:

1. Name of drug: Tylenol
2. Dose of drug (amount): 325 mg
3. Route of administration: PO (by mouth)
4. Time of administration (frequency): q4h (every 4 hours)
5. Qualifying phrase: prn (as needed) for pain

Component 1: Name

- *Generic name*—a generic drug is the same as a brand name drug in dosage, safety, strength, how it is taken, quality performance, and intended use. Generic names are not capitalized.
- *Brand name*—the general public usually knows the drug best by this name. The brand name is always capitalized. A trademark symbol (™ or ®) is usually stamped on the medication.

Component 2: Dosage

The dosage is the prescribed amount of medication to be taken, written in metric or apothecary system methods of weights and measures.

Note: The apothecary system is becoming obsolete.

Component 3: Route

The route of administration should always be included in a medication order; however, when in doubt, the route of administration should always be clarified. The following list contains the routes most frequently used in medication administration, with an example of each.

- **Oral (PO):** By mouth.
- **Sublingual** (subling): Under the tongue.
- **Inhalation:** Liquid medications are most commonly administered by the respiratory care department as part of its treatment procedure.

- **Instillation:** Administration of medication by spray, pump bottle, or dropper (as in eye or nose).
- **Rectal instillation**: Insertion into the rectum; for example, a **suppository,** a medicated substance mixed in a solid base that melts when placed in a body.
- **Topical:** Applied to skin or mucous membrane. Medications in this category may be available in the form of lotions, liniments, ointments, powders, sprays, solutions, suppositories, or transdermal preparations.
- **Parenteral routes** fluids or medications that are given by injection or intravenously (Fig. 13-4).
  - **Intradermal injection:** Injection between two skin layers. These injections are given principally for diagnostic testing.
  - **Subcutaneous injection (Sq or sub-q):** The medication is injected with a syringe under the skin into the fat or connective tissue.
  - **Intramuscular (IM) injection:** The medication is injected directly into the muscle.
  - **Intravenous or IV push (IVP):** A method of infusing a concentrated dose of medication over 1 to 5 minutes. This may also be referred to as a **bolus** *or a loading dose.*
  - **Intravenous or IV piggyback (IVPB):** A method of intermittent infusion of medication that has been diluted in 50 to 100 mL of a commercially prepared solution and is infused over 30 to 60 minutes through an established IV line. An IVPB may also be administered by using an IV access called a *saline lock* or *heparin lock* that is inserted into a vein and then capped off. This allows periodic access to the vein for medication administration. An IVPB may be attached to the saline lock every few hours and then disconnected once the medication has infused. The medication concentration in the IVPB is lower than the medication concentration in the IV push and is administered over a longer time (Fig. 13-5). Medication may also be included in an **admixture** added directly into a bag of IV solution.
  - **Volume control administration device:** Another method of infusing IV medications through 5 to 10 mL of compatible IV fluids. The fluid is placed within a secondary fluid container separate from the primary fluid bag (see the Evolve website).
  - **Heparin or Saline lock:** A device used for intermittent **intravenous infusion** of medication, also used to

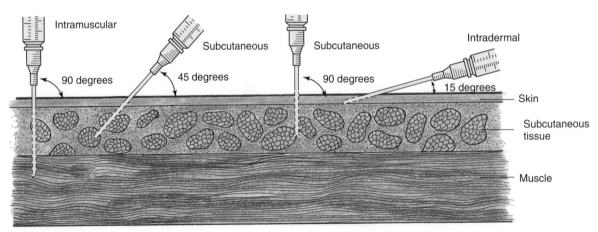

Figure 13-4 Angle of needle insertion for parenteral injections. (From Potter PA, Perry AG: *Fundamentals of nursing,* ed 6, St Louis, 2005, Mosby.)

maintain patent venous access for the infusion of medications in an emergency. A heparin or saline lock is an IV catheter with a small chamber covered by a rubber diaphragm or a specially designed cap (see Chapter 11, Fig. 11-12).

Component 4: Frequency of Administration

Each hospital maintains a schedule of hours for administration of medications. Table 13-2 lists examples of time frequencies used to administer medications, but these may vary among hospitals. Military time is usually used in place of standard time; prn orders are not assigned a time as they are given as needed by the patient.

Component 5: Qualifying Phrase

The qualifying phrase describes orders for specific conditions; prn orders require a qualifier such as the following:

> *For minor discomfort*
> *For severe pain*
> *For temp >101°*
> *For N/V*
> *For sleep if nec.*

Medication Resources

Many nurses carry a handheld device such as personal data assistant (PDA) or palm pilot with medical applications loaded on them, including a drug reference book. The *Physicians' Desk Reference* (PDR; published yearly by Medical Economics) and the *American Hospital Drug Information* (published by the

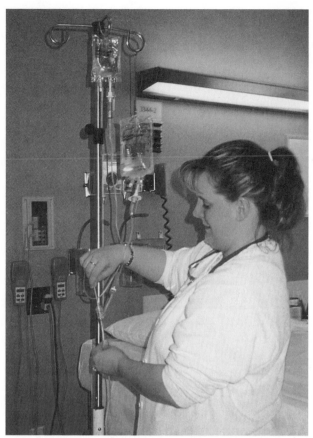

Figure 13-5 Piggyback setup. (From Potter PA, Perry AG: *Fundamentals of nursing*, ed 6, St Louis, 2005, Mosby.)

TABLE 13-2 Medication Time Schedule

Time Symbols	Meaning	Time Schedule	Military Time
q day	Once a day.	9:00 A.M.	0900
		(5:00 P.M. [daily] for anticoagulants—to allow for results of prothrombin time)	1700
		(7:30 A.M. [daily] for insulin, which must be administered before breakfast)	0730
bid	Two times a day during waking hours.	9:00 A.M. and 5:00 P.M. (9-5)	0900-1700
tid	Three times a day during waking hours.	9:00 A.M.-1:00 P.M.-5:00 P.M. (9-1-5)	0900-1300-1700
qid	Four times a day during waking hours.	9:00 A.M.-1:00 P.M.-5:00 P.M.-9:00 P.M. (9-1-5-9)	0900-1300-1700-2100
ac	One-half hour before meals. This varies according to when food cart arrives on unit.		
pc	One-half hour after meals. This varies according to when food cart arrives on unit.		
q3h	Every 3 hours.	9:00 A.M.-12:00 Noon-3:00 P.M.-6:00 P.M.-9:00 P.M.-12:00 Mid-3:00 A.M.-6:00 A.M. (9-12-3-6-9-12-3-6)	0900-1200-1500-1800-2100-2400-0300-0600
q4h	Every 4 hours.	9:00 A.M.-1:00 P.M.-5:00 P.M.-9:00 P.M.-1:00 A.M.-5:00 A.M. (9-1-5-9-1-5)	0900-1300-1700-2100-0100-0500
q6h	Every 6 hours.	9:00 A.M.-3:00 P.M.-9:00 P.M.-3:00 A.M. (9-3-9-3)	0900-1500 2100-0300
q8h	Every 8 hours.	9:00 A.M.-5:00 P.M.-1:00 A.M. (9-5-1)	0900-1700-0100
q12h	Every 12 hours.	9:00 A.M.-9:00 P.M. (9-9)	0900-2100

American Society of Hospital Pharmacists) are usually found on the nursing unit computers as well as stored on the units in hard copies.

DRUG GROUPS AND MEDICATIONS

The following drug groups and medications are frequently prescribed for hospitalized patients. There are many more groups and many more medications prescribed, and there are other uses for many of the medications than listed here.(Brand names of medications are capitalized and generic names are in parenthesis). It is beneficial for the HUC to have a basic knowledge of medications even if transcription of medications is no longer a HUC responsibility. There are some procedures that require that certain categories of medications the patient is receiving be noted during the ordering process. An example would be when ordering an arterial blood gas (ABG), it would be important to note if the patient is receiving an anticoagulant. The HUC would need to have knowledge of those categories and the medications included in those categories.

Drug Groups Commonly Used to Treat Cardiovascular Diseases and Conditions

Cardiovascular medications are used as a means to control or to prevent certain forms of heart disease. The number of cardiovascular drugs given to control or prevent certain forms of heart disease and even the number of categories are extensive. Doctors may use a combination of drugs depending on their action or what they treat. Many of these drugs also have effects on the kidneys or renal system.

Note: Specific cardiac medications, such as Lanoxin (digoxin), Cardizem (diltiazem), and Netro-Bid, Nitro-Dur, Nitrostat, Transderm-Nitro (nitroglycerin), would be noted when ordering cardiac studies such as an EKG.

Antianginals

Antianginals are used for treatment of chest pain caused by lack of blood to the heart.
Examples of Antianginals
Nitro-Bid, Nitro-Dur, Nitrostat, Nitroquick, Transderm Nitro (nitroglycerine)
Isordil (isosorbide dinitrate)

Antihypertensives

Antihypertensives are used for treatment of high blood pressure.
Examples of Antihypertensives
Aldactone (spironolactone)
Dyazide (triamterene)
Norvasc (amlodipine)
Vasotec (enalapril)
Zestril (lisinopril)

Antiarrhythmics

Antiarrhythmics are used for treatment of abnormal heart rhythms.
Examples of Antiarrhythmics
Lanoxin (digoxin)
Disopyramide, Norpace
Procainamide (procainamide hydrochloride), Procan, Procanbid, Pronestyl

Tenormin(atenolol)
Coreg (carvedilol)
Lopressor, Toprol (metoprolol)
Inderal (propranolol)
Quinidine (quinidine sulfate), Quinaglute, Quinidex, Cardioquin

HIGH PRIORITY

Emergency Antiarrhythmics
Antiarrhythmics that may be ordered stat for a patient in a cardiac emergency include amiodarone, bretylium, and lidocaine. These medications would be ordered and transcribed as a stat, one-time order, or they might be included under the emergency standing orders for a patient. An example of this type of order follows:
Amiodarone 300 mg IV push now. May repeat once at 150 mg in 3-5 min.

Diuretics

Diuretics are used for treatment of hypertension (high blood pressure). They induce urination, resulting in a decrease in pressure demand on the heart.
Examples of Diuretics
HydroDIURIL (hydrochlorothiazide)
Lasix (furosemide)

Potassium Replacements

Potassium replacements are used for treatment of low potassium levels.
Examples of Potassium Replacements
Potassium Chloride - Kaochlor, K-Lor, K-Lyte, Micro-K, Slow-K

Antiplatelet Drugs

Antiplatelet drugs reduce the ability of platelets to stick together, preventing the formation of blood clots in arteries.
Examples of Antiplatelet Drugs
Plavix (clopidogrel)
Aspirin (acetylsalicylic acid)
Aggrenox (dipyridamole plus aspirin)
Ticlopidine, Ticlid

Anticoagulants

Anticoagulants thin the blood and prevent clots from forming in the blood.

- Laboratory tests are ordered for patients taking anticoagulants (see Chapter 14).
- When ordering an invasive procedure such as an arterial blood gas (ABG) (see Chapter 16), it should be noted on the requisition that the patient is receiving an anticoagulant.

Examples of Anticoagulants
Coumadin (warfarin)
Heparin
Lovenox (enoxaparin sodium injection)
Innohep (tinzaparin)

Antihyperlipidemic Agents

Antihyperlipidemic agents are used for treatment of high cholesterol; they promote a reduction of lipid levels in the blood.

- Periodic liver function tests are ordered for patients taking antihyperlipidemic agents.

Examples of Antihyperlipidemic Agents
Lipitor (atorvastatin)
Vytorin (ezetimibe and simvastatin)
Crestor (rosuvastatin)
Zetia (ezetimibe)

Drugs Prescribed to Treat Infections
Antibiotics

The word *antibiotics* comes from the Greek *anti* ("against") and *bios* ("life"). An antibiotic is a drug that kills or slows the growth of bacteria. Antibiotics are one class of antimicrobials, a larger group that also includes antiviral, antifungal, and antiparasitic drugs. Antibiotics are often chemicals produced by or derived from microorganisms (i.e., bacteria and fungi.) Antibiotics are used to treat many different bacterial infections and work by killing or injuring bacteria. For the doctor to order the "right drug for the right bug"—to give the patient the best treatment possible—a culture of the eye, ear, nose, throat, or wound is obtained, or blood cultures often are drawn before antibiotic therapy is initiated. (*Note:* Many antibiotic names end in *-cillin*, *-oxacin*, or *-mycin*; this makes identification easier.)

- When ordering a blood culture, it is important to note on the requisition that the patient is taking an antibiotic. Note: Viral infections are treated with antiviral medications; yeast and fungal infections are treated with antifungal medications.

Examples of Antibiotics
Peni*cillin* (penicillin V, penicillin G, amoxi*cillin*, ampi*cillin*)
Erythro*mycin*
Vanco*mycin*
Tetracycline
Cipro (ciprofl*oxacin* hydrochloride)
Bacitracin
Tobra*mycin*
Trimox (amoxi*cillin*)
Zithromax (azithro*mycin*)
Keflex (cephalexin)
Augmentin (amoxi*cillin* and clavulanate)
Levaquin (levofl*oxacin*)
Veetids (peni*cillin*)

Drugs Administered to Treat Respiratory Disorders
Respiratory Drugs

Respiratory drugs are used to treat respiratory disorders, or lung diseases, such as asthma, bronchitis, pneumonia, and tuberculosis. There are many groups of drugs that treat respiratory disorders including bronchodilators, corticosteroid inhalers, leukotriene receptor antagonists, antihistamines, and antitussives.

Examples of Respiratory Drugs
Bronchodilator and corticosteroid inhalers, discussed in Chapter 17
Slo-Bid, Slo-Phyllin, Theobid, Theo-Dur, Theo-Dur Sprinkle (theophylline)
Singulair
Prednisone
Doxapram (doxapram hydrochloride)

Drugs Prescribed to Treat Convulsions
Anticonvulsants

Anticonvulsants are drugs used to prevent or reduce the severity and frequency of seizures (convulsions). Convulsions are involuntary spasms that cause a person's body to shake rapidly and uncontrollably. During convulsions, the person's muscles contract and relax repeatedly. A seizure is often referred to as a *convulsion*, although there are several types of seizures, some that have subtle or mild symptoms instead of convulsions. Seizures of all types are caused by disorganized and sudden electrical activity in the brain. When ordering a neurologic procedure such as an electroencephalogram (EEG), it is important to note that the patient is taking an anticonvulsant.

Examples of Anticonvulsants
Carbamazepine -CBZ
Neurontin (gabapentin)
Depakote (valproate)
Tegretol (carbamazepine)
Lamictal (lamotrigine)
Topamax (topiramate)

Drugs Used to Treat Diabetes

Antidiabetics (insulin and oral) are given to lower blood sugar. Diabetes mellitus, often referred to as *diabetes*, is a group of metabolic diseases in which a person has high blood sugar because the body does not produce enough insulin or because cells do not respond to the insulin that is produced.

Types of Insulin

Several types of insulin are available and are grouped according to how fast they work: rapid acting, short acting, intermediate acting and long acting.

Examples of Insulin
NPH (neutral protamine Hagedorn) — also known as Humulin N, Novolin N, Novolin NPH, NPH Iletin II insulin, and (isophane insulin)
Lente insulin
Novolin R
Humulin R
Lantus

A *standing order for insulin* is an order in which insulin is usually scheduled to be given ½ hour (ac) before breakfast. If the doctor is normalizing the amount of insulin required by the patient, the doctor may order insulin to be given on a sliding scale.

A *sliding scale insulin order* contains a set of instructions for administering insulin doses based on specific blood glucose readings. This insulin may be given in addition to the daily insulin as ordered and prescribed by the doctor.

Example of a Sliding Scale Insulin Order (Using Blood Glucose Monitoring)

Blood Sugar Level	Dosage or Action
200-249	5 Units of regular insulin
250-299	10 Units of regular insulin
300-349	15 Units of regular insulin
Over 350	Call the doctor

Not all diabetic patients have sliding scale orders or take insulin. Many diabetic patients control their illness through diet and exercise or use an oral medication to assist in controlling their blood glucose levels.

Examples of Oral Antidiabetic Drugs

Glucophage (metformin)
Diabinese (chlorpropamide)
Glucotrol, Glucotrol XL (glipizide)
Micronase, Glynase, Diabeta (glyburide)
Amaryl (glimepiride)
Actos (pioglitazone)

Medications Prescribed to Relieve Pain

Analgesics

An analgesic is either a nonnarcotic or a **narcotic** and is given to reduce pain. Pain can be sharp or dull, burning or numbing, minor or major, acute or chronic. Medications may stop the transmission of pain from the site of injury or may affect the brain directly. The effects of pain medication are different for different people, and the tolerance of pain varies greatly from one person to another. The right pain medication depends on the person experiencing the pain, not on the condition that is causing the pain.

Examples of Nonnarcotic Analgesics

Tylenol (acetaminophen)
Aspirin, Ascription (acetylsalicylic acid)
Ansaid (flurbiprofen)
Advil, Motrin (ibuprofen)
Anaprox (naproxen)

Examples of Narcotic Analgesics. Narcotics are controlled substances (Box 13-1, *Controlled Substances*).

Tylenol #1, #2, #3, or #4 (acetaminophen with codeine)
Lortab, Vicodin, (hydrocodone with acetaminophen)
Demerol (meperidine)
Roxanol (morphine sulfate)
OxyFast, OxyContin (oxycodone)

CODEINE IS A CONTROLLED SUBSTANCE

Numbers that are assigned to analgesics that contain codeine differentiate the amount of codeine found in the medications. The numbers represent the following:

#1 contains gr ⅛ (8 mg) codeine
#2 contains gr ¼ (15 mg) codeine
#3 contains gr ½ (30 mg) codeine
#4 contains gr 1 (60 mg) codeine

Patient-Controlled Analgesia

Patient-controlled analgesia (PCA) allows the patient to self-administer small doses of narcotics intravenously. A special IV infusion pump is used. The physician orders the number of

---

BOX 13-1	CONTROLLED SUBSTANCES

The federal government has categorized a class of medication as having a higher-than-average potential for abuse or addiction. Such medications, known as *controlled substances*, are divided into categories based on their potential for abuse or addiction. They range from illegal street drugs (Schedule I, or C-I) to medications with decreasing potential for abuse (C-II through C-V). Prescriptions containing narcotics or amphetamines are often classified as C-II because they have a relatively high potential for abuse or addiction.

The **Drug Enforcement Administration (DEA)** has a registration system in place by which medical professionals, researchers, and manufacturers are authorized to have access to Schedule I drugs, as well as Schedule II, III, IV, and V drugs. Authorized registrants apply for and, if authorization is granted, receive a DEA number. An entity that has been issued a DEA number is authorized to manufacture (drug companies), distribute, research, prescribe (doctors, nurse practitioners, physician assistants as state law allows) or dispense (pharmacy) a controlled substance.

Narcotics, analgesics with narcotics, hypnotics, and sedatives (tranquillizers) are controlled substances.

---

individual doses, the frequency of delivery, and the total dose permitted within certain time periods, called *lockout intervals*. The nurse receives the narcotic from the pharmacy in a syringe form or in a small cassette that fits into the PCA (Fig. 13-6).

An internal system within the PCA unit is programmed and does not permit the patient to overdose or self-administer the medication too frequently. The most common narcotics used in PCA systems are meperidine and morphine. Some conditions with which PCA is used include severe postoperative pain and the chronic pain of a terminal illness.

Medications Prescribed to Cause Relaxation and/or Induce Sleep

Sedatives or Tranquillizers

Sedatives or tranquilizers are drugs that cause relaxation and reduce restlessness without causing sleep. A sedative given in higher doses also may be called a *hypnotic*.

Examples of Sedatives or Tranquilizers

Valium (diazepam)
ProSom (estazolam)
Ativan (lorazepam)
Xanax (alprazolam)

Hypnotics

Hypnotics are stronger than sedatives and are commonly used to induce sleep. Drugs also may be classified as **sedative-hypnotics**, prescribed to relieve anxiety and induce sleep. In elderly patients they may cause dizziness, confusion, and ataxia. Drugs in this group have a high potential for abuse that often results in physical and psychologic dependence.

Examples of Sedative-Hypnotics. Sedative-hypnotics are controlled substances.

ProSom (estazolam)	Restoril (temazepam)
Dalmane (flurazepam)	Ambien (zolpidem)

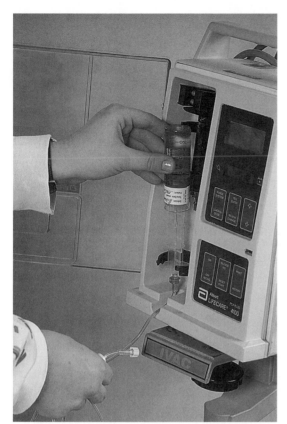

Figure 13-6 Patient-controlled analgesia (PCA) pump with syringe chamber. (From Potter PA, Perry AG: *Fundamentals of nursing,* ed 6, St Louis, 2005, Mosby.)

Medications Prescribed to Relieve Vomiting and Nausea

Antiemetics

Antiemetics are drugs that are effective against vomiting and nausea.

Examples of Antiemetics

Phenergan (promethazine hydrochloride)
Lorazepam (Ativan)
Xanax (Alprazolam)
Compazine (prochlorperazine)
Reglan (metoclopramide hydrochloride)

PARENTERAL NUTRITION

Total parenteral nutrition (TPN), partial parenteral nutrition (PPN), and *intravenous hyperalimentation* are orders written in order to provide nutrients to patients who are unable to receive food via the digestive tract (as discussed in Chapter 12). TPN is given when a patient requires an extended period of intensive nutritional support. It is usually administered through a central venous catheter. Some common types of long-term central venous catheters are Hickman, Broviac, Groshong, and Port-a-Cath. The type of catheter used is dependent on the length of treatment. Insertion of a central catheter requires informed consent; the catheter is surgically inserted under local anesthesia and sterile conditions. TPN solutions contain high concentrations of proteins and dextrose. Various components such as electrolytes, minerals,

trace elements, and insulin are added based on the needs of the patient. TPN provides the calories a patient requires and keeps the body from using protein for energy. Composition of TPN solution is complex and requires a written doctor's order; the solution is prepared by the pharmacist under sterile conditions using a laminar flow hood. The solution is kept refrigerated until 30 to 40 minutes before the time of infusion. The infusion rate is controlled by an infusion pump (see Chapter 11, Fig. 11-13).

The order for TPN is a preprinted form that is filled in by the doctor (Fig. 13-7). This form takes the place of the regular doctor's order form, and a copy is sent to the pharmacy. Because of the length and complexity of the TPN order, many hospitals transcribe only the date and TPN with rate and check the chart on the MAR. When the TPN solution is delivered from the pharmacy, the registered nurse checks it against the doctor's order on the preprinted form. Often the doctor uses the regular doctors' order form to make small changes in the composition of the original order. The original order on the MAR must be discontinued and the changed order rewritten. Some diseases that require TPN intervention are ileitis, bowel obstruction, massive burns, and severe anorexia. Patients who receive TPN require frequent (daily) blood tests for electrolyte and lipid levels (these laboratory tests are explained in Chapter 14).

> ⭐ **HIGH PRIORITY**
>
> The pharmacy should be notified immediately of any changes or pending changes to a patient's total parenteral nutrition (TPN) order. The TPN solution is very expensive and is wasted if any change is ordered in the formula after it has been prepared.

PPN is normally prescribed for patients who can tolerate some oral feedings but cannot ingest adequate amounts of food to meet their nutritional needs. PPN is a short-term therapy that usually lasts for less than 2 weeks. The dextrose or sugar content of the formula is lower than in the TPN that is given through a central line. PPN is administered via a peripheral intravenous catheter that is inserted into a large vein in the arm.

Both of these types of nutrition may be administered either in a medical facility or in the patient's home. Home parenteral nutrition normally requires a central venous catheter, which must first be inserted in a fully equipped medical facility. After it has been inserted, therapy can continue at home.

CATEGORIES OF DOCTORS' ORDERS RELATED TO MEDICATION ORDERS

Categories of doctors' orders are especially relevant to medication orders. For example, a standing medication order must have times assigned on the MAR, whereas the prn order does not have times assigned. To review, read the discussion of categories of doctors' orders in Chapter 9, then read and complete the following unit.

ADULT TPN ORDER FORM

	☐ Custom	☐ Standard Central	☐ Standard Peripheral
BASE SOLUTION			
g AA (60-120/d : 4 cal/g : 10 g/100 ml)	_____g	50 g/L	30 g/L
g Dextrose (200-700/d : 3.4 cal/g : 70 g/100 ml)	_____g	200 g/L	75 g/L
g Lipid (0-100/d : 9 cal/g : 20 g/100 ml)	_____g		40 g/L
ADDITIVES			
meq NaCl (60-150/d)	_____/bag	35/L or ____/L	35/L or ____/L
meq NaAcetate	_____/bag	_____/L	_____/L
meq KCl (30-100/d)	_____/bag	_____/L	_____/L
meq KAcetate	_____/bag	20/L or ____/L	20/L or ____/L
meq KPO4 (15-40/d)	_____/bag	15/L or ____/L	15/L or ____/L
meq NaPO4	_____/bag	_____/L	_____/L
meq CaGluconate (9-18/d)	_____/bag	4.5/L or ____/L	4.5/L or ____/L
meq MgSO4 (5-15/d)	_____/bag	5/L or ____/L	5/L or ____/L
mg ZnSO4	_____/bag	_____/L	_____/L
Multivitamin-12	_____/bag	Standard	Standard
Trace Elements (Zn, Cu, Mn, Cr)	_____/bag	Standard	Standard
Human Insulin R	_____/bag	_____/L	_____/L
Other: _____	_____	_____/L	_____/L
Other: _____	_____	_____/L	_____/L
Other: _____	_____	_____/L	_____/L
FINAL VOLUME to be infused over 24 hours	_____	_____	_____
RATE ml/hr	_____	_____	_____

_____ ml Iron Dextran/wk (0.5 ml = 25 mg Fe+ + q wk; incompatible with lipid-containing solutions. Lipids will be omitted from solution on the day iron is administered.)
_____ mg Vitamin K/wk (5 mg q wk)

IVPB Lipids _____ ml _____% Lipid q _____ . Run over _____ hrs.

LABORATORY
Daily: _____ Electrolytes _____ BUN _____ Creat _____ Glucose _____ CBC
Q Mon & Thurs: _____ SMA-20 _____Mg+ + _____ CBC
Q Week: _____ Protime _____Platelets
Other: _____
Other: _____
Other: _____

_____ Fingerstick glucose q _____ hrs.   Weight q _____

SLIDING SCALE:

Glucose	Sub Q Human Insulin R
Less than 80 mg%	Call M.D.
80 - 150 mg%	_____ units
151 - 200 mg%	_____ units
201 - 250 mg%	_____ units
251 - 300 mg%	_____ units
301 - 350 mg%	_____ units
Greater than 350 mg%	Call M.D.

Sign. _____

Date _____ Time _____

Phone or pager _____

IV Pharmacy Phone: X4557

ADULT TPN ORDER FORM

Figure 13-7 Total parenteral nutrition order form.

Standing Orders

Standing orders are in effect and administered as ordered until discontinued or changed by a doctor's order.

Example: *Carvedilol 25 mg PO q day*

Other Examples of Standing Medication Orders

Additional examples include the following.

Humalog Insulin units 40 q day

This medication is administered one time each day, such as at 0800, until discontinued.

penicillin VK 500,000 units IM q6h

This medication is administered every 6 hours, such as at 0900, 1500, 2100, and 0300, until discontinued.

hydroxocobalamin 1000 mcg IM twice a week

This medication is to be administered twice a week, such as on Monday and Thursday at 0900, until discontinued.

Fill in the following definition:
A standing order is _____.

SKILLS CHALLENGE

To practice transcribing standing medication orders, complete Activity 13-1 in the *Skills Practice Manual*.

Prn Orders

A prn order is administered according to patient needs until discontinued or changed by a doctor's order. Note: the abbreviation "prn" may not be included in the order. The qualifying phrase would make it a "prn" order (as shown in the example).

Example: *lorazepam 0.5 mg PO @ HS for sleep if nec.*

Other Examples of prn Orders

Other examples of prn orders are as follows.

morphine sulfate 10 mg IM q4h prn severe pain

The morphine sulfate may not be given to the patient more often than every 4 hours and then only if needed. In a prn order, it is impossible to set up a time sequence.

MOM 30 mL hs prn constipation

Milk of magnesia, a laxative, is given as needed, usually when the patient communicates to the nurse that he or she is constipated. This order is in effect until discontinued by the doctor. Laxatives are usually administered at bedtime.

lorazepam 0.5 mg po @ hs prn for insomnia due to anxiety

Lorazepam may not be given other than at bedtime, and only if the patient exhibits an inability to sleep because of anxiety.

Fill in the following definition:
A Prn order is _____.

SKILLS CHALLENGE

To practice transcribing prn medication orders, complete Activity 13-2 in the *Skills Practice Manual*.

One-Time or Short-Series Orders

One-time or short-series orders are administered one time or for a short time and then discontinued as ordered.

Example of one-time order: *Valium 10 mg IM one hour prior to 9 a.m. dressing change.*

Other One-Time or Short-Series Orders

Examples of one-time or short-series order medication orders are as follows.

ciprofloxacin hydrochloride 400 mg IV @ 6 P.M. today and at 6 A.M. tomorrow

This medication is given at the two times ordered and then is discontinued.

prochlorperazine 10 mg IM to be given 1 hr before therapy tomorrow

This medication is to be administered 1 hour before the patient is sent for therapy tomorrow, and then the order is discontinued.

Give bisacodyl supp tonight

This medication is to be administered on the evening the order was written; then it is discontinued.

Short-series example: *Prednisone 40 mg PO × 3 days, then 30 mg × 3 days, then 20 mg × 3 days, then 10 mg × 3 days.*

(All doses would be given PO as no other route is indicated, and the order would end in 12 days.)

Fill in the definition below:
A one-time or short-series order is _____.

SKILLS CHALLENGE

To practice transcribing one-time medication orders, complete Activity 13-3 in the *Skills Practice Manual*. To practice transcribing short-series order medication orders, complete Activity 13-4.

Stat Orders

Stat orders are administered immediately.

Example: *heparin 20,000 units IV push stat.*

Stat orders are to be communicated to the patient's nurse immediately; the nurse will read the order before administering the medication as a safety measure.

Other Examples of Stat Orders

Other examples of stat orders are as follows.

Tylenol #4 PO stat This order indicates that the Tylenol #4 should be given immediately. The order then is to be discontinued.

tetracycline hydrochloride 500 mg PO now and then q6h

This medication order consists of two parts. The first part calls for the antibiotic tetracycline hydrochloride to be given immediately. The second part of this order contains a standing order for the medication to be given four times a day, such as at 0900, 1500, 2100, and 0300. The standing order remains in effect until the doctor discontinues it.

Communication of Stat Medication Orders

When the EMR is in use, the medication order will be sent to the pharmacy automatically. If the EMR is not in use or if otherwise necessary, the medication must be ordered immediately from the pharmacy via phone, fax, or pharmacy copy. Immediately communicate the medication order to the nurse verbally. The nurse who is giving the medication then must review the order directly from the doctors' order sheet.

Fill in the following definition:
A stat order is _____.

SKILLS CHALLENGE

To practice transcribing and communicating stat medication orders, complete Activity 13-5 in the *Skills Practice Manual.* To practice transcribing and communicating IV medication orders, complete Activity 13-6 in the *Skills Practice Manual.*

REAGENTS USED FOR DIAGNOSTIC TESTS

The following diagnostic procedures are performed by the nursing staff. Supplies used to perform the tests are requisitioned from the pharmacy during the transcription procedure.

Skin Tests

Skin tests are administered intradermally or topically to detect allergens, to determine immunity, and to diagnose disease. Types and explanations of common skin tests follow.

Doctors' Orders for Skin Tests

Allergy Skin Testing by Dr. Dermat before Discharge
The most common method of skin testing involves the process of injecting small quantities of suspected allergens intradermally. Positive reactions (erythroderma) usually occur within 20 minutes in varying degrees. Other methods include the scratch, patch, conjunctival, Prausnitz-Küstner (PK), radioallergosorbent (RAST), and use tests.

PPD Today
This is a screening test for tuberculosis. The test agent that is administered to the patient is purified protein derivative (PPD).

Cocci 1:100 Now
This test is used to diagnose coccidioidomycosis (valley fever). The ratio 1:100 refers to the dilution of the test material. It may also be administered in a 1:10 dilution.

Histoplasmin 0.1 mL Today
This skin test is employed as an aid in diagnosing histoplasmosis, a fungal disease. ■

MEDICATION RENEWAL AND DISCONTINUATION ORDERS

Drugs such a narcotics and hypnotics, as well as other drugs controlled by federal or state laws, have an automatic stop date. Hospital medical committees may set stop dates on anticoagulants and antibiotics. When the EMR is in use, the drugs may be discontinued automatically and the nurse may leave a message via the computer for the doctor to renew the medication. When paper charts are used, the nurse may send a message via computer, or some hospitals use a renewal stamp as a reminder of the automatic stop date (Fig. 13-8). The information is stamped on the physician's order sheet by the HUC or the patient's nurse before the expiration date of the medication. When the doctor checks the yes or no box indicating to renew or discontinue and signs his or her name, it is regarded as an order and is transcribed as such. If the doctor fails to check a box and sign the order, the patient's nurse will send a message via computer or place a phone call to the doctor or his or her office for an order to renew or discontinue the medication. When a doctor discontinues a standing or prn order, a discontinue order is written on the doctor's order sheet: *DC Achromycin 500 mg PO tid or DC Demerol.*

SKILLS CHALLENGE

To practice transcribing medication orders with automatic stop dates, complete Activity 13-7. To practice renewing and discontinuing medication orders, complete Activities 13-8 and 13-9 in the *Skills Practice Manual.*

MEDICATION ORDER CHANGES

A patient's medication order may have to be changed for any number of reasons. The change may involve the dosage, route of administration, or frequency of a drug already ordered. When EMR is used; the order change is entered into the patient's computerized MAR. The original order is discontinued and the new order is entered. When paper charts are used the order change is written on the patient's order sheet and is transcribed by the HUC. Whenever this is done, it is considered a new order and should be written as such on the

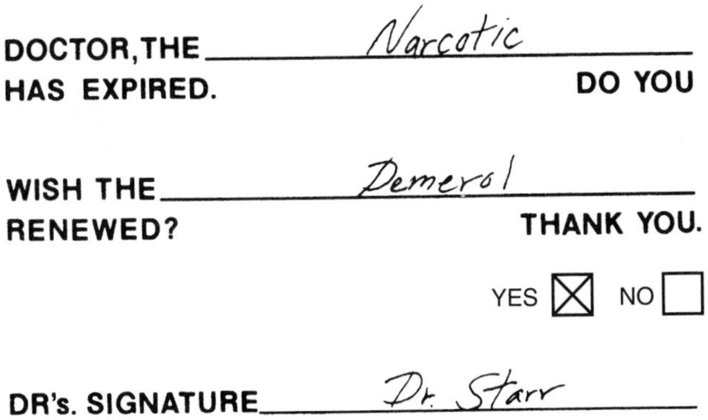

DOCTOR, THE _____ *Narcotic* _____

HAS EXPIRED. **DO YOU**

WISH THE _____ *Demerol* _____
RENEWED? **THANK YOU.**

YES ☒ NO ☐

DR's. SIGNATURE _____ *Dr. Starr* _____

Figure 13-8 Drug renewal stamp.

MAR. It is illegal to erase or cross out parts of an order, or to write over an order on the MAR, because this is a record of what medication has been administered to the patient. This may result in a serious medication error. The old order must be discontinued according to the policy and the new order written. (See Fig. 13-3, *A* for discontinuing medication on the MAR.)

Doctors' Orders for Medication Changes

- Change meperidine 50 mg *IM* q4h prn to Demerol 50 mg *PO* q4h prn (change in route of administration)
- Decrease ciprofloxacin *250 mg* IV q12h to *200 mg* IV q12h (change in dosage)
- Change lorazepam 1 mg PO *tid* to 5 mg PO *bid* (change in frequency of administration) ■

SKILLS CHALLENGE

To practice transcribing medication order changes, complete Activity 13-10 in the *Skills Practice Manual.*

To test your skill in transcribing a review set of medication orders, complete Activity 13-11

To test your skill in transcribing a review set of doctor's orders, complete Activity 13-12

To practice locating medications in the *Physicians' Desk Reference*, complete Activity 13-13 To practice recording telephone messages, complete Activity 13-14

KEY CONCEPTS

The implementation of the EMR and CPOE has changed the responsibilities of the HUC regarding the doctor's orders for medication. Even though the HUC does not transcribe the medication orders, it is beneficial for her or him to have a basic knowledge of medications. There are times when the HUC may need to relay a message regarding a medication. The HUC also has the responsibility of printing the medication prescription pamphlets for patients.

If the HUC has the responsibility of transcribing medication orders, extreme care must be taken. Errors may result in serious consequences to the patient and liability to the hospital and all involved personnel. The HUC must be careful not to omit any orders during the transcription procedure. Each order must be transcribed exactly as written by the doctor. Each order must be entered into the computer correctly or, if using a paper MAR, written legibly so it can be read easily by the nurse who is administering the medication.

Whenever there is any doubt regarding a medication order or any order, do not hesitate to check with the nurse and/or pharmacist. If requested by the patient's nurse, place a call to the ordering doctor so the nurse can clarify the order.

Websites of Interest

Rx.com: www.rx.com
PDR.net—Information regarding FDA-approved drug labeling: www.pdr.net
iHealthBeat—Newsletter reporting on technology and health care: www.ihealthbeat.org

REVIEW QUESTIONS

Visit the Evolve website to download and complete the following questions.

1. Define the following terms:
   a. adverse drug event
   b. over-the-counter drugs
   c. bolus
   d. patient-controlled analgesia
   e. oral
   f. topical
   g. intramuscular injection
   h. parenteral
   i. intravenous infusion
   j. skin test
   k. parenteral routes
   l. intravenous or IV push
   m. intravenous or IV piggyback
   n. intradermal

2. List four abbreviations that are included in The Joint Commission's "do not use" list.

3. Identify four causes of medication errors, and explain how the use of CPOE decreases the risk of errors.

4. Compare the HUC role regarding medication orders with and without EMR with CPOE.

5. Identify two types of medicine carts, and discuss their use.

6. List at least two over-the-counter medications that would be stored in the medication stock supply.

7. Discuss the use of the MAR when EMRs are used and when paper charts are used.

8. List five components of a medication order (in order).

9. List four routes by which medications may be administered.

10. Match the purpose (listed in column 2) for prescribing medications from the drug groups (listed in column 1).

a. Diuretic

b. Potassium replacement

c. Antiarrhythmic

d. Narcotic seizures (convulsions)

e. Hypnotic

f. Antibiotic

g. Anticoagulant

h. Antidiabetic

i. Antihyperlipidemic

j. Anticonvulsants

k. Analgesics

l. Antihypertensives

m. Antianginals in the blood

n. Antiplatelet drugs

o. Sedative (tranquillizer)

p. Respiratory drugs

1. treatment of chest pain

2. to induce urine flow— treats hypertension

3. treatment of high cholesterol

4. prevent or reduce the severity and frequency of

5. lower blood sugar

6. treatment of low potassium levels

7. treatment of abnormal heart rhythms

8. reduce the ability of platelets to stick together

9. kills or slows the growth of bacteria

10. treat upper respiratory, lung disorders

11. relieve anxiety and induce sleep

12. relieve minor aches and pains

13. thin the blood and prevent clots from forming

14. reduce severe pain

15. treatment of high blood pressure

16. relieve anxiety, stress

11. List four categories of medications discussed in this chapter that are controlled substances.

12. Why is it important to notify the pharmacy immediately if there is a change or a change pending in a patient's TPN orders?

13. Identify the following orders as standing, prn, short-order series, one-time, or stat.
   a. *meperidine 100mg IM now*
   b. *hydrocodone 5 mg po q4-6h for pain*
   c. *carvedilol 25 mg PO q day*
   d. *Ambien 10 mg this hs*
   e. *prednisone 40mg q day x 3 days, then 30mg q day x 3days, then 20mg q day x 3 days, then 10mg q day x 3 days.*

14. List three skin tests and give the purpose of each.

15. Discuss how medications are renewed, discontinued, and changed when the EMR is used and when paper charts are used.

SURFING FOR ANSWERS

1. Research common medication errors made in hospitals, and document four types of errors and at least two websites used.
2. Document two websites that discuss the benefits of e-prescribing, and list the benefits found.
3. Go to www.pdr.net and research two medicines that you or someone you know has been prescribed to take. Document the use and possible side effects of the medications.

Laboratory Orders

CHAPTER OBJECTIVES

On completion of this chapter, you will be able to:

1. Define the terms in the vocabulary list.
2. Write the meaning of each abbreviation in the abbreviations list.
3. List two general purposes of laboratory studies.
4. Name three major divisions and five other divisions of the laboratory.
5. Identify five specimens that may be studied in the laboratory, and list at least three specimens that would be obtained by an invasive procedure.
6. List six invasive procedures that would require a consent form signed by the patient.
7. Describe the health unit coordinator's responsibilities in ordering laboratory tests and sending specimens to the laboratory when EMR is used and when paper charts are used and describe how routine, stat, daily, and timed studies would be ordered and performed.
8. List three tests that would be performed at the bedside (POCT) to detect occult blood in gastric and stool specimens.
9. Describe the general purpose of the hematology division of the laboratory, and list six studies that would be performed in the hematology division.
10. Describe the general purpose of the chemistry division of the laboratory.

11. Identify at least three chemistry tests that would require the patient to be fasting, and explain the difference between fasting and NPO.
12. List four tests that are included in electrolytes.
13. Describe the general purpose of the toxicology department, and explain the procedure for ordering peak and trough drug levels.
14. Describe the general purpose of the microbiology division of the laboratory, and list six studies that would be performed in the microbiology division.
15. Describe the general purpose of the serology and immunology division of the laboratory, and list three tests performed in the serology and immunology division.
16. Describe the general purpose of the blood bank, and identify the steps that must be performed to obtain blood (packed cells) for transfusion.
17. Describe the general purpose of the urinalysis division of the laboratory, and identify three methods of obtaining urine specimens.
18. Identify the procedure that would be performed to obtain pleural fluid and cerebrospinal fluid (CSF), and explain the importance of accurate labeling and appropriate transportation of these specimens.
19. Describe the purpose of the pathology division of the laboratory, and identify and describe the purpose of two subdivisions of the pathology division.
20. Describe how errors may be avoided in recording telephoned laboratory results (critical or panic values).

VOCABULARY

Amniocentesis A needle puncture into the uterine cavity to remove amniotic fluid, the liquid that surrounds the fetus.

Antibody An immunoglobulin (protein) produced by the body that reacts with and neutralizes an antigen (usually a foreign substance).

Antigen Any substance that induces an immune response.

Biopsy Tissue removed from a living body for examination.

Clean Catch A method of obtaining a urine specimen using a special cleansing technique; also called a *midstream urine collection.*

Culture and Sensitivity The growth of microorganisms in a special medium (culture), followed by a test to determine the antibiotic to which they best respond (sensitivity).

Cytology The study of cells.

Daily Laboratory Test A test that is ordered once by a doctor and is performed every day until the doctor discontinues the order.

Differential (diff) Identification of the types of white cells found in the blood.

Dipstick Urine The visual examination of urine using a special chemically treated stick.

Electrolytes A group of tests done in chemistry, which usually includes sodium (Na), potassium (K), chloride (Cl), and carbon dioxide (CO_2).

Erythrocytes Red blood cells.

Fasting No solid foods by mouth and no fluids containing nourishment (e.g., sugar, milk).

Guaiac A method of testing stool for hidden (occult) blood using guaiac as a reagent (may also be called a *Hemoccult slide test*).

Lumbar Puncture A procedure used to remove cerebrospinal fluid from the spinal canal.

Nosocomial Infection An infection that is acquired by the patient while in the hospital. Also known as a *hospital-acquired infection* (HAI).

Occult Blood Blood that is undetectable to the eye.

Pap Smear A test performed to detect cancerous cells in the female genital tract; the Pap staining method can also be used to study body secretions, excretions, and tissue scrapings.

Paracentesis A surgical puncture and drainage of a body cavity.

Pathogens Microorganisms that cause disease.

Pathology The study of body changes caused by disease.

Plasma The fluid portion of the blood in which the cells are suspended; it contains a clotting factor called *fibrinogen.*

Postprandial After eating.

Random Specimens Specimens that can be collected at any time.

Reference Range Range of normal values for a laboratory test result.

Reflex Testing Additional tests done on a specimen subsequent to initial test results and used to further identify significant diagnostic information required for appropriate patient care.

Serology The study of blood serum or other body fluids for immune bodies, which are the body's defense when disease occurs.

Serum Plasma from which fibrinogen, a clotting factor, has been removed.

Sputum The mucous secretion from lungs, bronchi, or trachea.

Sternal Punctures Procedures to remove bone marrow from the breastbone cavity for diagnostic purposes; also called *bone marrow biopsies.*

Superbugs Pathogens that have become resistant to most of the antibiotics currently available and that often cause life-threatening infections that are extremely difficult to treat.

Thoracentesis A needle puncture into the pleural space in the chest cavity to remove pleural fluid for diagnostic or therapeutic reasons.

Timed Specimen A specimen that must be collected at a specific time.

Tissue Typing Identification of tissue types to predict acceptance or rejection of tissue and organ transplants.

Titer The quantity of substance needed to react with a given amount of another substance; used to detect and quantify antibody levels.

Type and Crossmatch Procedure in which the patient's blood is typed then is tested for compatibility with blood from a donor of the same blood type and Rh factor.

Type and Screen Procedure in which the patient's blood type and Rh factor are determined and a general antibody screen is performed.

Urinalysis The physical, chemical, and microscopic examination of the urine.

Urine Reflex Procedure in which urine is tested and if certain parameters are met, a culture is performed.

ABBREVIATIONS

Note: Most doctors' orders for laboratory tests are written on the doctors' order sheet as the abbreviation appears here; for example, *CBC* is the doctor's written order for complete blood (cell) count. Examples of doctors' orders are given only for those orders that require more than the abbreviation.

Abbreviation	Meaning	Example of Usage on a Doctor's Order Sheet
A1C	glycosylated hemoglobin (chemistry)	A1C today
Ab	antibody	HIV Ab
ACTH	adrenocorticotropic hormone (chemistry)	
ADH	antidiuretic hormone (chemistry)	
AFB	acid-fast bacillus (microbiology)	sputum for AFB Cx
Ag	antigen	CMV Ag
ALP *or* alk phos	alkaline phosphatase (chemistry)	
ANA	antinuclear antibody (serology)	
BC	blood culture (microbiology)	Blood cultures × 2-15 min apart
bili	bilirubin	

Abbreviation	Meaning	Example of Usage on a Doctor's Order Sheet
BMP	basic metabolic panel (chemistry)	
BNP	brain natriuretic protein (chemistry)	
BUN	blood urea nitrogen (chemistry)	
Bx	biopsy (cytology)	Liver needle Bx
Ca *or* Ca$^+$	calcium (chemistry)	
CBC	complete blood cell count (hematology)	
CC, creat cl, *or* cr cl	creatinine clearance (chemistry)	24 hr urine cr cl
C. diff	*Clostridium difficile* (microbiology and serology)	Stool × 3 for C. diff toxin and anaerobic cx
CEA	carcinoembryonic antigen (chemistry)	
Cl	chloride (chemistry)	
CMP	comprehensive metabolic panel (chemistry)	
CMV	cytomegalovirus (microbiology, serology)	CMV IgG and IgM
CO_2	carbon dioxide (chemistry)	
CPK *or* CK	creatine phosphokinase or creatine kinase (chemistry)	
CRP	C-reactive protein (chemistry)	
CRKP	carbapenem-resistant *Klebsiella pneumoniae* (microbiology and serology)	Bronch wash for G-stain, C&S and PCR for CRKP
C&S	culture and sensitivity (microbiology)	Sputum for C&S
CSF	cerebrospinal fluid (chemistry, hematology, microbiology, serology)	CSF Tube 1 C&S, Tube 2 prot & gluc
cult	culture (microbiology)	Blood cult × 2 sites
Cx	culture (microbiology)	Sputum Cx
diff	differential (hematology)	WBC c̄ diff
EBV	Epstein-Barr virus (serology)	
ESR *or* sedrate	erythrocyte sedimentation rate (hematology)	Westergren ESR
FBS	fasting blood sugar (chemistry)	FBS in am
Fe	iron (chemistry)	Fe c̄ TIBC
FPG	fasting plasma glucose (chemistry)	FPG q am
FS	frozen section (cytology)	Liver wedge Bx FS
GTT *or* OGTT	glucose tolerance test or oral glucose tolerance test (chemistry)	
H&H	hemoglobin and hematocrit (hematology)	

Abbreviation	Meaning	Example of Usage on a Doctor's Order Sheet
HbsAg	hepatitis B surface antigen (serology)	
hCG	human chorionic gonadotropin (test for pregnancy [chemistry])	
Hct	hematocrit (hematology)	
HDL	high-density lipoprotein (chemistry)	
Hgb	hemoglobin (hematology)	
HIVB$_{24}$Ag	human immunodeficiency virus antigen screen (serology)	
HSV	herpes simplex virus (serology)	
IgG, IgM	immunoglobulin G, immunoglobulin M (serology)	CMV IgG and IgM by RIA today
K	potassium (chemistry)	
LDL	low-density lipoprotein (chemistry)	
LP	lumbar puncture (also called *spinal tap*)	LP in am
lytes	electrolytes (chemistry)	
Mg *or* Mg$^+$	magnesium (chemistry)	CBC, CMP & Mg in AM
MRSA	methicillin-resistant *Staphylococcus aureus* (microbiology)	
Na	sodium (chemistry)	
NP	nasopharynx	NP smear for C&S
O&P	ova and parasites (parasitology)	Stool for O&P × 3
PAP	prostatic acid phosphatase (serology)	
PC	packed cells (blood bank)	Give 2 Units PC now
PCR	polymerase chain reaction (serology)	HIV Ab by PCR
PCV	packed-cell volume (hematology; same as hematocrit)	
PKU	phenylketonuria (chemistry)	
PO$_4$ *or* phos	phosphate or phosphorus (chemistry)	
POCT *or* PCT	point-of-care testing (performed on the nursing unit)	
PP	postprandial (chemistry)	2 hr PP BS
PSA	prostatic specific antigen (serology)	
PT/INR	prothrombin time and international normalized ratio (coagulation-hematology)	PT/INR qod while on warfarin

Abbreviation	Meaning	Example of Usage on a Doctor's Order Sheet
PTT *or* APTT	partial thrombo-plastin time or activated partial thromboplastin time (coagulation-hematology)	PTT qd until heparin DC'd
RBC	red blood cell count (hematology)	
RBS *or* BS	random blood sugar or blood sugar (chemistry)	BS today
RDW	red cell distribution width (hematology)	
retics	reticulocytes (hematology)	
RPR	rapid plasma reagin (serology)	
RSV	respiratory syn-cytial virus (microbiology)	
S&A	sugar and acetone (urinalysis)	
STO	specimen to be obtained (i.e., by nurse)	Urine C&S—STO
T$_3$, T$_4$, T$_7$	thyroid tests (chemistry)	
T&C *or* T&X-match	type and crossmatch (blood bank)	T&C for 2 Units of packed red cells
T&S	type and screen (blood bank)	
TIBC	total iron-binding capacity (chemistry)	
trig *or* TG	triglycerides (chemistry)	
TSH	thyroid-stimulat-ing hormone (chemistry)	
UA *or* U/A	(urinalysis)	
UC	urine culture	cath urine for UC
VRE	vancomycin-resistant *Enterococcus* (microbiology)	
WBC	white blood cell count (hematology)	
WNL	within normal limits	
XDR-TB	extensively drug-resistant tuberculo-sis (microbiology)	

★ HIGH PRIORITY

Most of the abbreviations listed previously apply to some commonly ordered laboratory tests. Many more abbreviations for laboratory tests are covered throughout this chapter. The words in parentheses indicate in which division of the laboratory the test is performed.

⊝ E X E R C I S E 1

Write the abbreviation for each term listed.

1. glycosylated hemoglobin
2. fasting blood sugar
3. ova and parasites
4. hemoglobin
5. erythrocyte sedimentation rate or sedimentation rate
6. potassium
7. acid-fast bacilli
8. red blood cell count
9. postprandial
10. cerebrospinal fluid
11. iron
12. culture and sensitivity
13. type and crossmatch
14. complete blood (cell) count
15. prostatic acid phosphatase
16. glucose tolerance test
17. packed cells
18. prothrombin time and international normalized ratio
19. urinalysis
20. alkaline phosphatase
21. hepatitis B surface antigen
22. frozen section
23. human immunodeficiency virus
24. magnesium
25. human chorionic gonadotropin
26. within normal limits
27. partial thromboplastin time or activated partial thromboplastin time
28. thyroid tests
29. thyroid-stimulating hormone
30. sugar and acetone
31. antigen
32. basic metabolic chemistry panel
33. cytomegalovirus
34. herpes simplex virus
35. type and screen
36. antibody
37. culture
38. respiratory syncytial virus
39. comprehensive metabolic panel
40. electrolytes
41. biopsy
42. point-of-care testing
43. packed-cell volume
44. random blood sugar or blood sugar
45. rapid plasma reagin
46. reticulocytes
47. prostatic specific antigen
48. differential
49. white blood cell count
50. phosphorus
51. total iron-binding capacity
52. hematocrit
53. lumbar puncture
54. sodium
55. nasopharynx
56. hemoglobin and hematocrit

57. carbon dioxide
58. antinuclear antibody
59. high-density lipoprotein
60. blood urea nitrogen
61. calcium
62. creatinine clearance
63. chloride
64. carcinoembryonic antigen
65. brain natriuretic protein
66. low-density lipoprotein
67. antidiuretic hormone
68. creatine phosphokinase or creatine kinase
69. Epstein-Barr virus
70. antibody
71. red cell distribution width
72. triglyceride
73. bilirubin
74. specimen to be obtained
75. immunoglobulin G and M
76. C-reactive protein
77. vancomycin-resistant *Enterococcus*
78. methicillin-resistant *Staphylococcus aureus*
79. extensively drug-resistant tuberculosis
80. adrenocorticotropic hormone
81. *Clostridium difficile*
82. carbapenem resistant *Klebsiella pneumoniae*

EXERCISE 2

Write the meaning of each abbreviation listed.

1. FBS	29. S&A
2. O&P	30. Ag
3. Hgb	31. BMP
4. ESR or sedrate	32. CMV
5. K	33. HSV
6. AFB	34. T&S
7. RBC	35. Ab
8. PP	36. Cx
9. CSF	37. RSV
10. Fe	38. CMP
11. C&S	39. lytes
12. T&X-match or T&C	40. Bx
13. CBC	41. POCT or PCT
14. PAP	42. PCV
15. GTT	43. RBS or BS
16. PC	44. RPR
17. PT/INR	45. retics
18. UA or U/A	46. PSA
19. ALP or alk phos	47. Diff
20. HbsAg	48. WBC
21. FS	49. PO_4 or phos
22. $HIVB_{24}Ag$	50. TIBC
23. Mg or Mg^+	51. Hct
24. hCG	52. LP
25. WNL	53. Na
26. PTT or APTT	54. NP
27. T_3, T_4, T_7	55. H&H
28. TSH	56. CO_2

57. ANA	70. RDW
58. HDL	71. trig or TG
59. BUN	72. bili
60. Ca or Ca^+	73. AiC
61. CC, creat cl, or cr cl	74. STO
62. Cl	75. IgG, IgM
63. CEA	76. C. diff
64. BNP	77. CRKP
65. LDL	78. XDR-TB
66. ADH	79. VRE
67. CPK or CK	80. MRSA
68. EBV	81. ACTH
69. Ab	82. CRP

★ HIGH PRIORITY

When the electronic medical record (EMR) with computer physician order entry (CPOE) is implemented, the physicians' orders are entered directly into the patient's EMR and are automatically sent to the appropriate departments. An additional requisition may be printed on the unit that may indicate a specimen to be collected by the nurse, who would then be notified by the HUC. The health unit coordinator (HUC) is responsible for sending labeled and bagged specimens to the laboratory department after they have been collected by nursing staff, residents, or doctors. Other HUC tasks may be indicated by an icon next to the appropriate patient's name on the computer census screen. An example of an additional task would be to hold a patient's tray for a glucose tolerance test.

INTRODUCTION TO LABORATORY PROCEDURES

Tests performed by the laboratory are ordered for diagnostic purposes and for evaluation of a prescribed treatment. See the Evolve website for a comprehensive list of the studies that are performed in a laboratory.

Hospital size determines the number of divisions within the laboratory and the types of tests performed in each division. For example, a large hospital may have a microbiology division with subdivisions such as bacteriology, serology and immunology, parasitology, virology, and mycology. In smaller hospitals, all the tests performed in the divisions mentioned previously may be done in the microbiology division or sent to outside laboratories. (Figure 14-1 is a laboratory divisional chart.) The divisions and some test names may vary among hospitals from those used in this book.

In this chapter, we will discuss three major laboratory divisions—hematology, chemistry, and microbiology—and five other divisions—toxicology, serology and immunology, pathology (including histology and cytology), blood bank, and urinalysis. The clinical laboratory may also perform tests related to nuclear medicine and gastroenterology when a hospital is not of sufficient size to maintain a separate nuclear medicine or the gastroenterology department.

When paper charts are used, it is necessary for the HUC to interpret terms used by the doctor to write laboratory orders.

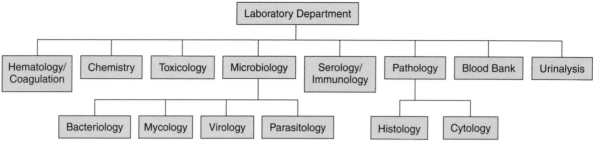

Figure 14-1 A laboratory divisional chart.

The word *routine* in a written laboratory order usually would indicate that the test will be performed within a 4-hour period because there is no urgency for the test results. For example, the doctor may write the order *Routine CBC*, meaning that the blood specimen for the complete blood count (CBC) may be drawn according to the hospital (laboratory) policy. *Routine* may also refer to the lab tests ordered routinely in the morning. Nursing personnel or laboratory personnel may draw blood specimens.

The doctor may use the word *daily* to indicate a **daily laboratory test,** as in the order *daily Hgb;* this means that the test is ordered once by the doctor but is requisitioned every day or entered into the computer for multiple days in advance by the HUC until the order is discontinued. Some hospitals have a policy that requires the doctor to renew daily laboratory orders every 3 days or discontinue the orders.

The word *stat,* as you recall, means "to be done immediately." Because of the urgency of a stat order, a different communication procedure is used. The procedure is to notify the laboratory by phone or verbally notify the appropriate nursing personnel on the unit. When calling the laboratory, supply the name of the patient, nursing unit, room number, and test ordered. The order is entered into the computer immediately if a laboratory technician is to draw the blood. The order would be entered when the specimen is collected if collected by nursing personnel. When placing an order for a test that must be drawn at a specified time such as drug levels or a 2-hr postprandial (PP) blood sugar, the term **timed specimen** is used.

Laboratory tests are communicated to the laboratory department by the HUC through the ordering step of transcription if computer physician order entry (CPOE) is not implemented. The physician will input the order directly if CPOE is being used, and the HUC may be responsible to further communicate the order to nursing or laboratory personnel. The HUC may be expected to telephone the lab in the case of stat laboratory orders regardless of whether the hospital uses paper or electronic medical records and CPOE.

Specimens

All laboratory tests require a specimen. Blood, the most commonly used specimen, is most often obtained by nursing or laboratory personnel through venipuncture (puncture into the vein), finger stick (puncture into a capillary), or peripheral arterial or venous lines (Fig. 14-2). An additional source of blood is the umbilical cord. A "cord blood" specimen may be ordered for patients in the labor and delivery unit and is collected by nursing personnel.

Blood specimens may have to be collected in different containers depending on the test ordered. For example, coagulation studies and chemistry studies must be taken in different tubes. Cultures performed on blood for different types of organisms (aerobic versus anaerobic bacteria) may require different tubes. Clear and complete information on all tests to be collected reduces the need for additional blood specimens to be drawn. When asked by a nurse to call the laboratory to inquire about amount or means of collecting a specimen; document the information and the name of the person providing the information. It may be helpful for the HUC to include additional information about routine tests whose specimens can be drawn at the same time as the specimen for a stat test in order to reduce the number of blood draws a patient may need to undergo.

Other specimens for testing include urine, stool, **sputum,** sweat, wound drainage, discharge from body openings, and gastric washings (lavage). Nursing staff members usually collect these specimens (Fig. 14-3).

The doctor usually obtains specimens by entering parts of the body or a body cavity. Types of specimens and the names of the procedures used to obtain them are listed in Table 14-1. A written consent is required to be signed by the patient before invasive procedures including any **paracentesis** (a surgical puncture and drainage of a body cavity), **amniocentesis, lumbar puncture,** or other invasive procedures listed are performed, except for pelvic examination. (Review "Preparing a Consent Form," Chapter 8.) It may be the HUC's responsibility to order trays, such as a lumbar puncture tray, or other equipment from the central service department (CSD) for the doctor to use to perform these procedures.

All specimens obtained by the nursing staff or doctor usually will be bagged and labeled (not always possible during an emergency) before they are handed to the HUC. It is recommended that the HUC keep plastic gloves in a drawer to use when specimens are not bagged and wash hands after handling specimens (even when placed in plastic bags). The label should include the date and time collected, along with the initials of the person who collected the specimen, in addition to patient information.

Requisitions for laboratory tests of specimens obtained by the nursing staff or doctor may be kept on the nursing unit until the specimen has been collected or the order has been entered into the computer when the specimen is sent. The requisition or computer printout of the order is attached to the specimen bag, and then it is sent to the laboratory. If CPOE is used, then a requisition or other document may need to be printed by the HUC. It is essential that the HUC check the patient name on the specimen and on the computer order screen and compare it with the doctor's order. Mislabeled specimens usually are discarded and the specimen redrawn, causing a delay in diagnosis and treatment and causing the patient additional discomfort.

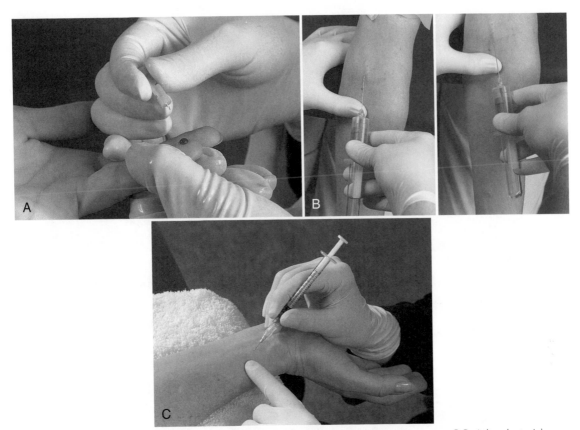

Figure 14-2   Methods of obtaining blood specimens. **A,** Finger stick. **B,** Venipuncture. **C,** Peripheral arterial draw. (From Sommer S, Warekois R: *Phlebotomy: worktext and procedures manual,* St Louis, 2001, Saunders.)

It is often the HUC's responsibility to take the specimen to the laboratory. This should be done as soon as possible. Some specimens (well wrapped) may be sent by the pneumatic tube system, especially when results are needed quickly (e.g., emergency department, surgery). Specimens that should *not* be sent by the pneumatic tube system are those that have been collected by an invasive procedure, such as cerebrospinal and amniotic fluids. When blood or urine is sent by the pneumatic tube system, specimens must be well wrapped and cushioned. Some facilities may have a policy that disallows any specimen from being transported via the pneumatic tube system because of possible loss or spilling of the specimen.

> ⭐ **HIGH PRIORITY**
>
> It is essential that the health unit coordinator check the patient's name on the specimen and computer order screen and compare it with the doctor's order. Mislabeled specimens usually are discarded and the specimen redrawn, causing a delay in diagnosis and treatment and causing the patient additional discomfort.

Point-of-Care Testing

Many laboratory specimens that were once collected and analyzed only in the laboratory department may now be performed on the nursing unit. A laboratory test whose specimen is collected and analyzed on the hospital unit by nursing personnel is called a *point-of-care lab test.* Because of point-of-care testing (POCT), the procedure for ordering a test may change.

Results are obtained via several methods. These include analysis by portable automated analyzers, the use of reagents (chemicals), and microscopic visualization.

Portable automated analyzers may be used in departments that require immediate results; these decrease the need for stat specimens to be sent to the laboratory. Some tests that may be done on the unit by this method include **electrolytes,** blood glucose, blood urea nitrogen (BUN), hemoglobin, and hematocrit. A test to evaluate pulmonary function (see Chapter 16), called *arterial blood gases* (ABGs), may be run by an automated analyzer on the unit.

Reagent-based tests may include a test for pregnancy or human chorionic gonadotropin (hCG) or activated clotting time (ACT), and a test for *Helicobacter pylori* (CLO - Campylobacter-like organism) test, a bacterium that has been indicated in ulcers of the gastrointestinal system. The CLO test actually uses a **biopsy** specimen obtained in the endoscopy department (see Chapter 16) and may yield positive results within 2 hours.

Some of the reagent-based tests that are considered point-of-care lab tests are those that are traditionally carried out by nursing personnel; these include blood and urine monitoring for the presence of ketones and for levels of glucose. Blood glucose monitoring is discussed in Chapter 10. The D-dimer coagulation study may be done with a finger stick specimen on the unit. **Guaiac,** Gastroccult, or Hemoccult tests, which use reagents to detect **occult blood** (undetectable to the eye) in gastric and stool specimens, are considered point-of-care tests in some health care facilities.

A test that uses both a reagent and microscopic visualization is the fern test, which is used to indicate the presence

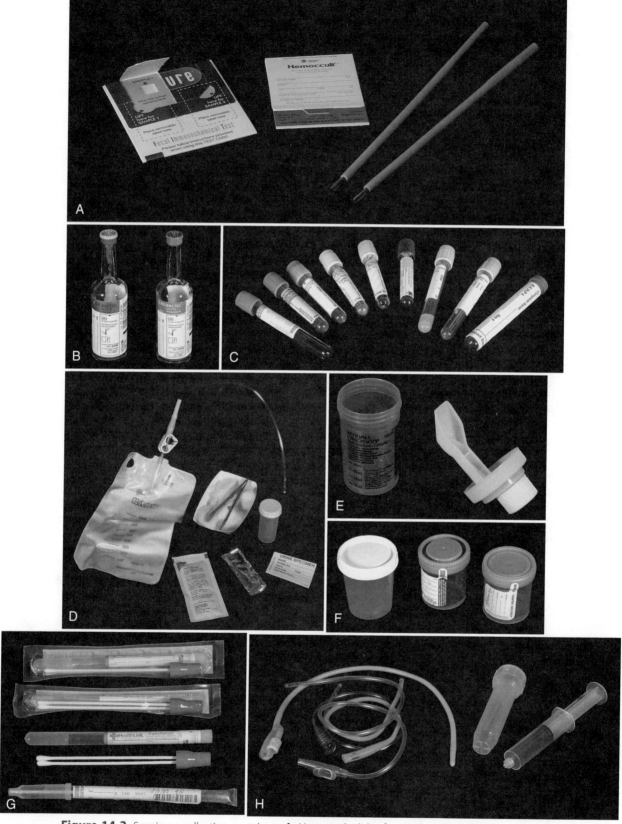

Figure 14-3 Specimen collection containers. **A,** Hemoccult slides for stool specimen. **B,** Containers for blood culture specimen. **C,** Various containers for blood specimen. **D,** Cath urine specimen container kit. **E,** Stool specimen container. **F,** Urine specimen containers: *Left,* voided specimen; *Right,* midstream specimen. **G,** Culturette and container for throat culture. **H,** Types of sputum collection containers.

TABLE 14-1 Types of Nonretrievable Specimens and Their Associated Procedures

Specimen	Procedure Performed to Obtain Specimen
Spinal fluid	Lumbar puncture; also called *spinal tap*
Bone marrow	Sternal puncture; also called *bone marrow biopsy*
Abdominal cavity fluid	Abdominal paracentesis
Pleural fluid	Thoracentesis or thoracocentesis
Amniotic fluid	Amniocentesis
Biopsy specimen	Biopsy of a part of the body
Cervical smear	Pelvic examination

of amniotic fluid (as a result of rupture of the amnion). The reagent portion uses a strip of paper that indicates acidity (pH paper), and the microscopic portion detects the characteristic fern pattern of crystallized amniotic sodium chloride (salt).

Reflex Testing

Reflex testing means that additional tests are done on a specimen indicated by and subsequent to the initial test results and used to further identify significant diagnostic information required for appropriate patient care. Reflex testing must be approved by the medical staff on an annual basis. Laboratory personnel must consult with the medical director, pathologist, or clinical consultant to determine the tests and criteria for reflex testing. Only tests documented as approved by the medical executive committee may be reflexed and must be medically necessary. Physicians must be informed of those tests that are reflexed and be given the option to order the test without the reflex test.

The CBC with automatic differential (CBC with auto diff) is the only example of a test that is "reflexed" and not considered a reflex test for billing purposes (the results of the auto diff indicate whether a manual diff needs to be performed).

★ HIGH PRIORITY

Some lab orders may include additional but important information, such as a specific method by which the test must be done (*Westergren Sed Rate, CMV IgG by PCR*). A physician may request that a test be sent to and performed by a specific outside laboratory or research facility. It is important that the health unit coordinator include all pertinent information on the requisition.

★ HIGH PRIORITY

Some lab tests (such as human immunodeficiency virus testing by **serology** or blood transfusion orders from the blood bank) may require a special consent form. It is the responsibility of the health unit coordinator (HUC) to recognize the need for the preparation of a consent even when it is not part of the written physician order. If computer physician order entry is used, the consent may be listed on the computer as an HUC task.

DIVISIONS WITHIN THE LABORATORY

It may be necessary to identify the division in which a test is performed in order to complete the correct requisition or enter it into the computer. This information is helpful in telephone communication when one is clarifying orders or requesting results.

Hematology

The hematology division performs tests related to physical properties of the blood and other body fluids (including blood cells and their appearance), tests related to clotting and bleeding disorders, and coagulation (clotting) studies done to monitor patients undergoing anticoagulant therapy.

Specimens

Most of these tests are done on a blood specimen. However, bone marrow and spinal fluid also may be studied in the hematology division.

Fasting

Fasting generally is not required for tests performed in the hematology division of the laboratory.

Communication with the Laboratory

Hematology studies are ordered by computer or by completing a downtime requisition form (Fig. 14-4).

Doctors' Orders for Hematology Studies

It is impossible to list all doctors' orders related to this division of the laboratory. However, we have listed the more common ones in their abbreviated forms, along with an interpretation for reference. Refer to the abbreviations list at the beginning of the chapter if necessary.

Note: Unless stated otherwise, all of the following tests are performed on blood specimens; therefore, as mentioned previously, nursing or laboratory personnel obtain the specimen, or point-of-care testing (POCT) is performed.

CBC (Complete Blood Cell Count) or Hemogram
A CBC or hemogram is composed of a number of tests, including RBC; Hgb; Hct; RBC indices; WBC count $\bar{c}$ diff, blood smear, and platelet count. These tests may be ordered separately. The number of tests included in a CBC may vary among hospitals.

RBC (Red Blood Cell Count)
The RBC is the number of red blood cells **(erythrocytes)** per cubic millimeter of blood.

Hgb (Hemoglobin)
Hgb is the oxygen-carrying protein of the red blood cell, and when oxygenated, gives blood its red color. This test may determine the need for additional blood, or it may aid in diagnosing types of anemia.

Hct (Hematocrit)
Hematocrit, also called *packed-cell volume* (PCV), is a measurement of the volume percentage of red blood cells in whole blood.

RBC (Red Blood Cell) Indices

Measurement of RBC indices is a method for determining the characteristics of red blood cells. The measurements are reported as MCH (content of hemoglobin in average individual red cell), MCHC (average hemoglobin concentration per 100 mL of packed red cells), MCV (average volume of individual red cells), and RDW (red cell distribution width—a distribution of red cell volume).

WBC (White Blood Cell Count)

A WBC (leukocyte count) is the count of the number of white blood cells that are present in the blood to fight disease-causing organisms. This test often is used in the diagnosis of infection.

Differential (Diff)

A **differential (diff)** reports the various types of white blood cells (or leukocytes) found in the blood specimen. Some of these types are lymphocytes (lymphs), monocytes (monos), neutrophils (neutros), eosinophils (eos), and basophils (basos). A diff is usually included in a WBC. The physician may request a "manual differential," which is done manually rather than by an instrument.

Blood Smear

A blood smear is an examination performed with special stains of the peripheral blood; it can provide a significant amount of information regarding drugs and diseases that affect red blood cells, white blood cells, and platelets.

Platelet Count (Plt ct)

Platelet count is the counting of clotting cells (platelets), which are essential for the coagulation process to take place.

ESR (Erythrocyte Sedimentation Rate)

An erythrocyte sedimentation rate, also called a *sedrate,* determines the rate at which red blood cells settle out of the liquid portion of the blood. This test is used to evaluate the progress of inflammatory and autoimmune diseases. The physician may request that the ESR be done

Doctor ordering ____________ ☐ Stat
Today's date ____________ ☐ Timed
Draw @ date ______ Time______ ☐ Routine
Collection date ______ Time______
Collected by ____________
Requested by ____________

Patient Label

Hematology, Serology, & Urinalysis / Urine Chemistry Requisition

Hematology	Serology	Urinalysis / Urine Chemistry
☐ Bleeding time, Ivy	☐ ANA	☐ Routine UA
☐ CBC c̄ diff	☐ ASO titer	☐ Reflex UA
☐ CBC c̄ manual diff	☐ CEA	☐ Amylase (2hr)
☐ Factor VIII	☐ CMV	☐ Bilirubin
☐ Fibrinogen	☐ IgG	☐ Calcium
☐ HCT	☐ IgM	☐ Chloride
☐ HGB	☐ Cocci screen	☐ Creatinine clearance 24 hour
☐ H & H	☐ EBV panel	☐ Glucose tolerance
☐ Eosinophil Ct absolute	☐ Enterovirus Ab panel 1	☐ Nitrogen
☐ Eosinophil smear	☐ Enterovirus Ab panel 2	☐ Occult blood
☐ ESR	☐ FTA	☐ Osmolality
☐ LE cell prep	☐ Hepatitis screen	☐ Phosphorus
☐ Platelet Ct	☐ HbsAb	☐ Potassium
☐ PT	☐ HbsAg	☐ Pregnancy
☐ PTT (APTT)	☐ HIV	☐ Protein
☐ RBC	☐ Monospot	☐ Sodium
☐ RBC Indices	☐ PSA screen	☐ Sp gravity
☐ Reticulocyte Ct	☐ RA factor	☐ Uric Acid
☐ Sickle cell prep	☐ RPR	
☐ WBC	☐ RSV	
☐ WBC c̄ diff	☐ Rubella screen	
☐ WBC c̄ manual diff	☐ Streptozyme	
☐ Other		

☐ Write in item ____________________

Figure 14-4 Downtime requisition for hematology, serology, and urinalysis or urine chemistry.

by a specific methodology, such as Wintrobe or Westergren.

Retics

The count of reticulocytes (immature red blood cells) determines bone marrow activity. It is used often in the diagnosis of anemia.

LE Cell Prep

LE cell prep is a diagnostic study for lupus erythematosus, an inflammatory disease.

Coagulation Studies

Studies related to clotting and bleeding are done in the hematology department. Tests may be done individually or as a panel.

PT/INR (Prothrombin Time with International Normalized Ratio)

A PT measures the clotting ability of blood. This test assists the doctor in determining the dosages of the drugs—usually warfarin (Coumadin)—prescribed in anticoagulant therapy. The HUC may be required to telephone the test results to the doctor. (Telephoned results require a "read-back" of the information and appropriate documentation.) How the results are reported depends on the testing method used, such as patient/control in seconds (e.g., 17 s/13 s); or patient/% of prothrombin activity (e.g., 14 s/70% activity).

In addition to the PT result, a result called the *international normalized ratio* (INR) is included. This is a calculation that uses the patient's PT result, the normal control result, and a coefficient factor that depends on the reagent used. The INR calculation is an attempt to standardize PT results.

APTT and PTT

The APTT (activated partial thromboplastin time) and PTT (partial thromboplastin time) are coagulation studies. These are performed individually and are commonly used to monitor heparin dosage. Actual levels of heparin (done in toxicology) may be performed in some hospitals to monitor an anticoagulant medication.

Bleeding Time

Bleeding time is the measurement of the time it takes for a standardized incision to cease bleeding. It differs from clotting time in that this test involves constriction of the smaller blood vessels. A standardized incision is an incision of specific length and depth. Several methods may be used, but template bleeding time (TBT), in which the incision is standardized by the use of a cutting device called a *template*, is preferred.

Clotting Time

Clotting time is the determination of the time it takes for blood to clot.

Coagulation Panel (Coag panel)

A coagulation panel usually consists of a PT/INR, APTT, and platelet count.

D-Dimer

The D-dimer (fragment d-dimer or fragment degradation product) may be done to diagnose deep vein thrombosis,

pulmonary embolism, or stroke. The test may not be useful if the patient has undergone invasive procedures or has an infection, has an inflammation, or is pregnant. ■

Refer to the Evolve website for other tests performed in the hematology division.

SKILLS CHALLENGE

To practice transcribing hematology and coagulation orders, complete Activity 14-1 in the *Skills Practice Manual*.

To practice transcribing daily laboratory orders, complete Activity 14-2 in the *Skills Practice Manual*.

Chemistry

The chemistry division performs tests related to the study of chemical reactions that occur in living organisms. When a disease process occurs, the levels of chemicals within the body fluids vary from normal. Any variance permits a diagnosis or evaluation of the patient's health status.

Specimens

Blood and urine are the specimens that are collected most commonly for study in this division of the laboratory. Whole blood, **plasma**, or **serum** may be used for chemistry tests. Many tests of the same name can be done on either blood or urine; therefore, often the doctor uses the word *serum* to indicate that the test is to be performed on blood and uses the term *urine* if the test is to be done on a urine specimen.

Specimens for urine chemistries may require that the urine be collected over a specified period, such as 24 hours. This is often referred to as a *24-hour urine specimen* (Fig. 14-5). It may be the HUC's responsibility to obtain the receptacle from the laboratory to be used for collection of the specimen. For some specimens that are to be kept for a period, a preservative is added to the collection bottle before it is sent to the unit. Other 24-hour specimens may have to be iced in the patient's bathroom until the collection is completed (see Box 14-1, *Chemistry Tests that May Require a 24-Hour Urine Specimen*).

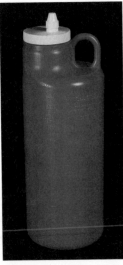

Figure 14-5 A 24-hour urine specimen container.

BOX 14-1	CHEMISTRY TESTS THAT MAY REQUIRE A 24-HOUR URINE SPECIMEN*

Albumin, quantitative and qualitative	Human chorionic gonadotropin (hCG)
Aldosterone	17-Hydroxycorticosteroids
Amino acids, quantitative-fractionated	5-Hydroxyindoleacetic acid, quantitative (5-HIAA)
Arsenic, quantitative	17-Ketogenic steroids
Calcium, quantitative	17-Ketosteroids
Catecholamines	Lactose†
Chlorides	Lead
Coproporphyrin, qualitative and quantitative	Metanephrines
Cortisol	Phosphorus
Creatine†	Porphobilinogen, quantitative
Creatinine clearance	Potassium
Epinephrine	Pregnanetriol
Epinephrine-norepinephrine	Protein, total
Estrogens, total	Sodium clearance
FIGLU (N-formiminoglutamic acid)	Uric acid†
Fluoride	Uroporphyrins, qualitative and quantitative
Follicle-stimulating hormone (FSH)	Vanillylmandelic acid (VMA)†
Glucose, quantitative†	Zinc
Homovanillic acid (HVA)	

*Check with your laboratory concerning these tests. Methods used may vary from hospital to hospital.
†Common test.

Fasting

Many blood chemistry tests require that the patient fast or be assigned NPO status. Fasting means that the patient is given nothing to eat for 8 to 10 hours before the specimen to be tested is collected; the patient may have water. NPO means nothing by mouth—food or fluid—after midnight. It may be the HUC's responsibility to notify the nutritional care department and to obtain bedside signs to be posted to remind personnel that the patient is being prepared for a test. Table 14-2 lists chemistry and other laboratory tests that require the patient to fast or be NPO. (Because some of these tests are not considered fasting by all laboratories, students should check with their instructor for the correct classification in specific hospitals.) Many fasting tests are ordered to be drawn during the routine morning draw time, because the patient is fasting naturally before breakfast.

Communication with the Laboratory

Chemistry tests are requisitioned by means of computer or by completing a downtime requisition form (Fig. 14-6).

Automated equipment permits many tests to be performed on a small sample of blood and in a short time. One requisition (or computer-entered laboratory request) is used to request a number of tests. Some of the automated instruments used are the Bayer Centaur, Dade RxL, Vitros, Paramax, Coulter (hematology), Stagos (coagulation), and Iris (urinalysis). In chemistry, these automated multicomponent studies are called *profiles, panels,* or *surveys.*

Doctors' Orders for Blood Chemistry Studies

Many chemistry tests are ordered as a group; these are called *panels* or *profiles* (see box, *Common Laboratory*

Panels). These profiles are standardized nationally according to Current Procedural Terminology (CPT) or Healthcare Common Procedure Coding System (HCPCS) guidelines so a facility may receive Medicare reimbursement. Custom panels may be designed by a facility and must be approved on an annual basis.

Note: Unless otherwise indicated, the specimen used for the following tests is serum, which is collected by nursing or laboratory personnel.

Standard Chemistry Panels
Lytes (Electrolytes)
Na, K, Cl, CO_2

BMP (Basic Metabolic Panel)
Na, K, Cl, CO_2, glucose, BUN, creatinine, and Ca

Renal Panel
Na, K, Cl, CO_2, glucose, BUN, creatinine, Ca, albumin, and phosphate

CMP (Comprehensive Metabolic Panel)
Na, K, Cl, CO_2, glucose, BUN, creatinine, Ca, albumin, total bilirubin, alk phos, total protein, AST, ALT. An outdated panel called an "SMA" or "SMAC" may still be written by some physicians, and the health unit coordinator (HUC) may need to verify exactly what chemistry tests the physician wants to be performed.

Lipid Panel
Chol, trig, HDL (HDL-C), LDL (LDL-C)

Hepatic (Liver) Function Panel
Alb, T. bili, D. bili, alk phos, T. protein, ALT (SGPT), and AST (SGOT)

TABLE 14-2 Fasting and/or NPO List for Laboratory Studies

Procedure	Fasting	NPO	Laboratory Division
Bromsulphalein (BSP)	Yes	No	Chemistry
Cholesterol	Yes	No	Chemistry
Chromosomes	Yes	No	Blood bank
Deoxycorticosterone	Yes	No	Chemistry
D-Xylose (blood or urine)	Yes	Yes	Chemistry
Electrophoresis, lipids	Yes	No	Chemistry
Electrophoresis, lipoprotein	Yes	No	Chemistry
Factor VIII assay	Yes	Yes	Coagulation
Fasting blood sugar (FBS)	Yes	No	Chemistry
Gastrin (serum)	Yes	Yes	Chemistry
Glucose, fasting (FBS)	Yes	No	Chemistry
Glucose tolerance test (GTT)	Yes	Yes	Chemistry
Insulin tolerance test (ITT)	Yes	Yes	Chemistry
Iron (Fe)	Yes	Yes	Chemistry
Iron-binding capacity (IBC)	Yes	Yes	Chemistry
Lipids	Yes	Yes	Chemistry or GI lab
Neutral fat (lipid profile fractionization)	Yes	Yes	Chemistry or GI lab
Orinase tolerance test	Yes	Yes	Chemistry
Parathyroid hormone (PTH)	Yes	Yes	Chemistry
Phenolsulfonphthalein (PSP) urine	Yes	Yes	Chemistry or GI lab
Phospholipids	Yes	Yes	Chemistry
Plasma cortisol	Yes	Yes	Chemistry
Renin	Yes	Yes	Chemistry
Schilling test	No	Yes	Chemistry
Serum lipids	Yes	Yes	Chemistry or GI lab
Testosterone	Yes	Yes	Chemistry
Total iron-binding capacity (TIBC)	Yes	Yes	Chemistry
Triglycerides	Yes	Yes	Chemistry

GI, Gastrointestinal.

COMMON LABORATORY PANELS

Electrolytes
Na
K
Cl
CO_2

BMP
Na
K
Cl
CO_2
BUN
Creat
Gluc
Ca

Renal Panel
Na
K
Cl
CO_2

Renal Panel, cont'd
BUN
Creat
Gluc
Ca
Alb
Phosphate

Hepatic Function Panel
Albumin
T. bili
D. bili
Alk phos
T. prot
AST
ALT

Cardiac Enzymes
CPK (CK)
CK-MB
Troponin
Myoglobin

CMP
Na
K
Cl
CO_2
BUN
Creatinine
Gluc
Ca
Alb
T. prot
AST
ALT
T. bili
Alk phos

Lipid Panel
Chol
Trig
LDL
HDL

CBC
RBC
WBC c̄ diff
Hb
Hct
RBC indices

Acute Hepatitis Panel
HA Ab IgM
HBcAb IgM
HBsAg
Hep C Ab

Epstein-Barr Virus Panel
EBV IgM
EBV IgG
EBV EA
EBNA

Doctor ordering _____	☐ Stat	Patient Label
Today's date _____	☐ Timed	
Draw @ date _____ Time _____	☐ Routine	
Requested by _____		

CHEMISTRY & TOXICOLOGY REQUISITION

CHEMISTRY

Panels
- ☐ Electrolytes
- ☐ BMP
- ☐ CMP
- ☐ Renal
- ☐ Hepatic
- ☐ Lipid

Tests
- ☐ Acetone
- ☐ Ace Level
- ☐ ACTH
- ☐ A/G Ratio
- ☐ Albumin
- ☐ Aldolase
- ☐ Alk Phos
- ☐ Amylase
- ☐ ALT (SGPT)
- ☐ AST (SGOT)
- ☐ Bilirubin, total
  - ☐ Direct
  - ☐ Indirect
- ☐ BNP
- ☐ BUN
- ☐ Calcium
- ☐ Carbon Dioxide
- ☐ Chloride
- ☐ Cholesterol
- ☐ Citrate
- ☐ CK (CPK)
- ☐ CKMB
- ☐ C-reactive protein
- ☐ Creatinine

CHEMISTRY CON'T

Tests cont'
- ☐ Cortisol
- ☐ Ferretin
- ☐ Folic Acid
- ☐ Folate
- ☐ FSH
- ☐ Glucose
- ☐ Glucose_____ Hr PP
- ☐ Glucose Tolerance
- ☐ Iron
- ☐ Lactic Acid
- ☐ LDH
- ☐ LH
- ☐ Lipase
- ☐ Magnesium
- ☐ Osmolality
- ☐ Osmolarity
- ☐ Phosphorous
- ☐ Potassium
- ☐ Protein
- ☐ Protein Electrophoresis
- ☐ Sodium
- ☐ TBG
- ☐ TIBC
- ☐ Triglycerides
- ☐ Troponin
- ☐ TSH
- ☐ T_3
- ☐ T_4
- ☐ Uric Acid
- ☐ VMA

TOXICOLOGY

- ☐ Acetaminophen
  - ☐ Peak
  - ☐ Trough
- ☐ Aminophylline
  - ☐ Peak
  - ☐ Trough
- ☐ Digitoxin
  - ☐ Peak
  - ☐ Trough
- ☐ Digitoxin
  - ☐ Peak
  - ☐ Trough
- ☐ Drug Screen
- ☐ Gentamycin
  - ☐ Peak
  - ☐ Trough
- ☐ Kanamycin
  - ☐ Peak
  - ☐ Trough
- ☐ Lidocaine
  - ☐ Peak
  - ☐ Trough
- ☐ Phenobarbital
  - ☐ Peak
  - ☐ Trough
- ☐ Tobramycin
  - ☐ Peak
  - ☐ Trough
- ☐ Vancomycin
  - ☐ Peak
  - ☐ Trough

☐ Write in item _____

Figure 14-6 Downtime requisition for chemistry and toxicology.

Custom Panel

An example of a custom panel is as follows.

Cardiac Enzymes or Cardiac Profile

CK (CPK) and CK-MB. A troponin I or troponin T may also be ordered. Additional tests may include isoenzymes, myoglobin, or a homocysteine level.

Each test in a panel may be ordered individually. Listed below are frequently ordered blood chemistry tests, written in abbreviated form as the doctor would write them on the doctors' order sheet. The full name of each test is given in parentheses. Normal values for common blood chemistry studies are given on p. 236.

Chemistry Tests

Alk phos (Alkaline Phosphatase)

The alkaline phosphatase level is used to evaluate bone and liver disease, among other uses.

ALT (Alanine Aminotransferase

Another name for ALT is serum glutamic-pyruvic transaminase (SGPT). This enzyme is released into the circulation by destroyed liver cells.

AST (Aspartate Aminotransferase)

Another name for AST is serum glutamic-oxaloacetic transaminase (SGOT). This enzyme is released into the circulation from destroyed skeletal or cardiac muscle, or the liver. The AST level is elevated in myocardial infarction, liver disease, acute pancreatitis, acute renal disease, and severe burns.

Serum Amylase

The level of amylase is elevated in acute pancreatitis, as well as in some other illnesses.

CPK (CK), and CK-MB

CPK (CK) and CK-MB are known as *cardiac enzymes*. These tests are ordered when a myocardial infarction (heart attack) is suspected.

CRP and hs-CRP

CRPs (C-reactive proteins) are indicators of inflammation and infections. The hs-CRP (high sensitivity C-reactive protein) can help identify cardiovascular disease and can be predictive of the future risk of heart attack, stroke, and peripheral arterial disease.

Bilirubin

This test measures liver function. Bilirubin is the result of red blood cells that have broken down and are excreted by the liver. In diseases in which a large number of red blood cells are destroyed (e.g., liver disease, obstruction of the common bile duct), a high concentration of bilirubin is found in the blood serum. The doctor may order this test as total bilirubin, using the direct or indirect method of testing.

BMP (Basic Metabolic Panel)

A BMP is a chemistry panel that consists of eight chemistry tests, including glucose, BUN, Ca, creatinine, Na, K, Cl, and CO_2.

BNP (Brain Natriuretic Peptide)

Increased levels of BNP are released when ventricular diastolic pressure rises; this may indicate congestive heart failure or increased risk of congestive heart failure or mitral valvular disease.

BS (Blood Sugar) or Glucose

A BS or glucose test is used to determine the amount of sugar in the blood. It is usually ordered at a specific time, as in *4 PM BS,* also called an *RBS.* The patient is not fasting when this test is performed.

BUN (Blood Urea Nitrogen)

This test is useful in diagnosing diseases that affect kidney function.

Cholesterol

Cholesterol levels may be used to measure liver function. The patient is usually in a fasting state for this test. It is believed that cholesterol may sometimes be responsible for causing high blood pressure and hardening of the arteries (atherosclerosis). It is important that the good blood lipids, or high-density lipoproteins (HDLs), be measured in relation to total cholesterol and low-density lipoproteins (LDLs).

CMP

A comprehensive metabolic panel consists of 14 chemistry tests, including glucose, BUN, creatinine, albumin, total bilirubin, Ca, alk phos, total protein, AST, Na, K, Cl, CO_2, and ALT.

CPK or CK (Creatine Phosphokinase or Creatine Kinase)

CPK or CK is an enzyme found mainly in the heart, brain, and skeletal muscle that is released when damage results from a disease process. Specific isoenzymes or types of CK may be ordered: CK-BB for brain, CK-MB for heart, and CK-MM for skeletal muscle damage.

Creatinine Clearance Test (12- or 24-hour Creatinine Clearance)

A creatinine clearance test is done to study kidney function. It requires testing the blood and a timed urine specimen collected for 12 or 24 hours.

Electrophoresis

Electrophoresis is a procedure performed to determine protein or fatty acid levels. The doctor may order any of three tests that result in a serum protein pattern. These tests are protein electrophoresis, lipoprotein electrophoresis, and immunoelectrophoresis.

FBS (Fasting Blood Sugar)

An FBS, also called *fasting glucose,* determines the amount of sugar in the bloodstream after the patient has not eaten for 8 to 10 hours. This test is used in the diagnosis of diabetes and monitoring of diabetes treatment.

GTT (Glucose Tolerance Test) or OGTT (Oral Glucose Tolerance Test)

A GTT (OGTT) is performed to detect abnormalities in glucose metabolism. The patient is in a fasting state. The patient has an FBS drawn to establish baseline data and then is given a large amount (75 g) of glucose solution to drink. A timed blood is taken 2 hours later. (The order has been communicated to the laboratory by requisition or computer to alert laboratory personnel to perform a fasting blood sugar test before administering the sugar solution.) An additional glucose tolerance test may include gestational diabetes screening.

A1C, HbA$_{1c}$, GHb, or GHB (Glycosylated Hemoglobin or Glycohemoglobin)

An A1C, HbA$_{1c}$, GHb, or GHB test shows the average amount of sugar in one's blood over a 3-month period. This test is used in monitoring patients with diabetes.

HDL (High-Density Lipoprotein)

An HDL "good" cholesterol level is thought to be important in the total cholesterol profile.

LDH (Lactate Dehydrogenase or Lactic Acid Dehydrogenase)

LDH is an enzyme that is released into the circulation after tissue damage to heart, liver, kidney, brain, or skeletal muscle.

Lytes (Electrolytes)

Electrolytes consist of four tests: sodium (Na), potassium (K), chloride (Cl), and carbon dioxide (CO_2). These four tests may be performed separately.

PSA (Prostatic Specific Antigen)

A PSA measures the body's level of prostatic specific **antigen.** Increased PSA levels may indicate the presence of prostate cancer.

Serum Creatinine (or Creatinine)

A serum creatinine test is performed to diagnose kidney disease. It studies the creatinine level in the blood serum.

TIBC (Total Iron-Binding Capacity)

A total iron-binding capacity test is useful in diagnosing anemia, some infections, and cirrhosis of the liver.

Troponin

Troponin is a test performed to diagnose acute myocardial infarction (AMI) from a few hours to as long as 120 hours after onset. It is more sensitive than CK-MB in detecting unstable angina with minor myocardial cell damage. Two subtypes may be ordered: troponin I and troponin T.

2-hr PP BS (2-hour Postprandial Blood Sugar)

A 2-hour **postprandial** blood sugar test is performed to assess the patient's response to carbohydrate intake. It is the HUC's responsibility to notify the laboratory when the patient has finished eating. The blood for this test may be drawn 2 hours after any meal and, if ordered for the laboratory to draw, is ordered as a "timed" draw at the specified time.

Triglycerides

Triglycerides are the principal lipids (greasy organic substances) in the blood. The patient is in a fasting state for this study, which is important in diagnosing heart disease, hypertension, and diabetes.

Uric Acid

Uric acid levels are used principally to diagnose gout. ■

NORMAL VALUES FOR FREQUENTLY PERFORMED HEMATOLOGY-COAGULATION STUDIES AND BLOOD CHEMISTRY STUDIES

Hematocrit (Hct)
- Male: 45-50 vol/dL
- Female: 40-45 vol/Dl

Hemoglobin (Hgb)
- Male: 14.5-16 g/dL
- Female: 13-15.5 g/dL

White blood cell count (WBC): 6000-9000/mm^3
Prothrombin time (PT): 12-15 sec
Sodium (Na): 132-142 mEq/L
Potassium (K): 3.5-5.0 mEq/L
Fasting blood sugar (FBS): 70-120 mg/dL

Additional Chemistry Studies

Many of the tests previously included in the special or nuclear chemistry division of the clinical laboratory or the nuclear medicine laboratory now may be performed through a non–radioisotope-based method and are now included in the chemistry division. The following studies are examples of those tests that are now performed by this division (see the Evolve website):

- CEA (carcinoembryonic antigen)
- An elevated level of CEA indicates liver, colon, or pancreatic cancer. CEA level also is used to monitor treatment of these conditions.

Examples of hormones that may be tested in chemistry include the following:
- ACTH (adrenocorticotropic hormone)
- Cortisol
- Folate
- FSH (follicle-stimulating hormone)—urine
- GH (growth hormone)
- hCG—a test for pregnancy
- LH (luteinizing hormone)
- PTH (parathyroid hormone)
- TBG (thyroxine-binding globulin)
- TSH (thyroid-stimulating hormone)
- T_3 (triiodothyronine)
- T_4 (thyroxine)
- T_7 (free thyroxine index)

⭐ **HIGH PRIORITY**

Laboratory Divisions
- Hematology: Study of physical properties of blood and other fluids, including blood cell studies and coagulation
- Chemistry: Study of changes in the levels of chemicals of the blood and other body fluids
- Toxicology: Study of poisons, their detection, their effects, and methods of treatment for conditions they produce; monitoring of drug use and detection of drug abuse
- Microbiology: Study of the organisms that cause disease; includes bacteriology, mycology, virology, and parasitology
- Serology and Immunology: Study of immunologic substances
- Pathology: Study of the nature and cause of disease, when changes in structure and function are noted
- Histology: Study of the microscopic structure of tissue
- Cytology: Study of cells obtained from body tissues and fluid
- Blood bank: Blood typing and crossmatching, storing blood and blood components for transfusion
- Urinalysis: Study of urine

 Doctors' Orders for Urine Chemistry Studies

Urine chemistry tests are listed here. Refer to the list presented earlier for tests that require a 24-hour urine collection.

Urine Glucose

Urine glucose is ordered in conjunction with blood glucose for a glucose tolerance test. Determines the amount of glucose in the urine.

Urine Creatinine

Urine creatinine usually is ordered in conjunction with the blood chemistry portion of the creatinine clearance test but may be ordered separately.

Urine Protein

An elevated urine protein is found in inflammatory diseases of the urinary system and the prostate gland.

Urine Osmolality

Urine osmolality determines the diluting and concentrating abilities of the kidneys. ■

Toxicology

Toxicology is the scientific study of poisons, their detection, their effects, and methods of treatment for conditions they produce. Tests for detecting drug and alcohol abuse and for monitoring drug usage also are performed in toxicology. Special consents, handling, and labeling may be required.

Specimens

Specimens include blood and urine.

Communication with the Laboratory

Toxicology studies are ordered by computer or by completion of a requisition form (see Fig. 14-6).

Doctors' Orders for Toxicology Studies

When doctors want to check levels of certain medications the patient is receiving, they order peak-and-trough levels (Fig. 14-7). Sometimes, toxic blood levels accumulate instead of being excreted. Antibiotics such as amikacin, gentamicin, kanamycin, and tobramycin are examples of medications ordered for peak-and-trough levels. Other medication levels may include Dilantin (random), digoxin

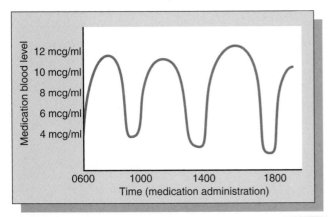

Figure 14-7 Graphic example of peak-and-trough levels of a medication.

(random), and tacrolimus (Prograf, trough level). For peak levels, the blood usually is collected 15 minutes after IV infusion and 30 to 60 minutes after IM injection. Trough levels usually require that blood be drawn 15 minutes before the next dose of medication is given to the patient. For peak-and-trough orders, the health unit coordinator (HUC) must work closely with the laboratory, nursing staff, and pharmacist to ensure proper scheduling of collections. When ordering peak-and-trough levels, the HUC would order them "timed," meaning that blood should be drawn stat at the specified time. In some cases, nursing staff will draw the peak level at the appropriate time.
- *Gentamicin peak and trough around third dose*
- *ETOH (alcohol) level now* ■

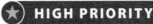

SKILLS CHALLENGE

For practice transcribing the following types of orders, please complete the following activities in the *Skills Practice Manual:*
- To practice transcribing blood chemistry orders, complete Activity 14-3.
- To practice transcribing stat laboratory orders, complete Activity 14-4.
- To practice transcribing fasting and NPO laboratory orders, complete Activity 14-5.
- To practice transcribing a review set of laboratory orders, including a toxicology order for peak and trough, complete Activity 14-6.

Microbiology

The terms *microbiology* and *bacteriology* sometimes are used interchangeably. However, large laboratories may use the broader term *microbiology* as a division name within the hospital, with areas in that division designated for bacteriology, parasitology, mycology, and virology, to name a few.

Microbiology is the study of microorganisms that cause disease. Specimens are cultured (grown in a reproducing medium) and identified with the use of biochemical tests. Identification of the causative organism of a specific disease is important because isolation procedures are based on the methods by which organisms are spread.

Bacteriology is often the largest division of microbiology. Specimens are cultured, grown in a reproducing medium, identified with the use of biochemical tests, and then tested for antibiotic sensitivity.

Parasites, organisms that live off other living organisms, are dealt with in *parasitology*. Fecal specimens are studied here for ova and parasites.

In *mycology*, cultures are set up to isolate and identify fungi. Because a fungus must grow to produce spores, these cultures may take several weeks.

Virology is the study of viruses that cause disease.

Infectious Diseases

There are many organisms with which we live that do not cause disease and are, in fact, beneficial to our health. An immunocompromised patient may, however, develop a life-threatening condition caused by an opportunistic infection with one of those organisms. Organisms that cause disease are called **pathogens.** There is an evolutionary trend of antibiotic resistance by many species of bacteria in response to exposure to antibiotics and their ability to share genetic material. A *superbug infection* or *superbug hospital-acquired infection* may be life-threatening and is difficult to treat because the pathogen has become resistant to most of the antibiotics currently available. An infection that a patient obtains while hospitalized is called a **nosocomial infection.** The HUC is an important part of the health care team in the prevention of the transmission of pathogens and may be required to post infection control precautions outside the patient's room and communicate those precautions to family members and visitors.

There are various ways in which a current infection with, past infection with, or exposure to a pathogen may be determined. The current presence of a pathogen may be determined by an attempt to grow the organism or by staining a specimen to see the actual organisms microscopically. These methods are primarily performed in the microbiology division of the clinical lab. One may study the body's reaction (antibodies) to an organism to determine if there is a current infection or if there has been a previous infection or exposure. Identification can also be done by testing for proteins specific to the pathogen or by doing special genetic tests for the pathogen's DNA or RNA. These are serologic or immunologic methods and are performed in the serology or immunology division of the lab.

 HIGH PRIORITY

The American Hospital Association analyzed and released data from the Healthcare Cost and Utilization Project (2007) and found that over 42,000 adult patients had acquired a nosocomial infection that year. These infections had extended the patients' stays by 19 days and had increased the cost of their hospital visits by over $43,000. Medicare may no longer reimburse hospitals for many of the additional costs according to the federal Deficit Reduction Act of 2005.

 HIGH PRIORITY

Superbugs, which cause superbug nosocomial infections, are pathogens that have become resistant to most of the antibiotics currently available; they often result in life-threatening infections that are extremely difficult to treat. Superbugs include the following:

MRSA	Methicillin-resistant *Staphylococcus aureus*
VRE	Vancomycin-resistant *Enterococcus*
CRKP	Carbapenem-resistant *Klebsiella pneumoniae*
C. diff	*Clostridium difficile*
MDR-TB	Multidrug-resistant tuberculosis
XDR-TB	Extensively drug-resistant tuberculosis

Specimens

Almost any type of specimen, including blood, stool, urine, sputum, bronchial washes or other body fluids, catheter tips, eye and ear drainage, and wound drainage, may be studied in the microbiology division.

Fasting

Fasting is not required for tests performed in the microbiology division of the laboratory.

Communication with the Laboratory

Microbiology tests are requisitioned via computer or by completion of a downtime requisition form (Fig. 14-8). The requisition form for the test may need to be printed by the HUC and remains on the unit until the specimen has been obtained. The physician may refer to the need to collect a specimen for a test as an "STO"—specimen to be obtained.

 Doctors' Orders for Microbiology Studies

Frequently ordered tests performed in the microbiology division, with an interpretation related to the health unit coordinator role, are listed here. For assistance with abbreviations, check the abbreviations list at the beginning of the chapter.

Bacteriology
Culture and Sensitivity (C&S)
Culture and sensitivity testing can be ordered on almost any specimen, including blood, urine, stool, sputum, wound drainage, pleural fluid, bronchial wash fluid, cerebrospinal fluid, intravenous and urinary catheters, and nose and throat specimens. The specimen is placed on an appropriate medium for growth. If organisms grow, they are tested for antibiotic sensitivity, which determines which antibiotics should be effective for treatment. Laboratory personnel, nursing staff, or the physician may be responsible for collection of the specimen.

Blood Culture (BC)
Blood culture specimens may be collected as multiple specimens (at different times or different sites) to ensure

Doctor ordering _____ ☐ Stat

Today's date _____ ☐ Timed

Collection date _____ Time _____ ☐ Routine

Collected by _____

Requested by _____

| Patient Label |

Antibiotics:

MICROBIOLOGY, FLUIDS, & CYTOLOGY REQUISITION

Microbiology

Specimen Source

☐ Abscess
_____
☐ Blood
☐ Body Cavity
_____
☐ CSF
☐ Ear Drainage
  ☐ Right
  ☐ Left
☐ Eye Drainage
  ☐ Right
  ☐ Left
☐ Nasal Smear
☐ Sputum
☐ Stool
☐ Throat
☐ Tissue
_____
☐ Urine
  ☐ Voided
  ☐ Clean Catch
  ☐ St Cath
  ☐ Foley Cath
☐ Wound Drainage _____
☐ Other _____

Test Requested

☐ AFB Culture
☐ AFB Stain
☐ C & S
☐ C & S Anaerobic
☐ C. Diff
☐ Fungal Culture
☐ GC Screen
☐ G-Stain
☐ Strep Screen
☐ Viral Culture
☐ Other
_____
☐ Stool
  ☐ Fat
  ☐ Fiber
  ☐ Occult Blood
  ☐ Ova & Parasites
    ☐ #1 of 3
    ☐ #2 of 3
    ☐ #3 of 3

Fluids

Specimen Source

☐ Abdominal
☐ Amniotic
☐ CSF
☐ Pericardial
☐ Peritoneal
☐ Pleural
☐ Synovial
☐ Other
# of Tubes _____

Test Requested

☐ Cell Count c̄ diff
☐ Glucose
☐ LDH
☐ Occult Blood
☐ Protein
☐ Sp Gravity
☐ RPR (CSF)
☐ Other
_____

Cytology

Specimen Source

☐ Amniotic
☐ Breast Bx
☐ Bronchial Asp
☐ Buccal
☐ Cervical Smear
☐ Cervical Bx
☐ Colon Bx
☐ CSF
☐ Gastric Fluid
☐ Lung Asp
☐ Pleural
☐ Pericardial
☐ Peritoneal
☐ Sputum
☐ Vaginal
☐ Other _____

Test Requested

☐ Pap
☐ Fungal
☐ Maturation Index
☐ Other
_____

Figure 14-8 Downtime requisition for microbiology, fluids, and cytology.

accurate isolation and identification of the causative organism.

AFB Culture (Acid-Fast Bacilli)
AFB culture is performed to detect the presence of acid-fast bacilli such as *Mycobacterium tuberculosis,* which causes tuberculosis. The nursing staff is responsible for collection of the specimen (usually sputum). A special stain may also be performed.

C. diff or C. difficile (Clostridium difficile) Toxin
Performed on stool specimens to identify an infection with *Clostridium difficile* bacteria. *C. diff* is transmitted easily, and infection often occurs while an individual is in the hospital (nosocomially). A patient may be placed in isolation until three consecutive results for *C. diff* toxin are negative. This

test may be ordered through microbiology or serology, because it is a swab test for the antigen.

Urine for CC (Colony Count)
The colony count is done to determine the quantity of bacteria present in a urine specimen.

Gram Stain
Gram staining is performed to classify bacteria into gram-negative or gram-positive groupings, thus allowing for differential diagnosis of the causative agent. Treatment can begin immediately, while awaiting the results of cultures.

Additional Culture Orders
Many cultures may be ordered to identify specific pathogens that cause infections. Some examples of

opportunistic organisms that may be cultured and studied include *Nocardia* and *Acinetobacter*.

Parasitology
Stool for O&P (Ova and Parasites)
This is an order that is usually ordered times three, which means that three different stool specimens (three requisition forms must be prepared) are required to determine the presence of ova (eggs) or parasites in the stool. The nursing staff is responsible for the collection of stool specimens.

Mycology
Mycology Culture
A mycology culture is performed to detect the presence of fungi. It may be performed on blood or spinal fluid specimens. Results may take several weeks to determine. Studies may be performed to determine the presence of fungi such as *Histoplasma, Coccidioides, Candida,* and *Pneumocystis jiroveci.*

Virology
Virus Culture and Virus Serology
Virus cultures may be done on any specimen; virus serology is done on a blood specimen to detect the presence of viruses or antibodies to viruses.

CMV (Cytomegalovirus) Cultures
CMV cultures are performed to detect cytomegalovirus infection. The virus is widespread and common and may be an opportunistic pathogen in an immunocompromised patient. For culture specimens, a blood (buffy coat), urine, sputum, or mouth swab may be used as a specimen. Fresh specimens are essential. The results may take about 3 to 7 days to attain. ■

SKILLS CHALLENGE

To practice transcribing microbiology and bacteriology orders, complete Activity 14-7 in the *Skills Practice Manual.*

Serology and Immunology

Serology is the study of antibodies and antigens useful in detecting the presence and intensity of a current infection. It also may be useful in identifying a previous infection or exposure to an organism. Autoimmune diseases may be studied, and pretransplant and posttransplant conditions evaluated and treated. Tests for syphilis, rheumatoid arthritis, human immunodeficiency virus (HIV), and some strains of influenza and **tissue typing** are a few of the studies done in this area.

Immunology

The response of the body to a foreign substance may include mobilization of leukocytes (white blood cells) against the foreign substance, as well as the production of certain proteins that neutralize the substance. These proteins are immunoglobulins (or more commonly antibodies) that circulate in the blood. Five main types of immunoglobulins have been identified: IgG, IgM, IgA, IgD, and IgE.

An important characteristic of antibodies is that much of the time they are produced specifically against a particular foreign substance, and they are ordered in reference to that substance. Any substance that elicits an immune response is called an *antigen.* Measurement of the **antibody** level may be ordered as a **titer.** Many serologic tests are done to detect antibody levels because antibodies are usually included in the serum portion of the blood. Serologic tests also can detect the presence of antigens.

Specimens

Most of these tests are done on the serum portion of a blood specimen. However, other body fluids such as spinal fluid and mucosal transudate (cheek swab) may be tested, along with biopsy specimens and secretions from wounds. Antigens also may be detected in stool specimens.

Fasting

Fasting is not required for tests performed in the serology division of the laboratory.

Communication with the Laboratory

Serology studies are ordered via computer or by completion of a laboratory requisition form (see Fig. 14-4).

 Doctors' Orders for Serology And Immunology

ANA (Antinuclear Antibody)
An ANA test detects the presence of certain autoimmune diseases such as systemic lupus erythematosus (SLE). There are additional tests for autoimmune diseases that determine the presence of antibodies against genetic material, such as the anti–DNase B test.

ASO Titer (Antistreptolysin O Titer)
An elevated ASO titer usually indicates the presence of a streptococcal infection, such as acute rheumatic fever.

CMV IgG (Immunoglobulin G) and IgM (Immunoglobulin M) Antibodies
Cytomegalovirus (CMV) IgG and IgM determine the levels of different types of antibodies (immunoglobulins) against cytomegalovirus. The presence of these antibodies may indicate exposure to or possible infection with cytomegalovirus.

EBV Panel (Epstein-Barr Virus)
An EBV panel determines various levels of antibodies (IgG and IgM) produced and directed against specific parts of the EBV, such as viral capsid antigen (VCA) and EBV nuclear antigen (EBNA). This can reveal whether the patient has had a recent or previous EBV infection. The specific tests in the panel are EBV VCA antibody IgM (EBV IgM); EBV VCA antibody IgG (EBV IgG); EBV early antigen antibody (EBV EA); and EBV NA antibody (EBNA).

FTA (Fluorescent Treponemal Antibody)
FTA is a serology test for syphilis.

HBsAG (Hepatitis B Surface Antigen)
HBsAg is a serum study undertaken to identify the presence of hepatitis B in the blood.

Acute Hepatitis Panel

The acute hepatitis panel includes HAAb IgM, hepatitis B core antigen (HBcAb) IgM, HBsAg, and HepC Ab. (RIBA - a method of testing used)

HIV-1 (Human Immunodeficiency Virus) Antibody Test

The HIV-1 antibody test uses oral mucosal transudate (OMT), a serum-derived fluid that enters saliva from the gingival crevice and across oral mucosal surfaces. This test is performed to screen for HIV. Additional tests (Western blot or p24 Ag) may be used for verification. A consent signed by the patient is required before HIV testing is conducted.

H. pylori AB

This is a test for the presence of antibodies against the bacterium *Helicobacter pylori,* which is implicated in the formation of gastric ulcers.

Heterophile Agglutination Test

A heterophile agglutination test is a diagnostic study for infectious mononucleosis.

RA (Rheumatoid Arthritis) Factor

An RA factor is a specific test for rheumatoid arthritis.

RPR (Rapid Plasma Reagin) Test

RPR tests are performed on blood and are screening tests for syphilis.

TB QFT-G

QuantiFERON-TB Gold is an immunologic screen for antibodies against tuberculosis *(Mycobacterium).* The results are available in a relatively short period of time, and the test may be done instead of tuberculin purified protein derivative (PPD) skin testing.

Many physicians will specify which method they prefer the serology division to use in performing this test. The method by which the physician would like a test performed should be included in the physician's order.

ELISA (Enzyme-Linked Immunosorbent Assay)

ELISA tests serum or plasma for antibodies and is widely used in the diagnosis of HIV and chlamydia. May also be called EIA (enzyme immunoassay).

RIA (Radioimmunoassay)

RIA tests serum or plasma for antibodies with the use of radioimmune reagents.

FIA (Fluorescent Immunoassay)

FIA tests serum or plasma for antibodies with the use of fluorescent reagents.

COMP FIX (Complement Fixation) or Complement Fixation Titers

Complement fixation titers are done to detect various viral, fungal, and parasitic diseases.

PCR (Polymerase Chain Reaction) or RT-PCR (Real-time Polymerase Chain Reaction)

PCR is a method by which relatively large quantities of DNA or RNA (nuclear material) may be produced from small amounts of original material. This test may be sensitive enough to detect very minute levels of antigen or antibody.

TITER

A titer is a measure of an antibody level. If the result is positive, the level of antibody present is expressed as a ratio that indicates the dilution achieved before antibodies are undetectable. An example of a low titer is 1:8; an example of a high titer is 1:2048.

Refer to Appendix F for other tests performed in the microbiology and serology divisions. ■

COMMON PATHOGENS, CAUSATIVE ORGANISMS, AND DISEASES

Bacteria
Staphylococcus (methicillin-resistant *Staphylococcus aureus* [MRSA])
Streptococcus
Group A β-hemolytic *Streptococcus* (GABHS)
Mycobacterium tuberculosis
    Mycobacterium pneumoniae
    Mycobacterium leprae (Hansen's disease)
Anthrax
Q fever
Enterococcus (vancomycin resistant enterococcus [VRE])
Escherichia coli
Nocardia
Salmonella
Clostridium
    Clostridium difficile
    Clostridium tetani
    Clostridium botulinum
Campylobacter
Borrelia (Lyme disease)

Viruses
Human immunodeficiency virus (HIV)
Hepatitis A, B, C, D, E virus (Hb, and so on)
Epstein-Barr virus (EBV)
West Nile virus (WNV)
Dengue fever
Eastern equine encephalitis virus (EEEV)
Cytomegalovirus (CMV)
Respiratory syncytial virus (RSV)
Varicella zoster virus (VZV)
Q fever

Yeast and Fungi
Candida
Aspergillus
Coccidioidomycosis (valley fever)
Tinea (ringworm)

Continued

COMMON PATHOGENS, CAUSATIVE ORGANISMS, AND DISEASES—cont'd

Protozoans
Amoeba
Plasmodium (malaria)
Giardia
Toxoplasmosis
Brucellosis
Trichomoniasis

Parasites
Scabies and lice
Tapeworms
Pinworms
Trichinosis (undercooked pork)
Botflies

Sexually Transmitted Diseases
Trichomoniasis (protozoan)
Chlamydia trachomatis (bacterium)
Neisseria gonorrhoeae (bacterium)
Syphilis (bacterium—*Treponema pallidum*)
Human papillomavirus (HPV)
Genital herpes (virus—herpes simplex virus type 2 [HSV-2])
Human immunodeficiency virus (HIV)

★ HIGH PRIORITY

It is important for the health unit coordinator (HUC) to be accurate when antibody levels are ordered. An immunoglobulin M (IgM) level generally checks for an acute or current infection, whereas an IgG level checks for "long-term" antibodies and may indicate immunity resulting from previous exposure or infection. (This is an important distinction for HUC students who may need to show immunity against certain diseases before a clinical class placement).

◎ SKILLS CHALLENGE

To practice transcribing serology orders, complete Activity 14-8 in the *Skills Practice Manual*.

Blood Bank

The blood bank, which is usually a part of the clinical laboratory, has the responsibilities of typing and crossmatching patient blood, obtaining blood for transfusions, storing blood and blood components, and keeping records of transfusions and blood donors.

Before whole blood, packed cells, and some other blood components are administered, the patient must undergo a **type and crossmatch**. This is a test that determines the patient's blood type and compatibility, and requires testing on each unit of the blood product being transfused.

The four major blood groups are A, B, AB, and O:

- Patients with type A blood may receive transfusions of types A and O.
- Patients with type B may receive transfusions of types B and O.
- Patients with type AB may receive transfusions of types A, B, AB, and O.
- Patients with type O may receive only type O blood transfusions.

This laboratory division also performs several other blood studies, including Coombs' tests. In a direct Coombs' test, which is also known as a direct antiglobulin test (DAT), a positive result is found in hemolytic disease of the newborn, hemolytic transfusion reactions, and acquired hemolytic anemia. The indirect Coombs' test detects the presence of antibodies to red blood cell antigens. This test is valuable in detecting the presence of anti-Rh antibodies in the serum of a pregnant woman before delivery. A **type and screen** is performed to determine the patient's blood type and Rh factor, and a general antibody screen is performed. Antibody screening is a test to detect atypical antibodies in the serum that may have been formed as a result of transfusion or pregnancy. Because the transfusion of blood and blood components is a treatment administered by nursing personnel, additional information on various types of blood transfusions (autologous, donor directed, and autotransfusion) is provided in Chapter 11.

★ HIGH PRIORITY

An order for transfusion of whole blood, packed red blood cells, and some other blood components automatically indicates that blood will be typed and crossmatched. Additional communication with the blood bank may be necessary when packed cells are ordered to verify if there is a current crossmatch (blood bank tube drawn within 3 days) for the patient. If there is a current crossmatch, it is not necessary to draw additional blood.

Specimen

A specimen of blood is used for blood bank orders.

Fasting

Fasting is not required for this procedure.

Communication with the Laboratory

Blood bank orders are requisitioned via computer or by completion of a downtime requisition form (Fig. 14-9). The number of units to be given and the names of the blood components are items that are included on this requisition.

Doctor ordering _____ ☐ Stat
Today's date _____ ☐ Routine
Collection date _____ Time _____
Collected by _____
Requested by _____

BLOOD BANK REQUISITION

☐ Routine   ☐ ASAP   ☐ Stat   ☐ For Hold

Patient Label

Date of Surgery _____   Date of Transfusion _____

Autologous Blood? ☐ Yes ☐ No   ☐ Whole Blood   # of Units _____
Donor Specific?   ☐ Yes ☐ No   ☐ Packed Cells   # of Units _____
☐ Type and X-match   ☐ Washed Cells   # of Units _____
☐ Type and Screen   ☐ Frozen Cells   # of Units _____
                                      ☐ Fresh Frozen Plasma   # of Units _____
☐ Coombs' Test   ☐ Platelet Concentrate   # of Units _____
☐ Other _____   ☐ Cryoprecipitate   # of Units _____
                                      ☐ Other _____

Comments _____
_____
_____
_____
_____

Figure 14-9 Downtime requisition for blood bank.

A blood transfusion consent must be signed before blood or blood products are administered. The patient may sign a refusal of blood transfusion form.

Doctors' Orders for Blood Bank

Listed here are examples of doctors' orders for blood component administration. (Refer to Chapter 11 for examples of blood, blood components, and plasma substitutes.)

- T&C for 2 Units packed cells
- Packed cells, 1 Unit (need type and crossmatching)
- FFP, 3 Unit stat (fresh frozen plasma)
- Give washed cells 1 Unit (need type and crossmatching)
- Cryoprecipitate (cryo) 1 Unit
- Give 2 Unit of platelets (plat or plts) (no crossmatching needed, but donor plasma and recipient red blood cells should be ABO (major human blood group system) compatible
- Normal serum albumin 5% (no crossmatching)
- T&C 6 U pc—hold for surgery in AM ■

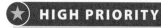

SKILLS CHALLENGE

To practice transcribing blood bank orders, complete Activity 14-9 in the *Skills Practice Manual.*

Urinalysis

The **urinalysis** division of the laboratory studies urine specimens for color, clarity, pH (degree of acidity or alkalinity), specific gravity (degree of concentration), protein (albumin), glucose (sugar), blood, bilirubin, and urobilinogen. Sediment is viewed microscopically for organisms, intact cells, and crystals.

Specimen

Urine is the specimen that is used for this test; however, the doctor may indicate that the nursing staff should follow a special procedure to obtain the specimen.

Procedures for Obtaining Urine Specimens

- Voided urine specimen: The patient voids into a clean container.
- **Clean catch**, or midstream, urine specimen: The nursing staff uses a special cleansing technique to obtain this type of specimen.
- Catheterized urine specimen: This specimen is sterile and is obtained by catheterizing the patient. This procedure is usually done for culture and sensitivity testing, which is performed by the microbiology department.

Urine specimens that are collected at an unspecified time are called **random specimens**. However, the preferred collection time for a urine specimen is early morning on arising.

Fasting

Fasting is not required for a urinalysis.

Communication with the Laboratory

Orders for urinalysis are entered into the computer, or a downtime requisition form (see Fig. 14-4) is used. Once again, the requisition is held on the nursing unit until the specimen has been collected, or the order is entered when the specimen has been obtained. The labeled specimen with the requisition or computer printout is sent to the laboratory.

 Doctors' Orders for Urinalysis

Listed here are examples of doctors' orders for urinalysis.
- Cath UA
- Clean catch UA
- **Dipstick urine** for ketones
- UA today
- **Urine reflex** (urine is tested in the laboratory; if certain parameters are met, the specimen is sent to the microbiology department to be cultured)

A urine specimen is sent to the laboratory. All regular urinalysis studies are performed, except that the specimen is not examined microscopically. ■

 HIGH PRIORITY

Points to Remember When Ordering Laboratory Studies
- Determine whether the test ordered is a point-of-care test or whether the specimen must be sent to the laboratory.
- All tests ordered require a specimen.
- Each specimen sent to the lab from the nursing unit requires a requisition and must be accurately labeled with the patient ID label and with the date, the time, and the initials of the person who collected the specimen written on the label.
- Include on the requisition the date and time of collection, the specimen source, and the name of the person who collected the specimen if collected by personnel on the unit.
- Order tests as efficiently as possible to avoid the necessity for specimens to be redrawn (e.g., routines with stats).
- Communicate stat laboratory tests immediately to the lab and/or nursing personnel, and include all pertinent information.

 SKILLS CHALLENGE

To practice transcribing urinalysis and urine chemistry orders, complete Activity 14-10 in the *Skills Practice Manual*.

The following tests may be sent to several of the laboratory departments for testing.

Studies Performed on Pleural Fluid

Studies are performed on pleural fluid to determine the cause and nature of pleural effusion, including hypertension, congestive heart failure (CHF), cirrhosis, infection, and neoplasms.

Specimen

Pleural fluid is obtained when the doctor performs a **thoracentesis**. The patient must sign a consent form for this procedure.

Fasting

Fasting is not required for tests performed on pleural fluid.

Communication with the Laboratory

The doctor orders tests to be done on the specimen, and the HUC enters the orders into the computer or completes a downtime requisition (see Fig. 14-8). As with any nonretrievable specimen obtained by invasive procedures, it should be labeled accurately, should be transported to the laboratory immediately, and should not be sent through a pneumatic tube system.

 Doctors' Orders for Pleural Fluid

Following are listed examples of doctors' orders for tests performed on pleural fluid:
- Thoracentesis, pleural fluid to lab for LDH, glucose, and amylase. Cl: Cancer
- Pleural fluid for cell count, diff
- Pleural fluid for C&S ■

Studies Performed on Cerebrospinal Fluid

Studies are performed on cerebrospinal fluid (CSF) to identify various brain diseases or injuries.

Specimen

Cerebrospinal fluid (CSF) is obtained when the doctor performs a lumbar puncture. The patient must sign a consent form before this procedure can be performed.

Fasting

Fasting is not required for tests performed on CSF.

Communication with the Laboratory

When cerebrospinal fluid (CSF) is obtained, it is inserted into three, possibly four (sterile) specimen tubes. The doctor orders tests to be done on each specimen tube. The HUC enters the respective tests into the computer or completes a requisition form. The doctor indicates in the orders the tube that should be used for each test (usually three or four tubes). The HUC enters this information into the computer or writes it on the requisition. It is sometimes the HUC's responsibility to transport these specimens to the laboratory or the transport department is called and an employee is sent to transport the specimens to the laboratory. It is important that the CSF specimen tubes are labeled accurately and transported to the laboratory immediately. Because they are difficult to obtain and gathering them again would cause the patient further pain, CSF specimens are never sent via pneumatic tube.

Doctors' Orders for Cerebrospinal Fluid

Following are examples of doctors' orders performed on cerebrospinal fluid (CSF):
- Lumbar puncture, fluid to lab for cell count and diff
- CSF for serology
- CSF to lab for tube 1-cell count, protein, and glucose; tube 2-AFB and fungal culture; tube 3-Gram stain ■

SKILLS CHALLENGE

To practice transcribing cerebrospinal fluid orders, complete Activity 14-11 in the *Skills Practice Manual.*

Pathology

Pathology is the study of the nature and cause of disease as seen in body changes. Histology and cytology are subdivisions of the pathology department. A pathologist is in charge of the pathology department.

Histology is the study of the microscopic structure of tissue. **Cytology** is the study of cells obtained from body tissues and fluids to determine cell type and to detect cancer or a precancerous condition.

Specimens

Organs, tissue, cells, and body fluids obtained from biopsies, centeses, **sternal punctures,** lumbar punctures, surgeries, and autopsies are studied in the pathology department. A **Pap smear** is a staining method developed by Dr. George Nicolas Papanicolaou that can be performed on various types of specimens to identify the presence of cancer. However, cells from the cervix are the most frequently studied specimens (cervical smear). During a pelvic examination, the doctor may remove tissue or cells from the cervix for study.

RECORDING LABORATORY RESULTS

The results of laboratory tests are a valuable tool for the doctor in the diagnosis and treatment of patients; therefore test result values are often communicated to the doctor before the computer report can be placed on the patient's chart. Stat and/or abnormal laboratory test results are communicated verbally or by telephone to the doctor by the HUC or nurse. The doctor may request on the doctors' order sheet that laboratory test results be communicated to him or her by telephone immediately on completion of the test.

To verbally communicate laboratory results, laboratory personnel call the HUC on the nursing unit, who records results on a telephone laboratory report sheet (Fig. 14-10). Laboratory results also may be accessed via computer and printed by the HUC. Results from an outside laboratory may be faxed to the nursing unit. Printed results include the **reference range,** or range of normal values, for each laboratory test (Fig. 14-11). The HUC should report values to the patient's nurse, who

may request that the results be called in to the doctor's office. Although the task may appear simple to perform, it demands great responsibility, because the doctor may prescribe treatment according to the laboratory values conveyed. Consider for a moment what the consequences could be should the value be recorded inaccurately. To avoid errors, the HUC should always read the laboratory values he or she has recorded back to the person in the laboratory. Always have the person taking information in the doctor's office repeat recorded values back to you. The written report should be placed in the patient's chart in a timely manner. Accuracy in selection of the correct patient's chart and of the appropriate location in the chart is very important.

★ HIGH PRIORITY

The health unit coordinator must notify the nurse or physician caring for the patient immediately when a *critical (panic) value is* called into the unit by laboratory personnel. The result of the lab test is such that it is outside of the normal limits (range) of acceptable values to the extent that it can be life-threatening without immediate medical intervention. (See message taking in Chapter 4).

SKILLS CHALLENGE

For practice transcribing the following types of orders, complete the following activities in the *Skills Practice Manual:*
- To practice transcribing a review set of laboratory orders, complete Activity 14-12.
- To practice transcribing a review set of doctor's orders, complete Activity 14-13.
- To practice recording telephone messages, complete Activity 14-15.
- To practice recording telephoned laboratory results, complete Activity 14-16.

KEY CONCEPTS

Laboratory studies are very useful in facilitating patient diagnosis and evaluation of treatment. Accuracy in ordering tests and sending specimens is of utmost importance because an error could result in a delay in diagnosis and/or treatment. It is imperative that all specimens be properly labeled according to hospital policy and sent or delivered to the laboratory in a timely manner.

One of the challenges for a HUC is to become familiar with the particular hospital's process of requisitioning laboratory orders. Become familiar with the various laboratory screens on the computer. It may be necessary to identify the division in which a test is performed before completing the correct requisition or entering the order into the computer. This information is helpful in telephone communication when one is clarifying orders or requesting results. Most hospital units have a written laboratory procedure manual. If this is not the case, call the hospital laboratory help desk to have your questions answered.

Websites of Interest

Staph SuperBugs and MRSA Super Bugs: www.staph-infection-resources.com/mrsa-superbugs.html

TELEPHONED LABORATORY RESULTS

Patient's name _____ Report called by _____
Room number _____ Report taken by _____
Date _____ Time _____

HEMATOLOGY	**CHEMISTRY**	**URINE**
RBC _____	GLUCOSE	COLOR _____
Hgb _____	Random _____	APPEARANCE _____
Hct _____	FBS _____	PH _____
WBC _____	E'LYTES	SP. GRAVITY _____
lymphs _____	Na _____	ACETONE _____
monos _____	K _____	GLUCOSE _____
neutros _____	Cl _____	BACTERIA _____
eos _____	CO_2 _____	WBC _____
basos _____	CARDIAC STUDIES	RBC _____
PLATELETS _____	SGOT _____	CASTS _____
RETICS _____	LDH _____	OCCULT BLOOD _____
SED RATE _____	CPK _____	OTHER
OTHER	BNP _____	
	Troponin _____	
	CALCIUM _____	
	PHOS _____	
	BUN _____	
	CREATININE _____	
	OTHER _____	

COAGULATION

BLEEDING TIME _____
COAGULATION TIME _____
PROTIME _____
  Patient _____
  Control _____
  % _____
PT
  Patient _____
  Control _____
  INR _____
PTT _____

TELEPHONED BLOOD GAS REPORT

Patient's name _____
Room number _____
Date _____ Time _____
Report called by _____
Report taken by _____

O_2 CONCENTRATION _____
O_2 TENSION _____
CO_2 TENSION _____
PH _____
ACT BICARB _____
BASE EXCESS _____
O_2 SAT _____

Figure 14-10 Telephoned laboratory test results form.

Guidelines for Laboratory Testing and Result Reporting of Antibody to Hepatitis C Virus: www.cdc.gov/mmwr/preview/mmwrhtml/rr5203a1.htm JCAHO Practice Alerts—"Blood Transfusion Errors": www.nysna.org/practice/alerts/alert29.htm
Healthline—"Nosocomial Infections": www.healthline.com/gale content/nosocomial-infections

⊖ REVIEW QUESTIONS

Visit the Evolve website to download and complete the following exercises.

1. Define the following terms:

   a. biopsy
   b. antibody
   c. pathogen
   d. lumbar puncture
   e. amniocentesis
   f. occult blood
   g. postprandial
   h. sputum
   i. sternal puncture
   j. urinalysis
   k. paracentesis
   l. dipstick urine
   m. plasma

2. List two general purposes of laboratory studies.

3. Name three major divisions and five other divisions of the laboratory.

4. List five specimens that may be studied in the laboratory, and list at least three specimens that would be obtained by an invasive procedure.

5. Identify six invasive procedures that would require a consent form signed by the patient.

Quest Diagnostics Incorporated

PATIENT INFORMATION
SPENCER, SUSAN

REPORT STATUS **Final**

Sonora Quest Laboratories, LLC
CLIENT SERVICE 602.685.5000

DOB: 07/25/1957 Age: 54
GENDER: F   Fasting: N

ORDERING PHYSICIAN
TURNER, JOSEPH
CLIENT INFORMATION
2017
TEMPE FAMILY PRACTICE
6655 S. RURAL RD., #3
TEMPE, AZ 85283

SPECIMEN INFORMATION
SPECIMEN: E45674008
REQUISITION: 20170293421
LAB REF NO:

ID: 10118513
PHONE: 4809219608

COLLECTED: 06/13/2012   14:31
RECEIVED: 06/14/2012   00:41
REPORTED: 06/14/2012   08:27

Test Name	In Range	Out of Range	Reference Range	Lab
CMP,CBC				
CMP,CBC				PAZ
WBC	5.8		4.0-11.0 k/mm3	
RBC	4.41		3.70-5.40 m/mm3	
HEMOGLOBIN	13.5		11.5-16.0 g/dL	
HEMATOCRIT	40.7		35.0-48.0 %	
MCV	92		78-100 fL	
MCH	30.6		27.0-34.0 pg	
MCHC	33.2		31.0-37.0 g/dL	
RDW(cv)	13.2		12.1-18.2 %	
RDW(sd)	44.6		36.0-55.0 fL	
PLATELET COUNT	268		130-450 k/mm3	
MPV	11.7		7.5-14.0 fL	
SEGMENTED NEUTROPHILS	60		40-85 %	
LYMPHOCYTES	31		10-45 %	
MONOCYTES	6		3-15 %	
EOSINOPHILS	2		0-7 %	
BASOPHILS	0		0-2 %	
ABSOLUTE NEUTROPHIL	3.5		1.6-9.3 k/uL	
ABSOLUTE LYMPHOCYTE	1.8		0.6-5.5 k/uL	
ABSOLUTE MONOCYTE	0.4		0.1-1.6 k/uL	
ABSOLUTE EOSINOPHIL	0.1		0.0-0.7 k/uL	
ABSOLUTE BASOPHIL	0.0		0.0-0.2 k/uL	
DIFFERENTIAL TYPE	Automated			
CMP,CBC				PAZ
GLUCOSE	79		65-99 mg/dL	

Glucose reference range reflects fasting state.

Test Name	In Range	Out of Range	Reference Range	Lab
UREA NITROGEN (BUN)	12		8-25 mg/dL	
CREATININE	0.79		0.60-1.40 mg/dL	
GFR ESTIMATED	85		>60 mL/min/1.73m2	

In African Americans, the calculated eGFR should be multiplied by 1.16.

Test Name	In Range	Out of Range	Reference Range	Lab
BUN/CREAT RATIO	15.2		10.0-28.0	
SODIUM	137		135-145 mmol/L	
POTASSIUM	4.2		3.5-5.2 mmol/L	
CHLORIDE	101		96-110 mmol/L	
CARBON DIOXIDE (CO2)	25		19-31 mmol/L	
ANION GAP	11		4-18	
PROTEIN,TOTAL	7.2		6.0-8.0 g/dL	
ALBUMIN	4.5		3.3-4.9 g/dL	
GLOBULIN	2.7		2.0-3.7 g/dL	
ALB/GLOB RATIO	1.7		1.0-2.0	
CALCIUM	9.0		8.4-10.6 mg/dL	

SPENCER, SUSAN - E45674008

Page 1 - Continued on Page 2

Figure 14-11 Laboratory results printout.

Continued

Quest Diagnostics Incorporated

Sonora Quest Laboratories, LLC

PATIENT INFORMATION
SPENCER, SUSAN

REPORT STATUS **Final**

ORDERING PHYSICIAN
TURNER, JOSEPH

REPORTED: 06/14/2012   08:27
COLLECTED: 06/13/2012   14:31

DOB: 07/25/1957 Age: 54
GENDER: F   Fasting: N
ID: 10118513

Test Name	In Range	Out of Range	Reference Range	Lab
CMP,CBC (Continued)				
CMP,CBC (Continued)				
ALKALINE PHOSPHATASE	57		39-170 IU/L	
ALT	17		2-46 IU/L	
AST	22		10-41 IU/L	
BILIRUBIN, TOTAL	0.4		0.2-1.3 mg/dL	
LIPID PANEL				PAZ
CHOLESTEROL		216 H	<200 mg/dL	
TRIGLYCERIDE	132		<150 mg/dL	
HDL CHOLESTEROL	71		>45 mg/dL	
NON-HDL	145		<160 mg/dL	
LDL CHOLESTEROL, CALC.	119		<130 mg/dL	

For moderately high risk and high risk cardiac patients reference
levels of <100 mg/dl and <70 mg/dl, respectively, should be
considered. Circulation 2004; 110:227-239.

VLDL CHOLESTEROL	22		0-29 mg/dL	
CHOL/HDL RATIO	3.0		<4.5	
THYROID CASCADE PROFILE				PAZ
TSH	2.36		0.45-4.50 mU/L	

Performing Laboratory Information:

PAZ Sonora Quest Laboratories 1255 W. Washington Tempe AZ 85281

SPENCER, SUSAN - E45674008

Page 2 - End of Report

Figure 14-11, cont'd Laboratory results printout.

6. Describe the health unit coordinator's responsibilities in sending specimens to the laboratory.

7. Describe how the following studies would be ordered and performed:
   a. routine
   b. stat
   c. daily
   d. timed

8. List three tests that would be performed at the bedside (POCT) to detect occult blood in gastric and stool specimens.

9. Describe the general purpose of the hematology division, and list six studies that would be performed in the hematology division.

10. Describe the general purpose of the chemistry division, and list six studies that would be performed there.

11. List six blood tests and four urine chemistry studies, and list four tests that are included in electrolytes.

12. Identify at least three chemistry tests that would require the patient to be fasting.

13. Explain the difference between fasting and NPO.

14. Explain the HUC responsibilities for ordering a 2-hr postprandial.

15. Describe the general purpose of the toxicology department, and explain the procedure for ordering peak and trough levels.

16. Describe the general purpose of the microbiology division of the laboratory, and list six studies that would be performed there.

17. Describe the general purpose of the serology and immunology division of the laboratory, and list three tests performed there.

18. Describe the general purpose of the blood bank, and identify the steps that must be performed to obtain blood (packed cells) for transfusion.

19. Describe the general purpose of the urinalysis division of the laboratory, and identify three methods of obtaining urine specimens.

20. Identify the procedure that would be performed to obtain pleural fluid and CSF, and explain the importance of accurate labeling and appropriate transportation of these specimens.

21. Describe the purpose of the pathology division of the laboratory, and identify and describe the purpose of two subdivisions of the pathology division.

22. Describe how errors may be avoided in recording telephoned laboratory results (critical or panic values).

SURFING FOR ANSWERS

1. Research the most common nosocomial infections and the associated costs to treat them, and identify the website used.
2. Research and document the number of deaths caused by nosocomial infections annually, and identify the website used.
3. Locate and document the most recent legislation related to reimbursement to hospitals for nosocomial infections, and identify the website used.
4. Locate and watch videos that demonstrate a physician performing a lumbar puncture, an amniocentesis, and a thoracocentesis, and identify the websites used.

CHAPTER 15

Diagnostic Imaging Orders

OUTLINE

CHAPTER OBJECTIVES

On completion of this chapter, you will be able to:

1. Define the terms in the vocabulary list.
2. Write the meaning of the abbreviations in the abbreviations list.
3. Explain how the health unit coordinator's responsibilities regarding diagnostic imaging orders differ with the implementation of the electronic medical record and computer physician order entry versus use of the paper chart.
4. List the information regarding the patient that the health unit coordinator must include when ordering procedures to be performed by the diagnostic imaging department.
5. Explain the respective roles of a radiographer and a radiologist.
6. Explain the benefits of picture archiving and communication systems for the patient and the doctor.
7. Name five patient positions that may be included in a diagnostic imaging order.
8. Identify diagnostic imaging orders that do not require routine preparation.

9. Explain when a patient would be required to sign an informed consent before a diagnostic imaging procedure.
10. Explain why contrast media are used, and list types commonly used.
11. Discuss sequencing or scheduling of multiple diagnostic imaging procedures ordered for the same patient.
12. Identify four diagnostic imaging procedures that would require routine preparation, and explain the importance of preparing the patient before these procedures.
13. Explain the purpose of special invasive x-ray and interventional procedures, and list at least three procedures performed in this division of the radiology department.
14. Describe an instruction the doctor would include when ordering computed tomography (CT), and list at least three CT procedures.
15. Describe the purpose of ultrasonography procedures, and list at least three procedures performed in the ultrasonography department.
16. Discuss the purpose of magnetic resonance imaging (MRI) procedures and the purpose of magnetic resonance angiography (MRA) procedures.

17. Discuss the importance of a patient's nurse completing the interview form before the patient undergoes MRI or MRA, and list contraindications that would exist for patients because of the strength of the magnet.
18. Discuss the purpose of nuclear medicine procedures, and list at least three nuclear medicine procedures.

VOCABULARY

C-Arm A mobile fluoroscopy unit used in surgery or at the bedside.

Cathartic An agent that causes evacuation of the bowel (laxative).

Clinical Indication Notation recorded when diagnostic imaging is ordered that indicates the reason for doing the procedure.

Computed Radiology Use of a digital imaging plate rather than film.

Computed Tomography A radiographic process that uses ionizing radiation to create computerized images (scans) of body organs in sections or that can be coronal, sagittal, or three-dimensional (referred to as *CT scans*).

Contrast Media Substances (solids, liquids, or gases) used in diagnostic imaging procedures that permit the radiologist to distinguish among various body soft tissue structures; may be injected, swallowed, inhaled, or introduced by rectum.

Fluoroscopy The direct observation of deep body structures made visible through the use of a real-time viewing screen instead of film; a contrast medium is required for this procedure.

Magnetic Resonance Angiography Use of magnetic resonance to study blood vessels.

Magnetic Resonance Imaging A technique used to produce computer images (scans) of the interior of the body with the use of a powerful magnetic field and radiofrequency waves.

Metastasis The process by which tumor cells spread to distant parts of the body.

Modality A method of application or employment of any therapeutic agent, limited usually to physical agents and devices.

Nuclear Medicine A branch of medicine that uses radioactive isotopes for the diagnosis and treatment of disease.

"On-Call" Medications Medications prescribed by the doctor to be given before a diagnostic imaging procedure is performed; the department notifies the nursing unit of the time the medication is to be administered to the patient.

Picture Archiving and Communication Systems (PACSs) Computers or networks dedicated to the storage, retrieval, distribution, and presentation of images. Full PACSs handle images from various modalities, such as ultrasonography, magnetic resonance imaging, positron emission tomography, computed tomography, endoscopy, mammography, and digital radiography.

Portable X-ray An x-ray study taken with a mobile x-ray machine that is moved to the patient's bedside.

Position Alignment of the body on the x-ray table that is favorable for taking the best view of the part of the body being imaged.

Radiography The process of obtaining film records (radiographs) of internal structures of the body.

Routine Preparation The standard preparation suggested by the radiologist to prepare the patient for a diagnostic imaging study.

Scan An image produced with the use of a moving detector or a sweeping beam; image is produced by computed tomography, magnetic resonance imaging, nuclear medicine, or ultrasonography.

Special Invasive X-ray and Interventional Procedures Procedures that involve diagnosing and treating patients using the least invasive techniques currently available in order to minimize risk to the patient and improve health outcomes.

Ultrasonography A technique that uses high-frequency sound waves to create an image (scan) of body organs (may also be referred to as *sonography* or *echography*).

ABBREVIATIONS

Abbreviation	Meaning	Example of Usage on a Doctor's Order Sheet
abd	abdomen, abdominal	US of abd
AP	anteroposterior	chest AP & Lat
BE	barium enema	BE in AM
CI	clinical indications	BE-CI: tumor
CT	computed tomography	CT scan of abd
CXR	chest x-ray examination	CXR today
DSA	digital subtraction angiography	cerebral DSA
F/U	follow-up	F/U CXR in AM
Fx	fracture	x-ray lt femur CI: fx
GB	gallbladder	US of GB
GI	gastrointestinal	GI study in am
H/O	history of	CXR H/O chronic asthma
IVP	intravenous pyelogram	
IVU	intravenous urogram; synonymous with IVP	IVU CI: Kidney stones
KUB (also called a *flat plate of abdomen*)	kidneys, ureters, and bladder	KUB today
L&S	liver and spleen	L&S scan tomorrow (nuclear medicine)
lat	lateral	PA & Lat chest today
LLQ	left lower quadrant	flat plate of abd att LLQ
LUQ	left upper quadrant	abd x-ray special attention to LUQ
LS	lumbosacral	x-ray LS spine (x-ray)

mets	metastasis	bone scan to determine mets
MRA	magnetic resonance angiography	MRA of cerebral arteries
MRI	magnetic resonance imaging	MRI of brain
PA	posteroanterior	PA & lat chest x-ray
PACS	picture archiving and communication system	The CXR may be viewed via PACS
PCXR	portable chest x-ray	PCXR stat
PET	positron emission tomography	PET scan tomorrow AM (nuclear medicine)
PTC or PTHC	percutaneous transhepatic cholangiography	PTC or PTHC tomorrow
RIS	radiology information system	x-ray report is available in RIS
RLQ	right lower quadrant	x-ray of abd: Compare c̄ preoperative x-ray
RUQ	right upper quadrant	Check RUQ and RLQ
SPECT or SPET	single-photon emission computed tomography	SPECT L/S spine CI: back pain
SBFT	small bowel follow-through	UGI c̄ SBFT
SNAT	suspected nonaccidental trauma	SNAT series CI: abuse
UGI	upper gastrointestinal	*UGI p̄ IVU*
US	Ultrasound	US of GB
VQ	Ventilation/perfusion (quotient)	VQ scan CI: shortness of breath

⊜ EXERCISE 1

Write the abbreviation for each term listed.

1. intravenous pyelogram
2. right lower quadrant
3. kidneys, ureters, and bladder
4. barium enema
5. posteroanterior
6. upper gastrointestinal
7. lateral
8. lumbosacral
9. left upper quadrant
10. anteroposterior
11. gastrointestinal
12. right upper quadrant
13. computed tomography
14. left lower quadrant
15. gallbladder
16. magnetic resonance imaging
17. small bowel follow-through
18. chest x-ray
19. digital subtraction angiography
20. portable chest x-ray
21. percutaneous transhepatic cholangiography
22. fracture
23. history of
24. follow-up
25. clinical indications
26. intravenous urogram
27. ultrasound
28. Picture Archiving and Communication System
29. positron emission tomography
30. liver and spleen
31. radiology information system
32. abdomen
33. metastasis
34. suspected nonaccidental trauma
35. single-photon emission computed tomography
36. ventilation/perfusion (quotient) scan

⊜ EXERCISE 2

The following is a list of orders for imaging procedures that may appear on patients' charts. Write the meaning of each underlined abbreviation.

1. BE tomorrow p̄ sigmoidoscopy
2. Stat LS spine x-ray
3. KUB this AM
4. US for fetal age
5. Abd x-ray c̄ attention to RLQ & LUQ
6. IVU & UGI tomorrow. Check with radiologist for prep.
7. CT of brain
8. GI study c̄ barium swallow
9. PA & lat chest now
10. MRI of brain
11. PCXR now
12. UGI c̄ SBFT
13. L & S scan in AM
14. PET scan in AM
15. CT c̄ DSA of head
16. SNAT series CI: abuse

COMMUNICATION WITH THE DIAGNOSTIC IMAGING DEPARTMENT

The diagnostic imaging department may also be called *medical imaging*. Many modalities, including **radiography**, **nuclear medicine**, **ultrasound**, **computed tomography** (CT), and **magnetic resonance imaging** (MRI), are included in the diagnostic imaging department. Diagnostic imaging procedures are performed to diagnose conditions and/or diseases (or to rule them out) and to assist the doctor in determining treatment. When the electronic medical record (EMR) with computer physician order entry (CPOE) is implemented, the doctors' diagnostic imaging orders are entered directly into the patients' EMR and are automatically

★ HIGH PRIORITY

When the electronic medical record (EMR) with computer physician order entry (CPOE) is implemented, the physicians' orders are entered directly into each patient's electronic record, and the diagnostic imaging order is automatically sent to the diagnostic imaging department. The health unit coordinator (HUC) may have tasks to perform, such as coordinating scheduling, ordering special diets, and so forth. An icon indicating an HUC task may appear, or the icon may signify a nurse request. The HUC will have to communicate with the nutritional care department (by e-mail or telephone) when ordering a diet for a patient who has completed a diagnostic procedure that required nothing by mouth (NPO) status.

Note: Some hospital nutritional care departments require that *all* diet orders be submitted in writing via computer.

Doctor ordering _____			Patient Label
Today's date _____	☐ Stat ☐ Routine ☐ ASAP		
Date to be done _____	Requested by _____		

RADIOGRAPHIC (X-RAY) PROCEDURES REQUISITION

Clinical indication _____

Transportation   ☐ Portable   ☐ Stretcher   ☐ Wheelchair   ☐ Ambulatory

O₂ ☐Yes /☐ No   Diabetic ☐Yes /☐ No   Hearing deficit ☐Yes /☐ No

IV ☐Yes /☐ No   Seizure disorder ☐Yes /☐ No   Sight deficit ☐Yes /☐ No

Isolation ☐Yes /☐ No   Non-English speaking ☐Yes /☐ No

Write out the entire doctor's order

Comments _____

☐ Abdomen _____
☐ Bone age study _____
☐ Bone x-ray order _____
☐ Chest order _____
☐ IVP _____
☐ KUB / flat plate of abdomen _____
☐ KUB order _____
☐ Mammogram _____
☐ Sinus series order _____
☐ SNAT series _____
☐ Spine order _____
☐ BE _____
☐ SBFT _____
☐ UGI _____
☐ Write in order _____

Figure 15-1 Downtime requisition for x-ray procedures.

sent to the diagnostic imaging department. When paper charts are used the diagnostic imaging orders are communicated by the ordering step of transcription via computer or by completion of a downtime requisition form (Fig. 15-1). Because the patient usually is transported to the diagnostic imaging department for the procedure, it is important to indicate the mode of transportation—wheelchair or gurney (stretcher). The patient may be transported by the diagnostic imaging department staff, transport service, or nursing department staff.

A portable or mobile x-ray examination is an exception to the standard transportation procedure. A request for a **portable x-ray** requires the radiographer to take the portable equipment to the patient's room. A portable x-ray examination is ordered when movement might be detrimental to the patient's condition. A written order from the patient's physician is required for a portable x-ray examination.

A **C-Arm** is a mobile fluoroscopy unit used at the bedside and also in surgery. It allows for lower x-ray doses to be used on patients by magnifying the intensity produced in the output image, enabling the viewer to easily see the structure of the object being imaged.

When ordering the diagnostic procedure, indicate the following information about the patient:

- reason for procedure (clinical indication)
- transportation required
- whether patient is receiving intravenous fluids

- whether patient is receiving oxygen
- whether patient needs isolation precautions
- whether patient has a seizure disorder
- if patient does not speak English
- whether patient is diabetic
- whether patient is sight or hearing impaired
- whether patient is pregnant or if pregnancy test results are pending

This information will assist personnel in the diagnostic imaging department to provide better care for the patient (see Fig. 15-1). The doctor may write the name of the radiologist who will perform an invasive procedure. The health unit coordinator (HUC) should include this information when entering the order or scheduling the test.

⭐ **HIGH PRIORITY**

Clinical indication (the reason the doctor is ordering the procedure) must be recorded by the HUC when a diagnostic imaging procedure is ordered. Insurance companies require this information before they will provide reimbursement to health care facilities. Diagnostic imaging departments will not perform procedures until they have received documented clinical indications. The clinical indication should be a symptom or complaint rather than a diagnosis.

HIGH PRIORITY

Downtime requisitions are included in this chapter for learning purposes. The Evolve website associated with the *Skills Practice Manual for Health Unit Coordinating* includes a simulated hospital computer program that may be used as well.

HIGH PRIORITY

A written order from the patient's physician is required to perform an x-ray stat or as a portable examination. The physician's original order for a routine x-ray study cannot be changed to "portable" or "stat" for convenience or because the original order was missed. If the nurse determines that the patient needs the x-ray examination stat or via the portable x-ray unit, the patient's physician would have to be called for a change to the original order.

BACKGROUND INFORMATION FOR RADIOLOGY

In 1895, Wilhelm Roentgen discovered a strange phenomenon that produced a photograph of the bones of his wife's hand. The exact mechanism for the production of these rays was unknown to Roentgen; therefore he used the algebraic symbol for the unknown, *x*, to title his discovery.

X-ray studies performed in the radiology area of the diagnostic imaging department are carried out by a *radiographer*, a person with special education in the area of radiography. X-ray images are developed in the department and are interpreted by a *radiologist*, a doctor who is a specialist in this field. Some studies are done by observing the path of contrast media in the body by means of **fluoroscopy**. Physicians' orders do not always include the word "x-ray." For example, "Chest PA & Lat" indicates a chest x-ray examination that includes two views (posteroanterior and lateral). Some procedures scheduled in the radiology area must be carried out in specific sequence so that the contrast medium necessary for one procedure does not block the image of another. **Computed radiology** is the use of a digital imaging plate rather than film. The digital image can be viewed and enhanced using software that has functions very similar to other conventional digital image–processing software, such as contrast, brightness, filtration, and zoom.

PICTURE ARCHIVING AND COMMUNICATION SYSTEM

Picture archiving and communication systems (PACSs) are computers or networks dedicated to the storage, retrieval, distribution, and presentation of images. Full PACSs manage images from various modalities, such as ultrasonography, MRI, positron emission tomography, CT, endoscopy, mammography, and radiography (plain x-ray images). PACSs replace hard copy–based means of managing medical images, such as film archives. PACSs provide off-site viewing and reporting (distance education, telediagnosis).

When a study has been reported by the radiologist, the PACS can mark it as read; this avoids needless double reading. Dictation of reports can be integrated into a single system.

The dictated recording is automatically sent to a transcriptionist workstation for typing; it also can be made available for access by physicians, avoiding typing delays for urgent results, or retained in cases of typing error. The report can be attached to the images and be viewable to the physician.

Physicians at various physical locations may access the same information simultaneously.

Global PACSs and other networks enable images to be sent throughout the world. These systems provide growing cost and space advantages over film archives. PACSs should interface with the existing hospital information system (HIS), the information technology (IT) department, and the radiology information system (RIS). An icon indicating a diagnostic medical image in a patient's medical record would allow the physician to view the image and the radiologist's report. Benefits for the doctor include faster results, ability to compare an image with a previous image (if applicable), ability to share with other physicians, and reduced risk of film loss. Benefits for the patient include reduction in treatment delays, reduced risk of film loss, and protection of confidentiality. An additional benefit is noted for the environment, in that x-ray photographic darkroom chemicals and toxins are eliminated from the process.

PATIENT POSITIONING

The doctor may wish an x-ray image to be taken while the patient is placed in a specific **position** on the x-ray table or erect (e.g., chest studies) to allow the best view of the area to be exposed. The HUC must be careful to include all of the x-ray order without making any changes, and to be absolutely accurate when transcribing such orders. For example, the HUC should not write AP (anteroposterior) when the order calls for PA (posteroanterior) positioning. The wrong abbreviation can cause the radiographer to film a different view, which may obscure an abnormality.

Following is a list of the positions used most frequently in the writing of x-ray orders:

- *AP position:* This view may be taken while the patient is standing or lying on the back (supine); the machine is placed in front of the patient.
- *PA position:* This view may be taken while the patient is standing or lying on the stomach (prone) with the x-ray machine aimed at the patient's back.
- *Lateral position:* This view is taken with the patient standing or lying on the side.
- *Oblique position:* This picture is taken with the patient standing or lying halfway on the side in the AP or the PA position.
- *Decubitus position:* In this view, the patient is lying on the side with the x-ray beam positioned horizontally.

HIGH PRIORITY

Examples of procedures performed in each of the modalities of diagnostic imaging are included in this chapter. They are too numerous to list, but the examples provided are a good representation of procedures that are performed in each **modality**.

RADIOGRAPHIC (X-RAY OR GENERAL DIAGNOSTIC) PROCEDURES

X-ray Examinations that Do Not Require Preparation (Plain Radiographs or Plain X-ray Images)

X-rays can penetrate solid material, such as bone; this in turn produces a shadow that is recorded on film. Procedures that require the filming of bone structures or that are ordered to determine the position of other organs in relation to these structures can be performed by qualified radiology personnel without the need for preparation for the procedure (Fig. 15-2).

Following are x-ray studies as they commonly are written on a doctors' order sheet.

Doctors' Orders for X-Ray Examinations that Do Not Require Preparation

Sinus Series CI: Sinusitis
X-ray examination of the paranasal sinus structures.
Purpose: Used to identify infection, trauma, or disease in the paranasal sinuses.

PA and Lat Chest CI: Pneumonia
Chest x-ray examination. (Frequently, *x-ray* is not written on the order because some terms in the order are recognized as directions used only in radiography. The terms *PA* and *lat* indicate the angles from which the doctor wishes the film to be taken.)
Purpose: Used to diagnose or assess patients with pneumonia, pneumothorax, or atelectasis, or to check for infiltrates. A chest x-ray image also is used to determine the size and position of the heart or for placement of invasive lines or tubes.

SNAT Series CI: Evaluate for Child Abuse
Purpose: X-ray examination of long bones, skull, and spinal column to evaluate for hairline fractures and untreated fractures to identify child or adult abuse.

Bone Age Study CI: FTT (Failure to Thrive)
Purpose: An x-ray examination of the wrist of an infant to evaluate the child's growth.

LS Spine Series CI: Possible Fracture
X-ray examination of the lumbosacral area of the spine.
Purpose: Used to detect and evaluate abnormalities of the lumbosacral region.

Mammogram CI: Lump 10 Degrees Lt Breast
X-ray examination of the breast.
Purpose: Used to detect cancer or cysts in the soft tissue of the breast.

X-ray of the Tibia with Close Attention to the Distal Portion CI: Fracture
X-ray of the bone in the patient's lower leg. *Distal* indicates that the radiologist is to observe a particular portion of the bone. Remember to include the entire order on the requisition.
Purpose: Used to identify fractures.

KUB (also called a *flat plate of abdomen*) CI: General Survey of the Abdomen
X-ray examination of the abdomen.
Purpose: Used to detect and evaluate any abnormalities in the abdomen.

Portable Film of Rt Femur CI: Fx
A radiographer takes a portable x-ray machine to the patient's bedside to film the right upper leg of the patient. It is important for the health unit coordinator (HUC) to write *portable* on the requisition form.
Purpose: Used to identify fractures.

Postreduction X-ray of the Lt Forearm
X-ray examination of the left forearm.
Purpose: Used to evaluate the alignment of a fracture after intervention. The clinical indication should be recognized as a "postreduction" study by the HUC.

AP and Lat Rt Hip CI: Postop Eval of Hip Replacement
X-ray of the right hip (*AP* and *lat* indicate the angles from which the doctor wishes the film to be taken).
Purpose: Used postoperatively to evaluate prosthetic replacement of the hip. Done at the bedside.

DEXA Scan (Bone Density) CI: Possible Osteoporosis
Dual energy x-ray absorptiometry imaging—an imaging system to assess bone mineral density.
Purpose: Used to measure the bone mineral density (BMD) in order to determine bone strength and the ability of the bone to bear stress. Another method of measuring bone density is quantitative computed tomography (QCT). Although significant patient preparation is not needed, the patient may need to skip certain bone-building medications the day of the examination. The patient must not have had a nuclear medicine or computed tomography study in the days before a DEXA scan. ∎

SKILLS CHALLENGE

To practice transcribing radiology (x-ray) orders that require no preparation, complete Activity 15-1 in the *Skills Practice Manual.*

Informed Consent and Other Forms

Diagnostic imaging procedures that are invasive and those that require the injection of contrast media are not performed until the patient has been informed about the procedure, risks, alternatives, outcomes, and so forth and has signed a consent form. It is the responsibility of the HUC to prepare the consent form for the patient's signature. Special invasive x-ray and interventional procedures require a signed consent. Other diagnostic imaging procedures that require a consent form may vary among health care facilities. Some studies (such as MRIs) require the completion of a "contraindications" form. Maintaining a list of procedures that require a signed consent form or contraindications form would assist the HUC in recalling them.

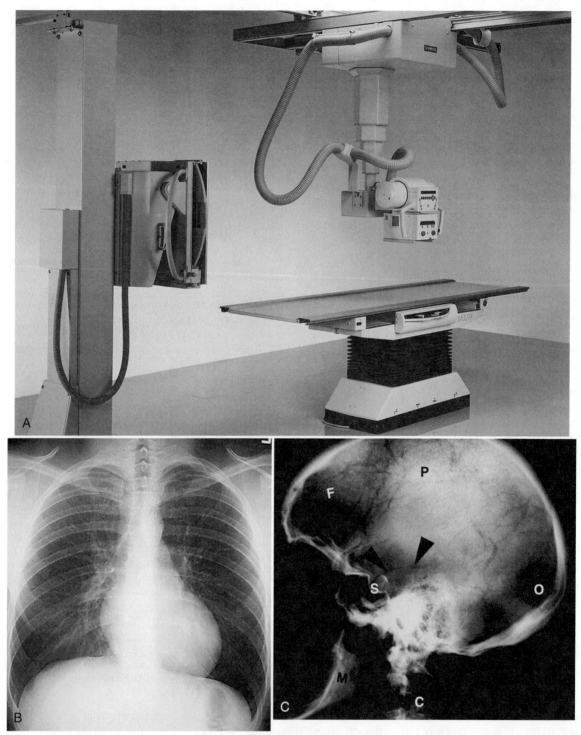

Figure 15-2 **A,** Radiographic table with chest unit. **B,** Chest x-ray image. **C,** Skull x-ray image, lateral view. Pointers indicate fracture line in temporal bone. *C,* Cervical vertebra; *F,* frontal bone; *M,* mandible; *O,* occipital bone; *P,* parietal bone; *S,* sella turcica. (**A** from Ballinger PW, Frank ED: *Merrill's atlas of radiographic positions and radiologic procedures,* ed 10, St Louis, 2003, Mosby. **B** from Bontrager KL, Lampignano JP: *Textbook of radiographic positioning and related anatomy,* ed 6, St Louis, 2005, Mosby. **C** from Pagana KD, Pagana TJ: *Diagnostic testing and nursing implications: a case study approach,* ed 4, St Louis, 1994, Mosby.)

X-ray Examinations that Require Preparation and Contrast Media

When an x-ray examination is performed, images of varying density appear on the exposed image. Differences in density are a result of the degree of absorption offered by different tissues and air to the radiation. It is easy to differentiate bony structures because the bones offer resistance and therefore appear light on the image. The lungs, however, which contain air, do not offer much resistance to radiation and appear black on the image. Certain organs and blood vessels within the body are difficult for the radiologist to see because there is little difference in density between them and their surrounding parts. To increase the contrast, it is necessary for a *contrast medium* to be given to the patient.

Contrast media consist of organic iodine compounds, barium preparations, air, water, gas, and, with nuclear medicine procedures, radiopharmaceuticals. Contrast media may be injected or taken into the body by mouth, inhalation, or rectum. Contraindications to the use of iodine compounds include allergy to shellfish and previous reactions to iodinated studies. For a contrast medium to prove most effective, the patient must be prepared for the procedure before it is scheduled. This process is known as a *routine preparation*, and the routine most often is established by the diagnostic imaging department.

The attending doctor may change the routine preparation if the patient's condition warrants. Specific changes to the routine preparation must be written on the doctors' order sheet by the patient's doctor. Sometimes a contrast medium used for one procedure may interfere with results obtained in another scheduled procedure. Therefore if multiple x-ray procedures are ordered, proper sequencing is necessary for clear results to be obtained. Sequencing is outlined by the diagnostic imaging department and varies among hospitals.

HIGH PRIORITY

If the patient is not properly prepared, the procedure will need to be canceled, causing a delay in diagnosis and treatment, perhaps a delay in discharge for the patient, and delays in the radiology department.

Sequencing and Scheduling

Following are typical guidelines for scheduling x-ray studies:

1. X-ray studies of the lower spine and pelvis should be ordered first, before a barium enema (BE) or an upper gastrointestinal (UGI) study is done. The presence of barium in specific parts of the body may obscure the portion of the body that is being studied.
2. Abdominal studies that use ultrasound or CT should precede studies that use barium.
3. Liver and bone scans and nuclear medicine studies may conflict with barium studies and should be done first.
4. Three x-ray studies that require contrast media frequently are ordered at the same time for diagnostic reasons. Only one or sometimes two can be done on the same day; thus studies may have to be scheduled

3 or more days in advance. The order of scheduling is as follows:
a. Intravenous urogram (IVU)
b. BE
c. UGI study or UGI and small bowel follow-through (SBFT)

HIGH PRIORITY

When transcribing diagnostic imaging orders, the health unit coordinator should do the following:
1. Record the clinical indication when entering the order.
2. Record the necessary mode of transportation when entering the order.
3. Record necessary patient information when entering the order.
4. Check whether a consent form is necessary; if so, prepare one for signature.
5. Check whether patient preparation is required; if so, communicate this to the appropriate nursing personnel.
6. Check whether scheduling is required; if so, schedule the procedure for the proper day and/or time.

Accuracy in performing these steps is vital for reaching the expected outcome.

Preparation Procedure

To visualize internal organs with the use of contrast media, **routine preparation** usually is required. Most of the preparation is done by the nursing staff, and preparatory steps may begin the day before the x-ray study is scheduled.

Following are examples of doctors' orders for x-ray examinations that require the patient to have some type of preparation. Each procedure and preparation is explained to help establish its relationship to the others and to clarify the role of the HUC.

Many hospitals have a computer system that automatically prints out the routine preparation when a procedure is entered. Some hospitals have preparation cards, that is, cards that list the tasks to be done to prepare the patient for the x-ray study. When a patient is scheduled for one of the x-ray procedures that require preparation, the computer printout or the preparation card usually is placed in the patient's Kardex form holder to remind the nursing staff of the tasks they need to perform.

Note: Preparation procedures vary among hospitals.

Table 15-1 provides an overview of the radiology procedures covered in this section, including both those that do not require preparation and those that do require preparation and contrast media.

📋 Doctors' Orders for X-Ray Procedures that Require Preparation and Contrast Media

BE CI: Lesion of the Colon

This procedure is used for visualization of the large intestine (Fig. 15-3). Barium contrast medium is introduced rectally in the patient for this test in the diagnostic imaging department. *Note:* This is not a therapeutic enema such as those discussed in Chapter 11.

TABLE 15-1 Overview of Radiology

X-rays are a form of electromagnetic radiation, similar to visible light. A computer or a special film is used to record the images that are created.

Examples of Radiology Procedures that Do Not Require Preparation or Contrast Media

Procedure	Purpose
Skeletal x-ray studies	To diagnose abnormalities, disease, and fractures of bones
Chest posteroanterior and lateral views (PA and lat)	To evaluate for surgery and diagnose obstructions, abnormalities, and disease
Kidneys, ureters, and bladder (KUB)	To diagnose abnormalities, obstructions, and disease within the abdomen
Suspected nonaccidental trauma (SNAT) series	To identify abuse (child or adult)
Bone age study	To assess development and growth of child

Examples of Radiology Procedures That Do Require Preparation or Contrast Media

Barium enema (BE)	To identify diseases of the large intestine (e.g., diverticula, cancer, ulcerative colitis)
Intravenous urogram (IVU) (or intravenous pyelogram [IVP])	To diagnose abnormalities, strictures, disease of the urinary system
Upper gastrointestinal (UGI) study	To detect hiatal hernia, strictures, ulcers, or tumors

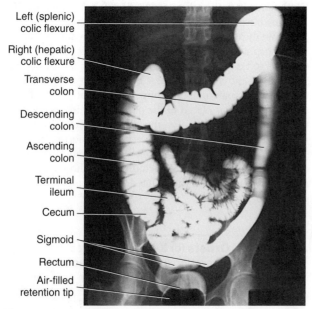

Left (splenic) colic flexure

Right (hepatic) colic flexure

Transverse colon

Descending colon

Ascending colon

Terminal ileum

Cecum

Sigmoid

Rectum

Air-filled retention tip

Figure 15-3 Barium enema showing contrast medium (barium) filling the intestines. (From Ballinger PW, Frank ED: *Merrill's atlas of radiographic positions and radiologic procedures,* ed 10, St Louis, 2003, Mosby.)

Purpose: Used to identify diseases of the large intestine such as diverticula, cancer, or ulcerative colitis.

Patient preparation:

- Cathartic PM and AM before the procedure
- Low-residue diet (Jello, simple broths) 8 to 12 hours before the examination
- NPO 2400 hours

Transcribing the order: In addition to transcribing the order for a barium enema, the health unit coordinator (HUC) would initiate diet changes and alert the nurse about any medications that are to be given in preparation. The doctor may wish to order an air contrast barium enema, which requires the same preparation as a barium enema but uses air as well as barium for the contrast medium.

Barium Swallow (Esophagogram) CI: Dysphagia

This procedure uses fluoroscopy, a viewing screen, and an x-ray machine to examine the esophagus after the patient drinks a barium solution.

Purpose: Used to detect strictures, ulcers, or tumors.

Patient preparation:

- NPO 8 to 12 hours before the procedure

Transcribing the order: The HUC would transcribe the order and initiate the diet change.

AN EXAMPLE OF A PREPARATION FOR A BARIUM ENEMA

Barium Enema

Citrate of Magnesia 1 bottle 2 PM on day before examination

Fleets enema HS day before examination, & repeat @ 6 AM on day of examination

NPO 2400 hours

IVU (synonymous with IVP; IVU is becoming the more common usage) CI: Ureterolithiasis

IVU is a procedure performed to outline the kidney, particularly the renal pelvis, ureters, and urinary bladder (Fig. 15-4). Contrast is established by injecting an iodinated contrast medium into the patient's vein. The injection takes place after the patient has been transported to the diagnostic imaging department.

Purpose: Used to determine the size, location, and function of the kidneys, ureters, and bladder and to identify the presence of abnormalities such as tumors or strictures.

Patient preparation:

- NPO 8 to 12 hours before the procedure is to be performed
- Some physicians write orders to hydrate the patient before the examination.

Transcribing the order: In addition to transcribing this order, the HUC would order the diet changes and prepare a consent form.

UGI c̄ SBFT CI: Peptic Ulcer

This procedure uses fluoroscopy, a viewing screen, and an x-ray machine to examine the distal portion of the esophagus, stomach, and small intestines after the patient drinks a barium solution.

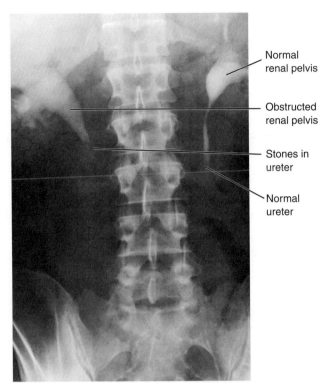

Normal renal pelvis

Obstructed renal pelvis

Stones in ureter

Normal ureter

Figure 15-4 Intravenous urogram (IVU) showing a distended urinary collecting system obstructed by a stone in the right ureter *(left side of figure)*. The left collecting system is normal in size and is unobstructed. (Intravenous pyelogram [IVP] and IVU are the same; IVU is used more commonly.) (From Pagana KD, Pagana TJ: *Mosby's manual of diagnostic and laboratory tests,* ed 3, St Louis, 2006, Mosby.)

Purpose: Used to detect hiatal hernia, strictures, ulcers, or tumors.

Patient preparation:
- NPO 8 to 12 hours before the procedure

Transcribing the order: The HUC would transcribe the order and initiate the diet change. ■

SKILLS CHALLENGE

To practice transcribing radiology (x-ray) orders that require preparation and contrast medium, complete Activity 15-2 in the *Skills Practice Manual.*

SPECIAL INVASIVE X-RAY AND INTERVENTIONAL PROCEDURES

Special invasive x-ray and interventional procedures are performed under the direction of a radiologist or are performed by an interventional radiologist. This division is also referred to as *interventional radiology* or *surgical radiology.* Special invasive x-ray and interventional radiology uses minimally invasive image-guided procedures to diagnose and treat diseases in nearly every organ system. The interventional radiologist combines expertise in performing procedures with knowledge of routine diagnostic imaging. A treatment procedure often immediately follows a diagnostic procedure (e.g., after a patient has undergone heart

catheterization, he or she may have stent placement immediately performed by an interventional radiologist specializing in cardiology). A request for the use of a special x-ray room or operating room must be submitted in advance by the doctor, or the procedure may be scheduled by computer as part of the transcription procedure. A downtime requisition is shown in Figure 15-5. The patient is required to sign a consent form, as procedures are invasive and contrast media are often used. (See Chapter 8 for use and preparation of a consent form.)

Special invasive x-ray and interventional procedures may be performed with or without a general anesthetic. When a general anesthetic is used, the nursing staff follows specific preoperative and postoperative routines (see Chapter 19). Preparations for these studies vary among hospitals.

The radiologist, interventional radiologist, and/or surgeon may prescribe preprocedure medications to be given at a specific time or "on call." When **on-call medications** are ordered, the doctor or department personnel, at the request of the radiologist and/or surgeon, notify the nursing unit to administer the medication.

Table 15-2 provides an overview of the special invasive x-ray and interventional procedures covered in this section. *Note:* There are many more diagnostic and treatment procedures than are listed in this table.

 Doctors' Orders for Special Invasive X-Ray and Interventional Procedures

PTC CI: Obstruction of the Bile Ducts
Visualization of the bile ducts through injection of iodine contrast directly into the biliary system.
Purpose: Usually done to determine the cause of obstruction, jaundice, or persistent upper abdominal pain after cholecystectomy.
Patient preparation: Special preparation may or may not be ordered.
Transcribing the order: Routine transcription

Carotid Angiogram CI: Aneurysm
An angiogram is a visualization of vascular structures within the body after injection of contrast medium (Fig. 15-6). The specific name given to the study is determined by the vascular structure to be studied (e.g., renal angiogram, cerebral angiogram).
Purpose: Used to diagnose vascular aneurysms, malformations, and occluded or leaking blood vessels.

Lower Abdominal Angiogram CI: Angiodysplasia
X-ray examination of a blood vessel after injection of contrast medium (Fig. 15-7). An angiogram may be identified according to its anatomic location (e.g., femoral angiogram).
Purpose: Used to detect obstruction or narrowing of a blood vessel or aneurysm.

Arthrogram of the Left Knee CI: Torn Ligament
X-ray examination of a joint after injection of contrast medium.
Purpose: Used to detect trauma, such as bone chips or torn ligamenta, resulting from an injury.

Doctor ordering _____

Today's date _____ ☐ Stat ☐ Routine ☐ ASAP

Date to be done _____ Requested by _____

Patient Label

SPECIAL INVASIVE X-RAY PROCEDURES REQUISITION

Clinical indication _____

Transportation ☐ Portable ☐ Stretcher ☐ Wheelchair ☐ Ambulatory

O₂ ☐ Yes / ☐ No   Diabetic ☐ Yes / ☐ No   Hearing deficit ☐ Yes / ☐ No

IV ☐ Yes / ☐ No   Seizure disorder ☐ Yes / ☐ No   Sight deficit ☐ Yes / ☐ No

Isolation ☐ Yes / ☐ No   Non-English speaking ☐ Yes / ☐ No

Write out the entire doctor's order

Comments _____

☐ Angiogram _____

☐ Arteriogram _____

☐ Arthrogram _____

☐ Cervical myelogram _____

☐ Cholangiogram _____

☐ Hysterosalpingogram _____

☐ Lymphangiogram _____

☐ PTC _____

☐ Spinal myelogram _____

☐ Venogram _____

☐ Voiding cystourethrogram _____

☐ Write in order _____

Figure 15-5 Downtime requisition for special invasive x-ray and interventional procedures.

Cholangiogram, Postoperative (T-Tube Cholangiogram) CI: Retained Stones

X-ray image taken 1 to 3 days after a cholecystectomy to examine the bile ducts. Examination is done after contrast medium has been injected through a T tube.

Purpose: Used to rule out residual stones in the biliary tract after a cholecystectomy. It is called *T-tube cholangiogram* because the catheter placed in the biliary ducts during surgery is called a *T tube.*

Hysterosalpingogram CI: Obstruction of Fallopian Tubes

X-ray examination of the uterus and fallopian tubes taken after injection of contrast medium.

Purpose: Used in fertility studies and to confirm abnormalities such as adhesions, fistulas, and so forth.

Lymphangiogram Left Leg CI: Lymphatic Obstruction

X-ray of the lymph channels and lymph nodes taken after injection of contrast medium.

Purpose: Used to identify metastatic cancer **(metastasis)** in the lymph nodes and to evaluate the effectiveness of chemotherapy.

Spinal Myelogram CI: Cord Compression Due to HNP (Herniated Nucleus Pulposus)

X-ray examination of the spinal cord after contrast medium has been injected between lumbar vertebrae into the spinal canal.

Purpose: Used to detect herniated disks, tumors, and spinal nerve root injuries.

Venogram of Left Leg CI: DVT (Deep Vein Thrombosis)

X-ray examination of a vein, usually in the lower extremities, after injection of contrast medium.

Purpose: Used to evaluate veins before and after bypass surgery and to investigate venous function when obstruction is suspected (Fig. 15-8).

Voiding Cystourethrogram (VCUG) CI: Bladder Dysfunction

X-ray films are taken to demonstrate the bladder filling then emptying as the patient voids.

Purpose: Used to demonstrate bladder dysfunction and urethral strictures.

Note: Endoscopies, including ERCP (endoscopic retrograde cholangiopancreatography), are covered in Chapter 16. ∎

SKILLS CHALLENGE

To practice transcribing orders for special invasive x-ray and interventional procedures, complete Activity 15-3 in the *Skills Practice Manual.*

TABLE 15-2 Overview of Special Invasive X-Ray and Interventional Procedures

Special invasive x-ray and interventional procedures are performed under the direction of the radiologist or performed by an interventional radiologist or a surgeon with a radiologist present. A signed consent is required for special invasive x-ray and interventional procedures, and contrast media are often used. "On-call" medication may or may not be ordered by the patient's doctor. There are many more diagnostic and treatment procedures than listed here.

Examples of Special Invasive X-Ray and Interventional Procedures

Procedure	Purpose
Arthrogram	To identify trauma, such as bone chips or torn ligaments, resulting from injury
Angiogram	To diagnose vascular aneurysms, malformations, and occluded or leaking blood vessels
Voiding cystourethrogram	To demonstrate bladder and urethral strictures
Venogram	To evaluate veins before and after bypass surgery and for obstruction
Spinal myelogram	To detect herniated disks, tumors, and spinal nerve root injuries
Hysterosalpingogram	To confirm abnormalities, such as adhesions and fistulas, and to be used in fertility studies
Lymphangiogram	To identify metastatic cancer in lymph nodes and to evaluate chemotherapy treatment

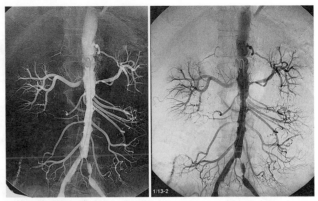

Figure 15-7 Lower abdomen angiogram, with digital subtraction angiogram (DSA) image on right. (From Bontrager KL, Lampignano JP: *Textbook of radiographic positioning and related anatomy*, ed 6, St Louis, 2005, Mosby.)

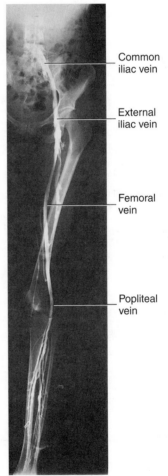

Common iliac vein

External iliac vein

Femoral vein

Popliteal vein

Figure 15-8 Normal venogram, lower left limb. (From Ballinger PW, Frank ED: *Merrill's atlas of radiographic positions and radiologic procedures*, ed 10, St Louis, 2003, Mosby.)

COMPUTED TOMOGRAPHY

Computed tomography uses a type of ionizing radiation (x-rays) to provide a computerized image that can generate multiple two-dimensional cross sections (slices) (Fig. 15-9). Spiral, helical, and three-dimensional rendering CT provides three-dimensional reconstructions. Contrast media

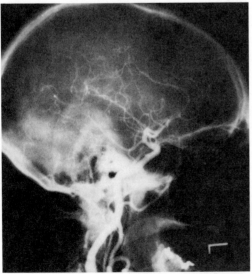

Figure 15-6 Carotid angiogram. (From Chipps E, Clanin N, Campbell V: *Neurologic disorders*, St Louis, 1992, Mosby.)

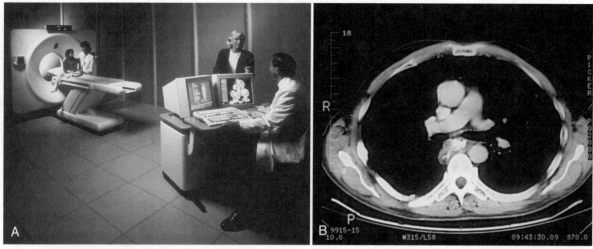

Figure 15-9 A, Computed tomography (CT) scanner. **B,** CT scan of the chest with intravenous (IV) contrast medium. (From Ballinger PW, Frank ED: *Merrill's atlas of radiographic positions and radiologic procedures,* ed 10, St Louis, 2003, Mosby.)

Doctor ordering			
Date to be done	☐ Stat	☐ Routine	☐ ASAP
Today's date	Requested by		

COMPUTED TOMOGRAPHY REQUISITION

Patient Label

Clinical indication _____

☐ With contrast ☐ Without contrast

Transportation ☐ Portable ☐ Stretcher ☐ Wheelchair ☐ Ambulatory

O₂ ☐Yes /☐ No   Diabetic ☐Yes /☐ No   Hearing deficit ☐Yes /☐ No
IV ☐Yes /☐ No   Seizure disorder ☐Yes /☐ No   Sight deficit ☐Yes /☐ No
Isolation ☐Yes /☐ No   Non-English speaking ☐Yes /☐ No

Write out the entire doctor's order
Comments _____

☐ CT scan of head _____
☐ CT scan of brain _____
☐ CT scan of abdomen _____
☐ CT scan of pelvis _____
☐ CT scan of spine _____
☐ CT of neck _____
☐ CT-guided liver biopsy _____
☐ DSA _____
☐ HIDA scan _____
☐ Write in order _____

Figure 15-10 Downtime requisition for computed tomography.

may or may not be used. If used, contrast media may include iodine-based agents given intravenously, gas or air introduced rectally for colon studies, or water given orally (e.g., for CT of the stomach). When writing the order, the doctor must indicate whether the procedure is to be performed with or without contrast. (Figure 15-10 shows a downtime requisition for CT.)

Table 15-3 provides an overview of the CT procedures covered in this section.

Doctors' Orders for Computed Tomography (CT) Scans

CT of Head DSA CI: Aneurysm
Combines angiography, fluoroscopy, and computer technology to visualize cerebrovascular structures without the interference of bone and soft tissue structures that may obscure the image.

TABLE 15-3 Overview of Computed Tomography (CT) Procedures

CT uses a type of ionizing radiation to provide a computerized image that can generate multidimensional sections (slices) of tissue. A contrast medium may or may not be used.

Examples of Computed Tomography Procedures

Procedure	Purpose
CT of head c̄ DSA	To evaluate postoperatively (e.g., endarterectomy) and to detect cerebrovascular abnormalities
Chest CT	To detect lung changes, pneumonia, cancer, pulmonary embolism, aortic dissection, and other conditions
Abdominal CT	To detect cancer, aortic aneurysm, bowel obstruction, and other conditions
Head CT	To diagnose brain tumor, infarction, bleeding, and hematoma
LS spine CT	To confirm spinal stenosis and changes in disks and vertebrae, and to confirm spinal infection
SPECT	To diagnose many structural and functional changes

DSA, Digital subtraction angiography; *LS,* lumbosacral; *SPECT,* single-photon emission computer tomography.

Purpose: Used to evaluate postoperatively (e.g., endarterectomy) and to detect cerebrovascular abnormalities.

CT Scan of Abd CI: Evaluate Carcinoma

A CT scan is often the preferred method for diagnosing many different cancers because the image allows a physician to confirm the presence of a tumor and to measure its size, its precise location, and the extent of its involvement with nearby tissue.

Purpose: Used to diagnose and determine stage of cancer and to follow its progress. CT also may be used to diagnose abdominal aortic aneurysm, bowel obstruction, and other conditions.

CT Scan of the Brain CI: Tumor

Computerized analysis of multiple images of brain tissue.

Purpose: Used to diagnose brain tumor, infarction, bleeding, and hematoma.

Patient Preparation: The patient is usually NPO for several hours before the procedure.

CT Scan of Abdomen and Pelvis CI: Retroperitoneal Lesion

CT images are obtained by passing x-rays through the abdominal organs from many angles.

Purpose: Used to diagnose tumors, abscesses, and bowel obstruction and to guide needles for biopsy.

Patient Preparation: Patient is usually NPO for 4 hours. These studies should be performed before barium studies are conducted.

CT of LS Spine CI: Spinal Stenosis

Scan of the lumbosacral area of the spine.

Purpose: Often ordered after myelogram. Used to confirm spinal stenosis or changes in the disks and vertebrae and to confirm spinal infection.

CT of the Neck CI: Tumor

Scan of the neck.

Purpose: Used to identify soft tissue masses and/or to evaluate the larynx.

CT of Chest CI: Lung Cancer

A CT scan of the chest requires special equipment to obtain multiple sectional images of the organs and tissues of the chest. A CT scan produces images that are far more detailed than those produced by a conventional chest x-ray examination.

Purpose: Used to diagnose pulmonary embolism or aortic dissection and to detect lung changes, pneumonia, and cancer.

64-Slice CT of the Heart CI: Possible ASHD

Note: ASHD is an abbreviation for arteriosclerotic heart disease

Three-dimensional scan of the heart that identifies structures as well as the vessels of the heart.

Purpose: Used to identify the risk of coronary artery disease and arterial occlusion. Does not replace cardiac catheterization with coronary angiography.

CT-Guided Liver Biopsies

Used to identify the location of tissue for a biopsy so that needle placement is precise.

Purpose: Used to obtain tissue from the liver for diagnostic purposes. CT-guided lung and breast biopsies also are performed. *Note:* Because these are invasive procedures done under CT guidance, a consent form must be prepared. ∎

ULTRASONOGRAPHY (SONOGRAPHY)

Ultrasonography, also called *sonography, ultrasound,* or *echo,* uses high-frequency sound waves to create an image of body organs. Ultrasonography is a technique that is used to visualize muscles, tendons, and many internal organs, and to assess their size, structure, and the presence of pathologic lesions (Fig. 15-11). Ultrasonography is useful in the detection of pelvic abnormalities and can involve techniques known as abdominal (transabdominal) ultrasound, vaginal (transvaginal or endovaginal) ultrasound in women, and rectal (transrectal) ultrasound in men. Ultrasound is used (1) to guide procedures such as needle biopsy, in which needles are used to extract sample cells from an abnormal area for laboratory testing, imaging of the breasts, and biopsy sampling for breast cancer, (2) to diagnose a variety of heart and vascular conditions, and (3) to survey damage after a heart attack or other illness. Ultrasonography is used to visualize a fetus during routine and emergency prenatal care, to date the pregnancy, and to check for the location of the placenta (afterbirth), the presence of multiple fetuses or physical abnormalities, the sex of the baby, and fetal movement, breathing, and heartbeat.

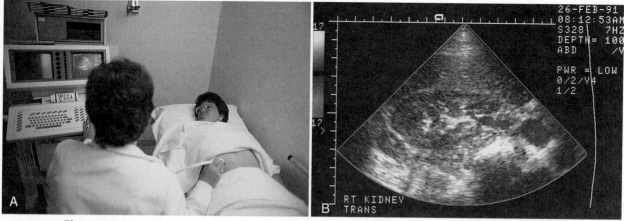

Figure 15-11 A, Ultrasound scanner. **B,** Ultrasound scan of the kidney. (From Brundage DJ: *Renal disorders,* St Louis, 1992, Mosby.)

Doctor ordering _____	
Today's date _____ ☐ Stat ☐ Routine ☐ ASAP	Patient Label
Date to be done _____ Requested by _____	

ULTRASONOGRAPHY REQUISITION

Clinical indication _____

Transportation ☐ Portable ☐ Stretcher ☐ Wheelchair ☐ Ambulatory

O₂ ☐Yes /☐ No   Diabetic ☐Yes /☐ No   Hearing deficit ☐Yes /☐ No
IV ☐Yes /☐ No   Seizure disorder ☐Yes /☐ No   Sight deficit ☐Yes /☐ No
Isolation ☐Yes /☐ No   Non-English speaking ☐Yes /☐ No

Comments _____

Write out the entire doctor's order

☐ Cardiac US _____

☐ Fetal US _____

☐ HIFU _____

☐ MRI guided focused US _____

☐ US of abd _____

☐ US of pelvis _____

☐ US of GB _____

☐ Write in order _____

Figure 15-12 Downtime requisition for ultrasonography.

Ultrasonography also has therapeutic applications (e.g., treating benign and malignant tumors, breaking up kidney stones [lithotripsy]) that can be highly beneficial when it is used with dosage precautions. High-intensity focused ultrasound (HIFU) (sometimes FUS or HIFUS) is a highly precise medical procedure used to heat and destroy pathogenic tissue rapidly. This typically is performed under computerized MRI guidance, at which time it is referred to as *magnetic resonance–guided focused ultrasound,* which often is shortened to MRgFUS. MRI is used to identify tumors or fibroids in the body before they are destroyed by ultrasound. See Figure 15-12 for an ultrasound downtime requisition.

Table 15-4 provides an overview of the ultrasonography procedures discussed in this section.

Doctors' Orders for Ultrasonography Studies

US of Abd

Ultrasound of abdomen

Purpose: Used to detect liver cysts, abscesses, hematomas, gallbladder disease (cholelithiasis, cholecystitis, obstructive jaundice), and tumors.

Patient preparation:

- NPO 8 to 12 hours before the procedure (for GB alone, may require only 4 to 6 hours NPO)
- If pelvis of female patient is included in abd study, full bladder, drink fluids—do not void
- No smoking AM of exam
- No gum chewing before exam

TABLE 15-4 Overview of Ultrasonography (Sonography)

Ultrasonography, also called *sonography* or *echography,* uses high-frequency sound waves to create an image of body organs. Female pelvic ultrasonography requires a full bladder.

Examples of Ultrasound Procedures

Procedure	Purpose
Renal ultrasound	To diagnose nephrolithiasis and nephritis and to identify tumors
Pelvic ultrasound	To identify ovarian cancer and other disorders and to identify ectopic pregnancy, multiple births, and fetal abnormalities
Abdominal ultrasound	To detect liver cysts, abscesses, hematomas, cholelithiasis, cholecystitis, obstructive jaundice, and tumors.

Ultrasonography is useful for examining other internal organs, including but not limited to the kidneys, heart and blood vessels, bladder, uterus, ovaries, unborn child (fetus) in pregnant patients, eyes, thyroid and parathyroid glands, and scrotum (testicles).

US of Pelvis

Ultrasound of pelvis
   Purpose: Used during pregnancy to identify ectopic pregnancy, multiple births, and fetal abnormality. Used otherwise to identify ovarian cancer and other disorders.
   Patient preparation:
   • Full bladder—drink fluids, do not void (usually only females)

US of Kidneys (Renal US)

Ultrasound of kidneys
   Purpose: Used to diagnose nephrolithiasis and nephritis and to identify tumors.
   Patient preparation:
   • No prep needed
   Note: Echocardiogram, echoencephalogram, and Doppler studies are covered in Chapter 16. ∎

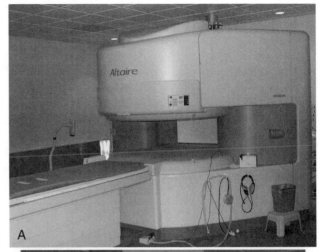

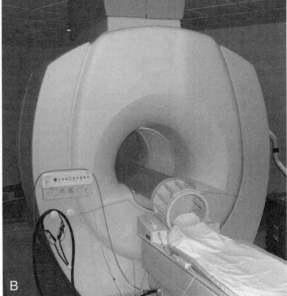

Figure 15-13 A, Open magnetic resonance imaging (MRI) machine. **B,** Closed MRI machine. Note that the tunnel is short and the edges are flared to minimize claustrophobia. (From Pagana KD, Pagana TJ: *Mosby's manual of diagnostic and laboratory tests,* ed 3, St Louis, 2006, Mosby.)

MAGNETIC RESONANCE IMAGING

Magnetic resonance imaging is a technique for viewing the interior of the body that uses powerful magnetic fields, radio waves, and a computer to produce images of body structures. **Magnetic resonance angiography** (MRA) uses magnetic resonance to study blood vessels.

For an MRI scan, the patient is securely placed on an imaging table within a large tube surrounded by a giant magnet (Fig. 15-13). The magnet creates a strong magnetic field that aligns the protons of hydrogen atoms, which then are exposed to a beam of radio waves. This excites the various protons of the body, producing a faint signal that is detected by the receiver portion of the MRI scanner. Receiver information then is processed by a computer, and an image is produced.

MRI scanners can generate multidimensional sections (slices) of tissue. MRI gives doctors the ability to view all sorts of body structures, including soft tissues. Bones do not obscure the image as they do in x-ray examinations. Studies are done on selected areas of the body, such as the brain, spinal cord, and bone. MRI frequently is used to detect cancers that otherwise would be difficult to diagnose and provides clinicians with the ability to detect cancers at early stages. Contrast media may or may not be used and may be as simple as water (taken orally, for imaging the stomach and small bowel), although substances with specific magnetic properties may be used, such as an agent called *gadolinium.* If a physician orders this type of contrast medium, an additional form such as a "contrast history information sheet" may need to be completed by the patient. When writing an MRI order, the doctor must indicate whether the procedure is to be performed with contrast. Many patients are claustrophobic, making it impossible to have an MRI in a *closed* MRI machine. The patient's doctor may choose to order the procedure with the use of an

Doctor ordering _____

Date to be done _____ ☐ Stat ☐ Routine ☐ ASAP

Today's date _____ Requested by _____

Patient Label

MAGNETIC RESONANCE IMAGING REQUISITION

Clinical indication _____

Transportation ☐ Portable ☐ Stretcher ☐ Wheelchair ☐ Ambulatory

O₂ ☐ Yes / ☐ No   Diabetic ☐ Yes / ☐ No   Hearing deficit ☐ Yes / ☐ No

IV ☐ Yes / ☐ No   Seizure disorder ☐ Yes / ☐ No   Sight deficit ☐ Yes / ☐ No

Isolation ☐ Yes / ☐ No   Non-English speaking ☐ Yes / ☐ No

Comments _____

Write out the entire doctor's order

☐ MRA _____

☐ MRI of brain _____

☐ MRI of spine _____

☐ MRI shoulder _____

☐ MRI knee _____

☐ Write in order _____

Figure 15-14 Downtime requisition for magnetic resonance imaging.

open MRI machine (may require that the patient be sent to another location for the procedure).

No adverse effects are associated because the procedure does not require radiation, but because of the strength of the magnet and the radiofrequency waves, MRI contraindications exist for patients with the following:

- Pacemaker or implanted cardiac defibrillator
- Implanted port device
- Neurostimulator
- Intrauterine device (IUD)
- Insulin pump
- Older metal plates, pins, screws, or surgical staples
- Ear implant
- Older metal clips from aneurysm repair
- Metal clips in eyes
- Retained bullets
- Pregnancy

Any other large metal objects implanted in the body (e.g., tooth fillings, braces) usually are not a problem.

Note: Only ferrous (iron-based) devices are attracted by a magnet. In all, 99.9% of devices used today for MRI are safe. (The physician should be consulted.)

The HUC, when transcribing MRI orders, would prepare an interview form for the nurse to complete before sending the patient for the MRI. The form lists any contraindications that may prevent the patient from having the procedure.

Dental bridgework may have to be removed before the scan is performed, but permanent fillings and inlays are acceptable because they are not made of ferrous metals. Before the examination is conducted, the patient is asked to remove metallic jewelry, a wristwatch, eyeglasses, hairpins, or a wig if metal clips are present. Credit cards, bankcards, and similar devices with magnetically coded strips should be removed as well. This

TABLE 15-5 Overview of Magnetic Resonance Imaging (MRI)

MRI is a technique that is used for viewing the interior of the body with the use of a powerful magnetic field, radio waves, and a computer to produce images of body structures. A contrast medium may or may not be used. A completed interview form is required.

Examples of Magnetic Resonance Imaging Procedures

Procedure	Purpose
MRI can be used to evaluate any part of the body	To diagnose internal injuries, conditions, or disease
	To monitor effects of medications and treatments inside the body

is especially important to remember in an outpatient diagnostic setting. Figure 15-14 shows a downtime requisition for MRI. Table 15-5 provides an overview of MRI procedures.

Doctors' Orders for Magnetic Resonance Imaging (MRI)

- MRI of brain (Fig. 15-15) and cervical spine CI: malignancy
- MRI lumbar spine CI: back pain and HNP
- MRI rt shoulder CI: rotator cuff injury
- MRI lt knee CI: posterior cruciate ligament tear
- MRA cerebral arteries CI: vertigo with possible arterial stenosis ■

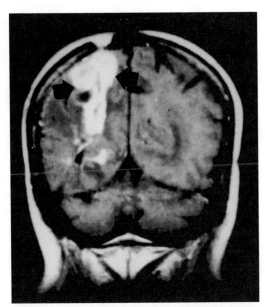

Figure 15-15 Magnetic resonance imaging (MRI) with arrows indicating a brain tumor accentuated by a Magnevist dye. (Courtesy Central Pennsylvania Magnetic Imaging, Williamsport, Pennsylvania; from Pagana KD, Pagana TJ: *Diagnostic testing and nursing implications: a case study approach,* ed 4, St Louis, 1994, Mosby.)

SKILLS CHALLENGE

To practice transcribing orders for computerized tomography scans, ultrasound, and magnetic resonance imaging, complete Activity 15-4 in the *Skills Practice Manual.*

NUCLEAR MEDICINE

Background Information

Nuclear medicine uses radioactive materials called *radiopharmaceuticals* to determine the functioning capacity of organs. Radioactive scanning materials are used to assist in diagnosing disease because of their ability to give off radiation in the form of gamma rays, which can be traced.

Depending on the study to be performed, the patient may take the radiopharmaceutical by mouth, or it may be injected into a vein. A gamma scintillation camera is the instrument used to form an image of the concentration of radioactive material within a specific organ of the body, thus producing a picture called a **scan** (Fig. 15-16, *A*). It is possible to perform organ scans on the bone (Fig. 15-16, *B*) with therapeutic doses of radiopharmaceuticals. Cancer of the thyroid and a blood condition called *polycythemia vera* respond to this treatment.

Radioactivity used in nuclear medicine differs from x-rays in that gamma radiation is transmitted from an outside source that passes the radiation through the body. In nuclear medicine, radioactive material is taken internally by mouth, by inhalation, or intravenously, and it emits gamma radiation from the specific organ that is being studied.

To communicate the doctor's order to the nuclear medicine department, the HUC must enter the order on the computer or complete a nuclear medicine downtime requisition (Fig. 15-17).

Preparation may be required before the procedure is performed. Check the health care facility's policy regarding preparation before scheduling the procedure.

Following are samples of nuclear medicine studies. Table 15-6 provides an overview of the nuclear medicine studies covered in this section.

Doctors' Orders for Nuclear Medicine Studies

Bone Scan—Total Body CI: Cancer, Prostate—Mets
Purpose: Performed to detect the presence of tumors, arthritis, or osteoporosis.

Bone Scan—Regional CI: Cervical Fx
Purpose: Performed to study a particular area of the body, such as vertebral compression fractures or unexplained bone pain.

Breast Scintigraphy (Breast Scan, Sestamibi Breast Scan) CI: Breast Cancer
Purpose: Used to identify breast cancer, especially in young women with dense breasts in whom the accuracy of mammography is diminished. Tracer doses of the isotope are used.
   Contraindications: (1) Patients who are pregnant, unless the benefits outweigh the risk of fetal injury; (2) patients who are lactating, because of the risk of contamination of breast milk.

★ HIGH PRIORITY

A DISIDA (diisopropyl iminodiacetic acid) scan is an exam of the gallbladder and the hepatobiliary system (the ducts connecting the gallbladder to the liver and the small bowel.

A HIDA (hepatobiliary iminodiacetic acid) scan is an imaging procedure that helps track the production and flow of bile from the liver to the small intestine.

A BRIDA (mebrofenin) scan is also an exam of the gallbladder and the hepatobiliary system—Mebrofenin has even higher hepatic extraction than DISIDA scan.

DISIDA, HIDA, or BRIDA Scans (Cholescintigraphy) CI: Gallstones
Purpose: Used to diagnose obstruction of the bile ducts (by a gallstone or tumor), disease of the gallbladder, and bile leaks. The DISIDA scan is most commonly ordered, but depending on the patient's serum bilirubin levels, a HIDA or BRIDA scan may be ordered instead.

L&S (liver and spleen) Scan CI: Cirrhosis
Purpose: Performed to evaluate injury to the spleen, chronic hepatitis, and metastatic processes. It should be done before barium studies are performed. Other body scans may be performed on the brain, heart, lungs, kidneys, gallbladder, and pancreas.

Gallium Scan—Total Body CI: Lymphoma (also may be ordered regionally)
Purpose: Performed to stage gallium avid tumors (those that attract high concentrations of gallium, e.g., lymphoma, lung cancer). It is used to locate infection or inflammation in

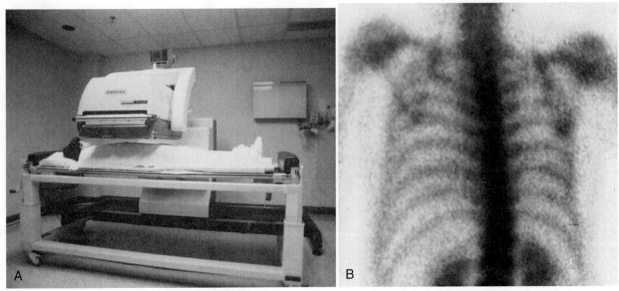

Figure 15-16 A, Patient prepared for bone scan. The patient's feet are tied to help maintain hips in position for maximal scanning uptake. **B,** Upper body bone scan. (**A** from Mourad LA: *Orthopedic disorders,* St Louis, 1991, Mosby. **B** from Pagana KD, Pagana TJ: *Mosby's manual of diagnostic and laboratory tests,* ed 3, St Louis, 2006, Mosby.)

Doctor ordering _____	
Date to be done _____ ☐ Stat ☐ Routine ☐ ASAP	Patient Label
Today's date _____ Requested by_____	

NUCLEAR MEDICINE REQUISITION

Clinical indication _____

Transportation   ☐ Portable   ☐ Stretcher   ☐ Wheelchair   ☐ Ambulatory

O_2 ☐Yes /☐ No   Diabetic ☐Yes /☐ No   Hearing deficit ☐Yes /☐ No

IV ☐Yes /☐ No   Seizure disorder ☐Yes /☐ No   Sight deficit ☐Yes /☐ No

Isolation ☐Yes /☐ No   Non-English speaking ☐Yes /☐ No

Comments _____

Write out the entire doctor's order

☐ HIDA scan _____

☐ Adenosine / thallium scan _____

☐ Bone scan (total) _____

☐ Bone scan (regional) _____

☐ Breast scintigraphy _____

☐ Cardiac scan _____

☐ Liver and spleen _____

☐ Gallium scan _____

☐ GI bleeding scan _____

☐ Thyroid uptake and scan _____

☐ DISIDA _____

☐ Neutrospec scan _____

☐ PET _____

☐ MUGA _____

☐ Scrotal nuclear imaging _____

☐ Thallium stress scan _____

☐ Sestamibi stress _____

☐ WBC scan _____

☐ Vent/Perfus (VQ) _____

☐ Write in order:

Figure 15-17 Downtime requisition for nuclear medicine.

TABLE 15-6 Overview of Nuclear Medicine

Nuclear imaging examines organ function and structure, whereas diagnostic radiology is based on anatomy. Contrast agents are used.

Example of Nuclear Imaging Procedures

Procedure	Purpose
Lung perfusion ventilation (VQ scan)	Study to diagnose pulmonary embolism
Liver and spleen scan	Performed to evaluate injury to the spleen, chronic hepatitis, and metastatic processes
Renal scan	Used to examine the kidneys and to detect any abnormalities, such as tumor or obstruction of renal blood flow
Thyroid scan	Used to evaluate thyroid function
Bone scan	Used to evaluate degenerative and/or arthritic changes in the joints, to detect bone disease and tumor, and/or to identify the cause of bone pain or inflammation
Gallium scan	Used to diagnose active infectious and/or inflammatory diseases, tumors, and abscesses
Brain scan	Used to investigate problems within the brain and/or in the blood circulation to the brain
Breast scan	Often used with mammograms to locate cancerous tissue in the breast
Octreoscan	Used to find primary and metastatic neuroendocrine tumors
DISIDA, HIDA, or BRIDA scan (cholescintigraphy)	Used to diagnose obstruction of the bile ducts, disease of the gallbladder, and bile leaks
NeutroSpec scan	Performed to identify abdominal, chest, or deep space infections that are otherwise not apparent clinically
Positron emission tomography (PET) scan	Used to obtain information about blood flow to the myocardium, metabolism, glucose usage, or schizophrenia
Scrotal nuclear imaging	Used to differentiate testicular torsion from other causes of pain
White blood cell (WBC) scan	Used to identify and localize occult inflammation or infection
Heart Scans	
Myocardial perfusion	Identifies ischemic or infarcted heart muscle
Myocardial function (MUGA)	Most accurate method used to measure cardiac ejection fraction
Cardiac flow	Performed in children with suspected cardiac anomalies
Nuclear ventriculography	Evaluates muscle wall activity
Cardiac stress test	Evaluates muscle wall activity during stress (physical or chemical)

Note: Exercise stress tests are discussed in Chapter 16.

patients with fever of unknown origin. It also is used to monitor response to treatment for infection, inflammation, or tumor.

Patient preparation: Usually, administer a **cathartic** or enema to minimize increased gallium uptake within the bowel.

SPECT (Single-Photon Emission Computer Tomography) CI: Pain L/S spine

Purpose: Performed to study structures in detail. It is similar to other nuclear medicine studies with the additional ability to visualize structures three-dimensionally and in thin slice images. SPECT scans may also be used to better determine functional problems in brain tissue in order to diagnose posttraumatic stress disorder, for example.

Thyroid Uptake and Scan CI: Check for Cold Nodules

Purpose: Performed to study thyroid gland performance. It demonstrates the ability of the thyroid gland to "take up" radioactive iodine.

Lung Perfusion/Ventilation Study CI: Embolism

Purpose: A diagnostic study for pulmonary embolism. The abbreviation *VQ scan* stands for ventilation/perfusion (quotient).

Scrotal Nuclear Imaging (Scrotal Scan, Testicular Imaging) CI: Rt Testicular Torsion

Scrotal imaging is helpful in the diagnosis of patients with sudden onset of unilateral testicular swelling and pain. Scrotal imaging can differentiate unilateral testicular torsion (twisting) from other causes of pain (e.g., torsion of the testicular appendage, orchitis, strangulated hernia, testicular hemorrhage). Tracer doses of isotopes are used.

Note: Testicular torsion is a surgical emergency that requires prompt surgical exploration to salvage the involved testicle. The surgeon must differentiate the condition from other causes of testicular pain that do not require surgery.

Gastrointestinal Bleeding Scan (Abdominal Scintigraphy, GI Scintigraphy) CI: GI Bleed

This study is used primarily to localize sites of GI bleeding.

PET (Positron Emission Tomography) Scan CI: Alzheimer's Disease

Purpose: Used to obtain information about blood flow to the myocardium, metabolism, glucose usage, and schizophrenia. Isotopes are used.

Patient preparation: Diet and medication adjustments are required before this procedure is performed.

WBC Scan (White Blood Cell Scan) CI: Osteomyelitis

Purpose: Used to identify and localize occult inflammation or infection in patients who have fever of unknown origin, suspected osteomyelitis, or inflammatory bowel disease. Tracer doses of the isotope are used.

NeutroSpec Scan CI: Chest Infection

NeutroSpec scanning is performed to identify abdominal, chest, or deep space infections that otherwise are not clinically apparent.

   Patient preparation: Encourage the patient to drink a lot of fluids, if possible, or administer increased intravenous fluids for patients who are NPO. ■

Doctors' Orders for Nuclear Cardiology Procedures

Cardiac nuclear scanning includes myocardial scan, cardiac scan, nuclear cardiac scanning, heart scan, thallium scan, multigated acquisition [MUGA] scan, isonitrile scan, sestamibi cardiac scan, and cardiac flow studies.

MUGA Scan (also called *gated pool imaging*) CI: CAD

Note: CAD is an abbreviation for coronary artery disease.

   Scanning of the heart using computers and synchronized electrocardiogram. MUGA (*multigated* acquisition) is the name of the computer machinery.

   Purpose: Used to calculate the cardiac ejection fraction.

Thallium Stress Scan CI: Infarction

A thallium stress test is a nuclear imaging method that provides a view of the blood flow into the heart muscle. A sestamibi stress test is the same test, but sestamibi is used as a radionuclide instead of thallium. Thallium and sestamibi tests also are called *MIBI stress test* and *myocardial perfusion scintigraphy;* these are used to evaluate how well the patient's heart is perfused (supplied with blood) at rest as compared with during activity.

   Stress is induced by use of the treadmill; if the patient cannot use the treadmill, medications are given to the patient to simulate the effects of exercise in the body. Drugs that simulate the effects of exercise are Persantine, adenosine, and dobutamine.

   Purpose: Used to monitor blood flow to the myocardium while at rest or after normal stress to diagnose coronary artery disease or to evaluate blood flow after a coronary bypass operation.

Adenosine/Thallium Scan or Persantine/Sestamibi Scan

Order for a thallium scan using medication (adenosine) to simulate the effects of exercise. Another combination is Persantine and sestamibi. Additional medications may be used to further pinpoint perfusion discrepancies and diseased or less functional vessels. Additional related tests include *stress resting cardiac (SR cardiac)* and *stress and nonstress cardiac (SANS).*

Octreoscan

Purpose: Octreoscan is an imaging agent that can reveal primary and metastatic neuroendocrine tumors.

Cardiac Flow CI: Cardiac Anomalies

This is most commonly performed in children with suspected cardiac anomalies.

   Purpose: Determines the direction of cardiac flow. ■

SKILLS CHALLENGE

For practice transcribing the following types of orders, complete the following activities in the *Skills Practice Manual:*
- For practice transcribing nuclear medicine orders, complete Activity 15-5.
- For practice transcribing a review set of doctor's orders, complete Activity 15-6.
- For practice recording telephone messages, complete Activity 15-7.

KEY CONCEPTS

The primary responsibility of the HUC in the transcription of diagnostic imaging orders, beyond ordering the requested study, involves communicating with the nursing staff about patient preparation and with the nutritional care department regarding diet changes. Accurate communication of the preparation procedure is vital to the expected outcome. An error may cause a procedure to be postponed or may result in an unclear diagnostic image or one in which the anatomy of interest is not visible; each of these outcomes is costly to the patient and hospital in terms of time and money. It is important to indicate, as part of the requisitioning process, the date on which the procedure is to be done. HUCs continue to have coordination responsibilities regarding scheduling of procedures when the electronic medical record is implemented.

Websites of Interest

"Who Are Interventional Radiologists?": www.sirweb.org/patients

"Interventional Cardiology and Radiology": www.ehow.com/facts 6936603interventional-cardiology-radiology.html

National Institutes of Health—"Nuclear Medicine Procedures": www.cc.nih.gov/drd/nucmed/patientinfo.html

Diagnostic Imaging—News and commentary: www.diagnosticimaging.com

REVIEW QUESTIONS

Visit the Evolve web site to download and complete the following exercises.

1. Define the following terms:
   a. cathartic
   b. fluoroscopy
   c. modality
   d. metastasis
   e. position
   f. on-call medication

2. Explain how the HUC responsibilities differ when EMR with CPOE is in use and when paper charts are in use.

3. List the information that the HUC must include regarding the patient when ordering a diagnostic procedure.

4. Explain the role of each of the following:
   a. radiographer
   b. radiologist

5. Explain the benefits of picture archiving and communication systems for the patient and the doctor.

6. Name five patient positions that may be included in an x-ray order.

7. Identify diagnostic imaging orders that would not require routine preparation.

8. Explain why contrast media are used, and list types of contrast media.

9. Discuss sequencing and scheduling of multiple diagnostic imaging procedures ordered on the same patient.

10. Identify four diagnostic imaging procedures that would require routine preparation, and explain the importance of preparing the patient before these procedures.

11. Explain when a patient would be required to sign a consent for a diagnostic imaging procedure.

12. Explain the purpose of special invasive x-ray and interventional procedures, and list at least three procedures performed in this division of radiology.

13. Describe an instruction that the doctor would include when ordering computed tomography, and list at least three computed tomography (CT) procedures.

14. Describe the purpose of ultrasonography procedures, and list at least three procedures performed in the ultrasonography area.

15. Discuss the purpose of magnetic resonance imaging (MRI) procedures and the purpose of magnetic resonance angiography (MRA) procedures.

16. Discuss the importance of the patient's nurse completing the interview form before the patient undergoes MRI or MRA, and list contraindications that would exist for patients as a result of the strength of the magnet.

17. Discuss the purpose of nuclear medicine procedures, and list at least three such procedures.

SURFING FOR ANSWERS

1. Research the most common routine preparations for the following tests: UGI, BE, abd US, cardiac catheterization, and IVU. Identify the website used.
2. Research and document the number of adverse reactions and deaths associated with diagnostic imaging examinations annually. Identify the website used.
3. Locate and document the cost of doing the following tests: MRI of the head without contrast; CT of the head without contrast; cardiac catheterization; and chest x-ray examination. Contrast the cost in an outpatient facility versus a hospital setting. Identify the website used.

CHAPTER 16

Other Diagnostic Studies

OUTLINE

CHAPTER OBJECTIVES

On completion of this chapter, you will be able to:

1. Define the terms in the vocabulary list.
2. Write the meaning of the abbreviations in the abbreviations list.
3. Describe the purpose of electrodiagnostics, and describe the indications that would initiate a doctor's order for a patient to undergo an electrodiagnostic procedure.
4. State the difference between a noninvasive procedure and an invasive procedure.
5. Describe the purposes of an electroencephalogram (EEG) and a quantitative electroencephalogram (QEEG).

6. State the category of medication (provide an example) that should be noted on the requisition when ordering an EEG.
7. Identify and describe the purpose of three evoked potentials.
8. Describe the purpose(s) of performing a caloric study, an electromyogram (EMG), and a nerve conduction study (NCS).
9. Explain the general purpose of cardiovascular electrodiagnostic procedures.
10. State the category of medication (provide an example) that should be noted on the requisition when an ECG is ordered.
11. List and describe three noninvasive cardiovascular electrodiagnostic procedures.

12. List and describe one cardiovascular nuclear medicine procedure and two cardiovascular ultrasound procedures.
13. Discuss the purpose of cardiac catheterization and the purpose of inserting a Swan-Ganz catheter and an arterial line (art-line or a-line).
14. Identify and discuss the purposes of at least three vascular plethysmography procedures.
15. Identify at least three vascular ultrasound studies, and discuss the purpose of each.
16. List at least six endoscopic procedures and the body parts visualized, and discuss the importance of patient preparation before a visual examination of the gastrointestinal system.
17. Identify three gastrointestinal studies that may be performed in the endoscopy department.
18. Discuss the general function of the cardiopulmonary (respiratory care) department, list at least four cardiopulmonary procedures, and identify the category of medication (provide an example) that would need to be noted when ordering arterial blood gas (ABG) monitoring.
19. Discuss the function of the sleep study department, and list a patient's symptoms that would initiate a doctor's order for a sleep study.

VOCABULARY

Ankle Brachial Index A noninvasive study to measure the difference in blood pressure between the upper and lower extremities.

Apnea The cessation of breathing.

Arterial Blood Gases A diagnostic study to measure arterial blood oxygen, carbon dioxide, base excess, bicarbonate, and pH (acidity) to assess and manage a patient's respiratory and metabolic status.

Arterial Doppler Ultrasound Type of ultrasound that uses the same method as vascular Doppler except that it is designed specifically for testing outer extremities such as arms and legs.

Arterial Plethysmography A manometric test that is usually performed to rule out occlusive disease of the lower extremities; may also be used to identify arteriosclerotic disease in the upper extremity.

Arterial Stiffness Index A noninvasive test that determines the flexibility and health of the arterial wall.

B-mode scanning An image made up of a series of dots, each indicating a single ultrasonic echo. The position of a dot corresponds to the time elapsed, and the brightness of a dot corresponds to the strength of the echo.

Caloric Study A test performed to evaluate the function of cranial nerve VIII. It also can indicate disease in the temporal portion of the cerebrum.

Capillary Blood Gases A diagnostic study performed primarily on infants. Blood is obtained from the infant's capillary arterial vessel, usually from the heel.

Capsule Endoscopy A noninvasive endoscopic study. A small capsule that is swallowed by the patient transmits and records pictures of the esophagus and small intestine.

Cardiac Stress Test A noninvasive study that provides information about the patient's cardiac function.

Color Doppler A form of sonography or echocardiology: colorization is used to identify the direction and speed (velocity) of blood flow.

Doppler Ultrasound A procedure used to monitor moving substances or structures, such as flowing blood or a beating heart.

Echo The reflection of an ultrasound wave back to the transducer from a structure in the plane of the sound beam.

Electrocardiogram (EKG or ECG) A graphic recording of the electrical impulses that the heart generates during the cardiac cycle.

Electroencephalogram (EEG) A graphic recording of the electrical activity of the brain.

Electromyogram (EMG) A record of muscle contraction produced by electrical stimulation. Used in the assessment of patients with diffuse or localized muscle weakness.

Electronystagmography A test used to evaluate nystagmus (involuntary rapid eye movement) and the muscles that control eye movement.

Electrophysiologic Study (EPS) A method of studying evoked potentials within the heart.

Endoscope A tubular instrument (rigid or flexible) with a light source and a viewing lens for observation that can be inserted through a body orifice or through a small incision.

Endoscopy The visualization of the interior of organs and cavities of the body with an endoscope. Biopsies may be obtained during an endoscopy. Endoscopic surgeries are discussed in Chapter 17.

Esophageal Manometry Performed in the endoscopy department and is used to identify and document the severity of disease that affects the swallowing function of the esophagus and to document and quantify gastroesophageal reflux (*also called esophageal function study* or *esophageal motility study*).

Evoked Potential (EPs) Tests used to evaluate specific areas of the cortex that receive incoming stimuli from the eyes, ears, and lower or upper extremities or sensory nerves.

Gastrointestinal (GI) Studies Diagnostic studies related to the gastrointestinal system. GI studies often are performed in the endoscopy department.

Holter Monitor A portable device that records the heart's electrical activity and produces a continuous EKG or ECG tracing over a specified period.

Impedance Cardiography A flexible and fast-acting noninvasive monitoring system that measures total impedance (resistance to the flow of electricity in the heart).

Impedance Plethysmography (IPG) A noninvasive study that is performed to estimate blood flow and quantify blood volumes.

Invasive Procedures Diagnostic or therapeutic techniques that require an incision and/or entry into a body cavity and/or interruption of normal body functions.

M-mode Echo Image obtained with M-mode echocardiography that shows the motion (M) of the heart over time. 2D M-mode would be a two-dimensional study.

Narcolepsy A chronic ailment that consists of recurrent attacks of drowsiness and sleep during the daytime.

Nerve Conduction Studies (NCSs) Studies performed to identify peripheral nerve injury in patients with localized or diffuse weakness, to differentiate primary peripheral nerve disease from muscular injury, and to document the severity of injury in legal cases; often performed with electromyography.

Noninvasive Procedures Diagnostic or therapeutic techniques that do not require the skin to be broken or a cavity or organ of the body to be entered.

Obstructive Sleep Apnea The cessation of breathing during sleep.

Occlusion A blockage in a canal, vessel, or passage of the body.

Quantitative Electroencephalogram (QEEG) A procedure that uses digital pattern recognition to identify functional problems such as attention-deficit/hyperactivity disorder (ADHD) (also called *brain-mapping*).

Real-Time Imaging An ultrasound procedure that displays a rapid sequence of images (like a movie) instantaneously while an object is being examined.

Rhythm Strip A cardiac study that demonstrates the waveform produced by electrical impulses from the electrocardiogram.

Spirometry A study conducted to measure the body's lung capacity and function.

Telemetry The transmission of data electronically to a distant location.

Tilt Table Test (TTT) A cardiovascular study done with the use of a "tilt table" to test for syncope.

Transesophageal Echocardiography A procedure used to assess the heart's function and structures. A probe with a transducer on the end is inserted down the throat.

Two-dimensional (2D) M-Mode Echocardiogram A technique used to "see" actual heart structures and their motions.

Vascular Doppler Ultrasound Ultrasound procedure that takes real-time video showing how the patient's blood is flowing through the arteries. This makes it easier to detect narrowing of the arteries, blockages, and blood clots. It also helps with monitoring the progression of arterial disease in a patient.

Vascular Duplex Scanning Type of scanning procedure; called "duplex" because it combines the benefits of Doppler with B-mode scanning.

Venous Plethysmography Procedure that measures changes in the volume of an extremity; usually performed on a leg to exclude DVT (deep vein thrombosis).

ABBREVIATIONS

Abbreviation	Meaning	Example of Usage on a Doctor's Order Sheet
ABG	arterial blood gases	ABG on RA
ABI	ankle brachial index	ABI today
ASI	arterial stiffness index	ASI
BAER	brainstem auditory evoked response; also called *auditory brainstem evoked potential* (ABEP)	BAER to evaluate hearing loss
CBG	capillary blood gases	CBG @ 10 AM
DVT	deep vein thrombosis	Admit Dx: poss DVT lt leg
ECG, EKG	electrocardiography	ECG before surgery; EKG today
EEG	electroencephalography	Schedule EEG
EGD	esophagogastroduodenoscopy	NPO for EGD
EMG	electromyography	EMG tomorrow
ENG	electronystagmography (electrooculography)	Schedule for an ENG
EPS	electrophysiologic study	EPS today
ERCP	endoscopic retrograde cholangiopancreatography	Schedule for ERCP in AM
ICG	impedance cardiography	Place on ICG today
IPG	impedance plethysmogram	IPG today
LOC	leave on chart (when it follows ECG/EKG)	ECG now, LOC
NCS	nerve conduction study	EMG NCS
OSA	obstructive sleep apnea	Sleep study to assess pt for OSA
PFT	pulmonary function test	PFT to evaluate COPD
QEEG	Quantitative electroencephalography	QEEG to evaluate ADHD
RA	room air	ABG on RA
SEP	somatosensory evoked potential	Schedule for SEP
TEE	transesophageal echocardiography	Schedule for TEE this afternoon
TTT	tilt table test	
VEP	visual evoked potential	Schedule VEP in AM

⊜ **EXERCISE 1**

Write the abbreviation for each term listed.

1. electroencephalography
2. electrocardiography (2)
3. electromyography
4. room air
5. leave on chart
6. arterial blood gases
7. capillary blood gases
8. endoscopic retrograde cholangiopancreatography
9. esophagogastroduodenoscopy

10. electrophysiologic study
11. nerve conduction studies
12. obstructive sleep apnea
13. brainstem auditory evoked response
14. electronystagmography
15. somatosensory evoked potential
16. visual evoked potential
17. deep vein thrombosis
18. transesophageal echocardiography
19. pulmonary function test
20. impedance plethysmography
21. impedance cardiography
22. tilt table test
23. quantitative electroencephalography
24. ankle brachial index
25. arterial stiffness index

EXERCISE 2

Write the meaning of each abbreviation listed.

1.	ABG	14.	ENG
2.	ECG or EKG	15.	SEP
3.	EEG	16.	VEP
4.	LOC	17.	DVT
5.	EMG	18.	TEE
6.	RA	19.	PFT
7.	EGD	20.	IPG
8.	ERCP	21.	ICG
9.	EPS	22.	TTT
10.	CBG	23.	ABI
11.	NCS	24.	ASI
12.	OSA	25.	QEEG
13.	BAER		

★ HIGH PRIORITY

When the electronic medical record (EMR) with computer physician order entry (CPOE) is implemented, physicians' orders are entered directly into the patient's electronic record, and the diagnostic procedure order is automatically sent to the appropriate department. The health unit coordinator (HUC) may have tasks to perform, such as coordinating scheduling, ordering special diets, and so forth. An icon may indicate an HUC task, or it may signal a nurse request. When paper charts are used, the doctors' orders are communicated by the ordering step of transcription via computer or by completion of a downtime requisition form. The HUC will have to communicate with the nutritional care department (by e-mail or telephone) when ordering a diet for a patient who has completed a diagnostic procedure that required him to be NPO (nothing by mouth).

Note: Some hospital nutritional care departments require that *all* diet orders be submitted in writing via computer.

★ HIGH PRIORITY

There are treatments and therapeutic procedures included in this chapter that may take place during diagnostic studies or that may be scheduled after these studies have been completed. These treatments and procedures are discussed in Chapter 17.

ELECTRODIAGNOSTICS

Background Information and Overview

Electrodiagnostics includes procedures used to evaluate the cardiovascular, nervous, and muscular systems to diagnose conditions and diseases. Indications to perform these procedures include numbness, tingling, weakness, muscle cramping, or pain. Most electrodiagnostic studies are performed with the use of electrical activity and electronic devices to evaluate disease or injury to a specified area of the body. Some type of electrode is applied to the patient to record electrical activity in most tests. Electrical impulses can be generated spontaneously or can be stimulated. The heart generates electrical impulses spontaneously during the cardiac cycle; these may be recorded by performing an electrocardiogram (ECG). Electrical impulses may be stimulated by an electrical shock applied to the body when an electromyogram (EMG) is performed. The most common electrodiagnostic procedures are discussed in this chapter and include tests done in various hospital departments.

Although electrodiagnostics are performed in several departments, other diagnostic tests visualize organs using sound waves; some tests are involve cameras to visualize the inside of hollow organs, and some tests include arterial blood draws or the use of specialized equipment. Many tests are noninvasive and do not require a consent form. Tests done in the cardiac cath lab (cardiovascular) or in the endoscopy department are invasive and may require a consent form and routine preprocedure preparation ("prep"). The tests discussed in this chapter are done in the following departments: neurodiagnostic studies (neurology), cardiovascular (cardiology), cardiopulmonary (respiratory), gastrointestinal (enterology), polysomnography (sleep studies), and endoscopy studies.

Noninvasive procedures involve a diagnostic or therapeutic technique that does not require that the skin be broken or a cavity or organ of the body be entered. Noninvasive procedures would not require the patient to sign a consent form. **Invasive procedures** involve a diagnostic or therapeutic technique that does require an incision or entry of a body cavity or organ. Invasive procedures require that the patient sign a consent form. Some invasive procedures require a routine preparation, an on-call medication, and/or a nothing-by-mouth (NPO) order or other dietary restriction orders, and some require sedation.

★ HIGH PRIORITY

Downtime requisitions are included in this chapter for learning purposes. The Evolve website associated with the *Skills Practice Manual for Health Unit Coordinating* includes a simulated hospital computer program that may be used as well.

NEURODIAGNOSTIC STUDIES (NEUROLOGY)

Neurologic and Neuromuscular System Electrodiagnostics

Electrodiagnostic tests involving the neurologic system include procedures involving the brain, cranial nerves, and sensory pathways of the eyes, ears, and peripheral nerves. Electromyography, often performed with electroneurography, is used to diagnose diseases or conditions of the neuromuscular system. Neurologic electrodiagnostic procedures that may be performed include those discussed in the following sections.

Electroencephalography

An **electroencephalogram (EEG)** is a recording of the electrical activity of the brain. The procedure is performed to identify and assess patients with seizures and to study brain function. Results of the study may be used to diagnose brain tumors, epilepsy, other brain diseases, or injuries and to confirm brain death or cerebral silence (Fig. 16-1). The role of the health unit coordinator (HUC) is to communicate the order to the electroencephalography department via computer or by completion of a downtime requisition. Anticonvulsant medications such as phenobarbital (Luminal) and phenytoin (Dilantin) should be noted when a procedure involving the neurologic system is ordered (Fig. 16-2).

Preparation of the patient by the nursing staff is usually required. The patient's hair is washed the night before the test is to be done. The use of cola drinks, cocoa, coffee, or tea is restricted because these liquids may act as stimulants; however, food and other fluids are permitted. Some hospitals have special preparation cards that contain information regarding preparation of the patient for an EEG. The HUC places the preparation card in the patient's Kardex holder during the transcription procedure.

An EEG may be ordered to be done via portable equipment (an EEG machine would be brought to the patient's bedside), or the patient may be transported to the neurology department for the test, which is performed by the EEG technician. To order an EEG, the doctor usually writes *EEG* on the doctors' order sheet.

Quantitative Electroencephalography (Brain Mapping)

A **quantitative electroencephalogram (QEEG)** uses digital pattern recognition to identify functional problems such as attention-deficit/hyperactivity disorder (ADHD).

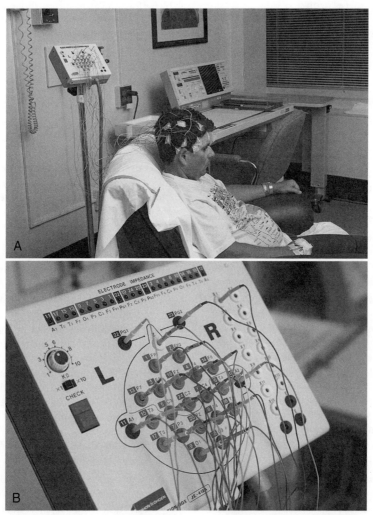

Figure 16-1 Electroencephalography. **A,** Electrodes are attached to the patient's head **(B)** with wires leading to corresponding areas on the equipment to record brain wave activity. (From Chipps E, Clanin N, Campbell V: *Neurologic disorders*, St Louis, 1992, Mosby.)

Doctor ordering _____

Date to be done _____ ☐ Stat ☐ Routine ☐ ASAP

Today's date _____ Requested by _____

| **NEUROLOGY DEPARTMENT REQUISITION** |

Patient Label

Clinical indication _____

Transportation ☐ Portable ☐ Stretcher ☐ Wheelchair ☐ Ambulatory

Anticonvulsant medication _____

O₂ ☐ Yes / ☐ No   Diabetic ☐ Yes / ☐ No   Hearing deficit ☐ Yes / ☐ No

IV ☐ Yes / ☐ No   Seizure disorder ☐ Yes / ☐ No   Sight deficit ☐ Yes / ☐ No

Isolation ☐ Yes / ☐ No   Non-English speaking ☐ Yes / ☐ No

Comments _____

Write out the entire doctor's order

☐ BAER _____

☐ Caloric study _____

☐ EEG _____

☐ EMG _____

☐ ENG _____

☐ Nerve conduction studies _____

☐ SEP _____

☐ VER _____

☐ Write in order _____

Figure 16-2 A neurology department downtime requisition.

Evoked Potentials

Evoked potentials (EPs) constitute a group of diagnostic tests that measure changes and responses in brain waves that are evoked from stimulation of a sensory (visual, auditory, or somatosensory) pathway. EPs are objective in that voluntary patient response is not needed. This makes EPs useful with nonverbal and uncooperative patients and permits the distinction of organic from psychogenic problems. The projected future of EPs is that they will aid in diagnosing and monitoring mental disorders and learning disabilities. Examples of EPs follow. These studies are performed by a physician in less than 30 minutes.

Visual Evoked Potential. The visual evoked potential (VEP) is a response to visual stimuli (e.g., a strobe light flash, reversible checkerboard pattern, retinal stimuli). It is also called *visual evoked response (VER)*. Abnormal results may be seen in patients with neurologic disease (e.g., multiple sclerosis, Parkinson disease). VEP may be used to detect lesions of the eye, disorders of neurologic development, and eyesight problems or blindness in infants. This test may be used during eye surgery to provide a warning of possible damage to the optic nerve.

Brainstem Auditory Evoked Response or Auditory Brainstem Evoked Potential. The brainstem auditory evoked response (BAER) or auditory brainstem evoked potential (ABEP) usually uses clicking sounds to stimulate the central auditory pathways of the brainstem. Either ear can be evoked to detect lesions in the brainstem that involve the auditory pathway without affecting hearing. This test is commonly used in low-birthweight newborns to screen for hearing disorders. Recognition of deafness enables infants to be fitted with corrective devices as early as possible, often preventing speech abnormalities. This test may be effective in the early detection of brain tumors of the posterior fossa.

Somatosensory Evoked Potential. Somatosensory evoked potentials (SEPs) usually are initiated by sensory stimulation of an area of the body. The time that it takes for the current of the stimulus to travel along the nerve to the cortex of the brain is measured. This test is used to assess patients with spinal cord injury and to monitor spinal cord functioning during spinal surgery. SEP is used to monitor treatment of diseases (e.g., multiple sclerosis), to evaluate the location and extent of areas of brain dysfunction after head injury, and to pinpoint tumors at an early stage.

Caloric Study (Vestibular Caloric Stimulation)

The **caloric study** is used to evaluate the function of the vestibular portion of the eighth cranial nerve (CN VIII). The external auditory canal is irrigated with hot or cold water to induce nystagmus (rapid eye movement). A caloric study also can aid in the differential diagnosis of abnormalities that may occur in the vestibular system, brainstem, or cerebellum. When results are inconclusive, electronystagmography may be performed. A caloric study is performed by a physician or a technician and takes approximately 15 minutes to complete. Most patients experience nausea and dizziness during this test.

Electronystagmography (Electro-oculography)

Electronystagmography is a test that is performed to evaluate nystagmus (rapid eye movement) and the muscles that control eye movement. Electrodes are taped to the skin around the eyes, and various procedures, such as pendulum tracking, changing of head position, and changing of gaze position, are used to stimulate rapid eye movement. This test is performed to evaluate patients with vertigo and to differentiate organic from psychogenic vertigo. The electronystagmogram (ENG) can be used to identify the site of a lesion if present and is used to evaluate unilateral deafness. The patient should avoid caffeine and alcohol for 24 to 48 hours before the test is performed. This procedure is performed by a physician or an audiologist and takes approximately 1 hour to complete.

Electromyography

An **electromyogram (EMG)** is used in the assessment of patients with diffuse or localized muscle weakness. An EMG often is combined with **electroneurography**; it can be used to identify primary muscle diseases and to differentiate them from primary neurologic pathologic conditions. A recording electrode is placed into a skeletal muscle to monitor its electrical activity. An EMG is performed by a physical therapist, a psychiatrist, or a neurologist and takes about 30 to 60 minutes. Slight pain may occur with insertion of the needle electrode.

Electroneurography (Nerve Conduction Study)

Nerve conduction studies (NCSs) are performed to identify peripheral nerve injury in patients with localized or diffuse weakness, to differentiate primary peripheral nerve disease from muscular injury, and to document the severity of injury in legal cases. It also is used to monitor nerve injury and response to treatment. This test is conducted by a physiatrist or a neurologist, takes about 15 minutes, and often is performed with an EMG. A mild shock that can be uncomfortable is required for nerve impulse stimulation.

Doctors' Orders for Neurologic and Neuromuscular Electrodiagnostics

- EEG tomorrow
- Schedule for ENG
- VER today
- EMG tomorrow AM
- Schedule BAER for tomorrow ■

SKILLS CHALLENGE

To practice transcribing neurologic and neuromuscular electrodiagnostics orders, complete Activity 16-1 in the *Skills Practice Manual*.

> **NEUROLOGIC AND NEUROMUSCULAR SYSTEM ELECTRODIAGNOSTIC TESTS**
>
> - Electroencephalography
> - Visual-evoked potential (VEP)
> - Brainstem auditory evoked response (BAER) or auditory brainstem evoked potential (ABEP)
> - Somatosensory evoked potential (SEP)
> - Caloric study (oculovestibular reflex study)
> - Electronystagmography (electro-oculography)
> - Electromyography
> - Electroneurography (nerve conduction study [NCS])

CARDIOVASCULAR DEPARTMENT (CARDIOLOGY)

Cardiovascular Electrodiagnostics

Electrodiagnostic tests of the cardiovascular system include procedures involving the heart and the vascular system. The results of electrodiagnostic tests and other cardiovascular studies aid the physician in making a diagnosis and prescribing treatment.

Electrocardiogram

An **electrocardiogram (EKG or ECG)** is a noninvasive procedure that measures the electrical impulses that the heart generates during the cardiac cycle. The ECG lead system is composed of several electrodes that are placed on each of the four extremities and a varying site on the chest. Each combination of electrodes is called a *lead*. The doctor may use the abbreviation *EKG* or *ECG* to order this study, which is performed at the bedside. *LOC* is a request to the ECG technician to leave a copy of the cardiac tracing on the patient's chart (Fig. 16-3). When ordering an ECG, the HUC should indicate whether the patient has a pacemaker or an automatic implanted cardiac defibrillator (AICD or ICD). Specific cardiac medications, such as digoxin (Lanoxin), diltiazem (Cardizem), and nitroglycerin (Nitro-Bid, Nitro-Dur, Nitrostat, Transderm-Nitro), should be noted when an ECG is ordered. An ECG usually is performed at the bedside by a technician, and in many hospitals it is routinely printed out and left on the chart. Some EMR systems automatically record an ECG into the patient's EMR or the HUC may scan it into the patient's EMR. It is important for the HUC to recognize that an order for an EKG or ECG is usually listed on the computer menu or paper requisition as a "*12-lead ECG.*"

A **rhythm strip** shows the waveforms produced by electrical impulses from the heart. One lead of the ECG is used (usually lead II) (Fig. 16-4). A rhythm strip may be printed from a continuous ECG when a patient is in a **telemetry** unit and is wearing a monitor. If the nurse or monitor technician detects an abnormality, or if the patient reports chest pain or discomfort, a rhythm strip may be printed for interpretation.

Impedance Cardiography

Impedance cardiography (ICG) is a noninvasive monitoring system that measures total impedance (resistance) to the flow of electricity in the heart. ICG is used to assess, plan, and individualize the treatment plan for patients with heart failure, severe trauma, or fluid management issues.

Holter Monitor

A **Holter monitor** is a portable continuous recording of the electrical activity of the heart for periods up to 72 hours. The patient's physician often orders this noninvasive test when a patient is c/o (complaining of) syncope, palpitations, atypical chest pains, or unexplained dyspnea. The ECG tape recorder is worn in a sling or holder around the chest or waist (Fig. 16-5). The ECG is recorded digitally during unrestricted activity, rest, and sleep. The Holter monitor includes a clock that permits accurate time monitoring on the ECG record. While wearing the monitor, the patient maintains a diary of activities and any symptoms experienced, including the time of occurrence.

Tilt Table Test

The **tilt table test (TTT)** (sometimes called *upright tilt testing*) is a noninvasive test that uses a "tilt table" to change the position of the patient from lying to standing while the ECG and blood pressure are measured. The TTT is used to assess patients who experience syncope (fainting).

Exercise Electrocardiography

An exercise ECG (also called a treadmill stress test) is a noninvasive study performed with the use of a treadmill or a stationary bicycle to evaluate cardiac response to physical stress. This study provides information on myocardial response to increased oxygen requirements and determines the adequacy of coronary blood flow. Occluded arteries are unable to meet the heart's increased demand for blood during testing (Fig. 16-6). *Note:* The use of caffeine is usually restricted for 24 hours before this test.

Electrophysiologic Study (Cardiac Mapping)

An **electrophysiologic study (EPS)** is an invasive procedure that is performed to study EPs within the heart. A small plastic catheter (wire) is inserted through the groin (or arm in some cases) and is threaded up into the heart with the use of a special type of x-ray examination, called *fluoroscopy*, which guides the catheter. Electrode catheters are used to pace the heart and potentially induce dysrhythmia. Mapping may be done to locate the point of origin of dysrhythmia.

Results of this study will help the physician select additional therapeutic measures, such as insertion of a pacemaker or defibrillator, or an additional diagnostic device such as an implantable loop recorder, which can record ECGs for up to 2 years. These procedures are performed by a cardiologist in a cath lab. Because this is an invasive procedure, the HUC may be required to prepare a consent form and communicate dietary and other routine preparations.

Note: Treatments or therapeutic procedures that may be performed during or scheduled after this study are discussed in Chapter 17.

CARDIOVASCULAR NUCLEAR MEDICINE STUDIES

Thallium and Sestamibi Stress Tests

Thallium and sestamibi stress tests are discussed in Chapter 15 because they are two-step procedures involving both the nuclear medicine and cardiovascular departments. The HUC

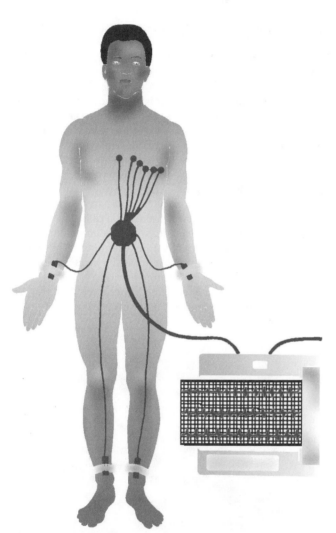

Figure 16-3 Electrode placement for a 12-lead electrocardiogram (ECG). (From Ignatavicius D, Workman L: *Medical-surgical nursing*, ed 5, Philadelphia, 2006, Saunders.)

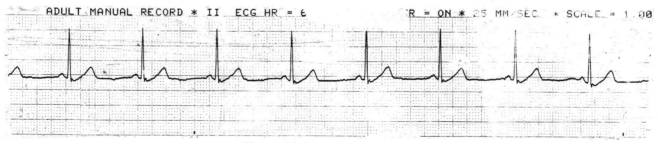

ADULT MANUAL RECORD * II ECG HR = 6   R = ON * 25 MM/SEC * SCALE = 1.00

Figure 16-4 A normal rhythm strip.

may have to coordinate procedures by communicating with both departments by phone, computer, or downtime requisition. The patient may be required to sign a consent form.

★ HIGH PRIORITY

When exercise testing is not advisable or the patient is unable to exercise to a level that is adequate to stress the heart, chemical stress testing is recommended. Chemicals that may be used include Persantine, adenosine, or dobutamine. Pacing is another method of stress testing. In patients with pacemakers, the rate of capture can be increased to a rate that would be considered a cardiac stress.

CARDIOVASCULAR ULTRASOUND (SONOGRAPHY, ECHOGRAPHY) STUDIES

Echocardiography

Echo refers to the reflection of an ultrasound wave back to the transducer from a structure in the plane of the sound beam. An *echocardiogram* is a noninvasive ultrasound procedure that is used to create a graphic recording of the internal structure of the heart and the position and motion of the cardiac walls and valves. This study, which is completed by sending ultra-high-frequency sound waves through the chest wall, usually includes **two-dimensional (2D) M-mode echocardiogram** recordings and a Doppler study. An **M-mode echo** is an image of a one-dimensional recording of the amplitude and rate of motion (M) of heart structures in real time, allowing the various cardiac structures to be located and studied during a cardiac cycle. The 2D mode moves the ultrasonic beam within one sector of the heart, producing a 2D image of the spatial

relationships within the heart. Color flow Doppler imaging demonstrates the direction and velocity of blood flow within the heart and great vessels. The procedure is performed by an ultrasound technician and may be performed at the bedside.

Intracardiac Echocardiogram

An intracardiac echocardiogram (ICE) is an invasive procedure that is performed to study the heart in pediatric patients. It is usually done during a repair of an atrial septal defect and is performed in the cath lab.

CARDIAC CATHETERIZATION AND INVASIVE CARDIOLOGY (CORONARY ANGIOGRAPHY, ANGIOCARDIOGRAPHY, VENTRICULOGRAPHY)

Cardiac catheterization is used to visualize the heart chambers, arteries, and great vessels. It is used most often to evaluate chest pain or abnormalities detected in a **cardiac stress test**. The procedure is used to locate the region of coronary **occlusion** (blockage) and to determine the effects of valvular heart disease. A catheter is passed into the heart through a peripheral vein (right-sided cardiac catheterization, or "right-heart cath") (Fig. 16-7) or artery (left-sided cardiac catheterization, or "left-heart cath"). Pressures are recorded, and radiographic dyes are injected through the catheter. With the assistance of computer calculations, cardiac output and other measures of cardiac function can be determined. The signed consent required for this procedure usually includes possible treatment or therapeutic procedure options.

Note: Treatments or therapeutic procedures that may be performed during or scheduled after this study are discussed in Chapter 17.

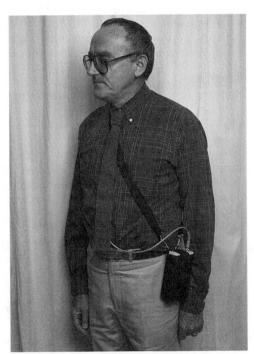

Figure 16-5 Patient wearing Holter monitor. (From Canobbio MM: *Cardiovascular disorders,* St Louis, 1990, Mosby.)

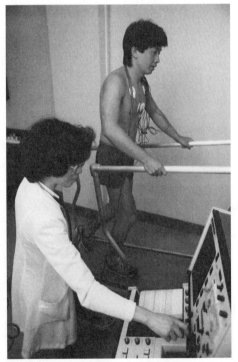

Figure 16-6 Patient taking an exercise stress test while the nurse monitors the electrocardiogram (ECG) response. (From Canobbio MM: *Cardiovascular disorders,* St Louis, 1990, Mosby.)

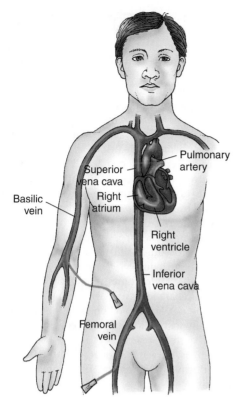

Figure 16-7 Right-sided cardiac catheterization. (From Ignatavicius D, Workman L: *Medical-surgical nursing*, ed 5, Philadelphia, 2006, Saunders.)

Swan-Ganz Catheter Insertion

The insertion of a Swan-Ganz catheter is a special procedure that is performed by a doctor in a critical care unit. A balloon-tipped catheter is inserted through the subclavian vein into the right side of the heart. The catheter goes through the right ventricle past the pulmonic valve and into a branch of the pulmonary artery. Measurements revealed by this procedure are used to guide and evaluate therapy.

Arterial Line (Art-Line or A-Line)

An **arterial line (art-line or a-line)** is a catheter that is placed in an artery and continuously measures the patient's blood pressure. It is most commonly used in intensive care and anesthesia to monitor the blood pressure in real-time (rather than by intermittent measurement). The arterial line may be used to obtain samples for arterial blood gas measurements.

VASCULAR PLETHYSMOGRAPHY STUDIES

Venous plethysmography is a noninvasive method of determining venous thrombosis and deep vein thrombosis (DVT). This test measures changes in the volume of an extremity and is usually performed on a leg to rule out DVT. Three blood pressure cuffs are applied to the proximal, middle, and distal portions of the extremity. A volume recorder (plethysmograph) attached to the cuffs then displays each pulse wave. Although this study may still be done in some facilities, it has largely been replaced by venous Doppler studies.

Note: Doppler studies also are used to identify DVT, but they are less accurate in evaluating the venous system below the knee.

Arterial plethysmography usually is performed to rule out occlusive disease of the lower extremities; it may also be used to identify arteriosclerotic disease in the upper extremity. Three blood pressure cuffs are applied to the proximal, middle, and distal portions of the extremity. A volume recorder (plethysmograph) attached to the cuffs then displays each pulse wave. Although this study may still be done in some facilities, it has largely been replaced by arterial Doppler studies.

Impedance plethysmography (IPG) is a noninvasive study that is performed to estimate blood flow and quantify blood volumes. Electrodes are applied to the leg, and electric resistance changes are recorded. This technique is not accurate in detecting the presence or absence of partially obstructive thrombi in major vessels.

DOPPLER ULTRASOUND: VASCULAR DOPPLER AND ARTERIAL DOPPLER ULTRASOUND STUDIES

Doppler ultrasound is a procedure used to monitor moving substances or structures, such as flowing blood or a beating heart. Doppler ultrasound is also used to locate vessel obstructions, to observe fetal heart sounds, and to image heart functions.

Arterial Doppler ultrasound is designed specifically for testing outer extremities such as arms and legs. An arterial Doppler ultrasound is used to evaluate the blood flow to and through the upper extremities (arms) and the lower extremities (legs). It records the patient's blood pressure of the arteries in the arms or legs along with taking ultrasound images. Arterial Doppler is used to evaluate the following:

- Numbness and tingling sensations in the hands, arms, feet, and legs
- Sensation of fatigue and heaviness in the arms and legs
- Possible thoracic outlet syndrome.

Vascular Doppler ultrasound is noninvasive and provides **real-time imaging** that displays how the patient's blood is flowing through the arteries. This makes it easier to detect narrowing of the arteries, blockages, and blood clots. It also helps with monitoring the progression of arterial disease in a patient.

Nicotine can cause vasoconstriction, so cigarette smoking before the Doppler studies must be avoided.

Duplex Scanning

Vascular duplex scanning is called "duplex" because it combines the benefits of Doppler with **B-mode scanning.** A computer provides a 2D image of the vessel, along with an image of blood flow. **Color Doppler** ultrasound can be added to arterial duplex scanning, which assigns color for direction of blood flow within the vessel. This provides an accurate representation of vessel anatomy and blood flow within the vessel.

Vascular ultrasound studies and vascular duplex scans that may be ordered include the following:

- *Carotid Doppler flow analysis:* A directional Doppler probe is used to detect the flow of blood in the major neck artery.

- *Carotid duplex scan:* A carotid duplex scan is a noninvasive ultrasound test that is used in the extracranial carotid artery to directly detect occlusive disease.
- *Vascular ultrasound studies (Doppler flow studies) on lower extremities:* In these procedures an ultrasound probe is placed over the major leg veins or arteries. A graphic tracing is produced, which shows flow changes caused by changes within the blood vessels.
- **Ankle Brachial Index:** This noninvasive study measures the difference in blood pressure between the upper and lower extremities.
- **Arterial Stiffness Index:** This noninvasive test determines the flexibility and health of the arterial walls.

CARDIOVASCULAR DIAGNOSTIC TESTS

Noninvasive
- Electrocardiogram (EKG or ECG)
- Impedance plethysmography (IPG)
- Holter monitor
- Cardiac stress test (exercise electrocardiogram or treadmill stress test)
- Thallium or sestamibi stress test (discussed in Chapter 15)
- Echocardiogram
- Plethysmography vascular studies
- Vascular ultrasound studies—arterial and venous Doppler studies
- Vascular duplex scans

Invasive (Usually Require Sedation of the Patient)
- Electrophysiologic studies (EPSs)
- Swan-Ganz catheter insertion
- Transesophageal echocardiogram
- Cardiac catheterization (coronary angiography, angiocardiography, ventriculography)
- Treatments that are done during cardiac catheterization such as radiofrequency ablation, coronary angioplasty, stent placement, and atherectomy are also done under sedation and are discussed with other therapies in Chapter 17.

See Figure 16-8 for a downtime requisition for noninvasive and invasive cardiovascular diagnostic procedures.

SKILLS CHALLENGE

To practice transcribing cardiovascular diagnostics orders, complete Activity 16-2 in the *Skills Practice Manual*.

Doctors' Orders for Cardiovascular Electrodiagnostics

- ECG stat LOC
- Schedule for heart cath 0800 in AM
- Arterial Doppler rt lower ext today
- 2D M-mode echo this afternoon ■

ENDOSCOPY PROCEDURES

Endoscopy is an invasive procedure that is performed to visualize and examine a body cavity or hollow organ. The procedure is usually named for the organ or body area to be visualized and is performed by a doctor. Most hospitals have an endoscopy department. The **endoscope** that is used to perform an endoscopy is a tubular instrument with a light source and a viewing lens for observation. Many endoscopic procedures now are performed with a video chip in the tip of a camera that is placed over the viewing lens. The color image then is transmitted to a nearby television monitor. Biopsies and surgical procedures often are performed during an endoscopy.

Note: Surgical procedures performed during endoscopy are discussed in Chapter 17.

In transcribing an endoscopy order, the HUC may call to schedule the procedure with the responsible department or may order the procedure via computer or downtime requisition (Fig. 16-9). Endoscopies require a patient to sign a consent form. Preparation varies according to the type of endoscopy to be performed. When ordering the procedure, the doctor usually will indicate if any preparation or "on-call" medication is required.

The following is a list of endoscopic examinations that are commonly performed in a hospital setting on an inpatient or outpatient basis:

- *Arthroscopy:* A visual examination of a joint interior with a specially designed endoscope. *Usual prep:* NPO 8 to 12 hours before examination because a general anesthesia usually is used to diminish pain.
- *Bronchoscopy:* A visual inspection of the bronchi by means of a bronchoscope (Fig. 16-10). *Usual prep:* NPO for 4 to 8 hours before the procedure to reduce risk of aspiration.
- *Colonoscopy:* A visual examination of the large intestine from the anus to the cecum by means of a fiberoptic colonoscope. *Usual prep:* cathartic and/or enemas and NPO before examination.
- **Capsule endoscopy:** Also called capsule enteroscopy, small bowel endoscopy, or the PillCam. A noninvasive visual examination of the esophagus and small intestine by means of a camera located in a small capsule swallowed by the patient. A sensor device is attached to the patient's abdomen in order to capture images sent by camera. *Usual prep:* NPO 10 to 12 hours before examination, possible cathartic and/or enemas.
- *Endoscopic retrograde cholangiopancreatography (ERCP):* This diagnostic procedure consists of inspection of the bile and pancreatic ducts and is performed with the use of a fiberoptic endoscope. *Usual prep:* NPO 8 to 12 hours before examination.
- *Esophagogastroduodenoscopy (EGD):* A visual examination of the esophagus, stomach, and duodenum. *Usual prep:* NPO for 8 to 12 hours before examination.
- *Sigmoidoscopy:* A visual examination of the sigmoid portion of the large intestine performed by means of a sigmoidoscope. *Usual prep:* cathartic and/or enemas and NPO 8 to 12 hours before examination.
- *Transesophageal echocardiogram (TEE):* **Transesophageal echocardiography** examines cardiac function and structure with the use of an ultrasound transducer placed

Doctor ordering _____

Date to be done _____ ☐ Stat ☐ Routine ☐ ASAP

Today's date _____ Requested by _____

┌─────────────────────────────┐
│   │
│   Patient Label   │
│   │
└─────────────────────────────┘

CARDIOVASCULAR DEPARTMENT REQUISITION

Clinical indication _____

Cardiac medications _____

Pacemaker? ☐ Yes / ☐ No   Type _____   Ht ___   Wt _____

Comments _____

LOC? ☐ Yes / ☐ No

Noninvasive Studies

☐ Arterial plethysmography   ☐ EKG c̄ rhythm strip

☐ Cardiac monitor   ☐ Holter monitor _____ hrs

☐ Carotid Doppler flow analysis   ☐ IPG

☐ Chemical stress test   ☐ Thallium stress test

☐ Doppler flow studies _____   ☐ Sestamibi stress test

☐ Echocardiogram 2DM-Mode   ☐ Trans-esophageal echocardiogram

☐ EKG / ECG /12-lead   ☐ Treadmill stress test

☐ Venous plethysmography   ☐ Vascular duplex scan

                                              ☐ Vascular us

Invasive Studies

☐ Cardiac catheterization   ☐ EPS

☐ Trans-esophageal echocardiogram   ☐ Write in order _____

Transportation   ☐ Portable   ☐ Stretcher   ☐ Wheelchair   ☐ Ambulatory

O₂ ☐ Yes / ☐ No   Diabetic ☐ Yes / ☐ No   Hearing deficit ☐ Yes / ☐ No

IV ☐ Yes / ☐ No   Seizure disorder ☐ Yes / ☐ No   Sight deficit ☐ Yes / ☐ No

Isolation ☐ Yes / ☐ No   Non-English speaking ☐ Yes / ☐ No

Figure 16-8 Cardiovascular diagnostic downtime requisition.

Doctor ordering _____
Date to be done _____ Time to be done _____
Today's date _____ Requested by _____

Patient Label

ENDOSCOPY DEPARTMENT REQUISITION

Clinical indication _____

Transportation ☐ Portable ☐ Stretcher ☐ Wheelchair ☐ Ambulatory

O_2 ☐ Yes /☐ No   Diabetic ☐ Yes /☐ No   Hearing deficit ☐ Yes /☐ No

IV ☐ Yes /☐ No   Seizure disorder ☐ Yes /☐ No   Sight deficit ☐ Yes /☐ No

Isolation ☐ Yes /☐ No   Non-English speaking☐ Yes /☐ No

Pre-op medication ☐ Yes /☐ No   Time given _____

Comments _____

☐ Arthroscopy   ☐ Esophagoscopy   ☐ Pelvioscopy
☐ Bronchoscopy   ☐ Fetoscopy   ☐ Peritoneoscopy
☐ Colonoscopy   ☐ Gastroscopy   ☐ Proctoscopy
☐ Colposcopy   ☐ Hysteroscopy   ☐ Sigmoidoscopy
☐ Cystoscopy   ☐ Laparoscopy   ☐ Sinus endoscopy
☐ Enteroscopy ERCP   ☐ Mediastinoscopy   ☐ Thoracoscopy
☐ EGD

☐ Write in order _____

Figure 16-9 Endoscopy downtime requisition.

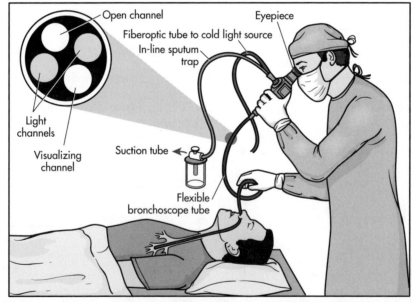

Figure 16-10 Bronchoscopy with the use of a flexible fiberoptic bronchoscope. The four channels consist of two that provide a light source, one vision channel, and one open channel that accommodates instruments or allows administration of an anesthetic or oxygen. (From Pagana KD, Pagana TJ: *Mosby's manual of diagnostic and laboratory tests,* ed 3, St Louis, 2006, Mosby.)

TABLE 16-1 Types of Endoscopies

All endoscopies require a signed consent. Preparations vary according to the procedure and the doctor and whether general anesthesia will be used.

Endoscopy	Area of Visualization	Preparation
Arthroscopy	Joints	NPO
Bronchoscopy	Larynx, trachea, bronchi, alveoli	NPO
Capsule endoscopy	Esophagus, small intestine	NPO
Colposcopy	Vagina, cervix	No
Cystoscopy	Urethra, bladder, ureters, prostate	Yes
Endoscopic retrograde cholangiopancreatography	Pancreatic and biliary ducts	NPO
Endourology	Bladder and urethra	No
Enteroscopy	Upper colon, small intestines	Yes
Esophagogastroduodenoscopy	Esophagus, stomach, duodenum	Yes
Fetoscopy	Fetus	No
Gastroscopy	Stomach	NPO
Hysteroscopy	Uterus	NPO
Laparoscopy	Abdominal cavity	Yes
Mediastinoscopy	Mediastinal lymph nodes	NPO
Sigmoidoscopy	Sigmoid colon	Yes
Sinus endoscopy	Sinus cavities	NPO
Thoracoscopy	Pleura, lung	NPO
Transesophageal echocardiogram	Heart	NPO

NPO, Nothing by mouth.

in the esophagus. The transducer provides views of the heart structure and its major blood vessels. This procedure may also be performed in the cath lab. See Table 16-1 for a list of types of endoscopies and their required preparation.

HIGH PRIORITY

The patient's intestinal tract is "cleaned out" (via cathartics or enemas) before gastrointestinal (GI) endoscopy is performed because the presence of stool would obscure visualization of the intestinal walls. Barium studies are performed after GI endoscopy because barium would obscure visualization of the intestinal walls. Gastrointestinal endoscopic studies cannot be done if the patient has not been properly prepared.

Doctors' Orders For Endoscopy

Sigmoidoscopy tomorrow AM.
- Fleet enema HS and repeat @ 0600
- NPO 2400 hours

Schedule for gastroscopy tomorrow AM.
- NPO $\bar{p}$ MN

Schedule ERCP for tomorrow.
- NPO $\bar{p}$ MN

Bronchoscopy tomorrow @ 9:30 AM
- Have consent signed.
- Demerol 50 mg
- Atropine 0.8 mg IM @ 8:30 AM

Schedule colonoscopy for 8 AM on Wednesday.

- Have consent signed.
- Clear liquids, NPO $\bar{p}$ MN
- Fleet enema HS and repeat @ 0600

Note: The doctor may or may not write an order for a consent to be signed. A consent is required for endoscopy. ■

SKILLS CHALLENGE

To practice transcribing endoscopy orders, complete Activity 16-3 in the *Skills Practice Manual*.

GASTROINTESTINAL STUDIES

Background Information

Some **gastrointestinal (GI) studies** are performed in the endoscopy department, usually on an outpatient basis, whereas others may be performed at the bedside by the nurse. The HUC may be asked to requisition the necessary equipment from the central service department for a bedside collection. Specimens collected by the nurse are sent to the hospital clinical laboratory for study, or they may be sent to a private laboratory.

GI studies are discussed in the following paragraphs.

Gastric Analysis

Gastric analysis is performed to measure the stomach's secretion of hydrochloric acid and pepsin and to evaluate the stomach and check for duodenal ulcers. This test takes

Doctor ordering _____

Date to be done _____ ☐ Stat ☐ Routine ☐ ASAP

Today's date _____ Requested by _____

Patient Label

| CARDIOPULMONARY (RESPIRATORY CARE) DEPARTMENT - DIAGNOSTICS REQUISITION |

Clinical indication _____

Anticoagulant medication? ☐ Yes Name of medication _____
☐ No

Room air ☐ Yes / ☐ No   Oxygen ☐ Yes / ☐ No   If yes, _____ L/min

Comments _____

☐ ABG   ☐ Pre-op teaching

☐ CBG   ☐ PFT: with bronchodilators ☐
                                     without bronchodilators ☐

☐ CPR Testing   ☐ Spirometry

☐ Pulse oximetry

☐ Write in order _____

Figure 16-11 A cardiopulmonary (respiratory care) diagnostics downtime requisition.

approximately 2½ hours to complete and may be performed in the endoscopy department.

Esophageal Manometry (Esophageal Function Study, Esophageal Motility Study)

Esophageal manometry (esophageal function study, esophageal motility study) is used to identify and document the severity of disease that affects the swallowing function of the esophagus. It also is used to document and quantify gastroesophageal reflux. The study includes measurement of the lower esophageal sphincter and a graphic recording of swallowing waves (motility). This study usually is performed in the endoscopy department. *Usual prep:* NPO 8 to 12 hours before examination.

Secretin Test

A secretin test evaluates pancreatic function after stimulation with the hormone secretin. The test measures the volume and bicarbonate concentration of pancreatic secretions. Lower than normal volume suggests an obstructing malignancy or cystic fibrosis. This test may be performed in the endoscopy department.

Note: Other GI studies are discussed in Chapters 14 and 15.

CARDIOPULMONARY (RESPIRATORY CARE) DEPARTMENT

Background Information

The cardiopulmonary (respiratory care) department evaluates, treats, and cares for patients with breathing or other cardiopulmonary (pertaining to the heart and lungs) disorders. The cardiopulmonary department also may perform presurgical evaluations. Patients who require respiratory care range from premature infants whose lungs are not fully developed to elderly people whose lungs are diseased. Cardiopulmonary diagnostic procedures are discussed in this chapter, and therapeutic options and treatments are discussed in Chapter 17.

The HUC communicates the doctors' order to the cardiopulmonary (respiratory care) department via computer or by completion of a requisition (Fig. 16-11).

No preparation is required for cardiopulmonary (respiratory care) tests unless the doctor has included special instructions with the order. For example, the doctor may discontinue respiratory medications before testing or may want the amount of oxygen adjusted or turned off before the patient's blood gas values are obtained. *Example:* DC O_2 at 10 AM, ABG at 11 AM.

Diagnostic tests commonly performed by the cardiopulmonary (respiratory care) department include those discussed in the following paragraphs. The division of the cardiopulmonary department that does testing may be called the pulmonary diagnostic lab.

Oximetry (Pulse Oximetry, Ear Oximetry, Oxygen Saturation)

Oximetry is a noninvasive method that is used to monitor arterial O_2 saturation levels (Sao_2) in patients at risk for hypoxemia. Oximetry typically is used to monitor oxygenation status during the perioperative period (before, during, and after surgery) in patients who have a compromised respiratory status caused by illness or disease, and in those receiving heavy sedation or mechanical ventilation. A monitoring probe or sensor is clipped to the finger or ear (see Fig. 10-3).

This study may be performed at the bedside by a respiratory therapist or nurse in a few minutes, or the device may be left in place to serve as a continuous monitor.

Arterial Blood Gases

Arterial blood gases (ABGs) are used to monitor patients on ventilators or critically ill nonventilated patients and to establish preoperative baseline parameters and regulate electrolyte therapy. The blood sample for this diagnostic study is obtained from the patient's artery by the respiratory care therapist (also called a *practitioner*). ABG measurements provide valuable information for assessing and managing a patient's respiratory (ventilation) and metabolic (renal) acid-base and electrolyte homeostasis. ABGs are also used to assess adequacy of oxygenation. Blood gases may be ordered for patients on room air (RA) or patients who are receiving oxygen.

When ordering ABGs, the HUC must note whether the patient is on RA or, if on oxygen, the flow rate (number of liters per minute). If anticoagulants are being administered to the patient, the names of medications (e.g., enoxaparin [Lovenox], heparin [Hepalean], warfarin [Coumadin]) should be noted as well. The arterial blood specimen must be placed on ice immediately and taken to the pulmonary laboratory for analysis.

Arterial Blood Gases with Lytes

A point-of-care (POC) ABG portable analyzer may be used to perform ABG tests as well as electrolyte (sodium, potassium, chloride, and bicarbonate) and hematocrit measurements (Fig. 16-12). The use of an analyzer requires that an arterial specimen be obtained from the patient.

Capillary Blood Gases

Measurement of **capillary blood gases** is performed primarily on infants. Blood is obtained from the infant's capillary arterial vessel, usually from the heel, by the respiratory care therapist. The blood is then analyzed in the pulmonary function laboratory. Measurement of CBGs provide valuable information for assessing and managing an infant's respiratory

(ventilation) and metabolic (renal) acid-base and electrolyte homeostasis. It is also used to assess adequacy of oxygenation.

Continuous Arterial Blood Gases with Lytes

A continuous ABG monitor may be used in a pediatric or intensive care unit (ICU) setting on patients for whom blood volume changes are critical. This type of monitor tests very small (negligible) amounts of blood while attached to an arterial or umbilical access and can take readings as often as every 5 minutes. Continuous ABG monitors perform the same measurements as POC tabletop analyzers or analyzers located in the cardiopulmonary department.

Pulmonary Function Tests

Pulmonary function tests (PFTs) are performed to detect abnormalities in respiratory function and to determine the extent of pulmonary abnormality. Tests usually include spirometry, measurement of air flow rates, and calculation of lung volumes and capacities. Other tests may be requested by the ordering physician.

 HIGH PRIORITY

Normal pH Values	Critical Values
Adult or child: 7.35 to 7.45	pH: <7.25 to >7.55
Newborn: 7.32 to 7.49	Pco_2: <20, >60
2 months to 2 years: 7.34 to 7.46	HCO_3: <15, >40
pH (venous): 7.31 to 7.41	Po_2: <40
	O_2 saturation: 75% or lower
	Base/Excess: ±mEq/L

Spirometry

Spirometry is a procedure that uses a spirometer with a time element that can determine air volume and air flow rates. Air flow rates provide information about airway obstruction. The patient breathes through a sterile mouthpiece into a spirometer, inhaling as deeply as possible and then forcibly exhaling as much air as possible. This test may be repeated with the use of bronchodilators, if values are deficient. The doctor may order a pre-bronchodilator and post-bronchodilator spirometry or PFT studies.

 Doctors' Orders for Respiratory Tests

- ABG on O_2 @ 2 L/min
- Bedside spirometry study
- Pre-bronchodilator and post-bronchodilator spirometry ■

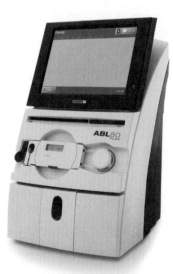

Figure 16-12 Radiometer's ABL80 FLEX point-of-care STAT analyzer measures blood gases as well as electrolyte and metabolite parameters. (Courtesy Radiometer Medical ApS, Westlake, Ohio.)

SKILLS CHALLENGE

- To practice transcribing cardiopulmonary (respiratory care) diagnostics orders, complete Activity 16-4 in the *Skills Practice Manual*.
- To practice transcribing a review set of doctor's orders, complete Activity 16-5 in the *Skills Practice Manual*.
- To practice recording telephone messages, complete Activity 16-6 in the *Skills Practice Manual*.

SLEEP STUDIES (POLYSOMNOGRAPHY, MULTIPLE SLEEP LATENCY TESTS, MULTIPLE WAKE TEST)

The sleep study department performs studies to assess a patient's sleep patterns. Sleep studies are ordered for patients who snore excessively, experience **narcolepsy** (excessive daytime sleepiness) or insomnia, or have motor spasms while sleeping, as well as in patients with documented cardiac rhythm disturbances limited to sleep time. Polysomnography is a comprehensive recording of the biophysiologic changes that occur during sleep. The polysomnogram (PSG) monitors many body functions including brain functions (EEG), eye movements (electro-oculogram [EOG]), muscle activity or skeletal muscle activation (EMG), heart rhythm (ECG), and breathing function or respiratory effort during sleep.

Inductive plethysmography is a noninvasive study that measures the patient's respiratory function and can differentiate central **apnea** from **obstructive sleep apnea** during a sleep study. Many hospitals have a sleep study department, and most sleep studies are performed on an outpatient basis. The doctor may order as follows: *Sleep study to assess patient for OSA.* During this procedure, electrodes for ECG, EEG, and EMG are applied to the patient. Excess hair may have to be shaved on male patients. Air flow, oximetry, and impedance monitors also are applied. The patient is allowed to sleep per normal routine and is monitored for respiratory disturbances such as apnea.

CARDIOPULMONARY (RESPIRATORY CARE) DIAGNOSTIC TESTS

- Oximetry (pulse oximetry, ear oximetry, oxygen saturation)
- Arterial blood gases (ABGs)
- Capillary blood gases (CBGs)
- Pulmonary function tests (PFTs)
- Spirometry
- Sleep studies (may be done in the polysomnography department)

KEY CONCEPTS

Recognition of the need for and proper scheduling of all diagnostic studies are of utmost importance to the patient, the doctor(s), and the hospital. Both the patient whose condition is as yet undiagnosed and the patient who is awaiting test results are dependent on the knowledge and communication skills of the individual who is coordinating activities on the nursing unit. The HUC who can identify and correctly order all appropriate diagnostic studies is an asset to the unit.

Websites of Interest

"Cardiac Catheterization": www.webmd.com/heart-disease/cardiac-catheterization

Doppler ultrasound exam of an arm or leg: www.nlm.nih.gov/medlineplus/ency/article/003775.htm

"Understanding Pulmonary Function Tests: www.healthguideinfo.com/asthma-management/p112306

"What Are Sleep Studies?" www.nhlbi.nih.gov/health/dci/Diseases/slpst/slpst_whatis.htm

---

 REVIEW QUESTIONS

1. *Visit the Evolve website to download and complete the following exercises:*
   a. arterial line (art-line)
   b. caloric study
   c. capsule endoscopy
   d. echo
   e. endoscope
   f. apnea
   g. endoscopy
   h. Holter monitor
   i. invasive procedure
   j. narcolepsy
   k. noninvasive procedure
   l. obstructive sleep apnea
   m. occlusion
   n. real-time imaging
   o. rhythm strip
   p. telemetry

2. Describe the purpose of electrodiagnostics and the indications that would initiate a doctor's order for a patient to undergo an electrodiagnostic procedure.

3. State the difference between a noninvasive procedure and an invasive procedure.

4. Identify and describe the purpose of three types of evoked potentials.

5. Describe the purposes of an electroencephalogram (EEG) and a quantitative electroencephalogram (QEEG).

6. State the category of medication and provide an example that should be noted on the requisition when ordering electroencephalograms.

7. Describe the purpose(s) of the following procedures:
   a. caloric study
   b. EMG
   c. NCS

8. Explain the general purpose of cardiovascular electrodiagnostic procedures.

9. State the category and provide an example of medication that should be noted on the requisition when ordering an ECG.

10. List and describe three noninvasive cardiovascular electrodiagnostic procedures.

11. List and describe one cardiovascular nuclear medicine procedure and two cardiovascular ultrasound procedures.

12. Discuss the purpose of each of the following:
   a. cardiac catheterization
   b. Swan-Ganz catheter
   c. arterial line (art-line or a-line)

13. Identify and discuss the purposes of three vascular plethysmography procedures.

14. Identify at least three vascular ultrasound studies, and discuss the purpose of each.

15. List at least six endoscopic procedures and identify the body parts visualized.

16. Discuss the importance of patient preparation for a gastrointestinal endoscopy, and explain why a barium enema would need to be scheduled after a GI endoscopy.

17. Identify three gastrointestinal studies that may be performed in the endoscopy department.

18. Discuss the general function of the cardiopulmonary (respiratory care) department.

19. List at least four cardiopulmonary (respiratory) tests, and identify the category of medication (provide an example) that would need to be noted when ordering ABG measurement.

20. Discuss the function of the sleep study department, and list patient symptoms that would initiate a doctor's order for a sleep study to be performed.

SURFING FOR ANSWERS

1. Research the most common medications that may need to be included when requisitioning tests from the cardiovascular, the cardiopulmonary, and the neurodiagnostic studies departments, and identify the website used.
2. Locate a video that demonstrates pulmonary function tests being performed, and identify the website used.
3. Locate and document the cost of doing an ECG, an EEG, and a colonoscopy, and identify the websites used.

Treatment Orders

CHAPTER OBJECTIVES

On completion of this chapter, you will be able to:

1. Define the terms in the vocabulary list.
2. Write the meaning of the abbreviations in the abbreviations list.
3. Discuss three methods that may be used to treat cardiovascular conditions, and identify three areas within the hospital where cardiovascular surgical and treatment procedures may be performed.
4. Identify the three commonly used procedures performed to repair obstructed coronary blood vessels.
5. Identify the name and location of a vein and an artery that may be used for grafts during a coronary artery bypass graft.
6. Discuss the reasoning for cardiovascular treatment procedures being performed in conjunction with diagnostic procedures, and list five treatment procedures performed in interventional radiology.
7. State the purpose of the cardiopulmonary (respiratory care) department pertaining to patient treatment orders, and list at least five cardiopulmonary (respiratory care) treatments.

8. Explain the importance of the health unit coordinator (HUC) including the entire doctor's order when communicating a cardiopulmonary (respiratory care) order (electronically, by requisition, or by telephone), and list the information that would be needed when sending an order for oxygen.
9. List four types of aerosol delivery devices, and identify at least two types of aerosolized drugs.
10. Explain the procedure and equipment needed to obtain an induced sputum specimen.
11. Discuss the purpose of incentive spirometry, chest percussion therapy, and noninvasive positive pressure ventilation, and explain the use of a mechanical ventilator.
12. State the purpose of the wound care department, and explain the purpose of hyperbaric oxygen therapy.
13. Identify the two basic types of traction and the traction setup used by patients to assist them to move in bed.
14. Identify three divisions that make up the physical medicine department.
15. Describe the purpose of the physical therapy (PT) division of physical medicine, and list four methods that would be used by PT personnel.

16. Describe the purpose of the occupational therapy (OT) division of the physical medicine department, and list three doctor's orders that would be sent to the OT department.
17. Explain the purpose of speech therapy, and describe the patients who would benefit from speech therapy.
18. Explain the need for dialysis, identify two types of dialysis, and discuss the process of each type.
19. Identify three areas in the hospital that may provide radiation treatments, and explain the HUC's role regarding doctors' orders for radiation.

VOCABULARY

Active Exercise Exercise performed by the patient without assistance as instructed by the physical therapist.

Activities of Daily Living Tasks that enable individuals to meet basic needs (eating, bathing, and so forth).

Aerobic Exercise Exercise that causes the heart and lungs to work harder to benefit the cardiovascular and circulatory system.

Aerosol Liquid suspension of particles in a gas stream for inhalation purposes.

Anaerobic Exercise Exercise that involves strengthening muscles by forcing them to work very hard for a brief time.

Angioplasty A medical procedure in which a balloon is used to open narrowed or blocked blood vessels of the heart (coronary arteries).

Auscultation The act of listening for sounds within the body to evaluate the condition of the heart, blood vessels, lungs, pleura, intestines, or other organs or to detect fetal heart sounds.

Cardiac Pacemaker An electronic device, temporary or permanent, that regulates the pace of the heart when the heart is incapable of doing it.

Certified Respiratory Therapist (CRT) Title granted after completion of an approved respiratory therapy program; graduates may become credentialed by taking an entry level examination to become CRTs.

Constraint-Induced (movement) Therapy (CI therapy) A therapy to treat a dysfunctional upper extremity that involves constraining the functional arm in a sling to improve the movement and use of the affected arm.

Crackles (rales) A common, abnormal respiratory sound that consists of discontinuous bubbling noises caused by fluid in the small airways or atelectasis and heard on auscultation of the chest during inspiration.

Débridement The process of removing dirt, foreign objects, damaged tissue, and cellular debris from a wound or a burn to prevent infection and to promote healing.

Defibrillation Application of an electric shock to the myocardium through the chest wall to restore normal cardiac rhythm. External defibrillators deliver the shock through the chest wall, whereas internal cardioverter-defibrillators (ICDs) deliver the shock via implanted electrodes within the heart.

Dialysis A mechanical process to remove from the blood toxic wastes that would normally be filtered out by the kidneys.

Dyspnea Difficult or labored breathing.

Endotracheal Tube A tube inserted through the mouth that supplies air to the lungs and assists breathing. The endotracheal tube is connected to a ventilator.

Extubation Removal of a previously inserted tube (such as an endotracheal tube).

Hemodialysis (extracorporeal dialysis) The removal of waste products from the blood through use of a machine through which the blood flows.

Hydrotherapy The use of water—including continuous tub baths, wet sheet packs, or shower sprays—to soothe pains and treat various conditions and diseases.

Hyperbaric Oxygen Therapy A treatment that involves breathing 100% oxygen while in an enclosed system pressurized to greater than one atmosphere (sea level).

Hypertonic A concentrated salt solution (>0.9%).

Hypotonic A dilute salt solution (<0.9%).

Induced Sputum Specimen A sputum specimen obtained by performing a respiratory treatment to loosen lung secretions.

Intervention Synonymous with *treatment*.

Intubation Insertion and placement of a tube within the trachea to maintain an open airway.

Isometric Of equal dimensions. Holding ends of contracting muscle fixed so that contraction produces increased tension at a constant overall length.

Nebulizer A gas-driven device that produces an aerosol.

Passive Exercise Exercise in which the patient is submissive and the physical therapist moves the patient's limbs.

Peritoneal Dialysis Process involving introduction of a fluid (dialyzing fluid) into the abdominal cavity; the fluid absorbs the wastes from the blood through the lining of the abdominal cavity or through the peritoneum; afterward, the dialysate is emptied from the abdominal cavity.

Positive Pressure Pressure greater than atmospheric pressure.

Range of Motion The range in which a joint can move.

Resistive Exercise Exercise that uses opposition. A T band or water may be used to provide resistance for patient exercises.

Splint An orthopedic device for immobilization, restraint, or support of any part of the body; may be rigid (metal, plaster, or wood) or flexible (felt or leather).

Spica Cast A cast that begins at the chest and includes one or both lower limbs.

Stent A tiny metal or plastic tube that is placed into an artery, blood vessel, or other duct to hold the structure open.

Stridor A high-pitched harsh sound heard during inspiration that is caused by obstruction of the upper airway; it is a sign of respiratory distress and therefore requires immediate attention.

Tank Room A room where hydrotherapy is performed.

Traction A mechanical pull to part of the body to maintain alignment and facilitate healing; traction may be static (continuous) or intermittent.

Ultrasound Therapy A deep heating modality using high-energy sound waves that is most effective for heating tissues or deep joints and is performed by a physical therapist.

Unit Dose Any premixed or prespecified dose; often administered with a small-volume nebulizer or intermittent positive pressure breathing treatments.

Ventilator A machine that is used to give the patient breaths through the ET or tracheostomy tube.

Wheezes Sounds that are heard continuously during inspiration or expiration or both and are caused by air moving through airways narrowed by constriction or swelling of airways or partial airway obstruction.

ABBREVIATIONS

Abbreviation	Meaning	Example of Usage on a Doctor's Order Sheet
AA	active assisted	AA exercises B/L LE
ADLS	activities of daily living	OT for ADLs
ADS	adult distress syndrome	The patient's dx is ADS
AKA	above-the-knee amputation	AKA protocol
BiPAP	bilevel positive airway pressure	
BiW	twice a week	PT 2 × a wk
BKA	below-the-knee amputation	consent for BKA
BLE	both or bilateral lower extremities	HBOT BLE
BUE	both or bilateral upper extremities	strengthening exercises BUE
CABG	coronary artery bypass graft	consent for CABG
CBNT	continuous bronchodilator nebulizer therapy	
CP	cold pack	CP L arm
CPAP	continuous positive airway pressure	CPAP 5 cm H_2O
CPM	continuous passive motion	CPM
CPR	cardiopulmonary resuscitation	CPR training for parents before child's discharge
CPT	chest percussion therapy	DC CPT
DPI	dry powder inhaler	instruct patient on use of DPI
EPC	electronic pain control	EPC
ES	electrical stimulation	ES
ET	endotracheal tube	CXR for ET tube placement
FWW	front-wheel walker	provide FWW
HA	heated aerosol	HA T-piece @ 60%
HBOT	hyperbaric O_2 therapy	HBOT qd 3 × wk for 8 wk
HD	hemodialysis	HD BiW × 3 h
HP	hot packs	HP to neck
ICD	implantable cardioverter-defibrillator	Have consent signed for ICD
IPPB	intermittent positive pressure breathing	IPPB q4h 0.5 mL Ventolin in 2 mL NS
IS	incentive spirometry	IS tid
ISOM	isometric	ISOM UE bid
lb or #	pounds	bucks traction 5# weight
LE	lower extremities	ROM LE qd
LLE	left lower extremity	passive exercises LLE
LLL	left lower lobe	CPT—LLL only
L/min	liters per minute	↑ O_2 to 4 L/min
LUE	left upper extremities	ROM LUE
LUL	left upper lobe	CPT to LUL
MDI	metered-dose inhaler	MDI puffs qid
NC or NP	nasal cannula or nasal prongs	02 40% by NC
NWB	non–weight bearing	Crutch-walking NWB
O_2	oxygen	O_2 6 L/min by mask
O_2 SAT	oxygen Saturation	Place on oximetry to monitor O_2 SAT
ORIF	open reduction, internal fixation	ORIF lt femur
OT	occupational therapy or occupational therapist	OT for ADLs
PD	peritoneal dialysis	Tenckhoff cath for PD
PDPV	postural drainage, percussion, and vibration	PDPV to LUL
PEP	positive expiratory pressure	IS PEP
PROM	passive range of motion	PROM LUE bid
PT	physical therapy or physical therapist	To PT for crutch walking
PTA	physical therapy assistant	PTA to assist patient in amb
PTCA	percutaneous transluminal coronary angioplasty	Have consent signed for PTCA
RLE	right lower extremities	ISOM to RLE
RLL	right lower lobe	CPT RLL
RML	right middle lobe	CPT RML
ROM	range of motion	ROM to upper extremities tid
RT	respiratory therapy or respiratory therapist	RT to obtain induced sputum specimen
RUE	right upper extremity	Hot pk to RUE
RUL	right upper lobe	CPT to RUL
SaO_2	arterial oxygen saturation (on pulse oximetry, not ABGs)	ABG now—notify resident of SaO_2
SpO_2	oxygen saturation via pulse oximetry	SpO_2 notify resident if O_2 SAT below 90%
SIDS	sudden infant death syndrome	The baby died of SIDS
STM	soft tissue massage	STM lt shoulder 20 min bid
SVN	small volume nebulizer	Δ SVN to bid

TENS	transcutaneous electrical nerve stimulation	Postop TENS
THR or THA	total hip replacement or arthroplasty	follow THR protocol
TKR or TKA	total knee replacement or arthroplasty	TKA protocol
TT	tilt table	PT for TT
TTOT	transtracheal oxygen therapy	Start TTOT today
Tx	traction	Buck's Tx
UD	unit dose	UD Ventolin now
USN	ultrasonic nebulizer	USN 15 min tid
WBAT	weight bearing as tolerated	amb, WBAT rt leg
WP	whirlpool	WP to L leg bid
>	greater than	Call hospitalist if pH >7.4
<	less than	Call Dr. Jones if O_2 Sats <70%

⊖ E X E R C I S E **1**

Write the abbreviation for each term listed.

1. left upper lobe
2. occupational therapy or occupational therapist
3. physical therapy or physical therapist
4. liters per minute
5. oxygen
6. intermittent positive pressure breathing
7. right upper lobe
8. range of motion
9. right lower lobe
10. activities of daily living
11. coronary artery bypass graft
12. right middle lobe
13. ultrasonic nebulizer
14. small-volume nebulizer
15. left lower lobe
16. pounds
17. non–weight bearing
18. whirlpool
19. hot packs
20. transcutaneous electrical nerve stimulation
21. electronic pain control
22. electrical stimulation
23. continuous passive motion
24. incentive spirometry
25. metered-dose inhaler
26. chest percussion therapy
27. active assisted
28. twice a week
29. above-the-knee amputation
30. soft tissue massage
31. lower extremities
32. hemodialysis
33. total hip replacement or arthroplasty
34. open reduction, internal fixation
35. traction
36. tilt table
37. isometric
38. below-the-knee amputation
39. endotracheal tube
40. heated aerosol
41. positive expiratory pressure
42. postural drainage, percussion, and vibration
43. oxygen saturation
44. unit dose
45. greater than
46. total knee replacement or arthroplasty /
47. less than
48. cold packs
49. cardiopulmonary resuscitation
50. hyperbaric oxygen therapy
51. transtracheal oxygen therapy
52. continuous positive airway pressure
53. both upper extremities
54. both lower extremities
55. right upper extremity
56. left upper extremity
57. right lower extremity
58. left lower extremity
59. physical therapist assistant
60. respiratory therapist
61. passive range of motion
62. weight bearing as tolerated
63. front-wheel walker
64. peritoneal dialysis
65. implantable cardioverter-defibrillator
66. adult distress syndrome
67. dry powder inhaler
68. sudden infant death syndrome
69. nasal cannula or nasal prongs
70. arterial oxygen concentration
71. continuous bronchodilator nebulizer therapy
72. percutaneous transluminal coronary angioplasty
73. bilevel positive airway pressure
74. oxygen concentration via pulse oximetry

⊖ E X E R C I S E **2**

Write the meaning of each abbreviation listed.

1. O_2
2. LUL
3. RLL
4. OT
5. PT
6. SIDS
7. ADL
8. lb or #
9. RUL
10. RML
11. NWB
12. ROM
13. L/min
14. SVN
15. LLL
16. IPPB
17. USN
18. HP
19. WP
20. CPM
21. ES
22. EPC
23. TENS
24. IS
25. CPT
26. MDI
27. ORIF
28. TT
29. SaO_2
30. AKA

31. UD
32. HA
33. ISOM
34. LE
35. STM
36. HD
37. Tx
38. PDPV
39. >
40. TKR or TKA
41. THR or THA
42. ET
43. BKA
44. <
45. BiW
46. PEP
47. CP
48. AA
49. CPR
50. HBOT
51. TTOT
52. CPAP
53. BUE
54. BLE
55. RUE
56. LUE
57. RLE
58. LLE
59. PTA
60. RT
61. PROM
62. WBAT
63. FWW
64. CABG
65. DPI
66. ADS
67. ICD
68. PD
69. NC or NP
70. CBNT
71. PTCA
72. O₂ SAT
73. BiPAP
74. SpO₂

★ HIGH PRIORITY

When the electronic medical record (EMR) with computer physician order entry (CPOE) is implemented, the physicians' orders are entered directly into the patient's electronic record, and the treatment order is automatically sent to the appropriate department. The health unit coordinator (HUC) may have tasks to perform, such as coordinating and scheduling procedures, ordering special diets and cathartics for preparation, and so forth. An icon may indicate a HUC task, or it may signify a nurse request. When paper charts are used, the doctors' orders are communicated by the ordering step of transcription via computer or by completion of a downtime requisition form.

★ HIGH PRIORITY

Downtime requisitions are included in this chapter for learning purposes. The Evolve website associated with the *Health Unit Coordinator Skills Manual* includes a simulated hospital computer program that may be used as well.

CARDIOVASCULAR

Cardiovascular conditions may be treated with medication and/or surgery, and/or placement of various therapeutic cardiac instruments. Some of the surgical procedures required and the placement of these therapeutic instruments are discussed in this chapter. An emergency procedure to correct life-threatening fibrillations of the heart is discussed in the High Priority box.

★ HIGH PRIORITY

Defibrillation
Defibrillation is a process in which an electronic device sends an electric shock to the heart to correct life-threatening fibrillations of the heart, which could result in cardiac arrest. This procedure should be performed immediately after identifying that the patient is experiencing a cardiac emergency, has no pulse, and is unresponsive. *External defibrillators* deliver the shock through the chest wall, whereas internal defibrillators (ICDs) deliver the shock via implanted electrodes within the heart.

Invasive Cardiovascular Therapies

Many cardiovascular therapies are invasive and are performed by an interventional cardiologist and/or an interventional radiologist. These procedures may be done in the cardiovascular laboratory (CV lab or cardiac cath lab), a special x-ray division of the radiology department, or the surgery department.

Insertion of a Cardiac Pacemaker

A **cardiac pacemaker** is an electric apparatus that is used in most cases to increase the heart rate in severe bradycardia by electrically stimulating the heart muscle. A pacemaker may be permanent or temporary, may emit the stimulus at a constant and fixed rate, or may fire only on demand. Permanent pacemakers are implanted under a chest muscle during surgery. With temporary pacemakers, wires from outside the body lead into the heart (Fig. 17-1).

★ HIGH PRIORITY

Pacemakers usually are used to correct bradycardia (a slow heart rhythm), whereas implantable cardioverter-defibrillators (ICDs) are used to correct various abnormal heart rhythms such as tachycardia (fast heart rhythm), cardiac fibrillation, and bradycardia.

Insertion of an Implantable Cardioverter-Defibrillator

An implantable cardioverter-defibrillator (ICD) may be referred to as an *automatic implantable cardioverter-defibrillator* (AICD); it

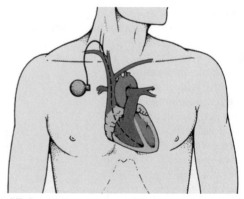

Figure 17-1 Pacemaker. (From Thibodeau GA, Patton KT: *Anatomy and physiology,* ed 6, St Louis, 2007, Mosby.)

is implanted in the chest. An ICD is an electric device that monitors and restores proper rhythm by sending low-energy shocks to the heart when the heart begins to beat rapidly or erratically (Fig. 17-2). Most ICDs are also capable of pacing the heart in response to bradycardia. Newer ICDs may be approved in the near future that do not require the placement of electrical leads into the heart.

Radiofrequency Ablation

Radiofrequency ablation is a treatment that is performed in conjunction with invasive diagnostic procedures such as electrophysiology studies (see Chapter 16). In this case radiofrequencies emitted from a catheter tip ablate (kill) abnormal heart tissue that is the source of cardiac dysrhythmia.

Angioplasty (Balloon Angioplasty, Coronary Angioplasty, Coronary Artery Angioplasty, Cardiac Angioplasty, Percutaneous Transluminal Coronary Angioplasty, Heart Artery Dilatation)

Angioplasty is a medical procedure in which a balloon is used to open narrowed or blocked blood vessels of the heart (coronary arteries). Although it is an invasive procedure and a consent form is required, it is not regarded as a type of surgery. An angioplasty usually is performed during a heart catheterization, when it is deemed necessary depending on the results of the coronary arteriography. Traditional angioplasty involves the use of a balloon catheter—a small, hollow, flexible tube that has a balloon near the end of it. The balloon catheter is moved into or near the blockage, and the balloon on the end is blown up (inflated) and then removed. This opens the blocked vessel and restores proper blood flow to the heart.

Stent

In most cases, a device called a **stent** is placed at the site of a narrowing or blockage in order to keep the artery open. Stenting (the implantation of a stent) is a common procedure. An intraluminal coronary artery stent is a small, self-expanding, metal mesh tube that is placed inside a coronary artery after balloon angioplasty to prevent the artery from reclosing (Fig. 17-3). A drug-eluting stent is coated with medicine (sirolimus or paclitaxel) that helps to further prevent the arteries from reclosing. Similar to other coronary stents, it is left permanently in the artery. Although most commonly used to treat

blockages in the coronary arteries, angioplasty and stent placement may be used to unblock arteries in the legs or arms to treat peripheral arterial disease (PAD) and vessel blockages in the kidneys, brain, and other organs. Additional procedures are discussed in the interventional radiology section of this chapter.

Atherectomy

In a small number of cases, a special catheter with a small, diamond tip is used to drill through hard plaque and calcium that is causing the blockage. This is called *rotational atherectomy.*

Atrial Septal Defect Repair

The repair of a congenital hole between the right and left atrium in newborns may be performed in the cath lab by insertion of the surgical instruments through the femoral vein. This is done with the aid of intracardiac echocardiogram (ICE).

Coronary Artery Bypass Graft

Coronary artery bypass graft (CABG; pronounced "cabbage") surgery has become a common treatment for blocked arteries when they are too severely blocked to be treated with angioplasty. Heart bypass surgery creates a detour or "bypass" around the blocked part of a coronary artery to restore the blood supply to the heart muscle (Fig. 17-4). After the patient has been anesthetized, the heart surgeon makes an incision in the middle of the chest and separates the breastbone. Through this incision, the surgeon can see the heart and the aorta (the main blood vessel leading from the heart to the rest of the body). After surgery, the breastbone is rejoined with wire, and the incision is sewn closed.

Artery and Vein Grafts

A vein from the leg, called the *saphenous vein,* may be used for the bypass; an incision is made in the leg, and the vein removed. The vein is located on the inside of the leg, running from the ankle to the groin. The saphenous vein normally does only about 10% of the work of circulating blood from the leg back to the heart. Therefore it can be taken out without harm to the patient or harm to the leg. The internal mammary artery (IMA) may also be used as the graft.

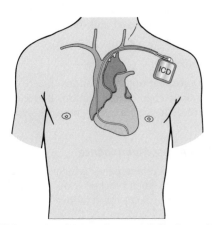

Figure 17-2 Implantable cardioverter-defibrillator. (From Lewis SM, Heitkemper MM, Dirksen SR: *Medical-surgical nursing,* ed 6, St Louis, 2004, Mosby.)

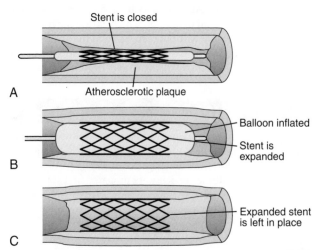

Figure 17-3 Coronary stent. (From LaFleur Brooks M: *Exploring medical language: a student-directed approach,* ed 6, St Louis, 2005, Mosby.)

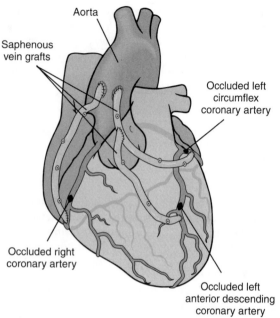

Figure 17-4 Coronary bypass (CBAG). (From Lewis SM, Heitkemper MM, Dirksen SR: *Medical-surgical nursing: assessment and management of clinical problems*, ed 5, St Louis, 2000, Mosby.)

The IMA provides the advantage of staying open for many more years than vein grafts, but in some situations it cannot be used. Other arteries also are being used now in bypass surgery. The most common of these is the radial artery. This is one of the two arteries that supply the hand with blood. It usually can be removed from the arm without resultant impairment of blood supply to the hand. Traditionally, the patient is connected to the heart-lung machine, or the bypass pump, which adds oxygen to the blood and circulates blood to other parts of the body during surgery.

Other surgical techniques for this procedure are being used more frequently. One popular method is called *off-pump coronary artery bypass*, or OPCAB. This operation allows the bypass to be created while the heart is still beating. Another alternative is the use of smaller incisions that avoid splitting the breastbone. This is referred to as *minimally invasive direct coronary artery bypass*, or MIDCAB. Coronary bypass surgery now can be performed with the aid of a robot, which allows the surgeon to perform the operation without even being in the same room as the patient. A surgical consent form is required, and the patient is admitted to the coronary intensive care unit after surgery.

⭐ HIGH PRIORITY

Usually, the consent form for heart catheterization includes all possible correction options, so the surgeon can proceed with the procedure or surgery as required. In other cases, multiple consents are prepared and signed.

 SKILLS CHALLENGE

To practice transcribing cardiovascular treatment orders, complete Activity 17-1 in the *Skills Practice Manual*.

INTERVENTIONAL RADIOLOGY

Background Information

Invasive diagnostic tests performed in the special procedures division of the diagnostic imaging department (see Chapter 15) or in the cardiac cath lab in the cardiovascular department (see Chapter 16) often result in concurrent treatment based on the findings at the time of the test. Because of the invasive nature and associated risks, it is expected that any treatment or **intervention** would occur in conjunction with the test itself.

As technology leads to an increasing ability to treat patients by a method other than open surgery, more techniques are being developed to treat patients with less invasive procedures while catheterized and under radiologic visualization and guidance. They tend to have less associated risk and quicker recovery of the patient. These treatment procedures may be done by an interventional radiologist and/or the interventional specialist.

Treatments
Embolization

Embolization is delivery of clotting agents (e.g., coils, plastic particles, gel, foam) through a thin catheter directly to an area. The procedure may be used to treat internal bleeding such as that caused by a ruptured aneurysm or a uterine fibroid tumor, and guided by angiography. It may also be used to block the supply of blood to affected blood vessels to prevent rupture, as in the treatment of arteriovenous malformations (AVMs) in the brain. Uterine artery embolization is done to stop life-threatening postpartum bleeding, potentially preventing hysterectomy. The same procedure is used to cut off the blood supply to fibroid tumors of the uterus, causing them to shrink and die, and is then called *uterine fibroid embolization* (UFE).

Biliary Drainage and Stenting

Biliary drainage and stenting involves use of a stent (small mesh tube) to open up blocked ducts and allow bile to drain from the liver.

Brachytherapy

Brachytherapy is radiation therapy performed by introducing radioactive pellets that travel and lodge in vessels of the targeted cancerous tissue.

Chemoembolization

Delivery of cancer-fighting medications directly to the site of a cancer tumor is chemoembolization. It is currently being used mostly to treat cancers of the endocrine system and liver cancers.

Hemodialysis Access Maintenance

Hemodialysis access maintenance is the use of catheterization and thrombolysis to open blocked grafts needed for hemodialysis, which is performed to treat kidney failure.

Stent Insertion

The small flexible tube made of plastic or wire mesh used to open coronary arteries (as discussed in Chapter 15) is also used to treat a variety of medical conditions in order to open blood vessels or other pathways that have been narrowed or blocked by tumors or obstructions. In some patients with high blood pressure (hypertension), the condition is caused by a narrowing of the arteries in the kidneys. The associated renal hypertension can often be treated with angioplasty and stenting.

Infection and Abscess Drainage

Patients with a variety of illnesses may develop an area of persistent infection (abscess) in the body. The infection can be drained by inserting a catheter through a small nick in the skin and to the site of the infection. This procedure is also used to treat complications of open surgery.

Needle Biopsy

Needle biopsy is a procedure to retrieve tissue from the breast, lung, and other organs to diagnose cancers; it is an alternative to surgical biopsy.

Radiofrequency Ablation

Radiofrequency ablation (RFA) is the use of radiofrequency (RF) energy to "cook" and kill cancerous tumors. The procedure is similar to the RFA used to treat abnormal heart rhythms during cardiac electrophysiology studies (see Chapter 15).

Endograft Insertion

Endograft insertion reinforces a ruptured or ballooning section of an artery (an aneurysm) with a fabric-wrapped flexible mesh tube (stent) used to "patch" the blood vessel. The procedure is also known as a *stent graft* or *endoluminal graft* (ELG). It is often used to treat abdominal aortic aneurysm (AAA).

Thrombolysis

Thrombolysis dissolves blood clots by injection of thrombolytic (clot-busting) drugs at the site of the clot. This procedure is used to treat blood clots in the brain to reverse the effects of stroke and to treat deep vein thrombosis in the leg to prevent permanent disability.

Transjugular Intrahepatic Portosystemic Shunt

Transjugular intrahepatic portosystemic shunt (TIPS) is a life-saving procedure to improve blood flow and prevent hemorrhage in patients with severe liver dysfunction.

Percutaneous Nephrostomy Tube Insertion

If the ureter becomes blocked by kidney stones or other obstructions causing a urinary tract obstruction, the interventional radiologist inserts a catheter through a small nick in the skin and into the blocked kidney to drain the urine.

Varicocele Embolization

Varicocele embolization is a treatment for "varicose veins" in the scrotum, which can cause male infertility and pain.

Varicose Vein Treatment

The saphenous vein is sealed shut through the use of a laser or radiofrequency treatment. Sufficient alternate venous return is verified by Doppler studies prior to this procedure.

Vena Cava Filter

A tiny cagelike device, the vena cava filter is inserted in a blood vessel to break up clots and prevent them from reaching and lodging in the heart or lungs. Prevents pulmonary embolism (PE).

Vertebroplasty

Vertebroplasty is a pain treatment for fractured vertebra in which medical-grade bone cement is injected into the vertebra.

CARDIOPULMONARY (RESPIRATORY CARE) DEPARTMENT

Background Information

Diagnostic tests performed in the cardiopulmonary (respiratory care) department are discussed in Chapter 16. The cardiopulmonary (respiratory care) department also evaluates patients with respiratory conditions and performs treatments to maintain or improve function of the respiratory system. Treatments usually are performed by a **certified respiratory therapist (CRT)** (also called a *respiratory practitioner*) at the patient's bedside. It is important that the health unit coordinator (HUC) enter all information regarding the order into the computer or onto the requisition form. The respiratory therapist then brings the needed equipment and medication to the unit, so the patient's treatment is not delayed while necessary items are obtained. The therapist reads the doctor's order before administering the treatment. On completion of treatment, the therapist documents the type of medication and treatment provided and other pertinent data on a respiratory therapy record sheet in the patient's chart.

In a hospital that uses computer physician order entry (CPOE), the physician will input the order directly to the cardiopulmonary department. To communicate the doctor's order to the cardiopulmonary (respiratory care) department, use the computer or complete a cardiopulmonary (respiratory care) treatment requisition (Fig. 17-5). The HUC may be required to notify nursing personnel or the cardiopulmonary department of stat orders.

Treatments

Before the doctor orders or the respiratory therapist administers respiratory treatment, the patient is evaluated by the doctor, who listens to the sounds within the body (**auscultation**) for detection of abnormal breath sounds such as **stridor, crackles (rales),** or **wheezes.**

Oxygen Therapy

Oxygen therapy is ordered to (1) treat hypoxemia (deficiency in the content of oxygen in arterial blood); (2) decrease the work of breathing for a patient with **dyspnea;** and (3) reduce myocardial (heart muscle) work. Oxygen is piped into the patient's room via a wall outlet and is administered under pressure (Fig. 17-6). A portable oxygen tank may be used when a patient is transported. Oxygen therapy may have a drying effect on the respiratory tract; therefore oxygen is commonly humidified during administration. Oxygen supports combustion, so no smoking is allowed in the room while oxygen is being administered. All hospitals and other health care facilities have a general "no smoking" policy for visitors and patients as well as employees.

An oxygen order contains the amount of oxygen (flow rate and/or concentration) the patient is to receive and the type of

Doctor ordering _____

Date to be done _____ ☐ Stat   ☐ Routine   ☐ ASAP

Today's date _____ Requested by _____

Patient Label

CARDIOPULMONARY (RESPIRATORY CARE) DEPARTMENT -TREATMENT REQUISITION

Clinical indication _____

Comments _____

☐ O_2 _____ L/M   ☐ NP   ☐ Mask   ☐ Type   ☐ Other _____

☐ Aerosol delivery type _____

☐ Bi-level press. vent. _____

☐ CPAP _____

☐ CPT _____

☐ IPPB _____

☐ IS _____

☐ SVN _____

☐ USN _____

Write in order _____

Ventilator orders

IMV mode _____ TV_____ FIO_2_____ PO_2_____ PS_____ Peep_____

☐ Write in order _____

Figure 17-5 Downtime requisition for cardiopulmonary (respiratory care) treatment.

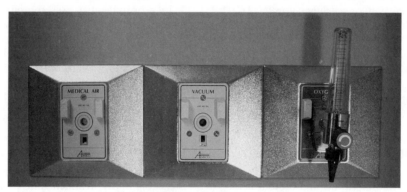

Figure 17-6 Wall outlet for oxygen.

delivery device to be used (mode of delivery). The flow rate is ordered in liters per minute.

Flow Rate or Concentration of Oxygen and Administration Devices. Oxygen may be administered with the use of a low-flow system, which provides only a portion of the total amount of gas the patient is breathing (the rest must be added from room air), or a high-flow oxygen system, which provides enough gas flow to meet all of the patient's ventilatory demands.

Low-flow oxygen administration devices include the following:

- A *nasal cannula (NC)*, frequently referred to as *nasal prongs (NPs)*, is the most commonly used method. Nasal cannulas should not be run over 6 L/min because this may cause excessive drying of the nasal mucosa.

- A *simple mask* is a device generally used for emergencies and short-term therapies that fits over the patient's nose and mouth and acts as a reservoir for the next breath. The simple mask should be run at a minimum of 5 L/min to ensure that the carbon dioxide the patient exhales is washed away and is not rebreathed.

- A *partial rebreathing mask* uses a simple mask connected to a bag reservoir with no valve between the bag and the mask. It is called a *partial rebreathing mask* because the first one third of exhalation enters the bag, mixes with source oxygen, and is consumed during the next inhalation.

- A *nonrebreathing mask* is designed to fit over the patient's nose and mouth as the simple oxygen mask does; however, a 500- to 1000-mL plastic bag is added to the mask, which has a series of one-way valves that permit the reservoir bag to fill only with pure oxygen (Fig. 17-7).

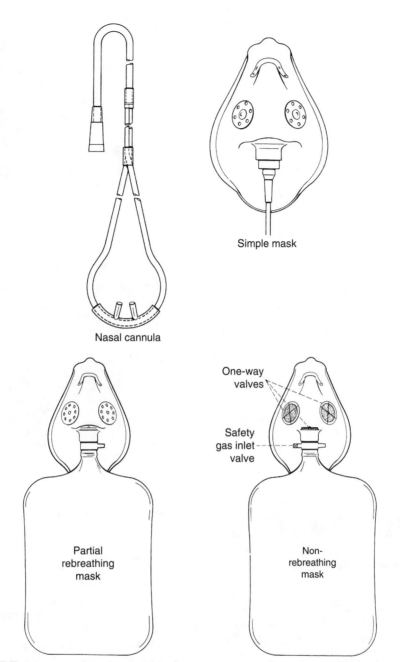

Figure 17-7 Devices used to administer low-flow system oxygen. (From Kacmarek RM: In-hospital administration of oxygen. In Kacmarek RM, Stoller JK, editors: *Current respiratory care*, Toronto, 1988, BC Decker.)

High-flow oxygen systems include the following:

- A *jet mixing mask*, also referred to as a *Venturi mask* (also known by brand name, *Ventimask*), delivers a total high flow by mixing oxygen with room air. The mask takes pure oxygen from the flow meter and mixes it with a certain proportion of room air to deliver a higher concentration of oxygen.
- A *large-volume* **nebulizer** is another example of a high-flow system. This device works much like the jet mixing mask, but it also provides bland (nonmedicated) **aerosol**

therapy and can be connected to a variety of devices, including an aerosol mask, a face tent for patients with facial burns or who cannot tolerate a mask, a T piece or Briggs adapter for intubated patients, or a tracheostomy mask (collar) for those with a tracheostomy (Fig. 17-8).

Plastic tubing is used to carry oxygen from the wall outlet to the patient. Although cardiopulmonary (respiratory care) department personnel usually set up, take down, and handle the equipment for oxygen administration, nursing staff members also monitor this treatment.

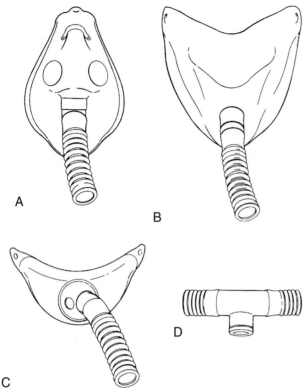

Figure 17-8 Various devices used to apply high-flow system oxygen. **A,** Aerosol mask. **B,** Face hood. **C,** Tracheostomy collar. **D,** Briggs T piece. (From Kacmarek RM: In-hospital administration of oxygen. In Kacmarek RM, Stoller JK, editors: *Current respiratory care,* Toronto, 1988, BC Decker.)

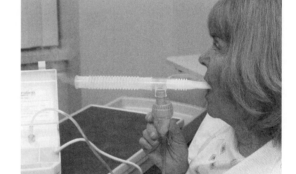

Figure 17-9 A metered-dose inhaler. (From Elkin MK, Perry AG, Potter PA: *Nursing interventions and clinical skills,* ed 3, St Louis, 2004, Mosby.)

Figure 17-10 Nebulization. (From Perry AG, Potter PA, Elkin MK: *Nursing interventions & clinical skills,* ed 5, St. Louis, 2012, Mosby.)

> ### ⭐ HIGH PRIORITY
>
> Orders for oxygen therapy include the amount of oxygen (flow rate and/or concentration) and the type of delivery device.
>
> It is important to recognize a new order for oxygen or a change in a previous order. An ABG on O_2 @ 4 L/min is *not* a new order for oxygen but is an arterial blood gas drawn while the patient's oxygen flow rate is at 4 L/min. It may be necessary to notify nursing staff or the cardiopulmonary (respiratory care) department of the requested oxygen flow rate.

Aerosol Treatments

Aerosol Delivery Devices

- *Metered-dose inhaler (MDI).* MDIs—small portable aerosol canisters filled with medication—are the most common type of aerosol treatment. One or two puffs of the medication is inhaled with a deep breath and an inspiratory hold for a few seconds. Usually MDIs are self-administered and require patient education and cooperation (Fig. 17-9).
- *Small-volume nebulizer (SVN) (handheld nebulizer [HHN]).* SVN treatments last 8 to 12 minutes and allow for numerous breaths to administer the medication. The ideal breathing pattern is for the patient to inhale deeply with an inspiratory hold for a few seconds. SVNs also may be called

spontaneous nebulizer treatments or *jet nebulizer treatments* or may be referred to by the brand name of the nebulizer device (Fig. 17-10).

- *Dry powder inhaler (DPI).* Dry powder inhalers (DPIs) are devices that provide the drug in powder form to be delivered into the lungs for absorption. A total of 1 or 2 puffs of the medication is inhaled with a deep breath and an inspiratory hold for a few seconds. An example of a DPI is Advair. Usually DPIs are self-administered and require patient education and cooperation (Fig. 7-11).
- *Hypertonic ultrasonic nebulizer (USN).* A USN with **hypertonic** solution often is used to induce a sputum specimen. It produces an aerosol that carries deep into the airways of the lung to loosen secretions so the patient may produce a sputum specimen. The solution used is a hypertonic (concentrated) salt solution of 10% sodium chloride (NaCl). This is called an **induced sputum specimen.**
- A *Lukens sputum trap* often is used by a respiratory therapist to collect a sterile induced sputum specimen (Fig. 17-12).
- *Intermittent* **positive pressure** *breathing (IPPB).* IPPB is a technique that is used to provide short-term or intermittent mechanical ventilation for the purpose of augmenting lung expansion, delivering aerosol medication, clearing retained secretions, or assisting ventilation. IPPB treatment usually is administered through the use of a pneumatically driven, pressure-triggered, pressure-cycled ventilator (Fig. 17-13).
- *Continuous bronchodilator nebulizer therapy (CBNT).* This is a nebulizer that introduces aerosolized bronchodilator with

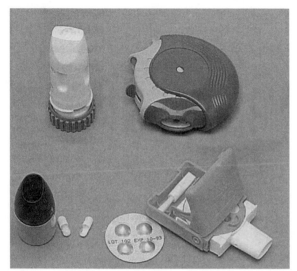

Figure 17-11 Dry powder inhalers. (Modified from Spiro S, MacCochran G: Delivery of medication to the lungs. In Albert R, Spiro S, Jett J, editors: *Comprehensive respiratory medicine,* St Louis, 1999, Mosby.)

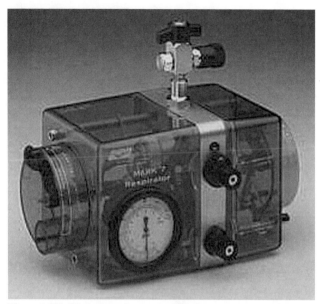

Figure 17-13 Bird Mark 7 intermittent positive pressure breathing machine. (From Kacmarek RM, Dimas S, Mack CW: *The essentials of respiratory care,* ed 4, St Louis, 2005, Mosby.)

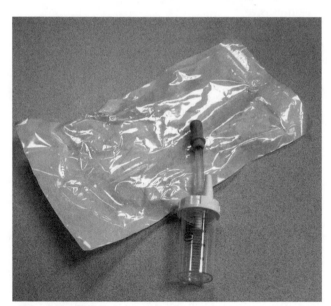

Figure 17-12 Lukens sputum trap, used to collect uncontaminated sputum specimens.

> ⭐ **HIGH PRIORITY**
>
> **Ultrasound diagnostic procedures** are performed in the ultrasound division of the diagnostic imaging department (see Chapter 15).
>
> An **ultrasonic nebulizer** is used as treatment by the cardiopulmonary (respiratory care) department. **Ultrasound therapy** is provided by the physical therapist. It is important to read the doctors' orders carefully so the order is sent to the appropriate department.

oxygen on a continuous basis (low or high flow), or while the patient is on a mechanical ventilator. This is usually ordered to treat severe exacerbation of asthma, respiratory distress, and chronic obstructive pulmonary disease (COPD).

Types of Aerosolized Drugs

- *Nasal decongestants.* Nasal decongestants are found primarily as over-the-counter (OTC) squeeze bottles that are sprayed into nostrils. These drugs are classified as vasoconstrictors. An example of a nasal decongestant is Neo-Synephrine.
- *Bronchodilators.* Bronchodilators enlarge the diameter of the airway, usually by relaxing the smooth muscle that surrounds the airways. Examples of bronchodilators include Ventolin, Atrovent, Maxair, and Serevent.
- *Antiasthmatics.* This is a relatively new category of drugs that desensitize the allergic response to prevent or decrease the incidence of asthma. Examples of antiasthmatics include cromolyn sodium and nedocromil sodium.
- *Corticosteroids.* Corticosteroids are used in moderate and severe asthma attacks to reduce the inflammatory response within the lung. They also are used on a standing basis to prevent inflammation. Examples of corticosteroids include AeroBid, Pulmicort, Vanceril, Flovent, and Azmacort.
- *Intranasal corticosteroids.* Corticosteroids introduced nasally are used to decrease vascular permeability and congestion. Examples of intranasal corticosteroids include Beconase, Rhinocort, Flonase, Nasacort and Nasonex.
- *Mucolytics.* Mucolytics break down secretions within the lungs to make it easier to expectorate and clear the lungs. Examples of mucolytics include Pulmozyme and Mucomyst.
- *Antimicrobials.* Antimicrobials are aerosolized antibiotics and antiviral agents that fight bacterial or viral infections involving the respiratory system. Examples of antimicrobials include gentamicin, tobramycin, amphotericin B, ribavirin, and pentamidine.

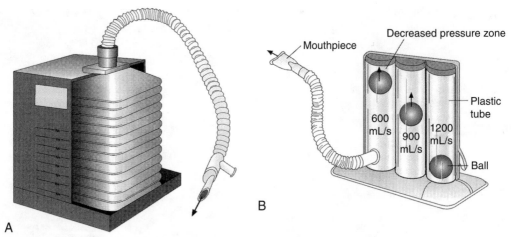

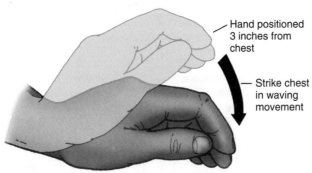

Figure 17-14 A, Volume-oriented incentive spirometer. **B,** Flow-oriented incentive spirometer. (From Eubanks DH, Bone RC: *Comprehensive respiratory care,* St Louis, 1985, Mosby.)

Figure 17-15 Movement of cupped hand at wrist to percuss chest. (From Wilkins RL, Stoller JK, Scanlan CL: *Egan's fundamentals of respiratory care,* ed 8, St Louis, 2003, Mosby.)

BOX 17-1	AN EXAMPLE OF SETTINGS FOR A MECHANICAL VENTILATOR

COPD: Initial Ventilator Settings
Noninvasive
Mode: Assist/control (pressure) or pressure support
Tidal volume (TV): 6 to 8 mL/kg ideal body weight (IBW)
Positive end-expiratory pressure (PEEP): 3 to 8 cm H_2O
Ventilating pressure: 8 to 12 cm H_2O
Inspiratory time: <1.0 s
Fio_2: to maintain Pao_2 >60 mm Hg
Backup rate: 8 to 10, actual patient rate determines baseline $Paco_2$

COPD, Chronic obstructive pulmonary disease.

Hypotonic Saline Solution. A **hypotonic** dilute salt solution (<0.9%) is used in humidifiers and continuous nebulizers to thin bronchial secretions and to induce sputum.

Other Respiratory Treatments

Incentive Spirometry. Incentive spirometry (IS), also known as *sustained maximal inspiration* (SMI), often is used postoperatively to encourage and reinforce the patient to take protracted, slow, deep breaths. The benefits of IS include improving inspiratory muscle performance, thereby reestablishing or simulating the normal pattern of pulmonary hyperinflation. The devices used provide patients with visual positive feedback when they inhale at a predetermined flow rate or volume and sustain the inflation for a predetermined length of time (Fig. 17-14).

Chest Percussion Therapy or Chest Physiotherapy. Chest percussion therapy (CPT) (also called *chest physiotherapy*), a technique of rhythmically tapping the chest wall with cupped hands (Fig. 17-15) or a mechanical device, is used to loosen secretions in the area underlying the percussion via the air pressure that is generated by the cupped hand on the chest wall. This treatment usually is performed in conjunction with postural drainage; a treatment of patient positioning that is designed to remove secretions from the lung. This may

also be referred to as *percussion and postural drainage* or *pummeling and postural drainage* (P&PD). High-frequency chest compression (HFCC) uses a mechanical vest that vibrates at high frequencies to loosen secretions and is often used for pediatric patients.

Mechanical Ventilator. A mechanical **ventilator** is a device designed to provide mechanical ventilation to a patient. Ventilators are used chiefly in intensive care medicine, home care, and emergency medicine (as stand-alone units), and in anesthesia as a component of an anesthesia machine. Mechanical ventilation is indicated when the patient's spontaneous ventilation is inadequate to maintain life. It also is indicated to prevent imminent collapse of other physiologic functions or ineffective gas exchange in the lungs (Box 17-1, *An Example of Settings for a Mechanical Ventilator*). Because mechanical ventilation serves only to provide assistance for breathing and does not cure a disease, the patient's underlying condition should be correctable and should resolve over time, although some conditions may warrant the use of mechanical ventilation for the duration of the patient's life. **Intubation,** or the insertion of an **endotracheal tube,** is necessary. The endotracheal tube may need to be changed and a new one ordered. *Weaning* is a term that is used to describe the gradual removal of mechanical ventilation from a patient. Arterial blood gas tests will be ordered at intervals to monitor ventilator settings. **Extubation** orders will be written when the patient is to be removed from the ventilator. Postextubation orders will be written to monitor respiratory status after the patient has been removed from the ventilator. In a hospital that has implemented CPOE, there may still be a requirement by the facility to process a written or printed set of ventilator orders.

Noninvasive Positive Pressure Ventilation. Noninvasive positive pressure ventilation (NIPPV), such as continuous positive airway pressure (CPAP) or bilevel positive airway pressure (BPAP), is the application of positive pressure by noninvasive means to a patient with acute or chronic respiratory failure, or while weaning a patient from ventilatory support. NIPPV enhances the breathing process by giving the patient a mixture of air and oxygen from a flow generator through a tightly fitted facial or nasal mask.

Doctors' Orders for Respiratory Treatments

The following orders include many instructions for the respiratory therapist. It is very important to be accurate in entering the order information into the computer or copying the information onto the cardiopulmonary (respiratory care) requisition, so the therapist will bring the correct equipment and/or supplies to carry out the order. The respiratory therapist also is required to read the physician's orders before administering treatment.

40% O₂ @ 4 L/min NC Cont

Four liters per minute of oxygen at 40% concentration is delivered continuously via nasal cannula.

SVN with UD albuterol tid c̄ CPT

This small-volume nebulizer (SVN) order includes a **unit dose** of albuterol and an order for chest percussion therapy three times per day.

SVN 1.25 mg Xopenex 3 mL NS tid

This treatment uses a simple device that produces an aerosol of medication and normal saline to be inhaled into the lungs.

⭐ HIGH PRIORITY

The health unit coordinator must notify the cardiopulmonary (respiratory care) department when the doctor writes an order for an induced sputum specimen. Small-volume nebulizer or hypertonic ultrasonic nebulizer treatment is given by a respiratory therapist to loosen lung secretions. A Lukens trap often is used by a respiratory therapist to collect a sterile sputum specimen.

IPPB 0.5 mL Ventolin & 3 mL NS tid

This IPPB order includes medication (Ventolin) and dosage (0.5 mL). IPPB orders must include frequency and medication; duration and pressure used are optional.

MDI Ventolin qid III puffs

MDI is a metered-dose inhaler, in which the medication is premeasured in the pharmacy.

HA @ 60% continuous via T piece

A heated mist (heated aerosol) is produced for the patient to breathe. It may be ordered for patients who are breathing through a tracheostomy or an endotracheal tube.

Incentive Spirometry (IS) 15 min tid

This incentive spirometry treatment will be performed for 15 minutes three times per day.

IS PEP @ 5 cm H₂O

This incentive spirometry treatment includes positive expiratory pressure (PEP), which supplies resistance against exhalation (keeps air from coming out) in order to reinflate the alveoli in patients with atelectasis. PEP also may be ordered with SVN treatments.

Bilevel Pressure I:10/ E:5

Bilevel pressure ventilation is a treatment that uses a machine to push air into the lungs during inspiration (such as IPPB) and expiration (such as CPAP) in order to treat severe atelectasis or sleep apnea.

CPAP 5 cm H₂O

This continuous positive airway pressure treatment provides continuous positive pressure in the airway throughout the entire respiratory cycle. This approach prevents the lungs from completely returning to resting level and may be used to treat patients with sleep apnea and other respiratory syndromes. CPAP usually is provided noninvasively through a facial apparatus. It also can be used in weaning patients from a mechanical ventilator, or in treating those with inadequate oxygen intake.

Cardiopulmonary (Respiratory Care) to Do Preoperative Teaching

The respiratory therapist will instruct the patient before surgery about incentive spirometry and other respiratory treatments that the doctor will order to be done after surgery. The patient will know then what to expect and will know what is expected in the performance of respiratory treatments.

Cardiopulmonary (Respiratory Care) to Do CPR Training with Parents before Child's Discharge

The respiratory therapist sometimes is asked to teach parents cardiopulmonary resuscitation (CPR) before a pediatric patient is discharged. ∎

SKILLS CHALLENGE

To practice transcribing cardiopulmonary (respiratory care) orders, complete Activity 17-2 in the *Skills Practice Manual.*

WOUND CARE DEPARTMENT OR CLINIC

Background Information

The wound care department or clinic specializes in the treatment of nonhealing, or slow-healing, wounds such as pressure sores caused by sitting or lying in one position and foot and leg ulcers associated with diabetes and burns. The healing process can be slowed or interrupted by any number of causes, including infection, poor diet, and other medical conditions, such as diabetes. The wound care department or clinic provides educational, medical, and supportive services to patients and their caregivers.

Hyperbaric Oxygen Therapy

Hyperbaric oxygen therapy is a treatment often performed in the wound care department or clinic in which the patient breathes 100% oxygen while in an enclosed system pressurized to greater than normal atmospheric pressure (three times normal); this is called a *hyperbaric chamber.* Hyperbaric oxygen therapy delivers oxygen systemically to injured areas quickly and in high concentrations. The increased pressure changes the normal cellular respiration process and causes oxygen to dissolve in the plasma. This stimulates the growth of new blood vessels, resulting in a substantial increase in tissue oxygenation that can arrest certain types of infections and enhance wound healing. Hyperbaric oxygen therapy generally is administered on an outpatient basis.

An Order for Hyperbaric Oxygen Therapy (HBOT)

• Hyperbaric oxygen therapy bid 3 × wk for 8 weeks

The patient will be enclosed in a hyperbaric chamber to breathe 100% oxygen twice a week for a period of 8 weeks.

TRACTION OR ORTHOPEDICS

The traction or orthopedic department provides for traction orders as well as the placement of casts when necessary. **Traction** is the process of putting a limb, bone, or group of muscles under tension with the use of weights and pulleys, to align or immobilize, to reduce muscle spasm, or to relieve pressure. It is used to treat patients with fractures, dislocations, and long-duration muscle spasms, and to prevent or correct deformities. Traction can be used in short-term or long-term therapy. Two basic types include skin traction and skeletal traction.

Apparatus Setup

Bed

The apparatus that is attached to the patient's bed may include pulleys, rope, weights, and metal bars. The weights (metal disks or sandbags) provide the "pull" to a part of the body. The pulleys, rope, and metal bars are assembled to suspend the weights. Each type of traction requires a different assemblage of these parts; thus a skilled person must perform this task. It is usually the responsibility of the nurse or an orthopedic technician to attach the traction apparatus to the bed. Physical therapy department personnel may assist with setting up traction equipment in smaller hospitals. The HUC communicates a traction order verbally by telephone or via computer or requisition to the person or department (such as the orthopedic equipment department) that is responsible for assembling the bed apparatus (Fig. 17-16).

Patient

The apparatus that is attached to the patient may consist of an external attachment, such as a halter, belt, or boot, or an internal attachment, such as a pin, tongs, or wires placed directly into the bone by the surgeon. The external apparatus is applied to the patient by the nursing staff, and sometimes the HUC must order necessary supplies from the central service department.

Although the types of supplies the HUC orders vary among hospitals, moleskin tape, slings, and sandbags commonly are requisitioned from the central service department. Some hospitals have designated nursing units for the treatment of patients with orthopedic conditions and for those who have traction orders.

Doctor ordering _____

☐ Stat   ☐ Routine   ☐ ASAP   Patient Label

Today's date _____ Requested by_____

ORTHOPEDIC/TRACTION EQUIPMENT REQUISITION

Diagnosis _____

Comments _____

Write out the entire doctor's order

☐ Write in order _____

☐ Bryant's _____

☐ Bucks _____

☐ Cervical _____

☐ Overhead frame and trapeze _____

☐ Russell's _____

☐ Skeletal tx _____

☐ Skin tx _____

☐ Split Russell's _____

Figure 17-16 Downtime requisition for orthopedic equipment.

Doctors' Orders for Traction

Traction Orders for Treatment of Bone Fractures

Two basic types of traction are used in orthopedics for the treatment of patients with fractured bones and for correction of orthopedic abnormalities. *Skin traction* applies pull to an affected body structure through straps attached to the skin surrounding the structure. Types include adhesive and nonadhesive skin traction. *Skeletal traction* is applied to the affected structure by a metal pin or wire inserted during surgery into the structure and attached to traction ropes. Skeletal traction often is used when continuous traction is desired to immobilize, position, and align a fractured bone properly during the healing process.

Skin Traction Orders
Skin Traction 5 lb to Left Arm

Skin traction uses 5- to 7-pound weights attached to the skin to indirectly apply the necessary pulling force to the bone. The doctor may give additional directions regarding positioning.

Skin Traction 7 lb to Pelvis

Pelvic traction is applied to the lower spine, with a belt around the waist. This procedure is noninvasive and is the preferred treatment if traction is temporary or if only a light or discontinuous force is needed. Weights usually are attached through moleskin tape or with straps, boots, or cuffs.

Left Unilateral Buck's Skin Traction 5 lb

A traction setup is used as temporary treatment of a patient with fractured hip, sciatica, or other knee or hip disorders (also may be called *Buck's extension*). *Unilateral* indicates that the traction is to be applied to one leg only

(Fig. 17-17). Bilateral leg traction indicates that traction is to be applied to both legs. Traction is produced by applying regular or flannel-backed adhesive tape to the skin and keeping it in smooth close contact through circular bandaging of the part to which it is applied. The adhesive strips are aligned with the long axis of the arm or leg, and the superior ends are about 1 inch from the fracture site. Weights sufficient to produce the required extension are fastened to the inferior end of the adhesive strips by a rope that is run over a pulley to permit free motion.

Russell's Traction rt Leg c̄ 10# Weight

Russell's traction is a combination of suspension and traction that is provided to immobilize, position, and align the lower extremity or extremities in the treatment of a fractured femur, hip and knee contractures, and disease processes of the hip and knee. Adhesive or nonadhesive skin traction may be used. *Split Russell's traction* suspends the traction weights from pulley-and-rope systems at the foot and head of the patient's bed. A jacket restraint often is incorporated to help immobilize the patient.

Spica Cast

A **spica cast** is one that begins at the chest and includes one or both lower limbs. It is usually placed during surgery on pediatric patients who have undergone repair for fractures of the hip or leg(s) or who have congenital hip or leg dysplasia.

Skeletal Traction Orders
Cervical Traction Crutchfield Tongs

Cervical traction is used in the treatment of fractures of the cervical vertebrae. Crutchfield tongs are attached to

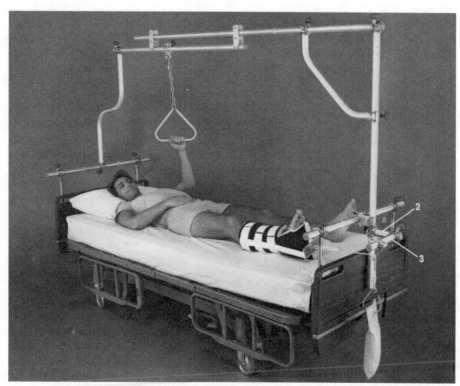

Figure 17-17 Unilateral Buck's traction.

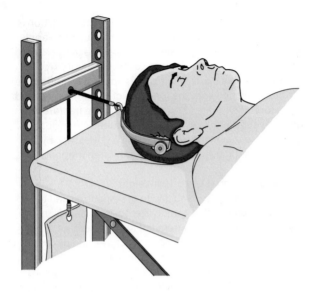

Figure 17-18 Crutchfield tongs. (From Phipps WJ, Monahan FD, Sands JK, et al: *Medical-surgical nursing,* ed 7, St Louis, 2003, Mosby.)

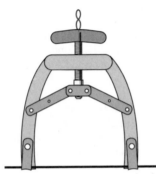

Figure 17-19 Steinmann pin. (From Elkin MK, Perry AG, Potter PA: *Nursing interventions and clinical skills,* ed 3, St Louis, 2004, Mosby.)

the skull to hyperextend the head and neck of patients with fractured cervical vertebrae for the purpose of immobilizing and aligning the vertebrae. The tips of the tongs are inserted into small burr holes drilled in each parietal region of the skull; the surrounding skin is sutured and covered with a dressing. A rope tied to the center of the tongs passes over a pulley at the head of the bed and is attached to a weight of 10 to 20 pounds, which hangs freely (Fig. 17-18). Other devices used for cervical traction include Gardner-Wells tongs and Vinke tongs. A special bed or Stryker frame may have to be obtained for the patient.

Thomas' Leg Splint Steinmann Pin 20 lb of Traction
A Thomas splint may be used to treat chronic joint disease through the use of a rigid **splint** constructed of steel bars curved to fit the involved limb that are held in place by a cast or a rigid bandage. A rigid metal splint that extends from a ring at the hip to beyond the foot may be used to treat a fractured leg and, in conjunction with various traction and suspension devices, to immobilize and position a fractured femur in a preoperative or postoperative patient. A Steinmann pin is a wide-diameter pin that is used for heavy skeletal traction; it is driven into the femur or tibia during surgery (Fig. 17-19).

Other Traction-Related Orders
Overhead Frame and Trapeze (Trapeze Bar)
An overhead frame and trapeze is used to help the patient move and support weight during transfer or position change. It also may aid in strengthening upper extremities (see Fig. 17-17). ∎

SKILLS CHALLENGE

To practice transcribing traction orders, complete Activity 17-3 in the *Skills Practice Manual.*

PHYSICAL MEDICINE AND REHABILITATION

Most hospitals have a physical medicine department that consists of physical therapy, occupational therapy, and speech therapy.

Physical Therapy
Background Information
Physical therapy is the division of the physical medicine department in the hospital that treats patients to improve and restore their functional mobility through methods such as gait training, exercise, water therapy, and heat and ice treatments. Patients include those injured in accidents, sports, or work-related activities. Children affected by cerebral palsy and muscular dystrophy are assisted toward normal physical development through physical therapy. Individuals who experience strokes, spinal cord injuries, and amputations are assisted back to their highest level of physical function through therapy. Exercises play a crucial role in the process of healing and recovering from injury or disease. **Aerobic exercise** causes the heart and lungs to work harder to benefit the cardiovascular and circulatory system. **Anaerobic exercise** involves strengthening muscles by forcing them to work very hard for a brief time.

Types of Exercises Performed by or with the Assistance of Physical Therapy
- **Passive exercise**—performed with the patient submissive; the physical therapist (PT) moves the patient's limbs.
- **Active exercise**—performed by the patient without assistance as instructed by the PT.
- **Resistive exercise**—use of opposition; a T band or water may be used to provide resistance for patient exercises.
- *Active assistive exercise*—involves a patient moving an extremity with assistance from the PT as required.
- *Progressive exercises*—gradually increasing the type of exercise.
- *Muscle reeducation exercise*—use of physical therapeutic exercises to restore muscle tone and strength after an injury or disease.
- *Coordination exercises*—designed to improve coordination and balance.
- *Relaxation exercises*—other types of exercises that may be ordered by the doctor.

The Physical therapist (PT), a person licensed to practice in this field, assesses the patient and initiates a plan of care. Physical therapy treatments may be carried out in the patient's

Doctor ordering _____		Patient Label
Today's date _____ Time to be done _____		
Date to be done _____ Requested by _____		

PHYSICAL THERAPY REQUISITION

Clinical indication _____

Transportation ☐ Portable ☐ Stretcher ☐ Wheelchair ☐ Ambulatory

O₂ ☐Yes /☐ No   Diabetic ☐Yes /☐ No   Hearing deficit ☐Yes /☐ No
IV ☐Yes /☐ No   Seizure disorder ☐Yes /☐ No   Sight deficit ☐Yes /☐ No
Isolation ☐Yes /☐ No   Non-English speaking ☐Yes /☐ No

Comments _____

Write out the entire doctor's order

☐ CMP _____
☐ Crutch training _____
☐ ES _____
☐ Exercise orders _____
☐ Evaluation _____
☐ Hot packs _____
☐ Hubbard tank _____
☐ Hyperbaric oxygen tx _____
☐ Shortwave diathermy _____
☐ TENs _____
☐ Ultrasound c̄ massage _____
☐ Walker training _____
☐ Whirlpool _____
☐ Write in order _____

Figure 17-20 Downtime requisition for physical therapy.

room or in the physical therapy department by the PT or by the physical therapy assistant (PTA). The PT reads the order before administering treatment. The PTA may perform certain treatment tasks as directed by the PT. After treatment, the PT records treatment details and other pertinent data for inclusion in the patient's chart.

To communicate the order to the physical therapy division, use the computer or complete a physical therapy requisition form (Fig. 17-20).

Doctors' Orders for Physical Therapy

Following are examples of doctors' orders for physical therapy. Brief descriptions are included to assist you in interpreting the orders.

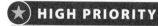

HIGH PRIORITY

Two errors that commonly occur when doctors' orders are read involve interpretation of the abbreviation "PT." This may be an order for physical therapy or for a prothrombin time, which is a coagulation study (see Chapter 14). "PT" also can be confused with "patient," as in the order "PT to ambulate daily," which could be interpreted as patient (pt) to ambulate daily rather than physical therapy (PT) to ambulate the patient daily. It is important to fully understand doctors' orders during transcription.

Hydrotherapy Orders
Hubbard tank 30 min qd T 100°F, active underwater exercises to elbows and knees débridement
This treatment is used for underwater exercises and for cleansing wounds and burns (Fig. 17-21). **Hydrotherapy** treatments may be ordered to be done with a sterile solution. The physical therapy department will select an appropriate substance to use. The whirlpool and the Hubbard tank would be located in the **tank room.**

Whirlpool bath LLE bid
The whirlpool is smaller than the Hubbard tank. It is used for the same purposes.

Exercise Orders
AA exercise lt shoulder and elbow daily
Active assisted exercises would involve the patient's moving an extremity with assistance from the physical therapist (PT), as required.

ROM bid to UE
Range-of-motion exercises frequently are ordered for bedridden patients; therefore they usually are performed in the patient's room. These exercises involve moving each joint of the upper extremities to the maximum extent in each direction.

PROM BLE bid
This passive range-of-motion exercise of both lower extremities would require the PT to move each joint of

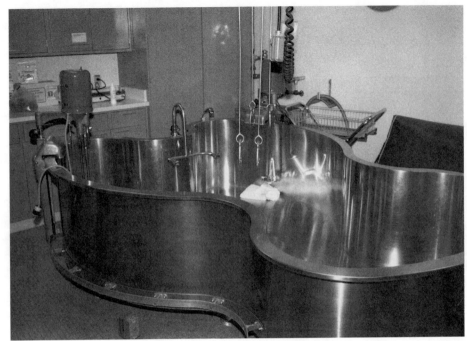

Figure 17-21 Hubbard tank.

both lower extremities the maximum distance in each direction.

Joint mobilization to lt shoulder bid
The PT will mobilize (move) the patient's left shoulder.

Strengthening of all four extremities
The PT will evaluate the patient's condition and will recommend a series of exercises designed to strengthen the patient's extremities. The physical therapy assistant (PTA) may help the patient with these exercises.

PT to amb pt with walker as tol
The physical therapy department often decides which equipment is best suited for the patient. For this order, the PT would assist the patient in using a walker for walking as tolerated.

PT to eval and treat
"PT to evaluate and treat" is the order most commonly written by the doctor. The PT will evaluate the patient and will initiate a plan of care.

ACL protocol per Dr. Melzer
Many physicians have preprinted courses of treatment (protocols) on file with the physical therapy department; these may be implemented throughout the patient's stay (precluding any complications). Programs of treatment include clinical pathways and goals that often are named after orthopedic surgery has been performed on the patient. Familiarity with orthopedic surgical procedures and abbreviations is helpful. An anterior cruciate ligament (ACL) protocol would follow an ACL repair.

Dr. Jen's BKA protocol
This preprinted protocol is used for rehabilitation after a below-the-knee amputation. Another physician's protocol may be different.

THA and TKA protocols
Many physicians have preprinted orders to be used when patients undergo total hip arthroplasty or total knee arthroplasty. The protocol is followed by physical therapy personnel.

Transfer training, wheelchair mobility
The PT teaches the patient how to transfer from the bed to the wheelchair and how to use the wheelchair; this training is ordered for patients who have had an amputation or a stroke or who have another physical disability.

Gait training with a walker, WBAT LLE
To carry out this order, the PT would train the patient to walk using a walker, with weight bearing on the left lower extremity as tolerated. Additional devices such as crutches and different types of canes may be used in patient ambulation.

Crutch walking, NWB daily
The PT instructs the patient to walk with crutches. Variations to this order may be noted regarding the amount of weight bearing permitted (such as full weight), any precautions that should be taken, or the type of crutch walking that should be taught to the patient (such as four-point gait). Additional variations in the amount of weight bearing may be addressed in the doctor's order.

CPM 0 to 45 degrees, progress to 0 to 90 degrees by day 5
A continuous passive motion machine is used after joint replacement or total knee arthroplasty. It may be

monitored by the PT or by nursing staff (Fig. 17-22). Additional motion orders may include active assistive **range of motion** (AAROM), active range of motion (AROM), and passive range of motion (PROM).

T-band exercises
With these exercises, a band of rubber or a Thera-Band is used for resistance.

Constraint-Induced (Movement) Therapy (CI Therapy)
These exercises involve improving upper extremity function by constraining and restricting the contralateral (functional) arm in a sling while training the affected one. This is used primarily for patients who have unilateral (single-sided) dysfunction owing to stroke or traumatic head injury.

Codman's exercises rt shoulder
These exercises for the shoulder are also called *pendulum exercises.*

Isometrics BUE (bilateral upper extremities)
Isometric exercises flex muscles without allowing actual movement of the limb. This order is performed on both upper extremities.

Heat and Cold Orders
- Ultrasound and massage to lower back
- Hydrocollator packs or hot packs to back bid
- Ice or cold packs to left leg bid

Pain Relief Orders
Postop TENS
Transcutaneous electrical nerve stimulation (TENS) is used to control pain by blocking transmission of pain impulses to the brain. Electrodes are applied to the skin surrounding the incision during surgery. Thin wires lead from the electrodes to a powered stimulator with a control. Usually the patient is taught before surgery how to use the device. For nonsurgical use, the PT attaches external electrodes to the skin (Fig. 17-23).

FES or ES
Functional electrical stimulation or electrical stimulation may be used to reduce pain or swelling, promote healing, or assist in exercising muscles. Different types of machines are used to deliver this treatment.

Other Physical Therapy Orders
Apply foam cervical collar
A foam cervical collar is applied to the patient's neck.

Use abduction pillow between legs during treatment
An abduction pillow is placed between the patient's legs. The pillow is designed to help patients recuperate from hip surgery with minimal discomfort while providing protection from hip dislocation.

Apply knee immobilizer to lt knee
A knee immobilizer is used to stabilize the knee after injury or surgery (Fig. 17-24).

Note: These orders are often included in physical therapy orders or may be addressed by nursing personnel. ■

Occupational Therapy
Background Information
Occupational therapy is the division of the physical medicine department in the hospital that works toward rehabilitation

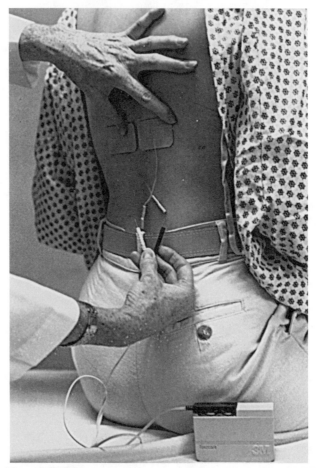

Figure 17-23 Transcutaneous electrical nerve stimulation (TENS). (From Ignatavicius DD, Workman ML, Mishler MA: *Medical-surgical nursing,* ed 2, Philadelphia, 1995, Saunders.)

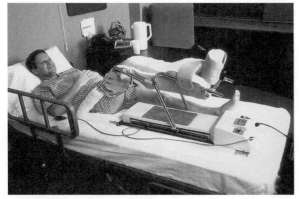

Figure 17-22 Continuous passive motion. (From Elkin MK, Perry AG, Potter PA: *Nursing interventions and clinical skills,* ed 2, St Louis, 2000, Mosby.)

of patients, in conjunction with other health team members, to return the patients to the greatest possible functional independence. Creative, manual, recreational, and prevocational assessments are examples of activities used in rehabilitation of the patient. Occupational therapy activities are ordered by the doctor and are administered by a qualified occupational therapist, an occupational therapy technician, or an occupational therapy assistant. To communicate the order to the occupational therapy division, use the computer or complete an occupational therapy requisition form (Fig. 17-25).

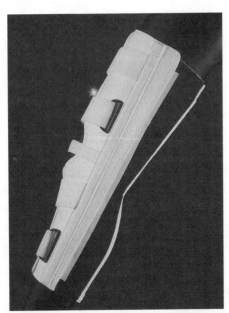

Figure 17-24 Knee immobilizer. (Courtesy Zimmer, Warsaw, Indiana; from Ignatavicius D, Workman L: *Medical-surgical nursing*, ed 5, Philadelphia, 2006, Saunders.)

 HIGH PRIORITY

Examples of basic skills to be achieved as a result of occupational therapy include toileting, bathing and dressing, cooking, and feeding oneself.

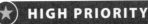 **Doctors' Orders** for Occupational Therapy

- OT for evaluation and treatment if needed daily
- Training in **activities of daily living** (ADLs)
- Supply and train in adaptive equipment such as button hooks and feeding utensils for ADLs
- OT to increase mobility
- Fabricate cock-up splint for left upper extremity ∎

 SKILLS CHALLENGE

To practice transcribing physical medicine and rehabilitation orders, complete Activity 17-4 in the *Skills Practice Manual*.

 HIGH PRIORITY

Physical therapy, occupational therapy, and speech therapy are used to improve and restore function and/or enhance patient independence. Restorative programs may be located in nursing homes and physical medicine and rehabilitation centers.

Doctor ordering _____

Date to be done _____ Time to be done _____

Today's date _____ Requested by _____

Patient Label

OCCUPATIONAL THERAPY REQUISITION

Clinical indication _____

Transportation ☐ Portable   ☐ Stretcher   ☐ Wheelchair   ☐ Ambulatory

O₂ ☐ Yes / ☐ No   Diabetic ☐ Yes / ☐ No   Hearing deficit ☐ Yes / ☐ No

IV ☐ Yes / ☐ No   Seizure disorder ☐ Yes / ☐ No   Sight deficit ☐ Yes / ☐ No

Isolation ☐ Yes / ☐ No   Non-English speaking ☐ Yes / ☐ No

Comments _____

Write out the entire doctor's order

☐ ADL _____

☐ Evaluation and treatment as needed

☐ Increase mobility

☐ Supply and train in adaptive equipment (e.g., Use ADL button hooks and feeding utensils)

☐ Write in order _____

Figure 17-25 Downtime requisition for occupational therapy.

Speech Therapy
Background Information
Speech therapy or speech language pathology is the evaluation and treatment of oral, motor, swallowing, cognitive-linguistic, speech, and language disorders. It is often needed to address a multitude of patient needs, including developmental problems related to the ability to speak and be understood as well as deficiencies that are a result of stroke, seizures, cancer, and other brain injuries.

Doctors' Orders for Speech Therapy

Speech therapy to evaluate motor speech disorder
A speech therapist or speech language pathologist will evaluate the patient to determine whether the problem with speech is related to brain function or to hearing loss.

Consult speech therapy for swallowing risk
The doctor may order a speech therapy consultation for recommendations for alternate nutrition based on risk of aspiration (choking) while swallowing. ■

DIALYSIS

The kidneys are essential organs in the removal of toxic wastes from the blood. When the kidneys fail to remove those wastes, medical **intervention** is necessary to sustain life. The kidneys may fail temporarily (acute renal failure), or they may be permanently damaged and may become nonfunctional (chronic renal failure and end-stage renal disease [ESRD]). Two main types of **dialysis** have been identified: hemodialysis and peritoneal dialysis.

- **Hemodialysis (extracorporeal dialysis)** is the removal of waste products from the blood through use of a machine through which the blood flows. This procedure is performed regularly in a special outpatient dialysis facility and is completed commonly for 3- to 4-hour periods over 3 days a week. For the hospitalized patient, hemodialysis usually is performed in a special unit in the hospital. If the patient is too ill to be moved, a portable hemodialysis machine may be used.
- **Peritoneal dialysis** is the introduction into the abdominal cavity of a fluid (dialyzing fluid) that then absorbs the wastes from the blood through the lining of the abdominal cavity, or peritoneum. The dialysate is then emptied from the abdominal cavity. This passive type of dialysis allows a greater level of freedom for the patient, as this fluid transfer may be performed outside of a health care facility. Some variations of peritoneal dialysis include continuous ambulatory peritoneal dialysis (CAPD), continuous cycling peritoneal dialysis (CCPD), and intermittent peritoneal dialysis (IPD).

Doctors' Orders for Dialysis

Hemodialysis 3 × wk for 2 hours
The patient will undergo hemodialysis for 2 hours per session three times a week.

Consent for Tenckhoff Catheter Placement for Peritoneal Dialysis
This procedure involves surgical placement of a long-term catheter or tube into the patient's abdomen so that peritoneal dialysis can be performed.

Consent for A-V Shunt
Hemodialysis requires vascular access. With this surgical procedure, a cannula is inserted into an artery, and another into a vein. Both of these are then connected to tubing that allows easier needle insertion for hemodialysis. ■

RADIATION TREATMENTS

The area in the hospital where radiation therapy is performed may be a division of the diagnostic imaging department, or it may be a totally separate department. Some new treatments are performed in the interventional radiology department as previously discussed in this chapter.

Many of those who undergo radiation therapy are outpatients. However, the HUC may be called on to schedule an appointment for an inpatient requiring treatment for a malignant neoplasm (cancer). Many hospitals require that units use a requisition form; others may schedule an appointment by telephone. After the initial visit the radiation therapy department usually notifies the nursing unit of the patient's treatment schedule.

SKILLS CHALLENGE

For practice transcribing the following types of orders, complete the following activities in the *Skills Practice Manual:*
- To practice recording a review set of doctors' orders, complete Activity 17-5.
- To practice recording telephone messages, complete Activity 17-6.

KEY CONCEPTS

Transcription of treatment orders involves communication of the order to the necessary department by computer or by requisition form, as well as communication of the order to the nursing staff verbally or through the Kardexing step of the transcription procedure. Professionals in their respective departments then execute the orders.

Websites of Interest

Treatments for respiratory infections - http://www.rightdiagnosis.com/r/respiratory_infections/treatments.htm Hyperbaric oxygen therapy for wound healing - http://www.worldwidewounds.com/2001/april/Wright/HyperbaricOxygen.html

MedicineNet.com—"Dialysis": www.medicinenet.com/dialysis/article.htm

REVIEW QUESTIONS

1. *Visit the Evolve website to download and complete the following exercises:*
   a. stridor
   b. isometric
   c. aerobic exercise
   d. tank room
   e. débridement
   f. crackles or rales
   g. auscultation
   h. dyspnea
   i. extubation
   j. stent
   k. nebulizer
   l. wheezes
   m. defibrillation
   n. intubation
   o. anaerobic exercise

2. Discuss three methods that may be used to treat cardiovascular conditions, and identify three areas within the hospital where cardiovascular surgical or treatment procedures may be performed.

3. Identify the three commonly used procedures performed to repair obstructed coronary blood vessels.

4. Identify the name and location of a vein and an artery that may be used for grafts during a coronary artery bypass graft.

5. Explain the purpose of a cardiac pacemaker and an implanted cardiac defibrillator.

6. Discuss the reasoning for cardiovascular treatment procedures being performed in conjunction with diagnostic procedures, and list two treatment procedures performed in interventional radiology.

7. State the purpose of the cardiopulmonary (respiratory care) department pertaining to patient treatment orders, and list at least five cardiopulmonary treatments.

8. Explain the importance of the HUC including the entire doctor's order when communicating a cardiopulmonary (respiratory care) treatment order electronically, by requisition, or by telephone.

9. Identify the information that is required when oxygen is ordered from the cardiopulmonary (respiratory care) department.

10. List four types of aerosol delivery devices and at least two aerosolized drugs.

11. Explain the procedure and equipment needed to obtain an induced sputum specimen.

12. Discuss the purpose of incentive spirometry, chest percussion therapy, and noninvasive positive pressure ventilation, and explain the use of a mechanical ventilator.

13. State the purpose of the wound care department, and explain the purpose of hyperbaric oxygen therapy.

14. Identify the two basic types of traction and the traction setup used by patients to assist them to move in bed.

15. Identify three divisions that make up the physical medicine department.

16. Describe the purpose of the physical therapy division of the physical medicine department, and list four methods used by physical therapy personnel.

17. Describe the purpose of the occupational therapy division of the physical medicine department, and list three doctor's orders that would be sent to the occupational therapy department.

18. Explain the purpose of speech therapy, and describe the patients who would benefit from speech therapy.

19. Explain the need for dialysis, identify two types of dialysis, and discuss the process of each type.

20. Identify three areas in the hospital that may provide radiation treatments, and explain the HUC role regarding doctors' orders for radiation.

SURFING FOR ANSWERS

1. Locate facilities in your area that have a da Vinci or other surgical robot. Identify the website used.
2. Research and describe procedures developed in the last 2 years that are now done via catheterization or endoscopy that were previously performed in surgery. Identify the website used.
3. Locate "interventional radiologists" and other interventional specialists who practice in your area. Identify the website used.

Miscellaneous Orders

CHAPTER OBJECTIVES

On completion of this chapter, you will be able to:

1. Define the terms in the vocabulary list.
2. Write the meaning of the abbreviations in the abbreviations list.
3. List seven points of information that should be communicated to the consulting physician's office when a consultation order is transcribed.
4. Explain the health unit coordinator (HUC) responsibilities regarding patient medical records from another facility (ordering, receiving, and scanning into a patient's electronic medical record [EMR] or filing into paper chart).
5. Discuss the procedure for photocopying, sending, or faxing patient medical records.
6. Describe the role of the case manager, and identify the types of patients that would require a case manager.
7. Name at least eight services rendered by the social services department.
8. Describe the process the HUC would follow when scheduling an appointment for a patient to be kept after discharge.

9. List six tasks the health unit coordinator may have to perform when arranging for a patient to leave the hospital on a temporary pass.
10. List at least six miscellaneous orders that would require action by the HUC.
11. Explain the purpose of a parent teaching room or transition room on a pediatric unit.

VOCABULARY

Consultation Order A request by the patient's attending physician for the opinion of a second physician with respect to diagnosis and treatment of the patient.

Microfilm A film that contains a greatly reduced photo image of printed or graphic matter.

Parent Teaching or Transition Room Many pediatric hospitals and/or units have a patient room with a bed so a parent can stay with the child 24 hours a day. Parents, after training, will assume full care of the child while they still have the support of the nursing staff. The child may then be discharged home to the parents' care.

ABBREVIATIONS

Abbreviation	Meaning	Example of Usage on a Doctor's Order Sheet
appt	appointment	Schedule an appt with dental clinic
DME	durable medical equipment	Contact DME supplier for hospital bed for home
DNR/DNI	do not resuscitate and do not intubate	DNR or DNI
NINP	no information, no publication	Pt requests NINP
Rx	treatment, therapy, prescription	Disch in a.m. c̄ Rx
wk	week	Disch, F/U appt in my office in 1 wk

⊜ EXERCISE 1

Write the abbreviation for each term listed.

1. week
2. no information, no publication
3. durable medical equipment
4. do not resuscitate
5. medication, pharmacy, prescription, prescribe, take
6. appointment

⊜ EXERCISE 2

Write the meaning of each abbreviation listed.

1. appt
2. DME
3. DNR/DNI
4. NINP
5. wk
6. Rx

CONSULTATION ORDERS

Background Information

The attending physician of a patient may wish to obtain the opinion of another doctor (specialist or surgeon) regarding diagnosis and/or treatment. The request for another doctor's opinion is written in the patient's electronic medical record (EMR) or on the doctors' order sheet by the patient's attending doctor or by a hospitalist, or resident (at the attending doctor's request); this is called a **consultation order.** The ordering doctor may specify that the consulting doctor is to consult only (write opinions and recommendations) or may also write orders.

⭐ HIGH PRIORITY

When the electronic medical record (EMR) with computer physician order entry (CPOE) is implemented, the physicians' orders are entered directly into the patient's electronic record. Many of the miscellaneous orders discussed in this chapter involve action to be taken by the health unit coordinator (HUC). When the doctor enters orders into the computer, an icon (usually a telephone) is displayed on the nursing unit census screen (next to the appropriate patient's name) to alert the HUC that there is a task to be performed. The most common doctors' orders that require HUC tasks when EMR is used include the following:

- Patient consultations
- Obtaining patient medical records from another facility
- Scheduling postdischarge appointments
- Surgical or procedure consent forms (covered in previous chapters)
- Discharge and transfer orders (covered in Chapter 20)

⭐ HIGH PRIORITY

Downtime requisitions are included in this chapter for learning purposes. The Evolve website associated with the *Health Unit Coordinator Skills Manual* includes a simulated hospital computer program that may be used as well.

Processing a consultation order usually requires that the health unit coordinator (HUC) notify the office of the requested doctor regarding the order. Prepare for the call to the doctor's office or answering service by writing the doctor's telephone number on a notepad; have the patient's chart close by so any additional requested information may be accessed easily. When you are speaking to the staff member in the doctor's office, the patient's insurance information may be requested. If the doctor's office is closed and the consultation is relayed to the answering service, the doctor's office secretary may call back for the patient's insurance information. It is important to document the time of the notification and the name of the person or operator number (answering service) spoken to. When EMR is used, the documentation is entered into the patient's EMR or the HUC communication screen and when paper charts are used, the documentation is written next to the order on the doctors' order sheet. In transcribing written orders in a patient chart, write this information next to the order on the doctors' order sheet, and initial it. The process in an EMR system usually requires timely updates in the computer when the office has been called and when the physician has actually been reached and returned the call. Documentation of calls, contact names, and times is as important with EMR and computer physician order entry (CPOE) as it is when transcribing paper-based charts. With the implementation of EMR, the time spent by the HUC making consultation and other telephone calls may be a significant portion of the tasks performed.

Note: Some hospitals may have a policy that requires the requesting doctor to notify the specialist personally, so patient history and additional information may be provided.

The following information should be communicated to the office of the consulting doctor:

- Hospital name
- Patient's name and age
- Patient's location (unit and room number)
- Name of the doctor requesting the consultation
- Patient's diagnosis
- Urgency of consultation and any additional information provided on the order
- Patient's insurance information, located on the patient's face sheet

After interviewing and evaluating the patient, the consulting doctor will dictate his or her findings and recommendations. A hospital medical transcriptionist will then compile the consultation report and send it to the nursing unit, and the HUC will file the report in the patient's chart (Fig. 18-1). When the EMR with CPOE is implemented, the physician will enter findings and recommendations directly into the patient's EMR via computer. The consulting doctor will take a copy of the patient's face sheet back to the office for billing purposes.

Doctors' Orders for Consultation

Doctors' orders for consultation may be expressed in writing on the doctors' order sheet as follows:
- Notify Dr. Cynthia Avery from Valley Anesthesia to eval for CABG surg
- Call Dr. Paul Reidy (Valley Surgeons) for consultation only
- Call Dr. Philip Vasquez to see patient re radiation therapy
- Have Dr. Jackson Williams Westside ENT see patient today—may write orders ■

HIGH PRIORITY

When calling a doctor's office or answering service for a consultation, document the time of the call and the name or the operator number of the person spoken to. Write this information next to the doctor's order on the doctors' order sheet and initial it, or enter the information in the patient's electronic medical record communication page.

Date of consultation: 5/17/XX

Name of consultant: John P. Rhine, MD

History: This 17-year-old woman was seen in consultation with her mother regarding problems referable to her nose. The patient has had progressive problems of congestion and sniffing, with difficulty moving air through her nose and sensation of pressure. She is a "mouth breather," and has history of allergy to pollens and dust. Patient feels these problems are becoming more severe. Her complaints are fairly consistent.

Examination: She presents with edema of her nasal mucosa, increase in the size of the turbinates, deviation of the nasal septum, and a rather narrow nasal airway.

Diagnosis:
1. Probable allergic rhinitis with hypertrophy of the turbinates.
2. Deviated nasal septum.
3. Narrow, inadequate nasal airway.

Comments:
1. I have discussed with this patient and with her mother the surgical approach to improving her nasal airway with septoplasty, and possible submucous resection of deviated portions of the septum, and possible reduction of the inferior turbinates. At the same time I would be performing a rhinoplasty procedure to smooth out the dorsal nose as well.
2. Because of the history of allergies to pollens, dust, and environmental pollutants, it is quite possible the patient will continue to have some sniffing, and consequently, the degree of improvement of her nasal airway with surgery cannot be precisely determined.

_____
J. P. Rhine, MD

DD:
DT:
jpr/ct

Figure 18-1 Dictated and typed consultation report.

SKILLS CHALLENGE

To practice transcribing a consultation order, complete Activity 18-1 in the *Skills Practice Manual*.

HEALTH INFORMATION MANAGEMENT SYSTEM ORDERS

Background Information

The health information management system (HIMS) department, also called *health information management, medical records,* or *health records,* stores the paper charts and manages the electronic charts of patients who have been treated at the health care facility in the past.

Ordering and Obtaining Patient Medical Records

Records from recent hospital admissions are sent to the unit on readmission of a patient automatically or when requested by the patient's doctor. The request is written on the doctors' order sheet, and the order is communicated to the HIMS department by telephone or via computer or telephone by the HUC. HIMS personnel will then send the old records or a printed hard copy if the record has been stored on **microfilm**. While old records are on the nursing unit, they are labeled with the patient's identification and stored in a designated area rather than in the current patient's chart holder.

★ HIGH PRIORITY

When the electronic medical record is implemented, the patient's current and previous medical records become accessible to the patient's doctor and appropriate health care personnel. In the future, the EMR will be electronically accessible by all of the patient's health care providers at all times.

The doctor may also request medical records from the patient's previous stay in another hospital. Because this information is confidential, the patient must give written permission for release of the information from one hospital to another. To transcribe a doctor's order to obtain medical records from another hospital, the HUC places a call to the HIMS department of the other hospital to request records and prepares a medical records release form (Fig. 18-2) for the patient to sign. When signed, this form may be faxed to the HIMS department in the other hospital, and the requested records are faxed to the nursing unit. The faxed records are usually placed in the patient's current chart if paper charts are used, or they are scanned into the patient's EMR if the EMR is used. After the records have been scanned into the patient's EMR, the original documents are stamped as "scanned" with date and time and are placed in a bin or a box to be picked up by HIMS.

The doctor or nurse may also ask the HUC to scan other documents and or graphs into the patient's EMR—for instance, electrocardiograms (ECGs), rhythm strips, handwritten histories and physicals, progress notes, and other documents. The HUC, after having scanned these documents, stamps the originals with a "scanned" stamp with the date and time, and places them in a bin or a box to be picked up by HIMS. In some EMR facilities, the electrocardiograph (machine) automatically sends the ECG to the electronic medical record. There may be a short delay between when the HUC scans a form into the EMR and when it becomes part of the record, as a result of a brief review by HIMS personnel to ensure accuracy.

★ HIGH PRIORITY

When the electronic medical record (EMR) is implemented, faxed patient records are scanned into the patient's EMR by the health unit coordinator. When paper charts are used, the faxed patient records are placed in the patient's current chart.

Photocopying, Sending, or Faxing Medical Records

When a patient is transferred to another facility or is sent to see another physician, the primary physician, hospitalist, or resident may write an order to have specific documents from the patient's medical record sent with the patient or faxed to the facility or doctor's office. The doctor's order must specify the documents to be copied. This may be the responsibility of the HUC, the patient's case manager, or HIMS. The policy for photocopying patient records is outlined in the hospital's policies and procedures. If the HUC is responsible and the EMR is used, the HUC would print the specified documents from the patient's EMR, and if paper charts are used, the HUC would photocopy the specified documents from the patient's paper chart. The HUC would prepare an information release form for the patient's nurse to have the patient sign. If hard copies of the medical record are being sent, the copied records would be placed in an envelope and labeled with the patient's ID label and would be handed to the transport person that arrives to transport the patient. The records could also be faxed to the receiving facility. When paper charts are used, the original documents are returned to their proper order in the patient's paper chart.

★ HIGH PRIORITY

Make certain that the "original" documents are returned to the the paient's chart and the "copies" are sent with the patient.

Doctors' Orders for Health Information Management Records

Doctors' orders for medical records may be expressed electronically or in writing on the doctors' order sheet as follows:

- Send old records from admission 5 years ago to floor
- Obtain old charts from all previous admissions

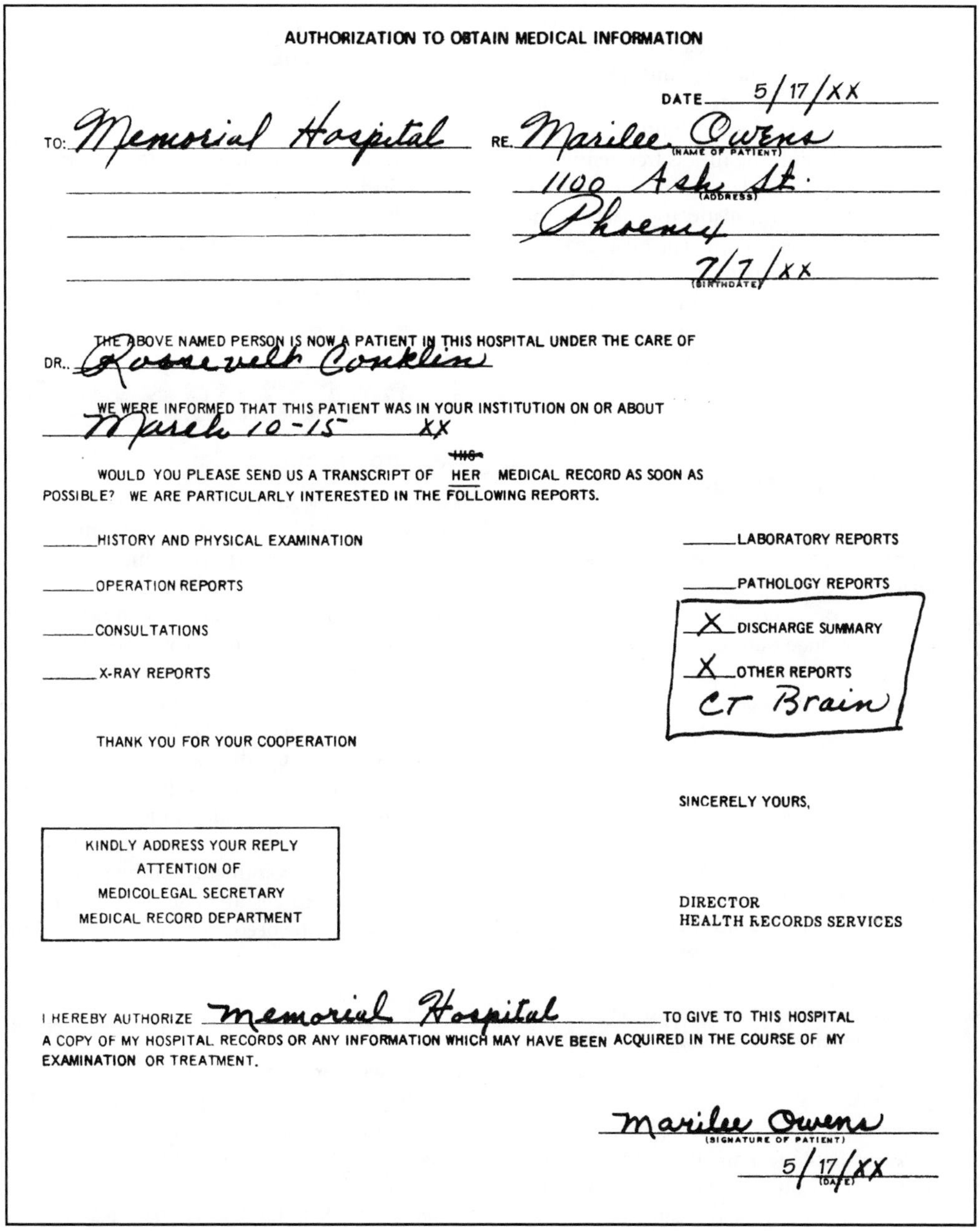

AUTHORIZATION TO OBTAIN MEDICAL INFORMATION

DATE _5/17/XX_

TO: _Memorial Hospital_   RE. _Marilee Owens_
(NAME OF PATIENT)

1100 Ash St.
(ADDRESS)

Phoenix

_7/7/XX_
(BIRTHDATE)

THE ABOVE NAMED PERSON IS NOW A PATIENT IN THIS HOSPITAL UNDER THE CARE OF
DR. _Roosevelt Conklin_

WE WERE INFORMED THAT THIS PATIENT WAS IN YOUR INSTITUTION ON OR ABOUT
March 10-15   XX

WOULD YOU PLEASE SEND US A TRANSCRIPT OF _HER_ MEDICAL RECORD AS SOON AS
POSSIBLE? WE ARE PARTICULARLY INTERESTED IN THE FOLLOWING REPORTS.

___ HISTORY AND PHYSICAL EXAMINATION   ___ LABORATORY REPORTS

___ OPERATION REPORTS   ___ PATHOLOGY REPORTS

___ CONSULTATIONS   X DISCHARGE SUMMARY

___ X-RAY REPORTS   X OTHER REPORTS
                                                CT Brain

THANK YOU FOR YOUR COOPERATION

                                              SINCERELY YOURS,

KINDLY ADDRESS YOUR REPLY
ATTENTION OF
MEDICOLEGAL SECRETARY
MEDICAL RECORD DEPARTMENT   DIRECTOR
                                              HEALTH RECORDS SERVICES

I HEREBY AUTHORIZE _Memorial Hospital_   TO GIVE TO THIS HOSPITAL
A COPY OF MY HOSPITAL RECORDS OR ANY INFORMATION WHICH MAY HAVE BEEN ACQUIRED IN THE COURSE OF MY
EXAMINATION OR TREATMENT.

                                        Marilee Owens
                                        (SIGNATURE OF PATIENT)
                                        _5/17/XX_
                                        (DATE)

Figure 18-2 Medical record release form to obtain records from another hospital.

- Obtain total body CT scan report from St. Joseph's Hospital (done 2/28/XX)
- Please copy all doctors' progress notes (last 3 days) and all diagnostic reports to be sent c̄ patient to Bryant's Rehab Center
- Please scan attached progress notes into Mr. Robert's EMR ∎

SKILLS CHALLENGE

To practice transcribing a health information management order, complete Activity 18-2 in the *Skills Practice Manual*.

CASE MANAGEMENT ORDERS

Background Information

Case management is a nursing care delivery model in which the case manager (a registered nurse [RN] or a social worker) coordinates the patient's care to improve quality of care while reducing costs. The case manager interacts on a daily basis with the patient, the patient's family, health care team members, and payer representatives. Case management is not needed for every patient and usually is requested for chronically ill, seriously ill, or injured patients, as well as for long-term high-cost cases. The case manager acts as the patient's advocate in getting home health services that best suit the patient's needs and in coordinating financial coverage through private insurers such as Medicare.

The doctor may write orders requesting that a case manager access and prioritize the patient's needs, coordinate care conferences between the patient's family and physicians, identify and coordinate available resources, and arrange for home care, admission to a long-term care facility, or hospice as needed. A patient with a life-limiting illness frequently can benefit from the services of hospice. *Hospice* is a multidisciplinary organization that stresses a holistic approach to the care of patients during the final stage of life. The hospice team comprises a physician, nurses, certified nursing assistants, social workers, a chaplain, and volunteers. Most hospice care can be rendered in the patient's home, although some hospice units are located in hospitals and freestanding hospice facilities.

 Doctors' Orders for Case Managers

- Case management for health assessment
- Case management to arrange home care with patient's family for discharge in 2 days
- Case management to arrange hospice care
- Case management to arrange transfer to Sunset Rehabilitation Center
- Case management to arrange patient care conference ■

 SKILLS CHALLENGE

To practice transcribing an order for case management, complete Activity 18-3 in the *Skills Practice Manual*.

SOCIAL SERVICE DEPARTMENT ORDERS

Background Information

The social service department provides much-needed information regarding resources available to patients and their families as they transition from the health care facility back to their home. Social workers provide many of the same services as case managers and may also work as case managers. Social workers assist with the following:

- Solving patients' care-related financial matters
- Transportation home
- Meals for patients' families who are staying at the hospital
- In-home meals for patients after discharge
- Teachers for long-term pediatric patients
- Living arrangements for families who stay with patients
- Finding custodial care or short-term care for patients
- Addressing psychosocial needs of patients
- Support for abuse victims, often by working with Protective Services
- Support for hospital staff after traumatic events (e.g., patient deaths, codes)
- Prepare and witness living will and advance directives for patient

 Doctors' Orders for the Social Services Department

- Contact family re plans to place in custodial care or short-term care facility
- Arrange for home-bound teacher for 1 month
- Social worker to call child protective services to evaluate home situation
- Have social worker evaluate patient's home caregivers
- Have social worker arrange for family to stay at Ronald McDonald House
- Consult social services for nursing home placement ■

SCHEDULING ORDERS

Background Information

Frequently while the patient is in a health care facility, the doctor may write an order to schedule the patient for various types of tests or examinations to be performed in specialized departments or outside of the health care facility. It is usually the HUC's task to notify the department or facility that performs the test or examination and schedule a time convenient for the involved department and the patient, as well as possibly arranging transportation to and from off-site testing. Often an order for scheduling with an outside office or facility is written (or entered by the doctor via CPOE) as part of the discharge orders. It is important to advise the patient's nurse to inform the patient and/or patient's family and to record the scheduled time on the patient's Kardex form and discharge instruction. In many hospitals, the HUC schedules post discharge appointments for the patient and also may place follow up calls to ensure patient follow up compliance. This is done to reduce the need for patient readmission to the hospital.

 Doctors' Orders that Require Scheduling

Following are examples of doctors' orders that require scheduling. These vary greatly among health care facilities, according to the services available.
- Schedule pt in outpatient department for radiation therapy
- Schedule pt for psychological testing
- Schedule pt for diabetic classes
- Schedule pt for VER Have pt see me in the office one wk $\overline{P}$ DC
- Schedule appt for dental clinic for evaluation and care ■

 SKILLS CHALLENGE

To practice transcribing an order to schedule a radiation appointment, complete Activity 18-4 in the *Skills Practice Manual*.

TEMPORARY ABSENCES (PASSES TO LEAVE THE HEALTH CARE FACILITY)

Most patients in an acute care facility are at a level of care that would not allow a temporary absence from the nursing unit or hospital. However, some long-term patients in skilled nursing facilities (SNFs) or rehabilitation units located at the hospital may be allowed to leave for 4 to 10 hours. Patients receive many benefits from visiting their homes or experiencing a recreational outing. A gradual return to society has therapeutic value for rehabilitating patients. A long-term patient also may be given a pass to attend a wedding, funeral, graduation, or similar event. A temporary pass requires the HUC to do the following:

- Arrange with the pharmacy for medications the patient is taking
- Note on the census worksheet when the patient leaves and returns
- Cancel meals for the length of the absence
- Cancel hospital treatments for the length of the absence
- Arrange for any special equipment that the patient may need
- Provide the nurse with a temporary absence release for the patient to sign (Fig. 18-3)

Doctors' Orders for Temporary Absence

- May have pass for tomorrow from 9 AM to 7 PM
- Temporary hospital absence from 8 AM to 6 PM Friday; arrange for rental of wheelchair
- May leave hospital from 10 AM to 1 PM today; have patient sign release

Note: Many insurance providers will not cover the patient's hospital stay if the patient is absent from the hospital for longer than 24 hours. ∎

OTHER MISCELLANEOUS ORDERS

Some orders do not relate to any department but are nevertheless deserving of mention. All should be Kardexed in their appropriate places or entered into the computer. A few of the orders are listed here.

- Call patient's family to come to the hospital

When a patient is terminal, the doctor or nurse may request that the HUC call the family to come to the hospital. Usually, this will be a situation in which the family would already be expecting the call.

- Diabetic nurse to do diabetic teaching with patient

Many hospitals employ nurses who specialize in diabetic teaching to work with newly diagnosed patients. The HUC notifies the diabetic nurse of the consultation.

- Have ostomy nurse work with and train patient in colostomy care

Many hospitals employ nurses who specialize in ostomy care and teaching. The HUC notifies the ostomy nurse of the consultation.

- Transfer patient to the parent teaching/transition room, and teach mother to change dressings; also, train in feeding tube care and feeding technique

Many pediatric hospitals and/or units have a patient room with a bed for a parent to stay with his or her child—the **parent teaching or transition room.** The parent, after training, will assume full care of the child. The child then may be discharged to the parent's care.

- Cardiopulmonary (resp care) to do pre-op and post-op teaching

This order is a request for a respiratory technician to inform a patient before surgery (preoperatively) what to expect and to demonstrate the use of an incentive spirometer. The order also requests that the respiratory technician follow-up with the patient after surgery (postoperatively) to assist the patient with breathing techniques and in using the incentive spirometer.

- Pre-op teaching

A preoperative teaching plan is designed for each patient's diagnosis and unique needs. This plan is reviewed and modified during the intraoperative and postoperative periods. Preoperative teaching may involve breathing exercises, as well as techniques for splinting an incision, moving in bed and transferring to a chair, and so forth.

- No visitors, limited number of visitors, or have visitors speak c̄ nurse before seeing pt

A sign should be posted on the patient's door telling visitors to see the nurse for further explanation. The switchboard and the information desk also should be notified.

- DNR/DNI (do not resuscitate/do not intubate) or no code

This order means that no resuscitative measures are to be performed. A "do not resuscitate/do not intubate" order may be requested by a patient on admission. This order is not a complete refusal of care; it simply states that a resuscitation code should not be performed in the event of cardiac or respiratory arrest. A verbal request by a patient or a patient's family member is not legal. If the physician writes an order for "do not resuscitate/do not intubate," the DNR/DNI status should be visible on the Kardex, written on the patient's chart and patient activity sheet, and noted in the computer if in an EMR facility. Some hospitals have DNR/DNI forms that specify the extent of resuscitative measures to be taken. This information is placed in the front of the patient's chart. The DNR/DNI order also must be written on the patient's order sheet by the doctor, and, depending on the hospital's policy, it must be rewritten or renewed if the patient is transferred to another unit or if there is a change in attending doctors.

- NINP (no information, no publication)

Various hospitals may use different abbreviations, but whatever words or abbreviations are used, this order means that the hospital staff denies that the patient is admitted when asked by visitors, in person or by telephone. This order may be extended to include family members. Often a code phrase or word is used for persons who are excluded from this restriction.

- Notify Dr. Avery of pt's adm to ICU

TEMPORARY ABSENCE RELEASE

The undersigned, being a patient of The Above Named Hospital, hereby confirms his (or her) agreement and understanding that neither the hospital, its employees, nor the attending physicians shall be responsible for his (or her) care or condition during any absences of the undersigned from the building or resulting from such absences.

Signed _____
PATIENT / PARENT / GUARDIAN

Date _____

Hour _____

Witness _____

09-0366   **TEMPORARY ABSENCE RELEASE**

Figure 18-3   Temporary absence release form.

This order is intended to inform the patient's primary physician of admission of the patient to the intensive care unit when another physician has admitted the patient.

- Notify hospitalist (covered in Chapter 2) if systolic BP >190

This order is to notify the hospitalist if the patient's systolic blood pressure is above 190.

SKILLS CHALLENGE

To practice transcribing a review set of doctors' orders, complete Activity 18-5 in the *Skills Practice Manual*.

KEY CONCEPTS

This chapter has discussed a variety of doctors' orders. It includes transcription practice for all classifications of doctors' orders. Monitoring the electronic medical records or transcribing handwritten or preprinted doctors' orders is a major HUC task. Repeated performance is necessary to gain expertise in this area.

When monitoring or transcribing doctors' orders on the nursing unit of the hospital, it will be helpful to use the procedures presented in this textbook as a reference.

Websites of Interest

Job description for a case manager: www.ehow.com/about_5208008_job-description-case-manager.ht
PreOp Patient Education: www.preop.com
Do Not Resuscitate Guide: www.rocketlawyer.com/document/do-not-resuscitate-guide.

REVIEW QUESTIONS

1. Define the following terms:
   a. consultation order
   b. microfilm
   c. parent teaching or transition room

2. The HUC is planning to call a doctor's office to notify the doctor of a consultation request. List the seven points of information to communicate to the consulting physician's office.

3. Explain the responsibilities of the HUC on receiving a request (electronic or handwritten doctor's order) to obtain a patient's medical records from another facility.

4. Discuss the process of scanning medical records received from another facility into a patient's EMR and the process of filing medical records into a patient's paper chart.

5. Explain the procedure the HUC would follow when photocopying, sending, or faxing a patient's medical record to another facility.

6. Describe the role of the case manager, and identify the type of patients that would require a case manager.

7. List at least eight services rendered by the social services department.

8. Describe the process the HUC would follow when scheduling an appointment for a patient to be kept after discharge.

9. List six tasks the HUC may need to perform for a patient who is given a 3-hour temporary pass.

10. List at least six miscellaneous orders that would require action by the HUC.

11. Explain why a patient or a patient's family member cannot verbally request that a DNR status be put into practice.

12. What is the purpose of a parent teaching or transition room?

SURFING FOR ANSWERS

1. Research "online doctor consultations." List five benefits, and document websites used.
2. Locate case manager responsibilities. List eight responsibilities, and document two websites used.
3. Locate outpatient organizations or facilities that provide the following; dialysis, radiation therapy, and home health care.
4. Locate three social support entities in your community that provide social services for homebound patients. Identify the website used.
5. Enter "phone etiquette for hospital staff." List at least five tips for phone communication, and document two websites used.

CHAPTER 19

Admission, Preoperative, and Postoperative Procedures

OUTLINE

CHAPTER OBJECTIVES

On completion of this chapter, you will be able to:

1. Define the terms in the vocabulary list.
2. Write the meaning of the abbreviations in the abbreviations list.
3. List four types of admissions and three types of patients.
4. Discuss who may admit a patient to the hospital and how the nursing unit and bed are assigned.
5. List 10 registration or admission tasks and eight patient interview guidelines.
6. Discuss the purpose of the admission forms.
7. Explain the purpose of advance directives, and discuss the types of advance directives that are available.
8. Discuss the purpose of patient identification (ID) labels and bracelets; explain the purpose of the three standard color-coded alert wristbands, and discuss other color-coded wristbands that may be used.
9. Explain the process of securing patient valuables, providing required information to the patient, and escorting the patient to the nursing unit.
10. List eight common components of a set of admission orders and 16 common health unit coordinator

(HUC) tasks regarding the patient's admission when paper charts are used.
11. Describe how a surgical patient's admission orders differ from a medical patient's admission orders, and discuss three options for the way in which patient surgeries are performed.
12. Explain the purpose of the preoperative care unit, and describe the patient preparation that may take place in the preoperative care unit.
13. List seven components that may be included in a set of preoperative orders (including anesthesiologists' orders) and seven HUC responsibilities regarding the preoperative patient's paper chart.
14. List seven records or reports that are usually required to be in the patient's electronic or paper chart before the time of the patient's surgery.
15. List nine components that may be included in a set of postoperative orders and four HUC responsibilities regarding the postoperative patients' paper chart.
16. Explain why it is important for the HUC to monitor the patient's electronic medical record (EMR) consistently.
17. Explain the purpose and the benefits of the electronic patient status tracking board for the patient's family and/or friends.

18. Explain what the HUC's responsibility would be regarding all medical records incuding, patient signed consent forms, handwritten progress notes, and reports faxed or sent from other facilities, or brought in by a patient when the EMR with computer physician order entry (CPOE) is implemented.

VOCABULARY

Admission Day Surgery Surgery scheduled on the day of the patient's arrival to the hospital; may be called *same-day surgery (SDS)* or *save-a-day surgery (SAD)*.

Admission, Discharge, and Transfer Log Book (ADT Log Book) A book used for a long-term record of admissions, discharges, and transfers for future reference. A patients' ID label is placed in the book with the date of admission entered next to it.

Admission, Discharge, and Transfer Log Sheet (ADT Log Sheet) A form used to record daily admissions, discharges, and transfers for quick reference and to assist in tracking empty beds.

Admission Orders Electronic or handwritten instructions provided by the doctor for the care and treatment of the patient on entry into the hospital.

Admission Service Agreement or Conditions of Admission Agreement (COA or C of A) A form signed on the patient's admission that sets forth the general services that the hospital will provide; also may be called *conditions of admission, contract for services,* or *treatment consent.*

Advance Directive Legal document that indicates a patient's wishes in the event that the patient becomes incapacitated and unable to make decisions regarding medical care.

Allergy Identification Bracelet A plastic band with an insert on which allergy information is printed, or a red plastic band that has allergy information written directly on it, that the patient wears throughout the hospitalization.

Allergy Information Information obtained from the patient regarding sensitivities to medications, food, and/or other substances (e.g., wool, tape).

Bariatric Surgery Surgery on part of the GI tract performed as a treatment for morbid obesity.

Blood Transfusion Consent A patient's written permission to receive blood or blood products.

Blood Transfusion Refusal A patient's written permission to refuse blood or blood products.

Census A list of all occupied (including patient name, age, and acuity and doctor's name) and unoccupied hospital beds.

Census Board A whiteboard located in the nurses' station area on which to record census information such as unit room numbers, admitting doctors' names, and the name of the nurse assigned to each patient. The patient's name intentionally may be omitted to maintain patient confidentiality.

Color-Coded Alert Wristbands Alert wristbands are used in many hospitals to quickly communicate a certain health care status or an "alert" that a patient may have. States have standardized colors. The three colors that are standard in most states include red, meaning "allergy alert"; yellow, meaning "fall risk"; and purple, meaning "DNR" (do not resuscitate). Other alerts that may have varying colors from state to state include seizure alert, diabetic, extremity restricted, and isolation.

Comorbidity The presence of one or more disorders (or diseases) in addition to a primary disease or disorder, or the effect of such additional disorders or diseases.

Direct Admissions Admissions of patients who were not scheduled to be admitted and are admitted from a doctor's office, clinic, or emergency room.

Elective Surgery Surgery that is not emergency or mandatory and can be planned at the patient's convenience.

Electronic Patient Status Tracking Board A viewing screen located in the surgical waiting areas, the hospital cafeteria, and other areas in the hospital designed to keep family and friends updated on the status of a surgical patient. Displays the status of surgical patients through the perioperative process from the patient's arrival in the perioperative suite through discharge from PACU.

Emergency Admission An admission necessitated by accident or a medical emergency; such an admission is processed through the emergency department.

Face Sheet A form initiated by the admitting department and included in the inpatient medical record that contains personal and demographic information, usually computer generated at the time of admission; also may be called the *information form* or *front sheet.*

Health Unit Coordinator Preoperative Checklist A checklist used by the health unit coordinator to ensure that the patient's paper chart is ready to be taken to surgery.

Hugs Infant Protection System An example of an alarm system that includes monitoring software and an ankle bracelet that contains a tiny radio transmitter designed to prevent infants from being removed from a health care facility without authorization.

Informed Consent Consent given by a patient after he or she has been given a description of the procedure, alternatives, risks, probable results, and anything else that is generally disclosed to patients before a signature of permission is obtained.

Inpatient Surgery Surgery performed that requires the patient to stay overnight or longer in the hospital.

Intraoperative Pertaining to the period during a surgical procedure.

Living Will A declaration made by the patient to family, medical staff, and all concerned with the patient's care, stating what is to be done in the event of a terminal illness; it directs the withholding or withdrawing of life-sustaining procedures.

Nonteaching Service The delivery of patient care without the involvement of providing clinical education and training to future and current doctors, nurses, and other health professionals.

Notary Public Someone who is legally authorized to certify the authenticity or legitimacy of signatures on a document.

Nursing Preoperative Checklist A checklist used to ensure that the paper or electronic chart and the patient are properly prepared for surgery.

Observation Patient A patient who is assigned to a bed on the nursing unit to receive care for a period of less than 24 hours; also may be referred to as a *medical short-stay* or *ambulatory patient.*

Outpatient Surgery Surgery performed that does not require an overnight hospital stay; also called *ambulatory surgery, same-day surgery (SDS),* or *save-a-day surgery (SAD).*

Patient Account Number A number assigned to the patient to access insurance information; usually a unique number is assigned each time the patient is admitted to the hospital.

Patient Health Information Management Number The number assigned to the patient on or before admission; it is used for records identification and is used for all subsequent admissions to that hospital; also may be called *health record number* or *medical record number.*

Patient Identification Bracelet A plastic band with a patient identification label affixed to it that is worn by the patient throughout hospitalization. In the obstetrics department, the mother and the baby would share the same identification label affixed to their ID bracelets.

Patient Identification Labels Self-adhesive labels used on the patient's identification bracelet to identify forms, requisitions, specimens, and so forth.

Perioperative Pertaining to the time of surgery (extending from admission for surgery until discharge).

Postoperative Orders Orders electronically entered or handwritten immediately after surgery. Postoperative orders cancel preoperative orders.

Power of Attorney for Health Care Written authorization by which the patient appoints a person (called a *proxy* or *agent*) to make health care decisions should the patient be unable to do so.

Preadmit The process of obtaining information and partially preparing admitting forms before the time of the patient's arrival at the health care facility.

Preoperative and Postoperative Patient Care Plan A plan that includes preoperative teaching, goals, and outcomes. This plan is reviewed and modified during the intraoperative and postoperative periods.

Preoperative Care Unit A unit within the surgery area where a patient is prepared for surgery.

Preoperative Orders Orders electronically entered or handwritten by the doctor before the time of surgery to prepare the patient for the surgical procedure.

Registrar The admitting personnel who registers a patient to the hospital.

Registration The process of entering personal information into the hospital information system to enroll a person as a hospital patient and create a patient record; patients may be registered as inpatients, outpatients, or observation patients.

Scheduled or Planned Admissions Patient admissions planned in advance; admission may be urgent or elective.

Surgery Consent A patient's written permission for an operation or invasive procedure.

Surgery Schedule A list of all the surgeries to be performed on a particular day; the schedule may be printed from the computer or sent to the nursing unit by the admitting department.

Teaching Service The delivery of patient care while providing clinical education and training to future and current doctors, nurses, and other health professionals.

Urgent Admission Admission of a patient not scheduled to be admitted, sent from a doctor's office or another facility and needing immediate care.

Valuables Envelope A container for storing the patient's jewelry, money, and other valuables that is placed in the hospital safe for safekeeping.

ABBREVIATIONS

Abbreviation	Meaning	Example of Usage on a Doctor's Order Sheet
BIBA	brought in by ambulance	Pt BIBA
DOA	dead on arrival	Pt was DOA
Dx	diagnosis	Dx: anemia
IVDU	intravenous drug user	Pt has hx of being an IVDU
MSSU	medical short-stay unit	Admit to: MSSU
OBS	observation	Pt to stay for 2 hr for OBS
OPS	outpatient surgery (ambulatory surgery)	Send pt to OPS
postop	after surgery	TCDB q2h postop
preop	before surgery	Call Valley Anesthesia for preop orders
SSU	short-stay unit	Pt to remain in SSU for 2°

⊜ EXERCISE 1

Write the abbreviation for each term listed.

1. medical short-stay unit
2. after surgery
3. observation
4. diagnosis
5. before surgery
6. outpatient surgery
7. short-stay unit
8. brought in by ambulance
9. dead on arrival
10. IVDU

⊜ EXERCISE 2

Write the meaning of each abbreviation listed.

1. OPS
2. preop
3. Dx
4. OBS
5. postop
6. MSSU
7. SSU
8. BIBA
9. DOA
10. IVDU

ADMISSION OF THE PATIENT

The health unit coordinator's (HUC's) role in the admission procedure is a very important one. Often the HUC is the first person the new patient encounters on the nursing unit. This is an opportunity to demonstrate the caring nature of the hospital by greeting the patient warmly and making him or her feel welcome. In some instances the HUC has the responsibility of admitting the patient. The ability to perform tasks in an efficient manner enables the health care team to provide the care and treatment ordered for the patient as soon as possible. The

HUC maintains a current record of all patients who are admitted, discharged, or transferred on an **admission, discharge, and transfer log sheet (ADT log sheet)** located at the nurses' station, and on the **census board** located in the nursing unit area for quick reference and to track empty beds. An **admission, discharge, and transfer log book (ADT log book)** is used for a long-term record of recently admitted, discharged, and transferred patients. A patient's identification (ID) label is placed in the book, with the date of admission entered next to it.

Types of Admissions

A person may be admitted to the hospital in a variety of ways. Types of admissions are discussed in the following sections.

Scheduled or planned admissions are admissions that are called into the admitting department in advance. Elective scheduled admissions occur when the patient and the doctor decide when to schedule a nonemergency or **elective surgery** or procedure. The scheduled admission patient enters the hospital through the admitting department and is usually admitted to the service of his or her primary doctor. A list of scheduled admissions may be available to print from the computer or may be sent to each nursing unit from the admitting department early in the day, allowing the nursing unit to plan for the admissions.

Direct admissions occur when a doctor sees a patient in the office, decides that the person should be admitted to the hospital, and places a call to the hospital to arrange the admission. An **urgent admission** occurs when a patient is determined to be in need of immediate care while at a doctor's office or another facility. An example of an urgent admission is a pregnant woman who goes to the hospital and, after evaluation by a doctor, is immediately admitted to labor and delivery. Admission of a patient who has been transported by ambulance or helicopter from another health care facility such as an extended care facility also would be called an urgent admission.

An **emergency admission** is unplanned and is the result of an accident, sudden illness, or other medical crisis. Patients enter the hospital through the emergency department (ED), are processed through the ED, and are referred to as *emergency admissions*. ED personnel prepare an ED record (Fig. 19-1). If the patient does not have an electronic medical record (EMR) available, his or her old records from prior admissions are often requested from the health information management services (HIMS) department. Should the patient's condition warrant admission to the hospital, the patient will be assigned to a nursing unit. The ED record is entered into the patient's EMR, or the paper form is sent to the nursing unit with the patient for placement into the patient's paper chart. The patient's old records also should be sent to the nursing unit with the patient and stored on the unit (if paper charts are used) until the patient is discharged or transferred. The HUC reviews the electronic or handwritten ED record to see whether all requested tests have been completed. For example, the ED doctor may have ordered a urinalysis that was not obtained in the ED. The HUC processes all tests that need to be completed.

Some life-or-death emergency patients are brought directly to an intensive care unit (ICU) and require immediate treatment. Patients brought directly to an ICU are not preregistered by the admitting department and may be unconscious and without ID. An example is a near-drowning victim transported by ambulance from a public swimming pool or lake.

The HUC would call admitting to request the patient be given an alias name and assigned a health record number. After the patient has been entered into the computer with an alias name, labels may be printed, tests ordered, and lab specimens sent to the laboratory. Family members will be sent to the admitting department on arrival so the patient can be admitted under the correct name. The patient's correct name will be entered into the computer, but the alias name will remain in the computerized record as well, for ID purposes. If an invasive procedure or surgery is immediately required to save the life of a patient who is unable to sign an **informed consent**, and no family member is present, two medical doctors would sign the consent.

HIGH PRIORITY

Types of admissions include scheduled, direct, urgent, and emergency.

Types of Patients

Patient type may be assigned according to the purpose and length of hospitalization. The three patient types consist of inpatient, observation patient, and outpatient.

An *inpatient* is a patient who has a doctor's electronic or handwritten order for admission to the hospital and is assigned to a bed on the nursing unit. The HUC will prepare a chart and process orders for the patient (see Chapter 8).

An **observation patient** is a patient who is assigned to a bed on a nursing unit to receive care for a period until deemed stable. An observation patient also may be referred to as a *continuing care, medical short-stay,* or *ambulatory patient*. Some hospitals may have a specific unit such as a medical short-stay unit (MSSU) or ambulatory care unit that provides short-term care. Some emergency rooms have an area furnished with recliner chairs and televisions designated for observation patients. The HUC may prepare a chart and process orders for the observation patient.

An *outpatient* is a patient who receives care in a hospital, clinic, or surgicenter. An outpatient usually is scheduled to receive surgery, treatments, therapies, or tests. The department that provides care for the outpatient processes the outpatient orders. Usually the assembly of a chart is not required, although patients on a routine basis may receive outpatient services that do require a chart.

The patient may be classified as receiving **teaching service** or **nonteaching service**, indicating whether residents and/or other health care students will be involved in the patient's care. Patients may also be classified according to the type of insurance coverage they have (e.g., Medicare, preferred provider organization [PPO], health maintenance organization [HMO]).

HIGH PRIORITY

Types of patients receiving medical care include inpatient, observation patient, and outpatient. Patients may also be classified as teaching or nonteaching or be classified according to type of health insurance coverage.

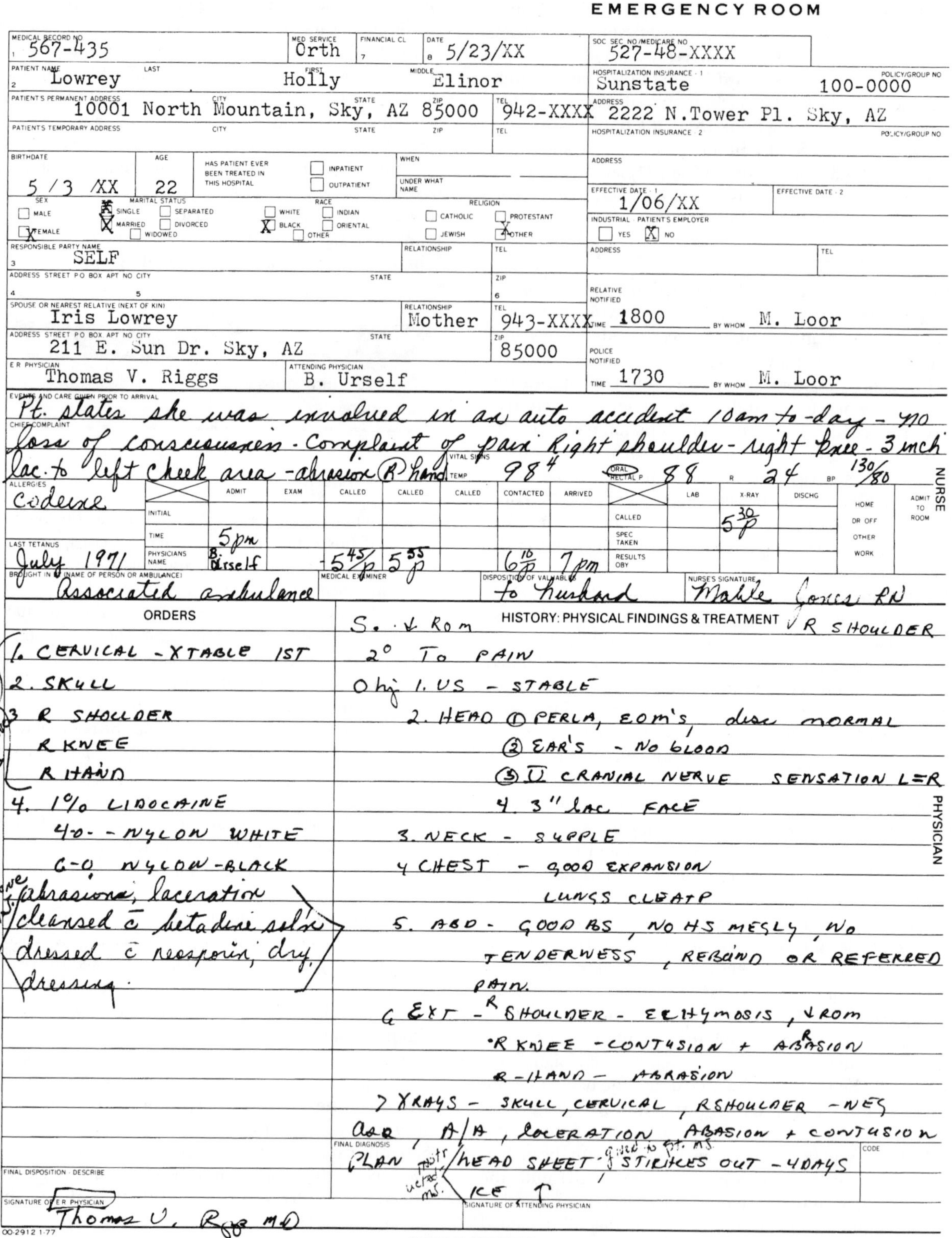

EMERGENCY ROOM

MEDICAL RECORD NO 1 567-435 | MED SERVICE Orth | FINANCIAL CL 7 | DATE 8 5/23/XX | SOC SEC NO/MEDICARE NO 527-48-XXXX

PATIENT NAME LAST 2 Lowrey | FIRST Holly | MIDDLE Elinor | HOSPITALIZATION INSURANCE - 1 Sunstate | POLICY/GROUP NO 100-0000

PATIENT'S PERMANENT ADDRESS 10001 North | CITY Mountain, Sky, | STATE AZ | ZIP 85000 | TEL 942-XXXX | ADDRESS 2222 N.Tower Pl. Sky, AZ

PATIENT'S TEMPORARY ADDRESS | CITY | STATE | ZIP | TEL | HOSPITALIZATION INSURANCE - 2 | POLICY/GROUP NO

BIRTHDATE 5/3/XX | AGE 22 | HAS PATIENT EVER BEEN TREATED IN THIS HOSPITAL ☐ INPATIENT ☐ OUTPATIENT | WHEN | UNDER WHAT NAME | ADDRESS

EFFECTIVE DATE - 1 1/06/XX | EFFECTIVE DATE - 2

SEX ☐ MALE ☒ FEMALE | MARITAL STATUS ☒ SINGLE ☐ SEPARATED ☒ MARRIED ☐ DIVORCED ☐ WIDOWED | RACE ☐ WHITE ☐ INDIAN ☒ BLACK ☐ ORIENTAL ☐ OTHER | RELIGION ☐ CATHOLIC ☐ PROTESTANT ☐ JEWISH ☒ OTHER | INDUSTRIAL - PATIENT'S EMPLOYER ☐ YES ☒ NO

RESPONSIBLE PARTY NAME 3 SELF | RELATIONSHIP | TEL | ADDRESS | TEL

ADDRESS STREET PO BOX APT NO CITY 4 5 | STATE | ZIP 6 | RELATIVE NOTIFIED

SPOUSE OR NEAREST RELATIVE (NEXT OF KIN) Iris Lowrey | RELATIONSHIP Mother | TEL 943-XXXX | TIME 1800 BY WHOM M. Loor

ADDRESS STREET PO BOX APT NO CITY 211 E. Sun Dr. Sky, AZ | STATE | ZIP 85000 | POLICE NOTIFIED

E R PHYSICIAN Thomas V. Riggs | ATTENDING PHYSICIAN B. Urself | TIME 1730 BY WHOM M. Loor

EVENTS AND CARE GIVEN PRIOR TO ARRIVAL / CHIEF COMPLAINT: Pt. states she was involved in an auto accident 10am to-day - no loss of consciousness - Complaint of pain Right shoulder - right knee - 3 inch lac. to left cheek area - abrasion (R) hand

VITAL SIGNS: TEMP 98⁴ | ORAL/RECTAL P 88 | R 24 | BP 130/80

ALLERGIES: Codeine

LAST TETANUS: July 1971

	ADMIT	EXAM	CALLED	CALLED	CALLED	CONTACTED	ARRIVED
INITIAL							
TIME	5pm						
PHYSICIANS NAME	B. Urself		5⁴⁵ p	5⁵⁵ p		6¹⁰ p	7pm

	LAB	X-RAY	DISCHG
CALLED		5³⁰ p	
SPEC TAKEN			
RESULTS OBY			

HOME / DR OFF / OTHER / WORK | ADMIT TO ROOM

NURSE

BROUGHT IN BY (NAME OF PERSON OR AMBULANCE) Associated ambulance | MEDICAL EXAMINER | DISPOSITION OF VALUABLES to husband | NURSE'S SIGNATURE Mable Jones RN

ORDERS
1. CERVICAL - XTABLE 1ST
2. SKULL
3. R SHOULDER
R KNEE
R HAND
(done MS)
4. 1% LIDOCAINE
4-0 - NYLON WHITE
6-0 NYLON - BLACK
abrasions, laceration cleansed c̄ betadine sol'n dressed c̄ neosporin, dry dressing. (done MS)

HISTORY: PHYSICAL FINDINGS & TREATMENT
S. ↓ Rom √ R SHOULDER 2° TO PAIN
Obj 1. VS - STABLE
2. HEAD ① PERLA, EOM'S, disc NORMAL
② EAR'S - NO BLOOD
③ Ⅱ CRANIAL NERVE SENSATION L=R
4. 3" lac FACE
3. NECK - SUPPLE
4 CHEST - GOOD EXPANSION
LUNGS CLEAR
5. ABD - GOOD BS, NO HS MEGLY, NO TENDERNESS, REBOUND OR REFERRED PAIN.
6 EXT - R SHOULDER - ECCHYMOSIS, ↓ ROM
R KNEE - CONTUSION + R ABRASION
R - HAND - ABRASION
7 XRAYS - SKULL, CERVICAL, R SHOULDER - NEG
A&R A/A, LACERATION, ABRASION + CONTUSION

FINAL DIAGNOSIS | CODE
PLAN (instr. given to pt. MS) HEAD SHEET (given to pt. MS) STITCHES OUT - 4DAYS, ICE ↑

PHYSICIAN

FINAL DISPOSITION - DESCRIBE

SIGNATURE OF E R PHYSICIAN Thomas V. Riggs MD | SIGNATURE OF ATTENDING PHYSICIAN

00-2912 1-77

MEDICAL RECORDS

Figure 19-1 Emergency department record.

Admission Arrangement

In all types of admissions, a doctor with admitting privileges to the hospital must authorize the patient's admission. One of the following is responsible to arrange for the admission of a patient: the attending or primary doctor; the emergency room doctor; the primary or attending doctor's office staff; or the HMO staff acting on instructions of the doctor. The doctor provides the admitting diagnosis or medical reason for admission. Many hospitals employ a *hospitalist* who may oversee the patient's care during the hospital stay. The hospitalist communicates with the patient's attending or primary doctor.

A doctor with admitting privileges to the hospital must authorize a patient's admission. In many hospitals, a hospitalist oversees the patient's care during his or her stay in the hospital.

Bed Assignment

Most hospitals are open for admissions 24 hours a day. The admitting department or registration staff performs many tasks in relation to the admission of the patient to the hospital. Usually, the hospital **census** is computerized and provides an accurate, up-to-date list of occupied and unoccupied hospital beds. Nursing unit assignments for scheduled admissions usually are determined in advance, and a specialized unit may be requested by the admitting doctor. A list of scheduled patient admissions may be made available on the computer or may be printed and sent to each nursing unit that receives patients. Nursing assignments generally are determined for scheduled admissions in the morning. Direct admissions or emergency admissions are assigned beds when the patient arrives at the hospital and is ready for a room. The admitting diagnosis and/or patient age usually determine the type of nursing unit that is suitable, and the nursing staff usually decides on the specific bed. In many hospitals, staff members on the nursing unit decide bed assignment. Nursing personnel are familiar with staffing and roommate issues and can best decide which bed is appropriate for the new patient. After receiving patient information such as name, diagnosis, age, and sex, the HUC or nurse may assign the bed number.

It is important to notify the admitting department of pending discharges in a timely manner, especially when the hospital is low on open beds. Delaying notification could cause a delay in another patient's admission and treatment.

Patient Admission and Registration

Registration is the process of entering personal information into the hospital information system to register a person as a hospital patient and create a patient record. A **registrar** in the admitting department or the HUC may assume the patient admission or registration responsibilities.

Patient Admission and Registration Tasks

Patient admission and registration tasks include the following:

1. Copy insurance cards.
2. Verify insurance (may be done in advance when admission is scheduled).
3. Ask patient or patient guardian to sign appropriate insurance forms.

4. Interview patient or family to obtain personal information.
5. Prepare admission forms (admission service agreement and face sheet) and obtain signatures.
6. Ask patient whether he or she has an advanced directives document or would like to create one (required in most states).
7. Prepare patient's ID bracelet and if necessary ID labels—patients may be asked to read and initial information on bracelet.
8. Secure patient valuables if necessary.
9. Supply and explain required information, including a copy of the Patients' Bill of Rights and hospital privacy laws (required by The Joint Commission [TJC]).
10. Include any test results, prewritten orders, or consents that were previously sent to the admitting department in the packet that accompanies the patient to the nursing unit.

Interview

When admissions are arranged in advance, preadmission information may be obtained by the registration staff by mail, by phone, or by computer. This information, including the patient's name, address, and telephone number; employer's name and address; insurance carrier; and doctor's name and diagnosis, is placed on a record called the *face sheet, information form, or front sheet* (see Chapter 8). If patient information was not obtained previously, this is done at the time of admission.

Interview Techniques. When interviewing a patient to obtain personal information, it is imperative to use the interpersonal skills discussed in Chapter 5. Being admitted to a health care facility is a stressful situation, and many patients may be experiencing physical discomfort. The following guidelines should be observed when patients are interviewed:

- Protect confidentiality.
- Ensure privacy when asking for personal information.
- Be proficient and professional.
- Asking whether the patient was hospitalized previously can hasten the registration process and reduce the risk of error in assignment of health information management and patient account numbers (demographics would have to be verified in case of possible changes).
- Treat each patient as an individual.
- Listen carefully.
- Project a friendly, courteous attitude.
- Include family or significant other in the process.

Patient registration tasks should be completed before orders are processed for the patient, unless a life-threatening emergency occurs.

Admission Forms

An **admission service agreement or conditions of admission agreement (COA or C of A)** lists the general services that the hospital will provide. It is an agreement between the patient and the hospital and includes a legal consent for treatment (see Chapter 8). This consent may specify financial responsibility also. The patient is to sign the form on admission. Patients who are unable to sign an admission service agreement may have a legal guardian sign for them. A copy of the admission service agreement is given to the patient after it has been signed, and the original becomes part of the patient's paper medical record or is scanned into the patient's EMR by the HUC.

The **face sheet**, *information form, or front sheet* is the form that is generated after patient information, such as address, telephone number, nearest of kin, insurance carrier, and so forth, is entered into the hospital information system. It is usually filed as the first page of the patient's paper medical record or is scanned into the patient's EMR by the HUC.

Advance Directives

Society now recognizes the individual's right to make decisions regarding care if he or she becomes incapacitated and to die with dignity rather than be kept alive indefinitely by artificial life support. As a result, most states have enacted "right to die" laws and laws dealing with advanced directives. The term **advance directive** refers to an individual's desires regarding care if she or he should become incapacitated and require end-of-life care. An adult witness or witnesses or a **notary public** must sign an advance directive. The notary public or witness cannot be the person named to make the decisions or the provider of health care. If there is only one witness, it cannot be a relative or someone who will be the beneficiary of property from the patient's estate if the patient dies.

Most states require that patients be asked if they have or would like to have an advance directive document when admitted to a hospital and most hospitals employ someone who is a notary public. See Chapter 8 for an example of an advance directive checklist, which provides documentation that the patient was asked and what decision was made regarding health care. Advance directives include the following documents:

- A **living will** is a declaration made by the patient to family, medical staff, and all concerned with the patient's care stating what is to be done in the event of a terminal illness. It directs the withholding or withdrawing of life-sustaining procedures. The patient may define what is meant by *meaningful quality of life*, a phrase commonly used in living wills to describe the level of functioning with which the patient would be comfortable.
- **Power of attorney for health care** allows the patient to appoint another person or persons (called a *proxy* or *agent*) to make health care decisions for him or her should the patient become incapable of making decisions. The proxy (agent) has a duty to act consistently with the patient's wishes. If the proxy does not know the patient's wishes, the proxy has the duty to act in the patient's best interests. Figure 19-2 is an example of a health care power of attorney and living will combined form. An advance directive becomes effective *only* when the patient can no longer make decisions for himself or herself. The patient may change or destroy any directive or living will at any time.

Routine admission patients may have had tests performed before their admission. Test results are forwarded to the hospital admitting department and are sent to the nursing unit with the other chart forms. Doctors may manually or electronically write orders or obtain consents in advance; these also are forwarded to the hospital admitting department and are sent to the nursing unit on admission.

At the time of admission or before admission, each patient is assigned a health information management number that is unique for that patient. The health information management number identifies the patient on all chart forms and is used for all future admissions to that hospital. The **patient account number** and the **patient health information management number** is assigned at the time of admission and is used to reference insurance information; it is usually unique to each admission. The patient account number also serves to identify all charges for equipment, supplies, and procedures. The business office uses the patient account number for billing purposes.

Patient Identification Labels

Patient identification labels are self-adhesive labels used on the patient's ID bracelet to identify forms, requisitions, specimens, and so forth (see Chapter 8). Patient ID labels may be prepared by registration staff members who enter the information into the computer, and then they can be printed from the computer on the nursing unit. Labels may also be printed by the HUC using a label maker. Some computer software programs print chart forms with patient information preprinted on them.

Patient Identification and Allergy Bracelets and Color-Coded Wristbands

A **patient identification bracelet** or band is prepared by registration staff on admission of the patient to the hospital. The bracelet is usually a plastic band with the patient's ID label affixed to it, or a cardboard insert may be used (Fig. 19-3). Identifying information may consist of (1) the patient's name, sex, age, and date of birth, (2) the patient's attending doctor's name, (3) the health information management number, and (4) the patient account number. The patient's room and bed numbers are usually written in pencil so they may be changed easily if the patient is moved to a different room and/or bed number. The health information management number serves as the main identifier because it is a unique number assigned to that patient. The bracelet is worn throughout the patient's hospitalization. All personnel who perform services for the patient must read the ID bracelet before administering any service, to ensure correct patient ID. An **allergy identification bracelet** is red; written on the band is the **allergy information** obtained from the patient or patient's family (if patient unable to provide information) or from the patient's medical history.

In an effort to meet TJC safety goals, hospitals across the United States have adopted **color-coded alert wristbands** that include unique alerts to help staff members quickly provide care. These bracelets are typically simple, color-coded strips that provide a visual cue to caregivers about a special need, condition or concern relating to the patient. Wristbands include such alerts as allergy alerts (red), fall risk (yellow), do not resuscitate (DNR) (purple), seizure alert, diabetic, extremity restriction, or isolation. Colors are mostly

HEALTH CARE POWER OF ATTORNEY & LIVING WILL
Combined Form

I, _____, as principal, designate _____ as my agent for all matters relating to my health care, including, without limitation, full power to give or to refuse consent to all medical, surgical, hospital, psychiatric and related health care. This power of attorney is effective whenever I am unable to make or to communicate health care decisions. All of my agent's actions under this power have the same effects on my heirs, devisees, and personal representatives as if I were alive, competent and acting for myself.

If my agent is unwilling or unable to serve or to continue to serve, I hereby appoint _____ as my agent.

In acting under this power, I want my agent to give great weight to the following statements: I am in favor of trial treatment. That means I want all necessary medical care to treat my condition until, and only until, my doctors and my agent reasonably decide that I am in an irreversible coma, or a persistent vegetative state, or a locked-in state, or that I cannot be expected to return to a fully conscious state. If, following the guidelines stated above, my doctors and my agent decide that further medical care is inappropriate:

1. **I want** only comfort care and **I do not want** to undergo artificial administration of food or fluids.
2. **I do not want** to be resuscitated in case I stop breathing or my heart stops beating.

If my doctors and my agent reasonably decide that I have a terminal illness, I want all decisions concerning my medical and surgical care to be made in light of the expected length and quality of life which would result from such care and the predictable effects on me of undergoing treatment. **If I cannot be expected to have a significant period of conscious life even after medical or surgical care, then I want comfort care only.** (Examples: I do not want any surgery or other care designed to prolong my life. I do not want artificially administered food or fluids and I do not want to be resuscitated.)

This combined health care directive is made under § 36-3221 and § 36-3261, Arizona Revised Statutes. It continues in effect for all who may rely on it, except those to whom I have given notice of its revocation.

_____   _____
Dated   Signature of Mark of Person Making Living Will or Granting Health Care Power of Attorney

Verification

I affirm that: (1) I was present when this living will was dated and signed or marked or (2) the person making this living will directly indicated to me that the living will expressed that person's wishes and that the person intended to adopt it at that time. The maker of this document appeared to be of sound mind and free from duress.

(If there is only one witness signing this document) I certify that: I have not been designated to make medical decisions for the person who signed this living will, I am not directly involved with providing health care to that person, I am not related to that person by blood, marriage, or adoption and I am not entitled to any part of that person's estate.

_____   _____   _____
Witness   Witness   Date

STATE OF ARIZONA   )
) ss.
County of   )

The maker of this document appears to be of sound mind and free from duress. It was subscribed and sworn to before me this _____ day of _____, 19_____.
_____   My Commission Expires _____
Notary Public

(A health care power of attorney and living will must be signed by a notary or by an adult witness or witnesses, who saw you sign or mark the document and who say that you appear to be of sound mind and free from duress. A notary or witness cannot be the person you name to make your decisions or your provider of health care. If you have only one witness, that witness cannot be related to you or someone who will get any of your property from your estate if you die.)

July 1995 • Arizona Hospital and Healthcare Association

Figure 19-2 Health care power of attorney and living will admission.

standard for allergies, fall risk, and DNR, but colors for other wristbands vary.

★ **HIGH PRIORITY**

When an ID or color-coded alert wristband slips off a patient's wrist or is cut off for any reason, the HUC will be asked to prepare a replacement.

Patients' Valuables

Patients who have a large quantity of money, expensive jewelry, or other items of value with them at the time of admission are requested to send them home with family or place them in the hospital safe. When the patient chooses to have the items placed in the safe, the items are put into a numbered **valuables envelope** (Fig. 19-4), and the patient is given a numbered claim check. The number is entered electronically

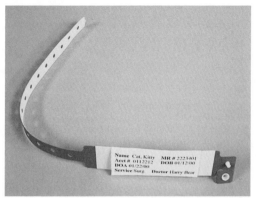

Figure 19-3 Patient identification bracelet.

or handwritten in the patient's chart, and the envelope is placed in the hospital safe. A clothing and valuables form is also prepared, which lists clothing, eyeglasses, false teeth, prosthesis, and any other items of value (Fig. 19-5). The form is signed by the patient, witnessed, and placed into the patient's paper chart or is scanned into the EMR. The clothing and valuables form is a reminder that there are valuables in the hospital safe.

Provided Patient Information

The registration staff or the HUC will explain the registration process and hospital rules to the patient and/or the patient's family. Because of various state laws, the hospital may be required to inform the patient of specific information. On admission, the patient usually is supplied with a copy of the patients' bill of rights and the hospital's privacy practices; other handouts may be provided regarding the hospital stay.

Escort to the Nursing Unit

Once the nursing unit and bed assignments have been made, a volunteer, a member of the hospital transportation department, or an admitting personnel staff member escorts the patient to the assigned unit. In some hospitals, the HUC may escort the patient to the room, advise him or her of visitation rules, and instruct the patient in use of the bed controls, the television control, and the Internet. If the patient has already been registered, the admitting papers are delivered to the receiving unit. The HUC greets the patient and tells the nurse who will be caring for the patient of the patient's arrival. The nurse completes the nurse's admitting record (see Chapter 8), which the HUC may use to complete the patient profile with information such as allergies, height, and weight.

⌖ SKILLS CHALLENGE

To practice preparing the newly admitted patient's chart and Kardex forms, complete Activity 19-1 in the *Skills Practice Manual.*

ADMISSION ORDERS

Admission orders are written directions provided by the doctor regarding the care and treatment of the patient on

Figure 19-4 Valuables envelope.

entry into the hospital. Most orders are written on the unit by the hospitalist, attending doctor, resident, or nurse practitioner, or they may be received by telephone immediately after the patient's arrival. However, at times, the admission orders arrive before the patient does. Doctors may have pre-printed order sets or clinical pathways for certain types of admissions, such as a patient admitted for a coronary artery bypass graft (CABG), **bariatric surgery,** or total hip or knee replacement surgery. Some patients with **comorbidity**—the presence of one or more disorders (or diseases) in addition to the primary disease or disorder—will need customized orders. Some doctors may write admission orders before the time of arrival of the patient and leave them on the nursing unit. The HUC must ensure that these orders are identified with the patient's name, which should be written on the order sheet in ink. The orders are labeled with the patient's ID label later, when the patient arrives on the nursing unit. When the EMR with computer physician order entry (CPOE) is implemented, the doctor enters the orders directly into the computer, or the preprinted order sets or clinical pathways may be computerized.

Admission Order Components

Common components of admission orders include the following:

- Admitting diagnosis
- Diet
- Activity
- Diagnostic tests and procedures
- Medications—Usually, medications are needed for the patient's disease condition, for sleeping, and/or for pain.

PATIENT VALUABLES

VALUABLES

QUANTITY   DESCRIPTION

☐ I have been informed that a safe is available in the Patient Accounts Department for the safekeeping of my valuables.

☐ I understand that the Hospital will assume responsibility for eyeglasses, bridgework, dentures and clothing (up to $50) lost or damaged due to negligence of Hospital personnel.

☐ I agree to assume full responsibility for any valuables not turned over to the Hospital for safekeeping in the Hospital safe by myself or my personal representative. I will hold the Hospital responsible for only those valuables listed above.

Signed: _____   Date _____ 20 _____
                    (Patient or Representative)

Witnessed by: _____
                         (Admission Representative)

Received by: _____   Deposit Envelope No. _____
                    (Cashier or Nursing Office Representative)

Verified by: _____
                    (Admissions Representative or Other Employee)

          Safe Deposit Envelope No. _____   Date of Deposit _____ 20 _____

          Comments: _____

                    _____

                                                            Patient Valuables

Figure 19-5 Clothing and valuables list. (Courtesy Rockford Memorial Hospital, Rockford, Illinois.)

PHYSICIANS' ORDER SHEET

DATE	TIME	SYMBOL	ORDERS
5/4/00	1300		Admit to med-surg unit
			DX: acute pulmonary edema
			BRP c̄ help
			VS q 2 for 8, then q4°
			1800 cal ADA NAS diet
			Daily wts
			I & O
			CBC, lytes & cardiac enzymes stat
			CMP in am
			ABG on RA now, then place on O₂ @ 2 L/M
			Repeat ABG in 2 hr—call me c̄ results
			Chest PA & lat today & in am: CI infiltrates
			EKG today & in am
			Lung perfusion/ventilation scan in am: CI embolism
			bepridil hydrochloride 300 mg qd
			bumetanide 2 mg PO now & qd
			Ambien 10 mg qhs prn for sleep
			Old records to floor
			Pt is a full code status
			Dr. John Stewart MD

Figure 19-6 Set of admission orders.

- Treatment orders
- Request for old records
- Patient alerts such as allergies, fall risk, or seizure risk (requiring bracelets to be worn by patient)
- Patient care category or code status—The patient care category or code status may be indicated on the patient's admission orders. The patient care category or code status refers to the patient's wishes regarding resuscitation. Code status may be written as full code, modified support, or DNR. The doctor must follow any state-specific statute and the hospital's policies and procedures when writing a DNR status.

Figure 19-6 is an example of a set of admission orders. HUC tasks performed during the admission procedure are listed in Procedure 19-1.

 SKILLS CHALLENGE

To practice transcribing a set of admission orders for a medical patient, complete Activity 19-2 in the *Skills Practice Manual.*

THE SURGERY PATIENT

Information

There are three options available for patients having surgery that include inpatient surgery, outpatient surgery, and admission day surgery. **Inpatient surgery** requires the patient to be admitted to the hospital before the surgery day. The procedure for admission of a medical or surgical patient is the same, except that diagnostic tests ordered by the doctor are performed on surgery patients as soon as possible after their arrival to the hospital. This allows the time needed to perform diagnostic studies and have the test results added to the patient's chart before surgery is performed. An abnormal blood test result or a chest radiograph that is abnormal may require that surgery be postponed pending further evaluation. Some surgeries, such as open heart surgery or organ transplant surgery may require additional diagnostic studies, patient preparation, preoperative teaching, and careful explanation of the procedure to the patient and the family. A tour of the ICU may be arranged so that the patient will be aware of surroundings and activities that will take place after surgery.

PROCEDURE 19-1

ADMISSION PROCEDURE

Tasks may vary among facilities, and many of the listed tasks also apply when using EMR. When CPOE has been implemented, tasks related to preparing a paper chart or transcribing orders would not apply.

TASK	NOTES
1. Greet the patient on his or her arrival on the nursing unit. Also applicable when using EMR.	Introduce yourself and give your status. Example: "I'm Olivia, the health unit coordinator for this unit."
2.	
a. Inform the patient that the nurse will be notified of his or her arrival.	
b. Notify the nurse who will be caring for the patient that the patient has arrived. Also applicable when using EMR.	
3. Notify the attending doctor and/or hospital resident or the hospitalist of the patient's arrival. Also applicable when using EMR.	
4. Move the patient's name from the admission screen on the computer to the correct bed on the nursing unit. Also applicable when using EMR.	
5. Record the patient's admission on the admission, discharge, and transfer sheet (ADT sheet) and the census board. Also applicable when using EMR.	
6. Check the patient's signature on the admission service agreement form. Also applicable when using EMR.	Compare the spelling of the patient's name on the face sheet, information form, or front sheet and the patient identification labels with the signature on the admission service agreement form. Also check to see that the doctor's name is correct.
7. Complete the procedure for preparation of the paper chart.	
a. Label all chart forms with the patient's identification labels (if paper charts used).	
b. Fill in all the needed headings (if paper charts used).	
c. Place all forms in the chart behind the proper dividers (if paper charts used).	
d. Label the outside of the chart (if paper charts used).	Identify the chart with the patient's and doctor's names and the room number.
8. Prepare any other labels or identification cards used by the facility. Also applicable when using EMR.	
9. Place the patient identification labels in the correct place in the patient's paper chart, or place in the nursing unit patient label book if EMR is used.	
10.	
a. Fill in all the necessary information on the patient's Kardex form, or enter it into the computer if Kardex is computerized (if paper charts used).	The information is obtained from the face sheet, information form, or front sheet prepared by the admitting department and the admission nurse's notes.
b. Place the Kardex form in the proper place in the Kardex file (if paper charts used).	
11. Enter appropriate required data into the computer (if this is an HUC responsibility), or scan required forms into the patient's EMR if the EMR is used. • May be the responsibility of the admitting nurse or the admitting department.	A patient profile requires information found on the face sheet screen, information form, or front sheet and the nurse's admission notes, such as name, address, nearest of kin, height, weight, and so on.
12.	
a. Place the allergy information in all the designated areas, or write "NKA" (if paper charts used).	**Allergy information** (the information obtained from the patient about any sensitivity to medication, food, or other substance) usually is placed on the front of the patient's chart, Kardex form, and medication record. The allergy information is obtained from the admission nurse's notes. Writing "NKA" indicates to the staff that the allergy information has been checked.
b. Prepare an allergy identification bracelet (red) or color-coded wristband with allergies written on it to be placed on the patient's wrist if necessary.	

Continued

PROCEDURE 19–1—cont'd

TASK	NOTES
13.	
a. Place alerts, such as fall risk, seizure risk, diabetic, extremity restriction, and isolation, in all designated areas.	**Risk information** (the information obtained from the patient's diagnosis, doctor's orders, or patient history) usually is placed on the front of the patient's chart, Kardex form, and medication record.
b. Prepare appropriate color-coded wristband to be placed on the patient's wrist as required.	
Also applicable when using EMR	
14.	
a. Note code status on front of chart and in all designated areas if necessary (if paper charts used).	The code status will most likely be written on the doctor's order sheet as DNR/DNI or Full Code.
b. Prepare appropriate code status information such as DNR/DNI or Full Code bracelet or color-coded wristband to be placed on the patient's wrist as required.	
Also applicable when using EMR.	
15. Place a label or a piece of red tape stating "name alert" on the spine of the chart if there is a patient on the unit with the same or a similar name (if paper charts used).	
16. Transcribe the admission orders according to hospital policy (if paper charts used).	
Monitor EMR for HUC tasks.	

Outpatient surgery may be performed in the outpatient department of a hospital, in a doctor's office, or in off-campus facilities such as a surgicenter, also called an *ambulatory surgical center (ASC)* or *outpatient surgical center.* Outpatient surgery does not require an overnight hospital stay. The purpose of outpatient surgery is to reduce costs and save the patient time that would be wasted with extra days spent in the hospital. **Admission day surgery** refers to patients who are scheduled for surgery on the day of their arrival to the hospital. The patient usually has completed a **preadmit,** which includes an interview and preparation of most of the needed admission forms. The patient will have all of the necessary preoperative laboratory tests, chest x-ray examination, and electrocardiogram (ECG) completed before the admission. After completion of the patient's surgery and some time spent in the postanesthesia care unit (PACU), the patient is admitted to a surgical nursing unit. Health insurance companies promote this type of admission because it eliminates a hospital day, which reduces the cost of the hospitalization. Other terms for this practice include *same-day surgery (SDS)* and *save-a-day surgery (SAD surgery).*

The doctor's office, the hospital admitting department, and the surgery-scheduling secretary usually coordinate the same-day surgery patient's admission. Laboratory tests, x-ray studies, and other diagnostic testing may be performed at the doctor's office, at an outside facility, or at the hospital on an outpatient basis before admission. The patient usually goes to the hospital admitting area to complete the registration process a few days before the actual admission day. An admitting staff member places the patient ID bracelet or band on the patient's wrist at that time.

On the day of surgery (several hours before the scheduled surgery), the patient reports to the registration desk and will be escorted to the preoperative care unit.

The patient's chart will contain the following:

- Doctors' orders
- All preadmission diagnostic reports that were performed

- Patient ID labels
- Admission forms

After spending time in surgery and the recovery room (PACU), the patient is assigned a bed and is transported to an inpatient surgical unit.

 HIGH PRIORITY

Usually, preoperative care, operating rooms, and the postanesthesia care unit (PACU) are contained in one complete area, separate from all inpatient activities.

Preoperative Care Unit

The **preoperative care unit** (located in the surgery area) is where a patient is prepared for surgery. This is also a waiting area for surgical patients. Preparation may include shaving the surgical area, insertion of a saline lock, starting of intravenous (IV) fluids, and/or inserting a catheter (may be done in the operating room). Preoperative breathing treatments may also be administered in this area. If the patient is a same-day surgery admission, the surgical consent form will also be signed and witnessed here. The anesthesiologist and surgeon will visit the patient in the preoperative area before surgery. The patient will be asked to repeat his or her name and a second identifier such as birth date by both doctors. The anesthesiologist will ask the patient to again state the last time he or she had anything to eat or drink and whether he or she has any allergies (even though this information has been documented by the nurse). The surgeon will ask the patient to state the surgery that is to be performed and will usually mark the operative area with a black marker. This is all done to avoid errors and provide a safe surgical experience.

Preoperative Orders

The doctor who will perform surgery on a patient writes orders (electronically or manually) relative to the surgery before the time the surgery is performed. For example, the surgeon who is performing an open heart surgery may wish the patient to receive preoperative teaching as provided by the cardiopulmonary (respiratory care) department on the evening before surgery. The doctor also may order a saline lock to be inserted or an intravenous (IV) line to be started before a patient leaves the nursing unit for surgery. The surgeon may also designate the anesthesiologist. The anesthesiologist will write preoperative orders that will include the time food and fluids are to be discontinued and the preoperative medication to be given to help relieve anxiety and aid in the induction of anesthesia.

The surgeon writes the surgical procedure for preparation of the surgery consent. If a discrepancy is found between the physician's written order for the consent, the **surgery schedule,** or information on the patient's chart, or if there is any confusion for the patient, the patient's nurse should be notified. The correct procedure must be verified by calling the doctor's office immediately. For example, the surgery consent as written by the physician may state that the patient is to have an "open reduction of the *left* femur," whereas the patient's diagnosis and physical examination indicate that the patient has a fracture of the *right* femur; obviously, such a discrepancy must be corrected before any orders are carried out. All charting rules must be followed when consent forms are prepared. The surgery consent must be written legibly in black ink and written exactly as the doctor wrote it, with the exception of abbreviations. Words cannot be added, deleted, or rearranged, and all abbreviations must be spelled out on the surgery consent. The first and last names of the patient and the doctor also are required. The patient must sign a **blood transfusion consent** or a **blood transfusion refusal** before surgery.

Preoperative Order Components

Orders related directly to the surgery have certain common components.

Surgeons' Orders

- *Name and description of surgery for surgery consent.* The consent must be signed before the patient receives any "mind-clouding" drugs. In the case of surgery that may result in sterility or in loss of a limb (amputation), two permits may be required.
- *Laxatives or enemas.* The order for a laxative or enema depends on the type of surgery. For surgeries within the abdominal cavity, all wastes must be removed from the intestines. This allows the surgeon more room for exploration and a clear field of vision, and it decreases the danger of contamination and infection.
- *Shaves, scrubs, or showers.* The site of the surgical incision must be prepared. This order requires the removal of body hair by shaving. The procedure is referred to as a *surgical prep.* The surgeon also may require a special scrub at the surgical site. In some facilities, the operating room staff members may do shaves and scrubs. Often the doctor writes an order for the patient to take a shower before surgery using an antibacterial soap such as Hibiclens.

- *Name of anesthesiologist or anesthesiology group.* It is necessary to know the anesthesiologist's name or specific anesthesiology group in the event that preoperative medication orders are not received. The HUC then may call the anesthesiologist, group, or person responsible for writing the **preoperative orders.** (In hospitals where nurse anesthetists administer the anesthesia, the surgeon may write the preoperative anesthesia orders.)
- *Miscellaneous orders.* Other orders may include T.E.D. hose, additional diagnostic studies, blood components to be given during surgery, or IV preparations to be started before surgery. Treatments and additional medications also may be ordered.

Anesthesiologists' Orders

- *Diet.* When surgery is to be performed during the morning hours, the patient is usually NPO at midnight. For a patient who is having late-afternoon surgery, an order may be written for a clear liquid breakfast at 0600 and then NPO. Food and/or fluids by mouth are not allowed for 6 to 8 hours before surgery in which an anesthetic is used that renders the patient unconscious. The NPO rule is maintained to lessen the possibility that the patient may aspirate vomitus while under anesthesia.
- *Preoperative medications.* The anesthesiologist or the surgeon usually writes an order for preoperative medication for the patient who is scheduled for surgery. The preoperative medication order may include a hypnotic to ensure that the patient rests well the night before surgery and an intramuscular injection to be given approximately 1 hour before surgery to relax the patient. Figure 19-7 is an example of preoperative orders. HUC tasks performed during the preoperative procedure are listed in Procedure 19-2.

 SKILLS CHALLENGE

To practice transcribing a set of preoperative orders, complete Activity 19-3 in the *Skills Practice Manual.*

The Surgery Patient's Electronic Medical Record or Paper Chart

The surgical patient's nurse usually completes a **preoperative and postoperative patient care plan** that integrates the nurse's knowledge, previous experience, and established standards of care. The plan usually includes preoperative teaching, goals, and outcomes. The plan is reviewed and modified during the **intraoperative** and postoperative periods. Outcomes established for each goal of care provide measurable evidence of the patient's progress. When the patient is involved in the development of the surgical care plan, surgical risks and postoperative complications are reduced.

It is the overall responsibility of the HUC to see that the surgical patient's paper chart is properly prepared to send to surgery with the patient. The registered nurse (RN) completes a preoperative checklist; however, the HUC is involved in preparing the patient's paper chart. It is often hospital policy that surgery cannot begin if any of the required reports are missing from the patient's EMR or paper chart. Therefore

PHYSICIANS' ORDER SHEET

DATE	TIME	SYMBOL	ORDERS
5/13/XX	1400		Full liq diet tonight
			T & X match 2 u PC & hold for surgery
			CBC, UA & chest x-ray PA & LAT Cl: pre-op
			ECG this pm
			Consent: partial gastrectomy, vagotomy
			& pyloroplasty
			Hibiclens shower this pm
			H & P by surgical resident
			Pre-ops per Dr. A. Sleep
			Start 1000mL5% D/W TKO prior to surg.
			Dr. G. Astro MD.
5/13/XX	1600		NPO 2400
			Restoril 15 mg hs tonight MR x 1
			Demerol 100 mg ⎫
			Vistaril 25 mg ⎬ IM @ 0700
			Dr. A. Sleep MD

Figure 19-7 Set of preoperative orders.

PROCEDURE 19-2

PREOPERATIVE PROCEDURE

Tasks may vary among facilities, and many of the listed tasks also apply when using EMR. When CPOE has been implemented, tasks related to preparing a paper chart or transcribing orders would not apply.

TASK	NOTES
1. Label the surgery forms with the patient's identification labels, and place them within the patient's paper chart (if paper charts used). Print consent forms and blood transfusion forms with patient ID from computer, or, if necessary, label the forms; after forms have been signed by patient, scan them into patient's EMR.	The surgery forms include the nurse's preoperative checklist, the operating room record, the anesthesiologist's record, the recovery room record, and so on. See the Evolve website for examples of operative records.
2.	
a. Check the patient's electronic or paper chart for the history and physical report (H&P).	If the history and physical report (H&P) is not found on the chart, call HIMS to check whether it has been dictated. Notify the patient's nurse and doctor if the report is not located.
b. Check the patient's electronic or paper chart for the following signed consent forms:	
• Surgical consent	Check the consent forms for patient and witness signatures and for the correct spelling of the surgical procedure.
• Blood transfusion consent or blood transfusion refusal form	
• Admission service agreement	
3. Check the patient's electronic or paper chart for any previously ordered diagnostic studies such as laboratory tests, x-ray studies, and so forth.	If the diagnostic test results are not on the patient's chart, locate the results on the computer, print them, and place in patient's chart. If unable to locate results, notify patient's nurse.

Continued

PROCEDURE 19–2—cont'd	
TASK	NOTES
4. File the current medication administration record in the patient's chart (if paper charts used).	
5. Print at least five face sheets to place in the paper chart. If the EMR is used, maintain five face sheets in a notebook to provide to consulting doctors and other health care providers as requested.	Face sheets are removed and are used by doctors and other health care providers to bill patients.
6. Place at least three sheets of patient identification labels in the patient's paper chart. If the EMR is used, maintain three sheets of labels in a notebook to label specimens as necessary.	Patient identification labels are used to label specimens.
7. Notify the appropriate nursing personnel when surgery calls for the patient. Also applicable when EMR is used.	Surgery personnel will call before transport is sent, to verify that the patient is prepared to be picked up.

the most important task is to have the following records on the chart:

- *Current history and physical record (H&P):* Essential in most health care facilities.
- **Surgery consent:** Before surgery is performed, an informed consent must be obtained that is accurate, includes patient's and surgeon's full names, is signed by the patient or legal guardian and dated, and includes a witness signature and date and time (see Chapter 8).
- *Blood consent:* A blood transfusion consent form must be signed to accept (see Chapter 8) or refuse (see Chapter 8) blood products.
- *Admission service agreement* (also called *conditions of admission):* Check to see whether this was signed on admission.
- **Nursing preoperative checklist:** Should be checked and signed by nursing personnel
- *Medication administration record (MAR):* Current MAR should be placed in chart before transport to surgery.
- *Diagnostic test results:* Results of preoperative tests, including laboratory, diagnostic imaging, and so forth, that were ordered by the doctor.

The HUC should closely monitor the surgical patient's electronic record before surgery to ensure that all orders have been processed. To ensure that each patient's paper chart is ready to be taken to surgery, an HUC may choose to create a **health unit coordinator preoperative checklist** (Fig. 19-8). This checklist should not be confused with the nursing preoperative checklist (Fig. 19-9), which is checked and signed by the patient's nurse to ensure proper patient preparation for surgery. The nursing preoperative checklist is a legal chart form in most facilities.

Each nursing unit will print from the computer a surgery schedule (Fig. 19-10) that lists all surgeries to be performed on the following day.

See Procedure 19-2 for HUC tasks required to prepare the patient's paper chart for surgery. Someone from surgery will call the nursing unit to determine whether the patient is ready to be picked up. After the HUC is given the okay from the patient's nurse and relays the message that the patient is ready,

transportation is sent to pick up the patient. The patient's paper chart is sent to surgery with transport when the patient is taken to surgery.

Examples of **perioperative** nurses' records may be found on the Evolve website.

 HIGH PRIORITY

Printing the day's surgery schedule for the nursing unit will assist the health unit coordinator in ensuring that the required reports and forms including a signed and dated surgery consent form are in the surgical patient's electronic medical record or paper chart.

Postoperative Orders and Routine

Immediately after surgery, most patients spend 1 or more hours in the recovery room or the PACU. A record of patient progress is kept on the recovery room record. This record, along with other surgery records, is included in the patient's chart. **Postoperative orders** (written by the surgeon to be carried out immediately after surgery) often are initiated here. For example, the recovery room staff may carry out the doctors' order for antiembolism elastic hose (or stockings) to be placed on the patient's legs. Recovery room personnel will indicate on the physicians' order sheet those orders that have already been executed (note order no. 7 on Fig. 19-11).

Postoperative Order Components

Postoperative orders that relate to the patient's treatment after surgery usually contain the following components:

- *Diet:* The patient may remain NPO or may be given sips of water or ice chips ("sips and chips"). The diet then is increased as tolerated.
- *Intake and output:* The patient's intake and output are closely watched for 24 to 48 hours (see Chapter 10).
- *IV fluids:* For most surgery patients, at least one bag of IV fluids is ordered after surgery. A record of the intake of IV fluids is maintained on a parenteral fluid sheet (see Chapter 8).

Surgical Patients		3-C						
Rm#	Patient	Surg Time	Service Adm Agreement	H & P	5 Sheets Pt ID Labels	5 Face Sheets	Surgical Consent	Dx Reports
305	Pack, Fanny	0730	X	X	X	X	X	X
311	Juniper, Jack	0800	X	X	X	X	X	X
312	Harris, Susan	1100	X	X	X	X	X	X

Figure 19-8 A preoperative checklist for the health unit coordinator.

PREOPERATIVE CHECK LIST   **DATE**

NURSING UNIT CHECK LIST

		YES	NO
1.	Pre-op bath/Oral hygiene given	✓	
2.	Make-up/Nail polish removed	✓	
3.	**Bobby Pins,** Combs, Hair Pieces Removed Disposition:	✓	
4.	Sanitary Belt removed	—	
5.	**Jewelry,** Rings, Religious Medals, or other items removed (May be worn during cardiac catheterization) when removed disposition is:	✓	
6.	Voided/Retention catheter	✓	
7.	Preoperative medicine given as ordered	✓	
8.	Addressograph with chart	✓	
9.	Pre-anesthetic patient questionnaire completed	✓	

10. Where family can be located during and immediately after surgery   *Surgery Waiting room*

NURSING UNIT AND OPERATING ROOM NURSES CHECK LIST

		UNIT NURSE		O.R. NURSE	
		YES	NO	YES	NO
11.	Surgical consent for: Rt. (Lt.) *Inguinal herniorrhaphy*	✓			
	as obtained from Doctor's Order sheet	✓			
12.	Consultation Special Consents				
13.	History and Physical Dictated On Chart	✓			
14.	Allergies Noted	✓			
15.	Hematology	✓			
16.	Urinalysis	✓			
17.	Surgical/Cardiac cath prep done	✓			
18.	Type and Cross Match *1* Units *P.C.*	✓			
19.	Culture site: Results:				
20.	Admission Chest X-Ray Report	✓			
21.	EKG Report if over 40 years	✓			

		REMOVED			
		YES	NO	YES	NO
22.	Prosthetic Teeth May be worn during cardiac catheterization				
	Permanent cap or caps				
	Permanent bridge				
	Removable bridge				
	Removable plate or plates				
	Loose teeth				
23.	Prosthesis and Disposition:				
	Artificial eye in out				
	Contact lens in out				
	Pacemaker				
	Other				

none
none

R.N. Signature

00-6015 Rev. 12-79

PATIENT IDENTIFICATION ON UNIT

A. **Person from surgery calling for patient**

 1. Ask for patient by name

 2. Check patient's chart

 3. Check patient's chart with call slip (not necessary with cardiac catheterization)

B. **Person from unit must accompany**

 1. Ask patient his/her name
    Ask patient his/her doctor's name

 2. Check chart face sheet for patient's name and hospital number with patient identiband

 3. Check call slip with identiband (not necessary for cardiac catheterization)

Winifred Marshall, R.N.
Signature Nursing Unit Personnel

Bill Standard, Ord.
Signature Surgery Personnel

SPECIAL COMMENTS TO OPERATING ROOM AND RECOVERY ROOM NURSES FROM NURSING UNIT: (PLEASE SIGN YOUR COMMENT)

B.P.:H.S. *130/70* a Pre-op *140/82* p Pre-op *136/80*

Pre-op TPR _____ NPO p *Mn* WT. *136*

Pertinent Drug Therapy:

Demerol 75 mg } *I.M.*
Atropine 0.4 mg } *8:30 am*

O.R. Nurse Signature

PREOPERATIVE CHECK LIST

Figure 19-9 Nurse's preoperative checklist.

SURGERY SCHEDULE FRIDAY JUNE 10, 0000

Time	Surgeon	Procedure	Patient's Bed Number
Operating Room 1			
0730	Dr. Singsong	Anterior Colporrhaphy; left Bartholin's cystectomy	412A
0930	Dr. Prossert	Dilatation & curettage; FS, possible vag. hysterectomy, bil. salpingo-oophorectomy	321
1130	Dr. Broad	Laparoscopy	621B
1330	Dr. Street	Rt. breast biopsy, FS, Poss. rt. radical mastectomy	416
Operating Room 2			
0730	Dr. Patellar	Arthrotomy lt. knee, open reduction, internal fixation with plateau medial meniscectomy	502B
0930	Dr. Home	Arthroplasty rt. elbow, insertion of prosthesis; reconstruction rheumatoid rt. hand	511
1330	Dr. Bowl	Bone graft lt. radius	516A
Operating Room 3			
0730	Dr. Branch	Cystoscopy, TURP	212
0930	Dr. Signe	Cystoscopy, manipulation ureteral stone	222A
1130	Dr. Blake	Circumcision	316B
Operating Room 4			
0730	Dr. Throat	Tonsillectomy	304A
0930	Dr. Ober	Hemorrhoidectomy	601
Operating Room 5			
0730	Dr. Love	Cholecystectomy, biopsy rib cage	617B
0930	Dr. Solano	Repair of lt. inguinal hernia	600

Figure 19-10 Surgery schedule.

- *Vital signs:* The patient's vital signs are monitored carefully after surgery—usually every 4 hours for 24 to 48 hours.
- *Catheters, tubes, and drains:* Postoperative patients may have a retention or indwelling urinary catheter. Other orders may pertain to intermittent catheterization of the patient, as necessary. Some patients may require suctioning when nasogastric or other tubes are in place.
- *Activity:* Activity after surgery may consist of only bed rest, and this may be increased as the patient continues to recuperate.
- *Positioning:* Some surgeons require that the patient's position be changed frequently. Elevation of the bed also may be very important.
- *Observation of the operative site:* It is imperative that the sites of the operation or the bandages be observed closely for bleeding, excessive drainage, redness, and swelling.
- *Medications:* Medications to relieve pain (narcotics) and nausea and vomiting (antiemetics) and to help the patient sleep or rest (hypnotics) may be prescribed for a period after surgery. Other medications are ordered as needed. (Figure 19-11 provides an example of postoperative orders.)

Postoperative orders usually cancel all previous orders. See Procedure 19-3, Postoperative Procedure, for HUC tasks that are involved in postoperative procedures.

When working in obstetrics, the health unit coordinator needs to be efficient in completing postoperative orders and also alert to visitors arriving on the unit. A **Hugs Infant Protection System** is an example of an alarm system that is used

in the newborn nursery to prevent infants from being removed from a health care facility without authorization.

Health Unit Coordinator Responsibilities Regarding Patients' Electronic Medical Records

It is important that the HUC monitor the patient's EMR consistently including admission, preoperative, and postoperative orders for tasks that may need to be performed. The surgical consent is usually entered into the patient's EMR for the HUC to prepare the consent for the patient's nurse to have the patient sign. It is equally important that the HUC scan all medical records including, signed consent forms, handwritten progress notes, and other reports and records faxed, sent, or brought in with the patient from other facilities.

Electronic Patient Status Tracking Board

An **electronic patient status tracking board** is a viewing screen that is located on the wall in the surgical waiting areas, in the hospital cafeteria, and other areas in the hospital. Each surgical patient is assigned a case number that is provided to family or friends waiting for the patient. The tracking board is designed to keep family and friends updated on the status of a surgical patient. The patient's case number is displayed on the board once the patient has arrived in the perioperative department. The location section of the board will display the patient's location (preoperative area, in surgery, PACU, and room), which is also color-coded as he or she moves from area to area. This allows the patient's family and friends the ability to leave the waiting area and get a meal or a cup of coffee

PHYSICIANS' ORDER SHEET

DATE	TIME	SYMBOL	ORDERS
6/7/03			*Post op*
			NPO
			NG tube to Low Suction
			Follow present IV c̄ 5% D/LR @ 125cc/h
			Demerol 75 mg IM q 4 h prn pain
			Compazine 10 mg IM q 4 h prn N/V
			Encourage to TCDB
			Knee length elastic hose ✓done / RR @1050
			May dangle this evening
			Dr. G. Astro

Figure 19-11 Set of postoperative orders.

without worrying about missing information about the surgical patient. The PACU personnel or the HUC working in the surgical area will also call the waiting areas and the patient's nursing unit to notify of the patient's progress. It is important that the patient's nurse be made aware of the patient's arrival in PACU and readiness to return to the room so that he or she may make plans and be prepared for the patient's arrival.

KEY CONCEPTS

For most patients, admission to the hospital is a stressful experience. The HUC can do much in the field of public relations for the hospital at this time. The HUC is usually the first person on the nursing unit with whom the new patient has contact. A warm welcome and a pleasant smile may help to relieve

PROCEDURE 19-3

POSTOPERATIVE PROCEDURE

Tasks may vary among facilities, and many of the listed tasks also apply when using EMR. When EMR with CPOE has been implemented, tasks related to preparing a paper chart or transcribing orders would not apply.

TASK	NOTES

1.
  a. Inform the patient's nurse of the patient's arrival to the PACU as soon as possible.
  b. Inform the patient's nurse of the expected arrival of the patient from the recovery room.
  Also applicable when EMR is used.
	PACU personnel usually notify the unit when the patient arrives from the operating room. The nurse then may plan and be prepared for the patient's return to the unit.
	PACU personnel will notify the nursing unit before returning the patient to the room and will give a report of the patient's condition to the appropriate nurse.

2. Place all operating records behind the proper divider in the patient's chart.	
3. Write the date of surgery and the surgical procedure in the designated places on the patient's Kardex form or in the computer.	
4. Transcribe the doctors' postoperative orders. Notify the nurse who is caring for the patient of stat doctors' orders.	All preoperative orders are automatically discontinued postoperatively. The HUC usually starts a new Kardex form for the patient.

★ HIGH PRIORITY

Postanesthesia care unit (PACU) personnel or a health unit coordinator working in surgery will call the surgery waiting room (where patients' families or friends are waiting) and the nursing unit to notify of the patient's arrival in the PACU, and they will call again when the patient is ready to return to the room. This will be done even when a tracking board is in use.

It is important to notify the patient's nurse of the patient's arrival in the PACU and of the time when the patent is to return to the nursing unit.

SKILLS CHALLENGE

To practice transcribing a set of postoperative orders, complete Activity 19-4 in the *Skills Practice Manual*.

---

anxiety. The expediency with which the patient's paper chart is prepared and the new orders are transcribed determines the ability of the health care team to initiate care and treatment sooner. When the EMR is used, it is important to monitor the nursing unit census screen for HUC tasks and to scan documents in a timely manner. Waiting for someone who is in surgery can also be very stressful for family members and friends. The HUC can assist them with information regarding where to wait, where the cafeteria is, and so on.

The HUC must be familiar with the common components in an admission, as well as with preoperative and postoperative order sets. As with all orders, quick, accurate, and thorough transcription is a must toward ensuring high-quality care for the patient.

Websites of Interest

Joint Commission Resources—"National Patient Safety Goals": www.jcrinc.com/National-Patient-Safety-Goals

Legacy Writer—Legal documents online: www.LegacyWriter.com

World Health Organization (WHO): www.who.int

Agency for Healthcare Research and Quality—"Having Surgery? What You Need to Know": www.ahrq.gov/consumer/surgery/surgery.htm

⊖ REVIEW QUESTIONS

1. Define the following terms:
   a. patient health information management number
   b. patient account number
   c. bariatric surgery
   d. perioperative
   e. census
   f. registration
   g. informed consent
   h. comorbidity
   i. elective surgery
   j. preadmit
   k. Hugs Infant Protection System
   l. electronic patient status tracking board
   m. admission, discharge, and transfer log sheet (ADT log sheet)
   n. admission, discharge, and transfer log book (ADT log book)
   o. census board

2. List four types of patient admissions and three types of patients,

3. Discuss who can admit a patient to the hospital and how the nursing unit and bed are assigned.

4. List 10 registration and admission tasks.

5. List eight interview techniques.

6. Discuss the following:
   a. face sheet (information form)
   b. admission service agreement or conditions of admission (COA or C of A)
   c. patient identification (ID) bracelet
   d. patient identification labels
   e. process of securing patient valuables

7. Explain the significance of three standard color-coded alert wristbands, and identify additional color-coded alert wristbands that may be used in hospitals.

8. Explain the purpose of advance directives, and discuss the types of advance directives that are available.

9. List at least eight common components of a set of admission orders.

10. List fifteen common HUC tasks regarding the patient's admission when paper charts are used.

11. Discuss how a surgical patient's admission orders differ from a medical patient's admission orders, and discuss three options for the way in which patient surgeries may be performed.

12. Discuss the purpose of the preoperative care unit, and describe the patient preparation that may take place there.

13. List seven components that may be included in a set of preoperative orders (including the anesthesiologist's orders).

14. List seven records or reports that are required to be in the patient's electronic or paper chart before surgery.

15. List seven HUC responsibilities that are related to a patient's preoperative orders when paper charts are used

16. List nine components that may be included in a set of postoperative orders.

17. List four HUC responsibilities related to a patient's postoperative orders when paper charts are used.

18. Explain the purpose and benefits of the electronic patient status tracking board for the surgery patient's family and friends.

19. Explain why it is important for the HUC to monitor the patient's EMR consistently.

20. Explain what the HUC's responsibility would be regarding patient signed consent forms, handwritten progress notes, and reports from other facilities faxed to the nursing station when the EMR with CPOE is implemented.

SURFING FOR ANSWERS

1. Find the definition of "Iatrophobia." Write out the definition and suggestions for dealing with it, and document the website used.
2. Research and document at least three surgical mistakes, and list two websites used.
3. Locate and explore the World Health Organization (WHO) Safe Surgery Saves Lives Checklist at www.safesurg.org.

CHAPTER 20

Discharge, Transfer, and Postmortem Procedures

CHAPTER OBJECTIVES

On completion of this chapter, you will be able to:

1. Define the terms in the vocabulary list.
2. Write the meaning of the abbreviations in the abbreviations list.
3. Discuss the purpose of patient discharge planning and patient care conferences, and identify personnel and individuals who would be involved in both.
4. List five types of discharges, and explain the importance of communicating pending discharge information and bed availability to the admitting department or bed placement in a timely manner.
5. List 12 tasks that may be required to complete a routine discharge when paper charts are used.
6. List six additional tasks that may be required when a patient is discharged to another facility and six additional tasks when a patient is discharged home with assistance when paper charts are used.
7. Describe six tasks necessary to prepare the discharged patient's medical record for the health information

management services (HIMS) department when paper charts are used.
8. Explain what the health unit coordinator (HUC) should do when a patient threatens to leave the hospital without a physician's discharge order.
9. Explain the HUC tasks that may be required and/or requested when a patient dies, and discuss the need for the patient's death to be verified and the time documented by a doctor or resident.
10. Discuss how the deceased patient is transferred to the morgue, and explain the possible HUC tasks related to the release of remains and organ donation.
11. Explain the usual circumstances regarding a patient's death that must be met for the patient to be accepted as an organ donor.
12. Explain why an autopsy would be performed and list the circumstances that would define a "coroners case."
13. List eight tasks performed by the HUC when a patient dies (postmortem) when paper charts are used.

14. List the two primary reasons a doctor would write an order for a patient to be transferred to another room or nursing unit.
15. List nine tasks that are performed when a patient is transferred from one unit to another when paper charts are used.
16. List seven tasks performed by the HUC when a patient is transferred from one room to another room on the same unit when paper charts are used.
17. List seven tasks that are performed by the HUC when a transferred patient is received on the unit when paper charts are used.
18. Discuss the importance of reading the entire set of discharge or transfer orders prior to the patient being discharged or transferred.
19. Describe additional tasks that the HUC may need to carry out to complete a routine discharge procedure when the electronic medical record with computer physician order entry is used.

VOCABULARY

Autopsy Examination of a body after death; it may be performed to determine the cause of death or for medical research purposes.

Clinical Death State in which no brain function is present.

Coroner A public officer whose primary function is to investigate by inquest any death thought to be of other than natural causes.

Coroner's Case A death that occurs because of sudden, violent, or unexplained circumstances, or a patient who expires unexpectedly within the first 24 hours after admission to the hospital (deaths investigated by a coroner).

Custodial Care Care and services of a nonmedical nature, which consist of feeding, bathing, watching, and protecting the patient.

Discharge Order A doctor's order that states that the patient may leave the hospital; a doctor's order is necessary for a patient to be discharged from the hospital.

Discharge Planning Centralized, coordinated, multidisciplinary process that ensures that the patient has a plan for continuing care after leaving the hospital.

Expiration Death.

Extended Care Facility A medical facility for patients who require expert nursing care or custodial care; may also be referred to as a *skilled nursing facility.*

Organ Donation Donating or giving one's organs and/or tissues after death; one may designate specific organs (e.g., only cornea) or may donate any needed organs.

Organ Procurement The process of removing donated organs; may also be referred to as *harvesting.*

Patient Care Conference A meeting that includes the doctor or doctors caring for the patient, the primary nurses, the case manager or social worker, and other caregivers (may include family) involved in the patient's care.

Postmortem After death (a postmortem examination is the same as an autopsy).

Release of Remains A signed consent that authorizes a specific funeral home or agency to remove the deceased from a health care facility.

Terminal Illness An illness ending in death.

Transfer Order A doctor's order that requests that a patient be transferred to another hospital room, another nursing unit, or another facility.

ABBREVIATIONS

Abbreviation	Meaning	Example of Usage on a Doctor's Order Sheet
AMA	against medical advice	Patient D/C AMA
Disch, DC	discharge	Disch today $\bar{p}$ chest X-ray
ECF	extended care facility	Please have case mgt arrange for transfer to ECF
SNF	skilled nursing facility	Arrange for ambulance transport to SNF (discussed in Chapter 2)
Trans	transfer	Trans to ICU

⊜ EXERCISE 1

Write the abbreviation for each term listed.

1. against medical advice
2. discharge
3. extended care facility
4. skilled nursing facility
5. transfer

⊜ EXERCISE 2

Write the meaning of each abbreviation listed.

1. AMA
2. Disch, DC
3. ECF

4. SNF
5. Trans

DISCHARGE PLANNING

Discharge planning is a centralized, coordinated, multidisciplinary process that ensures that the patient has a plan for continuing care after leaving the hospital. Discharge planning begins the moment a patient is admitted to the hospital and usually is handled by a case manager or a social worker who assist patients and their families with arrangements for post-hospitalization care. The case manager or social worker works with the patient and the patient's family, nurses, and physician(s) in developing a discharge plan of care that is tailored to meet the specific needs of the patient. Once the plan has been developed, the case manager secures the necessary posthospitalization services and can provide information about additional community resources when necessary.

A **patient care conference** is a meeting that includes the doctor(s) caring for the patient, the primary nurses, the case manager or social worker, and other caregivers (may include family) involved in the patient's care. The purpose of the conference is to review and evaluate the goals and outcomes of the patient's recovery progress and to modify the care plan as needed. Often a patient care conference is scheduled before the time of a patient's discharge so that a posthospitalization care plan can be developed. The health unit coordinator (HUC) should be made aware when the patient's paper chart is taken into the conference room.

DISCHARGE OF A PATIENT

Once a patient's doctor has entered a discharge order into the patient's electronic medical record (EMR) or has written a discharge order in the paper chart, the prompt attention of the HUC is required. Most patients prefer to leave the hospital as soon as possible after the discharge order has been written. When transcribing a **discharge order,** the HUC would enter the patient's name under "discharges" on the *admission, discharge, and transfer log sheet (ADT log sheet)* and would notify the admitting or bed placement department by telephone or computer. It is important to send or call a "pending discharge" to the bed placement or admitting department in a timely manner and to communicate when the bed is ready for another patient, especially when the hospital is full. Often there are patients waiting to be admitted, some for hours in the emergency department. Withholding notification of a discharge order will cause a delay in an incoming patient's admission and treatment. The HUC must also notify environmental services (housekeeping) when the patient has vacated the room, so the room can be cleaned and the room and bed prepared for the admission of a new patient. This notification may be done by phone or computer. The HUC would enter the date of discharge in the *admission, discharge, and transfer log book (ADT log book)* next to the patient's label (placed there when patient was admitted) with the date and type of discharge (e.g., Home, Sunset Assisted Living). The name is also erased from the nursing unit census board. This is done when using the EMR and when using paper charts.

When the EMR is implemented, the HUC may have the additional task of printing out the medication information sheets for medications that the patient will be taking after discharge.

When the EMR is used, the beds are color-coded on the computer census screen as follows:

Pink—female
Blue—male
Green—ready
Brown—dirty - needs cleaning

Types of Discharges

There are five types of discharges, as follows:

1. Discharge home
2. Discharge to another facility
3. Discharge home with assistance
4. Discharge against medical advice (AMA)
5. Expiration

All patient discharges require a doctor's order. When a patient insists on leaving AMA, the doctor usually writes a discharge order that documents that the patient is leaving AMA and the patient will be asked to sign a form stating that he or she is leaving the hospital against medical advice.

Routine Discharge Procedure

Most discharges from the hospital are routine in nature—that is, the patient is discharged alive to go home in the company of a family member or a friend or alone. See Procedure 20-1 and Figures 20-1 through 20-4.

Discharge to Another Facility

Insurance reviewers are employed by insurance companies to review hospitalized patients' charts to advise doctors regarding what the insurance will cover and how many hospital days will be covered. Insurance reviewers are required to show identification (ID) before having access to a patient's electronic or paper chart. When the patient no longer needs expert nursing care but still requires custodial care, the doctor is requested to transfer the patient from the hospital to an assisted living facility or nursing care home. **Custodial care** is care of a nonmedical nature, such as feeding, bathing, watching, and protecting the patient. The insurance reviewer places

---

PROCEDURE 20-1
ROUTINE DISCHARGE PROCEDURE

TASK	NOTES
1. Read the entire order carefully when transcribing the discharge order.	The discharge order may be indicated by an icon on the computer census screen next to the appropriate patient's name when the EMR is used or may be hand-written when paper charts are used. The order may be written on the doctor's order sheet the day before or the day of the expected discharge. Sometimes the doctor will write an order for a chest x-ray study or other diagnostic test(s) to be performed before discharge. Check for any prescription that may have been left on the chart by the doctor.

Continued

PROCEDURE 20-1—cont'd

TASK	NOTES
2. Notify the discharged patient's nurse when a discharge order has been written. When the EMR with CPOE is implemented, the HUC may print out the medication information sheets for medications that the patient will be taking after discharge (see Fig. 20-1).	The patient's nurse will provide the patient with discharge instructions.
3. Enter a "pending discharge" with the expected departure time into the computer.	Notification may be made by telephone or by computer. Entering a "pending discharge" with expected departure time notifies the business department to prepare the patient's bill. Some patients may be required to stop at the business office before leaving the hospital. The "pending discharge" notification also alerts the admitting department that a patient who is waiting to be admitted may be placed into a room slot. Holding notification of a discharge could delay another patient's admission and the start of treatment.
4. Explain the procedure for discharge to the patient and/or the patient's relatives.	Explanation of the discharge procedure may also be given by the nurse; however, many patients come to the nurse's station and ask the HUC for the explanation.
5. Hospital departments including nutritional care usually have access to certain portions of the patient's EMR and will be aware of the discharge order; if not, notify other departments that may be giving the patient daily treatments.	Departments such as physical therapy and cardiopulmonary (respiratory care) may have to be notified. Communication may be made by telephone or by computer. The HUC may need to cancel the patient's food tray or order an early tray.
6. Arrange for any appointments requested by the doctor.	Write out the appointment date and time on a piece of paper and give it to the patient's nurse. The appointment date and time may then be written on or typed into the discharge instruction sheet.
7. Arrange transportation if required.	Patients who do not have family or friends available to provide transportation may have to have a call made for a taxi. Many hospitals provide taxi vouchers for patients.
8. Prepare credit slips for medications returned to the pharmacy or equipment and supplies returned to the central services department (CSD).	Supplies specifically ordered for the patient from CSD but not used by the patient must be returned to CSD with a credit slip (see Fig. 20-2).
9. Notify nursing personnel or transportation service to transport the patient to the discharge area when the patient is ready to leave.	Patients should never be allowed to go to the discharge area without an escort from the hospital staff. Also, the patient should be transported via wheelchair.
10. a. Write the patient's name on the admission, discharge, and transfer log sheet (ADT log sheet). b. Erase the patient's name from the unit census board.	An example of an admission, discharge, and transfer log sheet is shown in Figure 20-3.
11. Notify environmental services to clean the discharged patient's room.	Notification may be made by telephone, by computer, or by informing environmental services personnel on the unit.
12. Prepare the patient's paper chart for the health information management services (HIMS) department. a. Check the summary or diagnosis-related group (DRG) worksheet for the doctor's summation and the patient's final diagnosis. It is important to have this information on patient discharge so that coding of DRGs may be placed on the chart by HIMS personnel. b. Check for the correct patient identification labels on chart forms. c. Shred all chart forms that have been labeled and have no documentation on them. d. Check for old records or split records and send with the chart to HIMS. e. Arrange chart forms in discharge sequence according to hospital policy. f. Send the discharged patient's chart to HIMS, along with any old records of the patient (must be sent on the day of discharge)	Many hospitals issue a discharge checklist (see Fig. 20-4) to prepare the chart for HIMS. (Applicable when paper charts are used.) After the patient's paper chart has been sent to HIMS, nurses, doctors, residents, and other health care providers will have to go there to complete charting or sign forms, if necessary.

DISCHARGE INSTRUCTIONS

DIAGNOSIS: _____

_____

SURGERY/PROCEDURE: _____

1. **ACTIVITY**	NO LIMIT	LIMIT
Bathing		
Driving		
Sexual		
Work		
Exercise		
Ambulation		

2. **MEDICATION:**

_____ Patient/family knows what medications are for.

_____ Prescriptions sent with patient or family.

NAME OF MEDICATION	**DOSAGE**	**FREQUENCY/TIMES**

3. **DIET:**

Your diet will be _____

Please call dietition at _____ if you have any questions.

4. **SPECIAL INFORMATION:** (include wound care, further treatments, referrals, equipment, etc.)

5. **RETURN VISIT TO PHYSICIAN:** Please call Dr. _____Phone: _____

to make an appointment in _____ days. Please call the doctor if you cannot take your medicine

or to answer any questions.

6. **INSTRUCTION SHEETS GIVEN:** (Please list pamphlets, written instructions or other standardized information.)

The above was discussed with me and
I understand all of the information.

_____
Signature of R.N.

_____
Date

_____
Signature of Patient/Guardian

Patient (original)   Medical Records (yellow)   Other (pink)   DISCHARGE INSTRUCTIONS

Figure 20-1 A, Discharge instruction sheet. (From Rockford Memorial Hospital, Rockford Illinois.)

Continued

Opportunity Medical Center - Pharmacy

DRUG: Zithromax 250 mg Tabs (Z- PAK)
INGREDIENT NAME: Azithromycin (az-ith-rie-MYE-sin)

COMMON USES: This medicine is a macrolide antibiotic used to treat bacterial infections.

BEFORE USING THIS MEDICINE: Some medicines or medical conditions may interact with this medicine. INFORM YOUR DOCTOR OR PHARMACIST of all prescriptions and over-the-counter medicine that you are taking. DO NOT TAKE THIS MEDICINE if you are also taking propafenone or pimozide. ADDITIONAL MONITORING OF YOUR DOSE OR CONDITION may be needed if you are taking anticoagulants (such as warfarin), digoxin, nelfinavir, cyclosporine, ergotamine, hexobarbital, phenytoin, rifampin, theophylline, triazolam, certain drugs for high cholesterol (such as lovastatin), medicines for irregular heartbeat (such as amiodarone, disopyramide, quinidine, or procainamide), or medicines that may affect your heartbeat. Ask your doctor if you are unsure if any of the medicines you are taking may affect your heartbeat. Inform your doctor of any other kidney problems, liver problems, allergies, pregnancy, or breastfeeding. Contact your doctor or pharmacist if you have any questions or concerns about taking this medicine.

HOW TO USE THIS MEDICINE: Follow the directions for using this medicine provided by your doctor. This medicine may be taken on an empty stomach or with food. DO NOT TAKE THIS MEDICINE within 1 hour before or 2 hours after aluminium- or magnesium–containing antacids. STORE THIS MEDICINE at room temperature, away from heat and light. TO CLEAR UP YOUR INFECTION COMPLETELY, continiue taking this medicine for the full course of treatment even if you feel better in a few days. DO NOT MISS ANY DOSES. Taking this medicine at the same time each day will make it easier to remember. IF YOU MISS A DOSE OF THIS MEDICINE, take it as soon as possible. If it is almost time for your next dose, skip the missed dose and go back to your regular dosing schedule. If you miss a dose, do not take 2 doses at once.

CAUTIONS: DO NOT TAKE THIS MEDICATION if you have had an allergic reaction to it or are allergic to any ingredient in this product. DO NOT TAKE THIS MEDICINE IF YOU HAVE HAD A SEVERE ALLERGIC REACTION to erythromycin or any macrolide or ketolide antibiotic. A severe reaction includes a severe rash, hives, breathing difficulties, or dizziness. If you have a question about whether you are allergic to this medicine, contact your doctor or pharmacist.

IF YOU EXPERIENCE difficulty breathing; tightness of chest; swelling of eyelids, face or lips; or if you develop a rash or hives, tell your doctor immediately. Do not take any more of this medicine unless your doctor tells you to do so. IF MODERATE TO SEVERE DIARRHEA OCCURS during or after treatment with this medicine, check with your doctor or pharmacist. Do not treat it with non-prescription (over-the-counter) medicines. BEFORE YOU BEGIN TAKING ANY NEW MEDICINE, either prescription or over-the-counter, check with your doctor or pharmacist. FOR WOMEN: IF YOU PLAN ON BECOMING PREGNANT, discuss with your doctor the benefits and risks of using this medicine during pregnancy. IT IS UNKNOWN IF THE MEDICINE IS EXCRETED in breast milk. IF YOU ARE OR WILL BE BREAST-FEEDING while you are taking this medicine, check with your doctor or pharmacist to discuss the risks to your baby.

POSSIBLE SIDE EFFECTS: SIDE EFFECTS that may go away during treatment include mild diarrhea, nausea, or stomach pain. If they continue or are bothersome, check with your doctor. CHECK WITH YOUR DOCTOR AS SOON AS POSSIBLE if you experience vomiting, hearing loss, or ringing in the ears. CONTACT YOUR DOCTOR IMMEDIATELY if you experience swelling of your hands, legs, face, lips, eyes, throat, or toungue; difficultly swallowing or breathing; hoarseness; irregular heartbeat; reddened blistered, or swollen skin; or severe diarrhea. An allergic reaction to this medicine is unlikely, but seek immediate medical attention if it occurs. Symptoms of an allergic reaction include rash, itching, swelling, dizziness, or trouble breathing. If you notice other effects listed above, contact your doctor, nurse,or pharmacist.

OVERDOSE: If overdose is suspected, contact your local poison control center or emergency room immediately. Symptoms of overdose may include nausea, vomiting, and diarrahea.

ADDITIONAL INFORMATION: DO NOT SHARE THIS MEDICINE with others for whom it was not prescribed. DO NOT USE THIS MEDICINE for other health conditions. KEEP THIS MEDICINE out of reach of children.

Figure 20-1, cont'd B, Prescription information printout.

a sticker on the cover of the patient's chart binder to indicate how many more days will be covered by the patient's insurance. If the doctor believes that the patient needs additional hospitalization, the reasons for the additional days will have to be documented.

Other patients may be discharged to an assisted living facility, a nursing care home, a rehabilitation facility, or an **extended care facility** (ECF) or skilled nursing facility (SNF). Frequently the hospital case manager or social service worker makes the arrangements for long-term care. The discharge of a patient to another facility is the same as a routine discharge but with additional steps (Fig. 20-5 and Procedure 20-2).

Discharge Home with Assistance

Many patients require care or assistance provided at home as part of their recovery process. Additional steps are required when a patient needs home health care. The HUC should notify the patient's case manager or the social worker when an order for discharge with assistance is written. The case manager or social worker will most likely be aware of the discharge order if involved in planning the patient's care. A follow-up notification by the HUC is recommended. The hospital case manager or social service worker arranges home health care and home health equipment. The case manager may perform all the required tasks; HUC responsibilities will vary among facilities (Procedure 20-3).

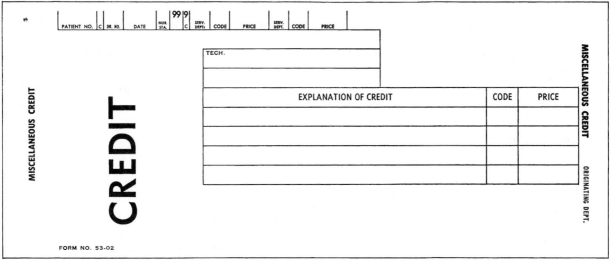

Figure 20-2 Credit requisition.

Admission/Discharge/Transfer Sheet

Nursing Unit _____   **Date** _____

Admissions   **Discharges**

103   Jackson, Henry   109   Pack, Fanny

110   Smith, Mary   102   Johnson, John

105   Packer, Penny

Transfers

101-1   Jones, Thomas to 303

Figure 20-3 Admission, discharge, and transfer log sheet.

Preparation of the Discharged Patient's Paper Chart for the Health Information Management Services Department

The following procedure would be used for all discharged patients' charts, including patients who have been transferred to another facility. Many hospitals have a discharge checklist to cover the steps of preparing the chart for the health information management services (HIMS) department.

- Check the summary or diagnosis-related group (DRG) worksheet for the doctor's summation and the patient's final diagnosis. It is important to have this information on patient discharge so that coding of DRGs may be placed on the chart by HIMS personnel.
- Check for the correct patient ID labels on chart forms.
- Shred all chart forms that have been labeled and have no documentation on them.
- Check for old records or split records, and send with the chart to HIMS.
- Arrange chart forms in discharge sequence according to hospital policy.
- Send the discharged patient's chart to HIMS, along with any old records of the patient (must be sent on the day of discharge).

DISCHARGE CHECKLIST

(To be completed and sent with chart to the Medical Records Department by end of shift on which the patient is discharged. Check Yes or No box.)

Date of Admission __12/4/XX__

Check List

HISTORY & PHYSICAL

Yes No

☒ ☐ 1. History and Physical on chart within 48 hours. Due _12/6/XX_
         (IF NO, ANSWER NUMBER TWO.)

☐ ☐ 2. History and Physical Notification Form # 00-0531 sent to Medical Records. Date sent _____

Health Unit Coordinator Signature _Iona Clerke_

Check List

FINAL DISPOSITION OF CHART

Yes No

☐ ☐ 1. All sheets labeled with correct patient master card and legible, and all reports are for this patient.

☐ ☐ 2. Portions of chart that have been removed are replaced in proper order, with chart dividers removed.

☐ ☐ 3. Reports are correctly inserted or attached.

        4. FRONT SHEET:

☐ ☐   a. Discharge diagnosis written on Front Sheet by Doctor. If No, answer 4b.

☐ ☐   b. Final diagnosis noted on Telephone Tentative or Final Discharge Diagnosis Form #00-0523 attached to chart and send to Health Information Systems Management with check list. If unable to complete, state reason on form.

☐ ☐ 5. Previous Medical Records returned to Health Information Systems Management Department.

☐ ☐ 6. Accordion folders used for sending records to Medical Record Department.

☐ ☐ 7. Discharge entered in Admission, Discharge, and Transfer Log.

Date of Discharge _____

Health Unit Coordinator Signature _____

☐ ☐ 8. Nurses notes are complete.

R.N. or L.P.N. Signature: _____

Figure 20-4 Discharge checklist.

The health unit coordinator should ask anyone entering the nursing station who is not known to him or her for identification. Visitors are not allowed in the nursing station, where computer screens or patent charts laying open may be in view. Insurance reviewers are required to show identification before having access to a patient's electronic or paper chart.

DISCHARGE AGAINST MEDICAL ADVICE

A patient may feel that the care being provided is not acceptable, or perhaps the patient believes that the care provided has not resulted in an improvement in their condition. Whatever the reason, the patient may decide to leave the hospital without the doctor's approval.

The patient may appear at the nurse's station and may announce, "I am not happy with the care I am receiving, and I'm going home now." The HUC should ask the patient to be seated until the nurse is advised. The hospitalist, resident, or admitting doctor may be called to speak with the patient. The patient may be advised that insurance probably will not cover

(Use Typewriter or Ballpoint Pen — Press Firmly)   *(See Instructions on back of Page 3)*

CONTINUING CARE TRANSFER INFORMATION

TO BE COMPLETED AND SIGNED BY NURSING SERVICE (Please attach a copy of the Nursing Care Plan)

PATIENT'S NAME Last First MI	DATE OF BIRTH	SEX	RELIGION	HEALTH INSURANCE CLAIM NUMBER

PATIENT'S ADDRESS (Street number, City, State and Zip Code)   ATTENDING PHYSICIAN   Name   Address

RELATIVE OR GUARDIAN   Name   Address   Phone Number

Name and Address of Facility Transferring FROM	Dates of Stay at Facility Transferring FROM		Facility Name and Address Transferring TO
	Admission	Discharge	

PAYMENT SOURCE FOR CHARGES TO PATIENT:

☐ Self or Family   ☐ Private Insurance ID Number _____   ☐ Blue Cross/Blue Shield ID Number _____   ☐ Employer or Union

☐ Public Agency _____   ☐ Other (specify) _____

PATIENT EVALUATION:

SPEECH:	HEARING:	SIGHT:	MENTAL STATUS:	FEEDING:
☐ Normal	☐ Normal	☐ Normal	☐ Always Alert	☐ Independent
☐ Impaired	☐ Impaired	☐ Impaired	☐ Occasionally Confused	☐ Help with Feeding
☐ Unable to speak	☐ Deaf	☐ Blind	☐ Always Confused	☐ Cannot Feed Self

DRESSING:	ELIMINATION:	BATHING:	AMBULATORY STATUS:
☐ Independent	☐ Independent	☐ Independent	☐ Independent
☐ Help with Dressing	☐ Help to Bathroom	☐ Bathing with Help	☐ Walks with Help
☐ Cannot Dress Self	☐ Bedpan or Urinal	☐ Bed Bath with Help	☐ Help from Bed to Chair
	☐ Incontinent	☐ Bed Bath	☐ Bed Bound

NURSING ASSESSMENT AND RECOMMENDATIONS:

TREATMENTS:

Last Medication: _____ /Dose: _____

Date: _____ Time: _____

APPLIANCES OR SUPPORTS: or check none ☐

Signature   Title   Date

TO BE COMPLETED AND SIGNED BY THE ATTENDING PHYSICIAN

ECF Admitting Diagnosis:

Please send a copy of the following records with patient:

☐ Summary Sheet (face sheet)
☐ Discharge Summary
☐ Physical Examination and History
☐ Consultation
☐ Other (specify) _____

Transfer by: ☐ Ambulance   ☐ Car   ☐ Other (specify) _____

Patient knows diagnosis: ☐ Yes   ☐ No

Surgical Procedures: (current admission)

Allergies: ☐ No   ☐ Yes (specify) _____

VDRL: ☐ Positive   ☐ Negative

Anticoagulant: ☐ Taking now   ☐ Previously

Orders: Diet, medication and special therapy   *(To be renewed in 48 hours)*

Chest X-Ray Diagnosis: _____

I will care for this patient after admission to new facility: ☐ Yes   ☐ No

Medication Regimen is stabilized: ☐ Yes   ☐ No

Anticipated length of stay for extended care _____ days

Physician's Signature   Date

If necessary, attach order sheet — The above constitutes valid temporary orders only if signed by a physician.

Address   Telephone Number

Figure 20-5 Continuing care transfer form.

PROCEDURE 20-2

ADDITIONAL STEPS REQUIRED TO DISCHARGE PATIENT TO ANOTHER FACILITY

TASK	NOTES
1. Notify case management or social service of the doctor's orders to discharge to another facility.	The case manager or social worker most likely was involved in planning for the discharge. • Follow up notification by the HUC is recommended.
2. Transportation usually will be arranged by the case manager or social worker.	The patient who is confined to bed or who has other special medical needs may require an ambulance.
3. Complete the continuing care or transfer form. (The case worker or social worker may complete the form.)	The continuing care form requires some information that the HUC may obtain from the face sheet. The nurse and the doctor must complete their sections of the form (see Fig. 20-5).
4. Print from the computer or photocopy patient chart forms as requested in the doctor's orders. Once the copies have been made, it is important to place the *original* paper chart forms back into the patient's chart in proper sequence.	Requirements for forms vary from facility to facility. The patient's doctor will write an order that indicates the specific forms to be printed from the computer or photocopied. Check hospital policy to determine who is responsible for printing or photocopying the requested chart forms (i.e., the HUC or HIMS).
5. Place continuing care form and requested chart form *copies* in a sealed envelope with the patient's identification label affixed on the outside of the envelope.	The envelope is given to the ambulance driver or a family member. This person delivers the envelope to the nurse at the nursing care facility. • When using paper chart, be certain copies are placed in envelope and originals are placed back in the chart.
6. Perform all routine steps as shown in Procedure 20-1.	

PROCEDURE 20-3

ADDITIONAL STEPS FOR DISCHARGE HOME WITH ASSISTANCE

TASK	NOTES
1. Notify case management or social service of the doctor's discharge to home with assistance order.	The responsible personnel will vary depending on patient type. The case manager or social worker will most likely be aware of discharge order if involved in planning patient's care. • Follow-up notification by HUC is recommended.
2. Prepare the continuing care form.	The HUC or the case manager will complete the personal information section.
3. Obtain a release of information signature from the patient.	This may be completed by the case manager or the patient's nurse. The HUC may prepare the release form.
4. Print from the computer or photocopy the chart forms as indicated in the doctor's order; replace *originals* in patient's chart.	This may be completed by the case manager or the HUC.
5. Place the continuing care form and *copies* of chart forms as required and give to appropriate family member.	This may be completed by the case manager or the HUC.
6. Perform all routine steps as shown in Procedure 20-1.	

the hospital bill if he/she leaves against medical advice. Everything possible is done to encourage the patient to remain in the hospital until treatment has been completed. However, if the patient does not pose a threat to self or others, he/she cannot be restrained from leaving, and usually the admitting doctor, resident, or hospitalist will write a discharge order to document that the patient is leaving against medical advice.

In the event that the patient is not convinced to stay, a release form (Fig. 20-6) is prepared by the HUC. This form is signed by the patient or his or her representative, and the signing is witnessed by an appropriate member of the hospital staff. The patient is then permitted to leave the hospital, and the discharge procedure is the same as for a routine discharge.

 HIGH PRIORITY

A patient may be restrained from leaving the hospital if two doctors certify that the patient poses a threat to self or others.

DISCHARGE OF THE DECEASED PATIENT

Patient Deaths

Not all patients who enter the hospital for care and treatment are discharged alive. Some patients who enter the hospital are

---

LEAVING HOSPITAL AGAINST ADVICE

Date_____

This is to certify that_____,
a patient in The Above Named Hospital, is leaving the hospital against the advice
of the attending physician and the hospital administration. I acknowledge that I
have been informed of the risk involved and hereby release the attending physician,
and the hospital, from all responsibility and any ill effects which may result from
this action.

_____
PATIENT

_____
OTHER PERSON RESPONSIBLE

_____
RELATIONSHIP

Witness_____

Witness_____

00-0434   **LEAVING HOSPITAL AGAINST ADVICE**

Figure 20-6 Form for discharge against medical advice.

well advanced in age. Other patients, in any age group, may have a **terminal illness** that results in expected death. Occasionally, death is unexpected, as in the case of complications from surgery, traumatic injuries, or sudden onset of a life-threatening condition, such as a heart attack. In other instances the patient's death is prolonged, and health care staff members have the opportunity to offer additional support to family members as time permits.

The HUC may be asked to call a member of the clergy from a specific religion to speak with the patient or to perform final rites. Most facilities have a list of representatives from various denominations and nondenominational groups who can assist patients and families. Many hospitals employ a chaplain to address the religious needs of patients. A notation should be made on the patient's Kardex form of any final rites that have been performed. It is important to remind clergy that a lighted candle may not be used when oxygen is in use in the patient's room.

Certification of Death

In cases in which a death is expected, the patient's nurse or family members may be with the patient at the time of **expiration** (death). At other times the patient may die unexpectedly. In either instance, the hospitalist, resident, or doctor must be notified to pronounce the patient dead and record the time of death. The patient is examined for any signs of life. If none can be detected, the patient is pronounced dead and the official time of death is recorded on the doctors' progress notes. The patient's doctor must complete a death certificate, and a report of the death must be filed with the Bureau of Vital Statistics.

Release of Remains

The patient's family or guardian must indicate the funeral home to which the body will be released. Usually the family must sign a form (see Evolve) before the patient can be released to the funeral home. The HUC would notify the funeral home of the expiration (when and if requested to do so). The HUC may also be asked to call the hospital morgue personnel to transport the deceased patient to the morgue. Most hospitals have a stretcher with a lower compartment that may be covered with a sheet to transport a deceased patient, making it unnecessary to close the doors to patient rooms on the unit when the patient is being transported to the morgue. Funeral home personnel may pick up the patient from the unit or the hospital morgue. A hospital security officer may have to accompany funeral home personnel.

Organ Donation

Many patients indicate their wishes for **organ donation** before the time of their death. The United Network for Organ Sharing operates an Organ Procurement and Transplantation Network. A 24-hour, 7-days-a-week computer system maintains the status of thousands of potential recipients, allowing for up-to-the-minute changes in patient status. In most cases, to be an organ donor the patient must be declared brain dead (referred to as **clinical death**) and be connected to a ventilator. Circumstances that can lead to brain death include head trauma injuries, anoxic injuries, cerebral bleeds such as strokes or aneurysms, and brain tumors. All of these events are injuries or insults to the brain that can cause swelling and ultimately cut off all blood flow to the brain, causing death. Brain death is declared by two physicians according to neurologic criteria approved by the American Medical Association. Most individuals who have died from cardiac arrest and have no cardiac or respiratory activity are potential donors for tissue but are unable to donate organs. However, there are some circumstances in which a patient can donate organs after cardiac death, termed *donation after cardiac death.*

A patient may designate specific organs (e.g., only cornea) or may indicate that any needed organs or tissues may be donated. Because of state laws, the nursing staff may be required to ask the family about organ donation. It will be necessary to check the hospital's policies regarding organ donation. Additional consent forms (see Evolve) are necessary for the harvesting of an organ (**organ procurement**). The HUC

would notify the morgue of the patient's death when and if requested to do so and would prepare all required forms for the patient's family to sign.

AUTOPSY OR POSTMORTEM EXAMINATION

An **autopsy,** or **postmortem** examination, of the body is performed to determine the cause of death or for medical research purposes (see Evolve). The family may ask that an autopsy be done, or the doctor may request it. Before an autopsy can be performed, however, the family must grant permission unless the death is declared a coroner's case. A consent for autopsy form must be signed by the next of kin.

Coroner's Cases

A **coroner's case** is one in which the patient's death is a result of sudden, violent, or unexplained circumstances, such as an accident, a poisoning, or a gunshot wound. Deaths that occur less than 24 hours after the start of hospitalization may also be called coroner's cases. State, county, and local governments have regulations that define a coroner's case in their particular localities. The law gives the **coroner** permission to study the body by dissection to determine whether evidence of foul play is present. A signed consent provided by the nearest of kin is not required when a death is ruled a coroner's case. See Procedure 20-4 for tasks related to the death of a patient that may be performed by the HUC.

TRANSFER OF A PATIENT

A variety of circumstances may necessitate a patient transfer. A patient's condition may change—it may improve, and the patient may be transferred out of intensive care, or it may deteriorate and an intensive care unit (ICU) stay may be required—or the patient may have to move to a specialty unit to receive a particular type of care (e.g., when an orthopedic patient develops cardiac problems). A patient may need a private room for infection control or isolation purposes. A patient may be transferred if a room he or she originally requested becomes available, for example, a private room. A patient may also be transferred because of roommate incompatibilities.

The duties performed in a series of tasks allow for an orderly transfer of the patient from one area to another. Transfer may occur from one unit of the hospital to another, or it may occur from one room to another on the same nursing unit. Tasks that may be performed for the transfer of a patient from one hospital unit to another are listed in Procedure 20-5. Tasks to be performed when a patient is transferred from one room to another on the same unit are listed in Procedure 20-6. Tasks to be performed when a transferred patient is received on a nursing unit are listed in Procedure 20-7.

DISCHARGE AND TRANSFER ORDERS

It is imperative that the HUC read the entire set of discharge or **transfer orders**. Additional orders included in a discharge or transfer order are often missed to be discovered after the patient has left the hospital. Discharge or transfer orders may include orders to be carried out before the time of a patient's discharge or information such as instructions for the patient to follow after leaving the hospital, requests for appointments for the patient, and so forth. In an effort to reduce patient

PROCEDURE 20-4

POSTMORTEM PROCEDURE

TASK	NOTES
1. a. Contact the attending doctor, hospitalist, or resident when asked by the nurse to do so, to verify the patient's death. b. The HUC will notify the attending or other doctors involved in patient's care when requested to do so.	When a patient expires during a code, the doctor presiding over the code will verify the patient's death. The resident or hospitalist may want to notify the attending physician in person. It is important to notify all doctors who were involved in the patient's care so they do not make a special trip to the hospital to see the patient.
2. Notify the hospital operator of the patient's death. 3. a. Prepare any forms that may be needed. b. Check the chart for a signed autopsy consent form.	These forms may consist of a release of remains or request for autopsy and/or consent for donation of body organs (see Evolve website). • A coroner's case does not require a signed consent— an autopsy will be required. Some hospitals use a postmortem checklist (Fig. 20-7) to ascertain whether all postmortem tasks have been completed.
4. Notify the mortuary that has been requested by the family.	If the family is not familiar with mortuaries in the area, a list of mortuaries is usually available from the hospital telephone switchboard operator. Nursing office personnel may notify the funeral home.
5. Check the chart or ask the patient's nurse to determine whether the body is to be taken to the morgue or is to remain there until the mortuary arrives. 6. The nurse or certified nursing assistant (CNA) will gather the clothes of the deceased and will place them in a patient belongings bag to be labeled with the patient's name, the room number, and the date. 7. Obtain the mortuary book from the nursing office, or have a mortuary form prepared when the mortician arrives.	Sometimes the family will request that the patient remain in the hospital room so that additional family members can see the deceased patient. The clothing is given to the family or to the mortician. A postmortem checklist is completed by the patient's nurse. The mortician who claims the body must also complete forms to show that he or she has claimed the body, the clothing, and/or any valuables (see Fig. 20-7).
8. Perform the routine discharge steps shown in Procedure 20-1.	

PROCEDURE 20-5

PROCEDURE FOR TRANSFER FROM ONE UNIT TO ANOTHER UNIT

TASK	NOTES
1. Transcribe the order for a transfer from one unit to another unit.	The transfer order may be indicated by an icon on the computer census screen next to the appropriate patient's name when the EMR is used or may be handwritten when paper charts are used.
2. a. Notify the nurse who is caring for the patient of the transfer order. b. Notify the admitting department of the transfer order to obtain a new room assignment. 3. a. Communicate new unit and room assignment to the nurse who is caring for the patient. b. Notify the receiving unit of the transfer by telephone or by computer. 4. Record the transfer on the unit admission, discharge, and transfer log sheet (ADT log sheet). 5. a. Send the patient's chart, Kardex form, and current medication administration record (MAR) with the patient to the receiving unit (if paper charts are used). b. Send all thinned records, old records (if paper charts are used), and x-ray films with the patient to the receiving unit.	An empty chart will be given by the receiving unit in exchange for the patient's chart (if paper charts are used).

Continued

PROCEDURE 20-5—cont'd

PROCEDURE FOR TRANSFER FROM ONE UNIT TO ANOTHER UNIT

TASK	NOTES
6. Erase the patient's name from the census board.	
7. a. Notify all departments that perform regularly scheduled treatments on the patient via computer.	
b. Notify the nutritional care department of the transfer via computer.	
8. Notify environmental services to clean the room.	Environmental services may be notified by telephone, by computer, or in person.
9. Notify the attending doctor and all other doctors involved with the patient's care	

PROCEDURE 20-6

PROCEDURE TO TRANSFER TO ANOTHER ROOM ON THE SAME UNIT

TASK	NOTES
1. Transcribe the order for the transfer to another room on the same unit.	The transfer order may be indicated by an icon on the computer census screen next to the appropriate patient's name when the EMR is used or handwritten when paper charts are used.
2. Notify the nurse who is caring for the patient of the request for transfer.	
3.	
a. Place the patient's chart in the correct slot in the chart rack after correcting the labels on the patient's chart and replacing patient ID labels with corrected labels (if paper charts are used).	
b. Place the Kardex form in its new place in the Kardex form file (if paper charts are used).	
4. Move the patient's name to the correct bed on the computer census screen. Send the change to the nutritional care department (if paper charts are used).	
5. Record the transfer on the unit admission, discharge, and transfer log sheet (ADT log sheet).	
6. Notify environmental services to clean the room (when EMR is used, the request will be sent to environmental services automatically).	Environmental services may be notified by telephone, by computer, or in person.
7. Notify the switchboard and the information center of the change (may not be necessary when EMR is used).	

readmissions as a result of noncompliance or lack of follow-up visits with physicians, some facilities require the HUC to schedule the follow-up appointments for the patient. The information is then entered into the computer and a copy is included in the discharge paperwork that the patient receives. Often a doctor will include other orders with a discharge order, such as the following: *discharge after a PA, LAT chest x-ray; disch, mother to have CPR training prior to disch; copy patient's last 3 days of labs and diagnostic studies and send with patient to Bryant's Rehab Center; discharge with Rx* (the prescription may be left in the patient's chart). In many EMR facilities, it is the HUC's responsibility to print a copy of related drug information in addition to the prescriptions that will be given to the patient on discharge.

If the doctor plans to transfer the patient to another room or another unit or to discharge the patient to home or to another facility, the doctor writes an order for such on the doctors' order sheet. In an EMR facility an icon will appear next to the patient's name on the computer to indicate that there are HUC tasks related to the patient's transfer or discharge.

The two primary reasons a doctor writes an order for a patient to be transferred are a change in status of acuity (for nursing care) or the need for an isolation room. The change in acuity for nursing care may be for more intensive nursing care (regular unit to ICU) or less intensive nursing care (ICU to regular unit). A transfer based on the need for isolation may include a requirement for airborne isolation in the case of a new diagnosis of tuberculosis, or a need for reverse isolation (to protect the patient) in the case of organ transplantation or the diagnosis of an immunosuppressive disease.

CHECK LIST
Post-Mortem Care

1) Telephone Notification
☐ Family
☐ ALL physicians involved in patient care
☐ Whether or not an autopsy is to be done
☐ Switch Board (name, room number, time, mortuary)
☐ Police in event of Coroner's Case (check to see if physician called)
☐ Mortuary if known - and if mortician is to come to the unit

2) Forms
Mortuary Form
When mortician comes to unit
☐ White copy to chart
☐ Yellow to mortician
☐ Pink to Business office with discharge requisition
☐ Patient Information Form remains on the unit
When patient goes to morgue
☐ Entire completed form goes with patient
☐ Patient Information Form attached to mortuary form
Autopsy
☐ Single copy remains on chart - send to Medical Records as soon as possible

3) Preparation of Body
When patient goes to Morgue
☐ Shroud and tag properly
☐ Mark on the shroud tag if patient is in isolation and causative organism, if known
☐ Complete #1 and 2
If a Coroner's Case
☐ Do not remove drains, IV's, etc., until police come. They may take the body with them.
☐ Notify mortuary of this
When patient goes to mortuary from the unit
☐ Do not shroud unless isolated
☐ Mark on tag causative organism

4) Transport Patient
☐ Patient elevator on E Wing 7:00 a.m. to 3:30 p.m., Mon. thru Fri.
☐ A, B, and C to 5th floor and cross to elevator #8 to 1st floor of S Building, S-4
☐ If body goes to refrigerator, mark 3 x 5 card on door
☐ Two people go with patient and their names are charted

5) Chart
☐ Complete all of Check List for Medical Records
☐ All of items noted in "Telephone Notification"
☐ Who takes body to morgue
☐ Name of mortuary
☐ Follow Discharge Procedure

6) Please refer to Procedure Book for clarification of any and all of the above points, especially in reference to Coroner's Case, fetal death and autopsy.

_____ R.N.
Signature

00-0585

Figure 20-7 Postmortem checklist.

PROCEDURE 20-7

PROCEDURE FOR RECEIVING A TRANSFERRED PATIENT

TASK	NOTES
1. Notify the nurse who is caring for the patient of the expected arrival of a transferred patient.	
2. a. Introduce yourself to the transferred patient upon his or her arrival to the unit.	
b. Notify the nurse who is caring for the patient of the transferred patient's arrival.	
3. a. Place the patient's chart in the correct slot in the chart holder, print corrected patient ID labels, and label the patient's chart (if paper charts are used).	Provide the empty chart to the unit from which the patient was transferred.
b. Place the Kardex form in the proper place (if paper charts are used).	
4. Record the receiving of a transfer patient on the unit admission, discharge, and transfer log sheet, and write the patient's name on the census board.	
5. Notify the nutritional care department of the patient's transfer.	
6. Move the patient's name from the unit the patient came from and place it in the correct bed on the computer census screen.	
7. Transcribe any new doctors' orders (if paper charts are used).	When the patient is transferred from an intensive care unit to a regular nursing unit or from a regular nursing unit to an intensive care unit, the doctor must write new orders. The previous orders are no longer valid.

Following are examples of how discharge or transfer orders may be expressed by the doctor on the doctors' order sheet.

Discharge

Home today
Discharge chest x-ray
Home Rx
Home, make appt to see me in 1 wk
Home crutches
Disch mother after car seat obtained
Arrange for CPR training for parents before the time of discharge

Transfer

Transfer patient to 3E please
Transfer patient to telemetry unit
Transfer patient to ICU after surgery
Transfer patient out of ICU to a medical unit
Transfer patient to airborne isolation room
Transfer patient to Rehab Center

⭐ **HIGH PRIORITY**

It is important to read a discharge order carefully before a patient leaves the unit. The doctor may write "discharge after chest x-ray" or other directions and/or may leave a prescription on the chart that must be given to the patient.

Changes in HUC Responsibilities with the Use of the Electronic Medical Record with Computer Physician Order Entry

The discharge, transfer, and postmortem procedures differ with the implementation of EMR with computer physician order entry (CPOE). Many of the tasks involving paper charts are eliminated, but the ADT documentation and the label book are used when EMR and paper charts are used. It may not be necessary to notify in-house departments of discharges and transfers when the EMR is implemented. Additional tasks include monitoring the patients' EMRs, printing forms from the computer, and scanning consents, handwritten progress notes, and other records or reports into the patient's EMR.

KEY CONCEPTS

The HUC's tasks for discharge and transfer procedures are many when the paper chart is used. Some tasks remain the same, and additional tasks may be required when the EMR is used. If the HUC memorizes these procedures in a particular order and does not deviate from the learned sequence, the tasks will always be performed thoroughly and completely.

Websites of Interest

Medical documentation standards: www.ehow.com/facts_6896 499_medical-documentation-standards.html.
Autopsy WebMD information and resources: www.webmd.com/a-to-z-guides/autopsy-16080.

Organ transplant information and facts: www.webmd.com/a-to-z-guides/organ-transplant-overview

⊖ REVIEW QUESTIONS

1. Define the following terms:
   a. autopsy
   b. clinical death
   c. terminal illness
   d. expiration
   e. postmortem
   f. custodial care
   g. organ procurement
   h. organ donation
   i. release of remains
   j. coroner's case
   k. extended care facility
   l. patient care conference
   m. discharge planning

2. Discuss the purpose of patient discharge planning and patient care conferences, and identify the personnel and individuals who would be involved in both.

3. List five types of discharges, and explain the importance of communicating pending discharge information and bed availability to the admitting department or bed placement in a timely manner.

4. List 12 tasks that are performed during a routine discharge of a patient from the hospital when paper charts are used.

5. List six additional tasks that may be required when a patient is discharged to another facility and six additional tasks when a patient is discharged home with assistance when paper chart are used.

6. Describe six HUC tasks involved in the preparation of the discharged patient's paper chart for HIMS.

7. What action should the HUC take if a patient approaches the nursing station desk and states, "I'm very upset with the care I'm receiving, and I'm leaving the hospital now!"

8. Explain the HUC tasks that may be required and/or requested when a patient expires, and discuss the need for the patient's death to be verified and the time documented by a doctor or resident.

9. Discuss how the deceased patient is transferred to the morgue, and explain the possible HUC tasks related to the release of remains and organ donation.

10. Explain the usual circumstances regarding a patient's death that must be met to be accepted as an organ donor.

11. Explain why an autopsy would be performed and list the circumstances that would define a "coroner's case."

12. List eight tasks performed on the death (postmortem) of a patient.

13. List the two primary reasons a doctor would write an order for a patient to be transferred to another room or nursing unit.

14. List nine tasks that are performed in the transfer of a patient from one unit to another unit.

15. Describe seven duties performed in the transfer of a patient from one room to another room on the same unit.

16. List seven tasks that are performed when a transferred patient is received on the unit.

17. Discuss the importance of reading the entire set of discharge or transfer orders before the patient is discharged or transferred.

18. Describe an additional HUC task that may be required for a routine discharge procedure when the EMR with CPOE is used.

SURFING FOR ANSWERS

1. Locate two websites that discuss patient discharge guidelines; document five guidelines and the websites used.
2. Research medical and legal problems that occur when patients leave the hospital AMA.
3. Perform a search for coroner duties and responsibilities; list at least five, and document two websites used.

CHAPTER 21

Reports, Infection Control, Emergencies, and Special Services

CHAPTER OBJECTIVES

On completion of this chapter, you will be able to:

1. Define the terms in the vocabulary list.
2. Write the meaning of the abbreviations in the abbreviations list.
3. Identify four categories of incidents that would initiate an incident report, and explain the purpose of completing an incident report.
4. Identify six components that constitute the chain of infection, and list four types of personal protective equipment used as barriers between the practitioner (health care worker) and the patient's body fluids.
5. List four examples of diagnosed infections that would require a patient to be placed in airborne isolation.
6. Identify the most common way to confirm and identify microorganisms and to determine which antibiotic will destroy the identified microbes.
7. Identify three circumstances that would cause a patient to become immunocompromised and in need of being placed in reverse or protective isolation.
8. Discuss ways in which an individual working in the hospital environment can reduce his or her risk of infection.
9. Discuss four primary ways that the human immunodeficiency virus (HIV) may be transmitted from one person to another, and identify two opportunistic diseases related to acquired immunodeficiency syndrome (AIDS).
10. Identify a highly contagious virus transmitted through blood and body fluids and an airborne pathogen that would require health care providers to take extra precautions such as blood and fluid precautions and to use special personal protective equipment (PPE).
11. Discuss the pathogenic microorganisms that are frequently responsible for nosocomial infections and the best way for health care providers to stop the spread of these hospital-acquired infections.
12. Discuss health unit coordinator (HUC) tasks related to prevention of infection in the hospital work environment.
13. Identify the meaning for each of the following color emergency call codes: red, blue, orange, pink, gray, and silver.
14. Identify the communication tool that provides details on chemical dangers and safety procedures.

15. Explain the RACE system, and describe what the responsibilities of the HUC would be during a fire code and a disaster procedure.
16. List six guidelines that should be followed for electrical safety.
17. Identify events that would activate the hospital disaster procedure.
18. List nine tasks that the HUC may perform in a medical emergency.
19. Describe how to handle flowers and mail delivered to the unit.

VOCABULARY

Airborne Precautions (Isolation) Transmission-based precautions; require use of a mask and a private room with monitored negative air pressure and high-efficiency filtration, in conjunction with standard precautions.

Cardiac Arrest State in which the patient's heart contractions are absent or insufficient to produce a pulse or blood pressure (may also be referred to as *code arrest*).

Centers for Disease Control and Prevention (CDC) Division of the U. S. Public Health Service that investigates and controls diseases that have epidemic potential.

Chemical Code A term used when medical intervention only (such as medication) will be used in a cardiac or respiratory arrest.

Code Blue (Code Arrests) A term used in hospitals to summon additional help for a patient who has stopped breathing and/or whose heart has stopped beating (cardiac arrest).

Code or Crash Cart A cart stocked by the nursing and pharmacy staff with emergency medication, advanced breathing supplies, intravenous solutions and appropriate tubing, needles, a heart monitor and defibrillator, an oxygen tank, and a suction machine; used in emergency situations.

Communicable Diseases Diseases that may be transmitted from one person to another.

Disaster Procedure A planned procedure that is carried out by hospital personnel when a large number of people may have been injured or exposed to hazardous materials.

Epidemiologist Physician who coordinates with health officials with regard to reporting and monitoring incidents of infectious diseases that may lead to epidemic outbreaks. *Epidemiology* is the branch of medicine that deals with the study of the causes, distribution, and control of disease in populations.

Hepatitis B Virus An infectious blood-borne disease that is a major occupational hazard for health care workers.

Hepatitis C Virus A hepatitis infection that is blood-borne and that may also be an occupational hazard for health care workers.

Human Immunodeficiency Virus (HIV) The virus that causes acquired immunodeficiency syndrome.

Incident An episode that does not normally occur within the regular hospital routine and may involve patients, visitors, physicians, hospital staff, or students.

Isolation The placement of a patient apart from other patients for the purpose of preventing the spread of infection, or protecting a patient whose immune system is compromised.

Material Safety Data Sheet (MSDS) A basic hazard communication tool that gives details on chemical dangers and safety procedures.

Medical Emergencies Emergencies that are life-threatening.

Methicillin-Resistant Staphylococcus aureus (MRSA) A variation of the common bacterial species *Staphylococcus aureus*. It has evolved the ability to survive treatment with β-lactam antibiotics, including penicillin and methicillin.

Nosocomial Infections Infections that are acquired from within the health care facility.

Occupational Safety and Health Administration (OSHA) A U.S. governmental regulatory agency that is concerned with the health and safety of workers.

Pathogenic Microorganisms Disease-carrying organisms too small to be seen with the naked eye.

Respiratory Arrest Condition that is present when the patient ceases to breathe or when respirations are so depressed that the blood cannot receive sufficient oxygen and therefore the body cells die (also may be referred to as *code arrest*).

Reverse or Protective Isolation A precautionary measure taken to prevent a patient with low resistance to disease from becoming infected.

Risk Management A department in the hospital that addresses the prevention and containment of liability regarding patient care incidents.

Standard Precautions The creation of a barrier between the health care worker and the patient's blood and body fluids (also may be called *universal precautions*).

Tuberculosis A disease caused by *Mycobacterium tuberculosis*, an airborne pathogen.

ABBREVIATIONS

Abbreviation	Meaning
AIDS	acquired immunodeficiency syndrome
ARC	AIDS-related complex
CDC	Centers for Disease Control and Prevention
HBV	hepatitis B virus
HCV	hepatitis C virus
HIV	human immunodeficiency virus
MRSA	methicillin-resistant *Staphylococcus aureus*
OSHA	Occupational Safety and Health Administration
PPE	personal protective equipment
RACE	rescue individuals in danger. alarm: Sound the alarm. confine the fire by closing all doors and windows. extinguish the fire with the nearest suitable fire extinguisher.
TB	tuberculosis

EXERCISE 1

Write the meaning of each abbreviation listed.

1. OSHA	7. AIDS
2. MRSA	8. HCV
3. ARC	9. TB
4. CDC	10. HIV
5. PPE	11. HBV
6. RACE	

EXERCISE 2

Write the correct abbreviation for each term listed.

1. Occupational Safety and Health Administration
2. methicillin-resistant *Staphylococcus aureus*
3. AIDS-related complex
4. Centers for Disease Control and Prevention
5. personal protective equipment
6. *Rescue* individuals in danger, *Alarm*—Sound the alarm, *Confine* the fire by closing all doors and windows, *Extinguish* the fire with the nearest suitable fire extinguisher
7. acquired immunodeficiency syndrome
8. hepatitis C virus
9. tuberculosis
10. human immunodeficiency virus
11. hepatitis B virus

INCIDENT REPORTS

An **incident** is an event that does not normally occur within the regular health care facility routine and may involve patients, visitors, physicians, hospital staff, or students. The incident may be the result of an accident, such as a patient's falling while on the way to the bathroom, or it may involve a situation such as spilled liquids in a hospital corridor that cause someone to slip and sustain an injury. Events other than accidents that occur within the hospital or on hospital property are also reportable.

Incidents that require written reports include the following:

- Accidents
- Thefts from persons on hospital property
- Errors of omission of patient treatment or errors in administration of patient treatment, including medication
- Exposure to blood and body fluids, as may be caused by a needle stick

When an incident or event occurs, the health unit coordinator (HUC) prepares an incident report form for the person who is reporting the incident or event. Many facilities use computer programs by which incident or event reports are generated electronically.

An incident report form (Fig. 21-1) should be completed for all incidents that occur to anyone, no matter how insignificant they may seem. Documentation of all incidents is important in identifying hazards and preventing continuing problems, and in the case of a lawsuit that may arise from them. The names and home addresses of witnesses are required in case the incident should result in a lawsuit and the witnesses are no longer employed at the hospital when the case is brought to court.

The attending doctor, hospitalist, or resident may be called to examine the patient involved in an incident. All incidents involving patients are reported to the attending doctor. Copies of the incident report are sent to the nurse manager, to risk management, and to quality assurance. If the incident involves another department, a copy is sent to the manager of that department. The incident report never becomes a part of the patient's permanent record.

Employee hospital incidents must be documented and the employee seen by the employee health nurse or evaluated by a doctor to be eligible for coverage by the state Workers' Compensation Commission. Hospital employees who fail to put into writing something that may appear trivial, such as a finger puncture with a needle, have no evidence to present should an infection develop after the injury. Exposure to blood and body fluids as may be caused by a needle stick may require the employee to be tested for human immunodeficiency virus (HIV) if the patient who is involved has not been tested.

Risk management personnel may interview witnesses to a patient incident in preparation for a lawsuit. Risk management staff also study patient incidents to look for trends and to prevent future similar incidents.

★ HIGH PRIORITY

Patient incident reports are not a part of the patient's permanent record.

The HUC is responsible for maintaining a supply of incident report forms for the nursing unit.

INFECTION CONTROL

For statistical purposes, records of infectious diseases must be maintained. A report should be submitted to the infectious disease department or to personnel in the hospital (Fig. 21-2). Most hospitals employ an **epidemiologist** or an infection control officer who maintains all infection records and investigates all hospital-acquired infections. Infection control is essential for providing a safe environment for patients and health care workers. Patients are at risk for acquiring infection because of lowered resistance to infectious microorganisms and increased exposure to numbers and types of disease-causing microorganisms, and because they must often undergo invasive procedures. The presence of a pathogen does not mean that an infection will begin. Development of an infection depends on six components called the *chain of infection*, as follows (Fig. 21-3):

1. Infectious agent or pathogen (bacteria)
2. Reservoir or source in which pathogen can live and grow (e.g., human body, contaminated water or food, animals, insects)
3. Means of escape (e.g., blood, urine, feces, wound drainage)
4. Route of transmission (air, contact, and body excretions)
5. Point of entrance (mouth, nostrils, and breaks in the skin)
6. Susceptible host (individual who does not have adequate resistance to the invading pathogen)

Confidential Information
INCIDENT REPORT
(Patient or Visitor)
Not a Part of Patient's Permanent Chart

1. Date of Admission

2. Diagnosis

3. Date of Incident _____ Time _____ M | Room No., Name, Age, Sex, Hospital Number, Attending Physician

4. Were Bed Rails up? _____ | 5. Hi Lo Bed Position
   (YES OR NO) _____ | (UP OR DOWN)

6. Were a Safety Belt or Restraints in use? _____
   DESIGNATE SPECIFICALLY

7. Activity (Complete Bed Rest, Bathroom Privileges, Etc.)

8. Sedatives _____ Dose _____ Time _____ M
9. Narcotics _____ Dose _____ Time _____ M   Given within 12 hours previous to incident
10. Tranquilizers _____ Dose _____ Time _____ M

11. Nurse's Account of Incident (State incident, where discovered, condition of patient, etc.)

12. History of Incident as related by Patient

13. List Witnesses or Persons Familiar with Details of Incident (Include roommate's name and hospital number.)
    Name _____ Address _____
    Name _____ Address _____
    Name _____ Address _____

14. Time Doctor was called _____ AM _____ PM | 15. Time Doctor Responded _____ AM _____ PM

16. Time Supervisor called _____ AM _____ PM

17. Date of Report _____

18. _____
    SIGNATURE OF PERSON REPORTING
19. _____
    SIGNATURE OF DEPARTMENT SUPERVISOR
20. _____
    SIGNATURE OF DEPARTMENT HEAD

A

Complete **IMMEDIATELY** for **EVERY** incident and send to Administrator via Department Head.

Figure 21-1 An incident report **A,** General information.

If infection is to be prevented, the chain must be broken. By following infection prevention and control techniques, health care workers can prevent the spread of microorganisms to patients and can also protect themselves. Infections can be prevented or controlled through hand hygiene, disinfection or sterilization, and the use of barriers. Proper hand hygiene is the most important method of prevention because the hands of health care workers are the primary site through which disease is transmitted from patient to patient. The **Centers for Disease Control and Prevention (CDC)** recommends a ban on artificial fingernails for health care professionals when they are caring for patients at high risk for infection.

PHYSICIAN'S STATEMENT

21. State injuries or other result, if any, from this incident _____
_____
_____

22. How, if at all, did the results of this incident affect the patient's original condition?_____
_____
_____

23. What treatment was given?_____
_____

24. Were X-rays or other tests ordered (specify)_____
_____
_____

25. Results of X-ray or other tests_____
_____
_____

26. Patient Examined: Date _____ Hour_____AM _____PM

27. Signed_____ M.D. (House Physician)

28. Signed_____ M.D. (Attending Physician)

B

Figure 21-1, cont'd B, Doctor's statement.

⭐ **HIGH PRIORITY**

Hand hygiene is the most important intervention in preventing infection because health care workers' hands are the primary means by which disease is transmitted from patient to patient. Most hospitals have a policy that bans artificial fingernails for all health care professionals.

Standard Precautions

In 1987 the CDC developed and presented a concept to protect health care workers from blood-borne pathogens such as HIV, hepatitis B virus (HBV), and hepatitis C virus. At that time a quiet panic arose among health care workers. They were not sure of how HIV was spread or how they could protect themselves. The CDC called this new concept "universal precautions" (for blood and body fluids). Nationwide, hospitals and other health care facilities accepted and taught this new concept to their employees. "Universal precautions" are now usually referred to as "standard precautions."

Standard precautions involve the creation of a barrier between the practitioner (health care worker) and the patient's body fluids. Standard precautions are used with all patients in health care settings, under the assumption that all body excretions and secretions are potentially infectious. Standard precautions now apply to nonintact skin, mucous membranes, and body fluids including blood, semen, vaginal secretions, peritoneal fluid, pleural fluid, pericardial fluid, synovial fluid, cerebrospinal fluid (CSF), amniotic fluid, urine, feces, sputum, saliva, wound drainage, and vomitus.

The barrier in standard precautions is created by the wearing of personal protective equipment (PPE), consisting of such items as gloves, gown, mask, goggles or glasses, pocket masks with one-way valves, and moisture-resistant gowns (Fig. 21-4 shows a nurse with PPE). *Every health care employee should practice standard precautions as required with every single patient.*

Airborne Precautions (Isolation)

Airborne precautions (isolation) are *transmission-based precautions* used for patients in whom infections such as tuberculosis (TB) are transmitted through the air. Airborne precautions reduce the risk that droplet nuclei or contaminated dust particles may travel over short distances (less than 3 feet) and land in the nose or mouth of a susceptible person. The patient is placed in a private room with monitored negative air pressure

---

Report # _____

REPORT OF INFECTION

COMPLETE ALL BLANKS IN TOP SECTION   UNIT

1. Diagnosis is: _____
_____
_____

2. Date of admission: _____

3. Evidence of Infection on admission?
     Yes ☐   No ☐

4. Date of last previous admission here:
_____

5. Hospitalized at another hospital?
     Yes ☐   No ☐
If yes, name hospital?
_____

     Date: _____

6. Date of surgery/delivery _____

7. Procedure done: _____
_____

8. Culture sent?   Yes ☐   No ☐
     (If yes, what was cultured?)
_____ Blood
_____ Urine
_____ Sputum
_____ Drainage from _____
_____ Other(specify) _____

9. *Fever?   Yes ☐   No ☐
NOTE: *Fever = temp. greater than
100.4°F (38°C) Oral
101°F (38.4°C) Rectal

10. Pt. Isolated?   Yes ☐   No ☐
If yes, enter date next to type initiated
_____ a. Limited
_____ b. Respiratory
_____ c. Wound & Skin
_____ d. Enteric
_____ e. Strict
_____ f. Protective

11. Date of Discharge: _____

CHECK <u>ALL</u> <u>THAT</u> APPLY:

DIARRHEA:
_____ Over 3 stools/24 hrs. for more than 2 days s̄ laxatives, enemas, x-rays preps, cardiac drugs or antibiotics

PHLEBITIS: Location _____

     Non-Suppurative:
_____ Mechanical Intracath
_____ Drug
_____ Possible focal site of infection
_____ Observed by Nurse
_____ Diagnosis by Physician

     Suppurative:
_____ Purulent drainage

POST PARTUM:
_____ *Fever(exclude 1st PP day)
_____ Purulent vaginal discharge
_____ Diagnosis by Physician

POST-OP:
_____ Continuous *Fever for 2 consecutive days
_____ Abscess(usually documented at time of surgery)

RESPIRATORY TRACT:
Upper
_____ Coryza(profuse nasal drainage)
_____ Pharyngitis
_____ Diagnosis by Physician

Lower:
_____ Sudden on set of cough
_____ Purulent sputum
_____ Suppuration of trachea
_____ X-ray Dx - Pneumonia
_____ Diagnosis by Physician

SKIN:
_____ Abscess
_____ Boil
_____ Cellulitis
_____ Purulent decubiti
_____ Suppuration

BLOOD:
_____ HAA Pos.
_____ HAA Neg.
_____ Positive Culture

URINARY TRACT:
Asymptomatic:
_____ No clinical symptoms
_____ Positive bacteriology X 100,000/ml
_____ Positive bacteriology X 10,000/ml c̄ previous urine culture negative
_____ Pyuria X 10 WBC

Symptomatic:
_____ Frequency
_____ Burning
_____ Urgency
_____ CVT(costo-vertebral tenderness)

WOUND:
_____ Abscess(usually documented at surgery time)
_____ Continuous *Fever for 2 consecutive days
_____ Stitch abscess
_____ Suppuration of wound
_____ Diagnosis by Physican
_____ Other _____

Report completed by: _____   Date: _____

COMMENTS: _____
_____
_____

(DO NOT WRITE IN THIS SECTION. FOR USE BY INFECTION CONTROL OFFICER ONLY)

Figure 21-2 Infection report.

---

and high-efficiency filtration. The room usually has a door, an entryway or ante-room with a sink, and another door, with both doors remaining closed. Individuals who enter the room are required to wear masks, gloves, and gowns. Hand washing is also required. Linen and trash are bagged to prevent contamination.

Examples of patients who would be placed in airborne isolation are those diagnosed with infections such as active TB, measles, chickenpox, or meningitis. A culture is the primary method used to confirm and identify microorganisms; sensitivity testing determines which antibiotics will destroy the identified microbes. See Chapter 14 for more information regarding

cultures and sensitivities, as well as serological tests (such as polymerase chain reaction) used to identify pathogens and patient's immunological response to exposure or infection.

Reverse or Protective Isolation

Reverse isolation or *protective isolation* is used to protect patients with decreased immune system function by reducing their risks of exposure to potentially infectious organisms. Reverse isolation is also known as *immunocompromised isolation*. Patients who are immunocompromised include organ transplant recipients, burn victims, and those receiving chemotherapy.

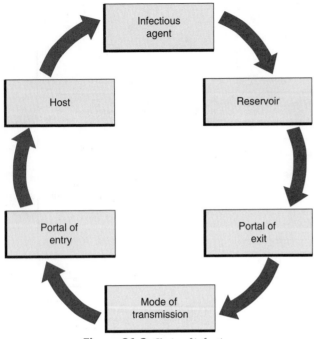

Figure 21-3 Chain of infection.

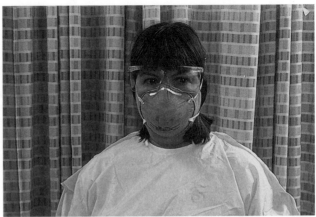

Figure 21-4 A nurse wearing a fitted tuberculosis (TB) mask, gown, and goggles. Gloves also would be worn (personal protective equipment [PPE]). (From Potter PA, Perry AG: *Fundamentals of nursing*, ed 6, St Louis, 2005, Mosby.)

⭐ **HIGH PRIORITY**

Hand washing is the most important precaution against infection and may be more effective against some pathogens than alcohol-based wipes or gels. Hands should be washed when one arrives at work, before and after personal breaks, and after any patient specimen is handled (even if bagged). Use soap, and scrub between the fingers. Rinse each hand thoroughly with running water from the wrists down to the fingertips. Dry with a clean paper towel, and use the towel to turn off the faucet. Microorganisms also can be transmitted through the handling of objects in the nursing station. Clean the telephone receiver with an antiseptic wipe on arrival and periodically throughout the day. Use antiseptic solution frequently throughout the day. Avoid putting your hands on your face, in your eyes, or in your mouth while on the nursing station.

DISEASES TRANSMITTABLE THROUGH CONTACT WITH BLOOD AND BODY FLUIDS

HIV/AIDS

AIDS stands for *acquired immunodeficiency syndrome*. AIDS is caused by a virus called **human immunodeficiency virus (HIV)**. This virus attacks the immune system and thereby reduces the body's ability to defend itself against infection and disease. Persons who have AIDS become susceptible to many opportunistic infections that are not usually a threat to persons with a normally functioning immune system. These infections are called *opportunistic* because the organisms take advantage of the patient's weakened immune system. As the immune system becomes weaker, these opportunistic illnesses may overwhelm the patient with AIDS and cause death.

HIV is transmitted by blood, vaginal fluids, and semen and is not spread through casual contact; it is spread in four primary ways. The first is by sexual contact. The second is by the use of needles that were previously injected into someone who carried the virus. The third is from an infected mother to her infant during pregnancy, birth, or breast feeding. The fourth is by transmission of the virus through blood transfusions; this mode is especially common if the patient received the transfusion before blood was routinely tested for the virus (before the late 1980s). Surgical patients, hemophiliac patients, and mothers who received transfusions during or after birth have contracted the HIV virus in this way. HIV also may be transmitted through the blood of an infected person that enters another person's bloodstream through a cut, an open sore, or blood that is splashed into the mouth or the eye. Appropriate PPE must be worn when one is coming into contact with body fluids from all patients.

An HIV carrier is a person who carries the virus in the blood but who may stay healthy for a long time. Some may never get sick. The only indication of HIV infection in the carrier may be a positive blood test for antibodies to the virus or a positive result of a test for the virus (antigen) itself. Once infected with the HIV virus, a person remains infected for life.

Months or years after initial infection, some people who carry the virus develop symptoms that may include tiredness, fevers, night sweats, swollen lymph glands, or mental deterioration resembling Alzheimer disease. Often the symptoms are recurrent and disable the person. This person is said to have AIDS-related complex (ARC).

AIDS is the most severe form of the infection. A full-blown case may not appear until months or years after the initial infection. ARC symptoms may or may not have appeared. The two most frequent opportunistic illnesses that may overtake the AIDS patient are (1) *Pneumocystis jiroveci* pneumonia (PCP) (pneumonia caused by *P. jiroveci*); and (2) Kaposi sarcoma (KS), an otherwise rare skin cancer.

Hepatitis B, C Virus

Hepatitis B is an inflammation of the liver that is caused by the **hepatitis B virus (HBV).** It was formerly called *serum hepatitis.* Similar to HIV, hepatitis B is spread by body fluids, but it is even more contagious than HIV. Health care providers are at risk for exposure. Standard blood and body fluid precautions must be practiced. **Hepatitis C virus** is also a blood-borne pathogen for which there is currently no immunization and was previously called *non-A, non-B hepatitis.*

The **Occupational and Safety and Health Administration (OSHA)** mandates that employers provide hepatitis B vaccine for all employees who have an occupational exposure risk. The vaccines are given in three doses over a 6-month period. An employee has the right to refuse the hepatitis B vaccine but must sign a form that states this refusal. There is no vaccine currently available for hepatitis C.

Tuberculosis

Tuberculosis is caused by *Mycobacterium tuberculosis,* an airborne pathogen. Working with patients who have TB requires the use of special PPE, such as special masks fitted to the individual health care worker, so that one can avoid inhaling the tiny droplets that carry the virus through the air. TB has increased in the United States, and some viruses have become resistant to drug therapy—for example, extensively drug-resistant tuberculosis (XDR-TB), for which there are few antibiotic treatments available.

Nosocomial Infections

Nosocomial infections are infections acquired from within the health care facility that often are transmitted to the patient by health care workers. Several genera of **pathogenic microorganisms** that are frequently responsible for hospital-acquired infections include *Streptococcus, Staphylococcus, Clostridium, Enterococcus,* and *Pseudomonas.* **Methicillin-resistant *Staphylococcus aureus* (MRSA)** is a variation of the common bacterial species *S. aureus.* It has evolved the ability to survive treatment with β-lactam antibiotics, including penicillin and methicillin. Patients with open wounds and weakened immune systems are at greater risk of infection than the general public. Excellent hand-washing technique is the best way for health care workers to stop the spread of nosocomial infection. Additional resistant pathogens are discussed in the chapter on laboratory orders (see Chapter 14).

HEALTH UNIT COORDINATOR TASKS PERFORMED TO CONTROL INFECTION

The HUC tasks for infection control and **isolation** vary from institution to institution. It is necessary in any health care facility for the HUC to have a basic understanding of infection control policies and standard precautions. *Accurate* information must be given to inquiring visitors. If the HUC is unable to answer a question or is unsure of what to say, a nurse should be asked to speak with the visitor. All infectious or **communicable diseases** on the unit must be reported to infection control. Nurses will ask the HUC to order PPE and isolation packs as needed. The HUC should wear gloves when handling or transporting specimens and should practice good hand-washing technique throughout the working day. Eating, drinking (open cups), and handling of contact lenses should not be done at the nursing station. Food should not be stored in refrigerators with specimens. The HUC transcribes laboratory orders that pertain to infection control. Following is a list of doctors' orders and the division of the laboratory to which they are sent.

Cerebrospinal fluid (CSF) for the following:
Cell count—hematology
Protein and glucose—chemistry
Lactate dehydrogenase (LDH)—chemistry
Potassium hydroxide (KOH) smear and/or Gram stain—microbiology
Culture and sensitivity (C&S), fungal culture, acid-fast bacilli (AFB), and tuberculosis (TB)—microbiology
Lyme titer, syphilis serology—serology
(Possible) C-reactive protein, lactic acid, chloride—chemistry

Another area of institutional policy about which the HUC must be fully aware involves disclosure of information, such as in cases of AIDS. Laws regarding AIDS and confidentiality vary from state to state, as do laws regarding disclosure of HIV-positive persons. When in doubt, *do not disclose information.* In many health care facilities, guidelines have been established to assist the health care worker. Examples of some of these guidelines include the following:

One does not put "diagnosis of AIDS" or "rule out AIDS" on the computer; the primary diagnosis is the infection, symptoms, or cancer. AIDS or HIV infection becomes the secondary diagnosis and appears on the medical record but not in the computer.

Family, friends, and other persons may not know about the AIDS diagnosis and must not be told by any health care employee unless so advised by the doctor. Confidentiality and knowledge of the health care facility's policies and guidelines are essential if the HUC is to complete tasks and offer high-quality patient care in the area of infection control.

EMERGENCIES

Emergency Call Codes

An issue recently identified as a potential problem is the fact that there is no standardized national list of emergency call codes. Each hospital has developed its unique list of codes that every employee must memorize and use. Because many physicians are on staff at several hospitals with different call codes, the need for a common list of codes has become apparent. The American Hospital Association has made recommendations for a standard list of emergency call codes, but it has been up to state hospital associations and participating individual hospitals in those states to identify and implement a standard set of emergency codes. A review of the current but evolving list reveals that the most commonly used codes include the following:

- Code Blue (cardiac or respiratory arrest)
- Code Red (fire)
- Code Orange (hazardous material spill)

- Code Pink or Amber Alert (infant or child abduction)
- Code Gray (combative person)
- Code Silver (person with a weapon or hostage situation)

Additional codes may include External Triage (external disaster), Internal Triage (internal emergency), Rapid Response Team (rapid response team), Tornado Watch or Tornado Warning, and Code Name Clear (to clear a code when ended).

It is of the utmost importance that the HUC become familiar with the emergency codes used at a facility because the HUC is usually the primary communicator in calling the emergency codes and directing emergency personnel who respond on the unit. There is usually a specific telephone extension used to quickly reach the hospital operator in calling an emergency. It is becoming more common to outline all emergency procedures on the hospital website rather than in a printed policy and procedures manual.

Chemical Safety

During orientation all employees will receive chemical safety training regarding OSHA requirements for hazardous chemicals. Chemicals must be labeled with a statement of warning and a statement of what the hazard is, to eliminate risk and facilitate first aid measures undertaken in the event of a spill or exposure. A **material safety data sheet (MSDS)** is a communication tool that provides details on chemical dangers and safety procedures. Chemicals should not be stored above eye level or in unlabeled containers. Never add water to acid or mix chemicals indiscriminately. Never use chemicals in ways other than intended. Appropriate PPE should be worn when chemicals are used. Spill kits must be available and must comply with OSHA guidelines. It is unlikely that a HUC will be handling chemicals, but it is important to be informed so you will know what to do in case of a spill or an employee incident involving chemicals. Again, many hospitals use "Code Orange" to denote a hazardous material spill.

Fire and Electrical Safety

Fire and electrical safety is also a part of employee orientation. The term *fire* is not used because it may trigger responses that could be fatal to a patient or could create panic among patients. In some hospitals a code number such as Code 1000 may be called, but more often a "Code Red" is announced by the hospital telephone operator to alert all hospital personnel when a fire or fire drill is taking place. It is essential that all employees be aware of the location of fire extinguishers. The HUC may be expected to assist with the evacuation of patients who are endangered by the fire. If the fire is not on the unit, the HUC may help nursing personnel to close the doors to patient rooms. All hospital units or sections of the hospital are separated by fire doors. These doors are constructed to help contain the fire in one area. They also must be closed during a fire. Most hospitals teach the RACE system because it is easy to remember:

R	Rescue individuals in danger.
A	Alarm: Sound the alarm.
C	Confine the fire by closing all doors and windows.
E	Extinguish the fire with the nearest suitable fire extinguisher.

Classes of Fire

Class A: wood, paper, clothing
Class B: flammable liquids and vapors
Class C: electrical equipment
Class D: combustible or reactive metals

The HUC often is asked to call maintenance when electrical equipment used for patient care needs repair. Electrical equipment used in the nursing station must be well maintained for safety purposes.

Guidelines for Electrical Safety

- Avoid the use of extension cords.
- Do not overload electrical circuits.
- Inspect cords and plugs for breaks and fraying.
- Unplug equipment when servicing.
- Unplug equipment that has liquid spilled in it.
- Unplug and do not use equipment that is malfunctioning.

Disaster Procedure

A **disaster procedure** is a planned procedure that is carried out by hospital personnel when a large number of persons have been injured. All hospitals in the United States have developed disaster or emergency preparedness plans that outline chains of command, communication procedures, and other important protocols to keep the hospital running in a crisis. A disaster manual is maintained on nursing units that outlines the hospital's disaster procedures. When an event occurs such as a multiple injury car accident, train or airplane accident, a bombing, earthquake, infectious disease outbreak, or a group of people exposed to hazardous chemicals, rapid access to information is critical. It can sometimes mean the difference between life and death.

Disaster drills are held once or twice a year to keep hospital personnel informed and in practice. Announcing a code such as "Code 5000" or more commonly "External Disaster or External Triage" on the hospital public address system activates the disaster procedure. An "Internal Disaster or Triage" may be called for an event that requires the assistance of all hospital personnel if it is limited to a situation that affects the current patient population in the hospital, such as the need to move a large number of patients owing to a power outage.

Wireless technologies are becoming part of hospital disaster preparedness plans. Examples of wireless technologies include; *Vocera's 802.11 voice devices* that can be integrated with data event notification and escalation applications, critical alert and alarm systems. *Everbridge Aware* that allows one person to communicate critical information to tens, hundreds, or thousands of individuals, anywhere, anytime, and on any device. The Aware Emergency Notification System contacts individuals based on their preferences and stops sending messages after a recipient confirms receipt. Other wireless technologies include *REACT Systems (Critical Response Notification Systems) AtHoc IWSAlerts solution.*

The HUC usually is designated to handle communication and if necessary, call off-duty health care personnel to assist in caring for hospital patients and disaster victims and in handling communications. The role of the HUC may vary among hospitals.

Medical Emergencies

Two **medical emergencies**—that is, life-threatening situations—that require calm, swift action and good communication on the part of the HUC are cardiac arrest and respiratory arrest. (It is common hospital terminology to refer to these as *code arrests* or, more commonly, **code blue.**) When either of these conditions occurs, the hospital telephone operator is notified immediately to announce the code so that personnel who need to respond will also be notified. Most hospitals have a call system installed in patients' rooms that allows hospital personnel to alert the hospital operator, as well as the nursing station and even nursing staff directly, of a patient's code (Fig. 21-5). In **cardiac arrest,** the patient's heart contractions are absent or are grossly insufficient, and no pulse and no blood pressure are detected. In **respiratory arrest,** the patient may cease to breathe, or respirations may become so depressed that the patient does not receive enough oxygen to sustain life. Both conditions require quick action by hospital personnel and the use of emergency equipment. Treatment must be instituted within 3 to 4 minutes because brain cells deteriorate rapidly from lack of oxygen. When it has been determined that medical treatment (such as medication) will be done in response to cardiac or respiratory arrest, but not chest compression or more invasive intervention, then it is called a **chemical code.** If a patient becomes unstable but is not yet in a code blue status—some hospitals have a "rapid response team" that may be called to assist in early intervention.

Each hospital nursing unit and department maintains a **code or crash cart** (Fig. 21-6). This is taken to the code arrest patient's room immediately. It is important for HUCs to know the location of the code or crash cart and any other emergency equipment so it can be brought quickly to the nursing unit when needed.

Hospitals have designated hospital personnel who report to each code arrest. These individuals are members of the code arrest team. They may be employed in various hospital departments, such as intensive or coronary care, other nursing units, the cardiopulmonary (respiratory care or pulmonary functions) department, the cardiovascular department, the clinical laboratory, diagnostic imaging, surgery, and so forth. The code team members will usually be carrying out stat orders such as lab work, electrocardiograms (ECGs), portable chest x-ray examinations, and arterial blood gases as

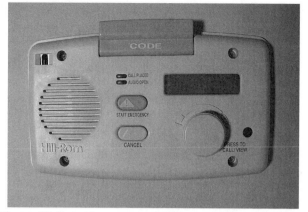

Figure 21-5 A call system installed in patients' rooms to alert the hospital operator and the nursing station of a patient's code.

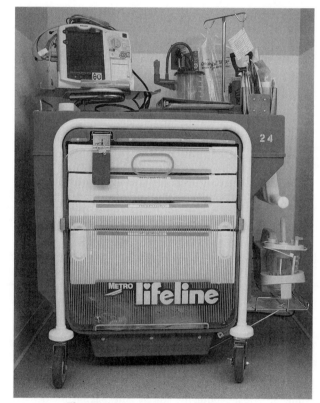

Figure 21-6 An example of a crash cart.

well as nursing and physician interventions. The HUC must be prepared to assist nonclinically in the activities of the code team to help ensure the best outcome for the patient.

As a member of the health care team, the HUC may be asked to perform the tasks outlined in Procedure 21-1.

SPECIAL SERVICES

Flowers

When a health care facility is large enough to include a specific area where all flowers are delivered, the task of delivering flowers to patients may be assigned to a hospital volunteer. In this case, the HUC may need only to direct the volunteer to the correct room.

PROCEDURE 21-1

PROCEDURE FOR PERFORMING TASKS RELATED TO MEDICAL EMERGENCIES

TASK	NOTES
1. Notify the hospital telephone operator to announce the code.	Notification is made by pressing a special button on the telephone, stating "code blue," and giving the location. Be very specific when stating unit, such as 4A-Apple, 4B-Boy, 4C-Charlie, or 4D-David. Code blue is used to designate a cardiac or respiratory arrest regardless of patient age.
2. Direct the code arrest team to the patient's room.	
3. Remove the patient information sheet from the patient's chart, and take or send the chart to the patient's room.	
4. Notify all doctors connected with the patient's case (attending doctor, consultants, and residents).	
5. Notify the patient's family of the situation if requested to do so.	If the HUC does communicate with the family, the conversation should be carried on in as controlled a manner as possible, so as to not cause panic. The dialogue might be, "Mr. Whetstone, your brother's condition has changed, and the doctor thought you would like to know. The doctors are with him now. Will you be coming to the hospital?"
6. Label laboratory specimens with the patient's identification (ID) label, enter the test ordered in the computer, and send the specimen to the laboratory stat.	
7. Call the appropriate departments for treatments and supplies as needed.	Usually, cardiopulmonary (respiratory care), diagnostic imaging, cardiovascular services, clinical laboratory, and the central services department (CSD) are the departments involved.
8. Alert the admissions department and the intensive care unit (ICU) about the possibility of a transfer to ICU.	If the code procedure is successful, the patient is usually transferred to ICU or the critical care unit (CCU), where he or she can be closely monitored.
9. For a successful code, follow Procedure 20-5 regarding transfer to another unit.	See Chapter 20, p. 355.
10. For an unsuccessful code procedure, follow Procedure 20-4 regarding postmortem care.	See Chapter 20, p. 355.

In hospitals in which the representative from the florist delivers the flowers directly to the unit, the HUC should ascertain that the patient is still on the unit or within the hospital before signing for and accepting the flowers. After signing the delivery slip, the HUC may deliver the flowers to the patient's room.

The HUC must be aware of any restrictions—for example, flowers are not allowed on some nursing units, such as intensive care or cardiopulmonary (respiratory care) units, and latex balloons are not allowed in most hospitals (especially not on pediatric units). If family members are present, flowers and balloons may be sent home with them.

Mail

Mail is delivered to the nursing unit daily. The mail is checked and the patient's room and bed numbers are written on each envelope. In the event that the patient has been discharged, the HUC would write "Discharged" in pencil on the envelope and return it to the mailroom. The mail may be distributed to patients as time allows, or the task may be designated to a hospital volunteer.

KEY CONCEPTS

It is very important to know the routines and to be able to perform the tasks related to medical emergencies, fires, and disasters. When emergencies occur, there is no time to look in a book for directions about what should be done. The other tasks discussed in this chapter may not be part of the HUC's regular routine; therefore the procedures for these can be reviewed in the hospital as time permits.

⊖ REVIEW QUESTIONS

An electronic download of these review questions is available on the Evolve website.

1. Define the following terms:
   a. cardiac arrest
   b. respiratory arrest
   c. communicable disease
   d. code or crash cart

e. pathogenic microorganisms
f. medical emergency
g. isolation
h. incident
i. epidemiologist
j. risk management
k. disaster procedure
l. nosocomial infections

2. Identify four categories of incidents that would initiate an incident report, and explain the purpose of completing an incident report.

3. Identify six components that constitute the chain of infection, and list four types of personal protective equipment used as barriers between the practitioner (health care worker) and the patient's body fluids.

4. List four examples of diagnosed infections that would require a patient to be placed in airborne insolation.

5. Identify the most common way to confirm and identify microorganisms and to determine which antibiotic will destroy the identified microbes.

6. Discuss ways in which someone working in the hospital environment can reduce his or her risk of infection.

7. Identify three circumstances that would cause a patient to become immunocompromised and in need of being placed in reverse or protective insolation.

8. Discuss four primary ways that the human immunodeficiency virus (HIV) may be transmitted from one person to another, and identify two opportunistic diseases related to acquired immunodeficiency syndrome (AIDS)

9. Identify a highly contagious virus transmitted through blood and body fluids and an airborne pathogen that would require health care providers to take extra precautions such as blood and fluid precautions and special PPE.

10. Discuss the pathogenic microorganisms that are frequently responsible for nosocomial infections.

11. Discuss the best way for health care providers to stop the spread of these hospital-acquired infections.

12. Discuss HUC tasks related to prevention of infection in the hospital work environment.

13. Identify the meaning for each of the following color emergency call codes:
a. red
b. blue
c. orange
d. pink
e. gray
f. silver

14. Identify the communication tool that provides details on chemical dangers and safety procedures.

15. Explain the "RACE system."

16. Describe what the responsibilities of the HUC would be during a fire code and during a disaster procedure.

17. List six guidelines that should be followed for electrical safety.

18. List nine tasks that the health unit coordinator may perform in a medical emergency.

19. Identify events that would activate the hospital's disaster procedure.

20. Describe how to handle flowers and mail delivered to the nursing unit.

SURFING FOR ANSWERS

Following the guidelines for surfing the Web (see Box 1-9) provided in Chapter 1, find the following information and list the websites used. If necessary, use a school computer or go to a library.

1. Locate two websites that outline standard precautions and good hand-washing technique. Identify the most recent nosocomial infection that could have been prevented by implementing standard precautions. The following websites may be of help:
Centers for Disease Control and Prevention: www.cdc.gov
OSHA: www.osha-slc.gov

2. Find three websites (probably Hospital Association websites) that discuss emergency call codes, including one that is being implemented in your state (if applicable). Compare and contrast the call code lists on these websites.

CHAPTER 22

Medical Terminology, Basic Human Structure, Diseases, and Disorders

UNIT 1
Medical Terminology: Word Parts, Analyzing, and Word Building

OUTLINE

UNIT OBJECTIVES

On completion of this unit, you will be able to:

1. Identify the three main origins of medical terms.
2. Name and define the four word parts that are commonly used in building medical terms.
3. List three guidelines to follow when connecting word parts to form a medical term.
4. Define *analysis of medical terms.*
5. Given a list of medical terms and a list of word parts, divide the medical terms into their component parts—that is, word roots, prefixes, suffixes, and combining vowels—and identify the types of word parts present in each term by name.
6. Define *synthesis of medical terms.*
7. Given a description of a medical term and a list of word parts—that is, word roots, prefixes, suffixes, and combining vowels—write out the medical term that represents a stated medical condition.

INTRODUCTION TO MEDICAL TERMS

Most medical terms are made up of Greek (e.g., *nephrology*) and Latin (e.g., *maternal*) words; however, some terms, such as *triage* and *lavage*, have been adapted from modern languages such as French. Two other sources of medical terms include acronyms and eponyms. An acronym is a word formed from the first letters of major terms in a descriptive phrase, such as laser (*l*ight *a*mplification by *s*timulated *e*mission of *r*adiation). An eponym is a name given to something that was discovered by or is identified with an individual. The Pap smear (Dr. Papanicolaou) and Lou Gehrig disease (amyotrophic lateral sclerosis [ALS]) are two examples of eponyms.

Although a background in Greek or Latin is not necessary to learn the meaning of medical terms, it is necessary to learn the English translation of the Greek or Latin word parts. In this course of study, the parts of the word are memorized rather than the whole word. By learning word parts, one will be able to build words according to a given definition and break down words into word parts to determine their meaning. For example, in the medical term

nephr / ectomy

nephr is the word part that means "kidney" and *-ectomy* is the word part meaning "surgical removal." Thus, *nephrectomy* means "surgical removal of the kidney." Once one has memorized the meanings of the word parts (*nephr-* and *-ectomy*), one will know their meanings when they appear in other medical terms.

In the preceding example, one can define the term by literally translating it. However, a few medical terms have implied meanings.

For example, the word

an / emia

literally translated means "without" *(an-)* "blood condition" *(-emia)*. However, the correct interpretation of anemia—an implied meaning—is a deficiency of red blood cells (RBCs). Knowledge of the meanings of the word parts for a medical term with an implied meaning takes one almost, but not quite, to the exact meaning of the term.

Medical terms are used instead of English words because one medical word says what it would take many English words to say. For example, *nephrectomy* means "surgical removal of the kidney." Medical terms are efficient and factual, they save space, and they often describe a situation or procedure more exactly.

Pronunciation of medical terms varies. What is acceptable pronunciation in one part of the country may not be used in another part of the country; therefore flexibility is necessary in the pronunciation of medical terms.

Correct spelling is absolutely necessary to avoid the incorrect use of a term. *Ileum* (portion of small intestine) and *ilium* (one of the bones of the hip) are two examples of terms close in spelling, yet anatomically diverse in meaning.

As you begin working with medical terminology, you may feel overwhelmed at the task of learning this new language. However, repeated use of the word parts will assist you in building your vocabulary, and soon you will be using medical terms fluently in your everyday speech. Many students employ the use of mnemonics (memory-aiding devices) to remember the word parts. For example, *entero* is the word part for "intestine." One might think of "digested food *entering* the intestine" and more easily recall the meaning of *entero*. Similarly, *ileum* of the small intestine is spelled with an *e* and one might associate "eating" with the intestine and not mistake this term with *ilium*, the bone in the hip.

This unit deals with word parts and how they are used together to form medical terms. *Remember:* It is important for you to master Unit 1 before proceeding to Unit 2, and so forth, because each unit is a continuation of the previously studied units.

WORD PARTS

In this course of study, the development of a medical vocabulary is based on memorizing parts of words rather than whole words. *Word part* is the term that will be used to describe the components of words. To build or analyze (divide into parts) medical terms, you first must learn the following four word parts:

1. Word root
2. Prefix
3. Suffix
4. Combining vowel

Word Root

The word root is the basic part of the word; it expresses the principal meaning of the word. For example, in the medical term

gastr / ic

gastr (stomach) is the word root.

Prefix

The prefix is the part of the word that is placed before the word root to alter its meaning. For example, in the medical term

intra / gastr / ic

intra- (within) is the prefix.

Suffix

The suffix is the part of the word that is added after the word root to alter its meaning. For example, in the medical term

gastr / ic

-ic (pertaining to) is the suffix.

Combining Vowel

The combining vowel, usually an *o*, is used between two word roots or between a word root and a suffix to ease pronunciation. Three guidelines are followed in using a combining vowel.

1. When a word root is connected to a suffix, a combining vowel usually is not used if the suffix begins with a vowel. For example, in the word [*gastr / ectomy*], *ectomy* (surgical removal) begins with the vowel *e*; thus the combining vowel *o* is not used.
2. When two word roots are connected, the combining vowel is usually used even if the second root begins with a vowel. For example, in the word [*gastr / o / enter / itis*], the second word root *enter* (intestine) begins with the vowel *e*, but the combining vowel *o* is still used.
3. A combining vowel is not used when a prefix and a word root are connected. For example, in the medical term [*sub / hepat / ic*], a combining vowel is not used between the prefix, *sub-*, and the word root, *hepat*.

Note: A combining form, not a true word part, is simply the word root separated from its combining vowel with a slash mark. For example, *gastr / o* is a combining form. Although *o* is the most commonly used combining vowel, *a, e,* and *i* also may be used. Throughout this chapter, the word roots are listed in combining forms.

Word Root	Meaning
cardi / o	heart
cyt / o	cell
electr / o	electricity, electrical activity
enter / o	intestine
gastr / o	stomach
hepat / o	liver
nephr / o	kidney

Prefixes	Meaning
intra-	within
epi-	upon
sub-	under, below
trans-	through, across, beyond

Suffixes	Meaning
-ectomy	excision, surgical removal
-gram	record, x-ray image
-ic	pertaining to
-itis	inflammation
-logy	study of

ANALYZING MEDICAL TERMS

To analyze medical terms, divide the term into word parts with the use of vertical slashes and identify the word part by labeling it as follows:

P	prefix
WR	word root
S	suffix
CV	combining vowel

After labeling and identifying, simply define the medical term according to the definitions of the word parts.

EXERCISE 1

Analyzing medical terms: Analyze the following medical terms by dividing each into word parts and writing *P, WR, S,* or *CV* above the appropriate part, as in the following examples. Use the earlier list to help you identify word parts.

Example 1: gastroenteritis

WR	CV	WR	S
gastr /	o /	enter /	itis
stomach		intestine	inflammation of

Example 2: intragastric

P	WR	S
epi /	gastr /	ic
upon	stomach	pertaining to

1. cytology
2. gastrectomy
3. subhepatic

4. electrocardiogram
5. cardiology
6. transhepatic

SYNTHESIS OF MEDICAL TERMS (WORD BUILDING)

Synthesis is the process of creating a medical term by using word parts. In building medical terms from a given definition, keep in mind that the beginning of the definition usually indicates the suffix that is needed to build the term.

EXERCISE 2

Synthesis: Build medical terms from the following definitions. Use the earlier list to assist you.

Example: study of the kidney—nephrology

1. study of the heart
2. study of cells
3. surgical removal of the stomach
4. inflammation of the stomach and intestines
5. pertaining to the stomach
6. pertaining to within the stomach
7. surgical removal of the kidney

REVIEW QUESTIONS

1. Name the three main origins of medical terms, and give an example for each.

2. List the four word parts. Define and give an example of each.

3. List the guidelines followed in connecting the following:
   a. prefix and word root
   b. word root and word root
   c. word root and suffix

4. Define:
   a. analysis of medical terms
   b. synthesis of medical terms

UNIT 2
Body Structure, Integumentary System, and Oncology

OUTLINE

UNIT OBJECTIVES

On completion of this unit, you will be able to:

1. Describe the function and structure of body cells.
2. Identify and describe the function of four types of tissue
3. Explain the structure of an organ and the structure of a system.
4. List five body cavities, and name a body organ contained in each cavity.
5. List the four quadrants and nine regions of the abdominopelvic cavity.
6. Define the *anatomical position* and the directional terms outlined in this unit.
7. List four functions of skin.
8. List the seven signs of cancer, and describe first-, second-, and third-degree burns.
9. Define *abscess, laceration, abrasion, gangrene, infection,* and *decubitus ulcer.*
10. Read the objectives related to medical terminology, and demonstrate ability to meet the objectives by completing Exercises 1 through 6.
11. Define the unit abbreviations.

BODY STRUCTURE (ANATOMY) AND FUNCTION (PHYSIOLOGY)

Body Cells

The cell is the basic unit of all living things (Fig. 22-1). The human body is made up of trillions of cells. Cells perform specific functions, and their size and shape vary according to function. Bones, muscles, skin, and blood are all made up of different types of cells. Body cells are microscopic; approximately 2000 are needed to make an inch (although a single nerve cell may be several feet long). Cells are constantly growing and reproducing. Such growth is responsible for the development of an embryo into a child and a child into an adult. This growth is also responsible for the replacement of cells that have a relatively short life span and cells that are injured, diseased, or worn out.

To visualize the structure of a cell, we can diagrammatically compare the three main parts of the cell with the three parts of an egg: the eggshell, the egg white, and the egg yolk.

Cell Membrane

The cell membrane (eggshell), the boundary of the cell, is porous, flexible, and elastic. The protective cell membrane actively or passively regulates the movement of a substance into and out of the cell. The cell membrane keeps the cell intact. The cell dies if the cell membrane can no longer carry out these functions.

Cytoplasm

Cytoplasm (egg white) is the main body of the cell in which are found various organelles, such as the mitochondria, which are specialized structures that carry out activities necessary for the cell's survival. For example, in the muscle cell, basic contracting is done by the sarcomere within its cytoplasm, called *sarcoplasm.*

Nucleus

The nucleus (egg yolk), a small structure, is located near the center of the cell. It is the control center of the cell and plays an

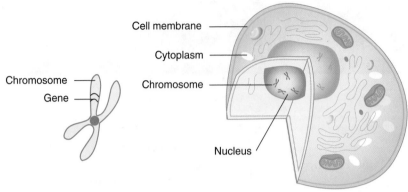

Figure 22-1 Parts of a body cell.

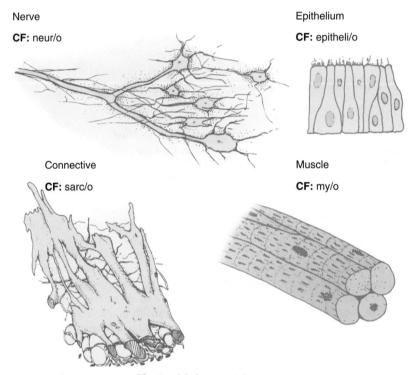

Figure 22-2 Types of tissues.

important role in reproduction. Chromosomes located in the nucleus contain the genes that determine hereditary characteristics. Not all cells contain a nucleus—for instance, the mature RBC. Some other cells, such as certain bone cells and skeletal muscle cells, contain several nuclei.

Body Tissues

A tissue is made up of a group of similar cells that work together to perform particular functions (Fig. 22-2). Tissues may be categorized into the following types:

- *Epithelial tissue:* Epithelial tissue forms a protective covering (skin) or lines body cavities (e.g., digestive, respiratory, and urinary tracts).
- *Connective tissue:* The main functions of connective tissue are to connect and hold tissues together, to transport substances, and to protect against foreign invaders.

Connective tissue forms and protects bones, fat, blood cells, and cartilage and provides immunity.
- *Muscle tissue:* Muscle tissue makes up the muscles of the body that contract and relax to produce movement.
- *Nerve tissue:* Nerve tissue forms parts of the nervous system; it conducts electrochemical impulses and helps to coordinate body activities.

Body Organs

An organ is made up of two or more types of tissues that perform one or more common functions. The stomach is an organ that is made up of muscle, nerve, connective, and epithelial tissue.

Body Systems

A *body system* is made up of a group of organs that work closely together in a common purpose to perform complex body

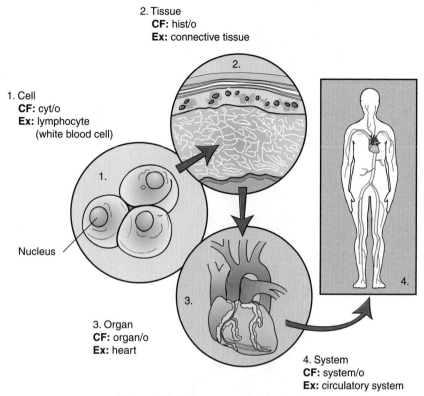

2. Tissue
CF: hist/o
Ex: connective tissue

1. Cell
CF: cyt/o
Ex: lymphocyte
(white blood cell)

Nucleus

3. Organ
CF: organ/o
Ex: heart

4. System
CF: system/o
Ex: circulatory system

Figure 22-3 Organization of the body.

functions (Fig. 22-3). For example, the urinary system is made up of the following organs: kidneys, ureters, urinary bladder, and urethra. Its main function is to remove wastes from the blood and eliminate them from the body. Other body systems include the digestive, musculoskeletal, nervous, reproductive, endocrine, circulatory, respiratory, sensory, and integumentary systems. Some organs are a part of more than one system. The pharynx, for example, is part of both the digestive and the respiratory systems. In the digestive system the pharynx allows for the passage of food; in the respiratory system it allows for the passage of air.

Homeostasis is the maintenance of a stable, relatively constant environment within body cells and tissues. Stability of the body's normal volume, temperature, and chemicals is effected by the successful harmony of the organ systems and is regulated by the nervous and endocrine systems. Failure to keep the body systems in homeostasis results in disease.

Body Cavities

Large spaces within the body that contain internal organs, or viscera, are called *body cavities* (Fig. 22-4). The two major body cavities are the *dorsal cavity* (near the back) and the *ventral cavity* (near the front).

Dorsal Cavity

The dorsal cavity is composed of the cranial cavity and the spinal cavity, which form a continuous space.

- *Cranial cavity:* Space in the skull that contains the brain
- *Spinal cavity:* Space in the spinal column that contains the spinal cord

Ventral Cavity

The ventral cavity is composed of the thoracic (or chest) cavity and the abdominopelvic cavity.

- *Thoracic cavity:* The chest cavity contains additional spaces, including right and left pleural cavities and the mediastinum. Organs within the thoracic cavity include the heart, lungs, trachea, esophagus, thymus gland, and major blood vessels.
- *Right and left pleural cavities:* Double-walled sacs that create spaces that surround the lungs.
- *Mediastinum:* Space that contains the heart, trachea, esophagus, thymus gland, and major blood vessels.
- *Abdominopelvic cavity:* This space is divided into the abdominal cavity and the pelvic cavity.
- *Abdominal cavity:* Upper portion of the abdominopelvic cavity. This space contains the stomach; most of the intestines; and the kidneys, ureters, liver, pancreas, gallbladder, and spleen. The abdominal cavity is separated from the thoracic cavity by a muscle called the *diaphragm.*
- *Pelvic cavity:* Lower portion of the abdominopelvic cavity. This space contains the bladder, urethra, reproductive organs, part of the large intestine (sigmoid colon), and the rectum. The abdominopelvic cavity is divided into four quadrants and nine regions (Fig. 22-5). You will frequently encounter these descriptive terms during your health care employment.

Directional Terms Pertaining to the Body

Directional terms, which are used to describe a location on or within the body, refer to the patient in the *anatomical position.*

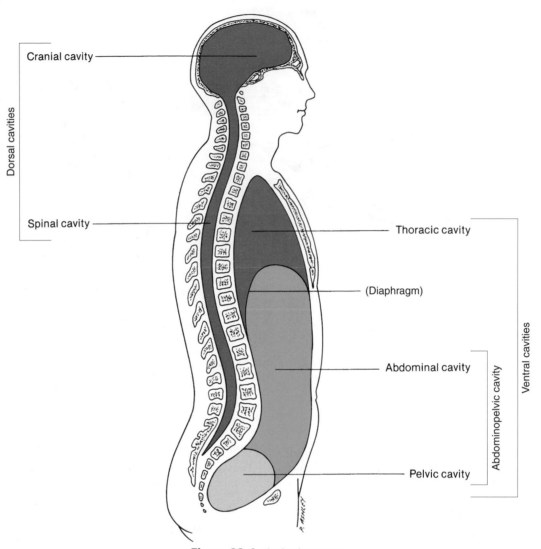

Cranial cavity

Dorsal cavities

Spinal cavity

Thoracic cavity

(Diaphragm)

Abdominal cavity

Ventral cavities

Abdominopelvic cavity

Pelvic cavity

P. ASHLEY

Figure 22-4 The body cavities.

Anatomical position is the point of reference that ensures proper description: body erect, face and feet forward, arms at side, and palms facing forward. In Figure 22-11 (in Unit 3 of this chapter), the skeletal orientation is in the anatomical position.

- *Superior (cranial):* Pertaining to *above.* (The eye is located superior to the mouth.)
- *Inferior (caudal):* Pertaining to *below.* (The mouth is located inferior to the nose.)
- *Anterior (ventral):* Pertaining to *in front of.* (The eyes are located on the anterior of the head.)
- *Anteroposterior (AP):* Pertaining to *front to back.* (Directionally moving from the front to the back.)
- *Posterior (dorsal):* Pertaining to *in back of.* (The gluteus maximus is posterior to the navel.)
- *Posteroanterior (PA):* Pertaining to *back to front.* (Directionally moving from the back to the front.)
- *Lateral (lat):* Pertaining to the *side.* (The little toe is lateral to the big toe.)
- *Bilateral (bilat):* Pertaining to *two (both) sides.* (Bilateral otitis media [ear infections].)

- *Medial:* Pertaining to the *middle.* (The nose is medial to the ears.)
- *Abduction:* Pertaining to *away from.* (Spreading the fingers wide apart is an example of abduction.)
- *Adduction:* Pertaining to *toward.* (Bringing the fingers together from being spread out shows adduction.)
- *Proximal:* Pertaining to *closer than* another structure to the point of attachment. (The elbow is proximal to the wrist.)
- *Distal:* Pertaining to *farther than* another structure from the point of attachment. (The fingers are distal to the elbow.)
- *Superficial:* Toward the surface. (Hair follicles are superficial structures.)
- *Deep:* Farther from the surface. (The femur is deep to the skin.)
- *Prone:* Lying with the face downward. (The patient is placed in a prone position for suturing of the back of her head.)
- *Supine:* Lying on the back. (Supine positioning was required for his sternal puncture.)

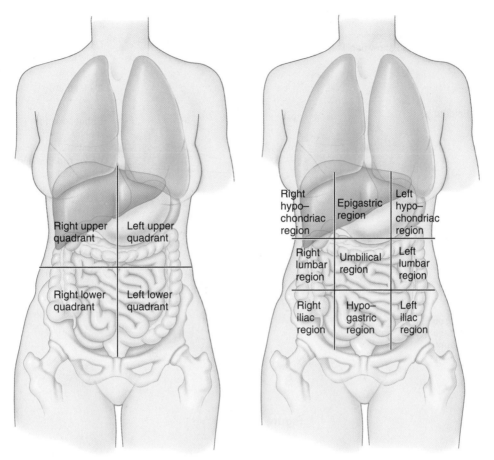

Figure 22-5 Division of the abdominopelvic cavity into four quadrants and nine regions.

INTEGUMENTARY SYSTEM

The integumentary system consists of the skin (the largest organ of the body) and accessory structures (hair, nails, and sweat and oil glands) (Fig. 22-6). The skin of an adult may weigh 20 pounds or more. The skin has many functions. The main one is to protect underlying tissues from pathogenic (disease-causing) microorganisms and other environmental hazards. The skin also assists in the regulation of body temperature and the synthesis of vitamin D. As a sensory organ, the specialized receptors of the skin pass messages of pain, temperature, pressure, and touch to the brain.

The thin outer layer of skin is called the *epidermis* and is composed of epithelial tissue. The cells of the innermost layer produce themselves. As they move toward the surface, the outermost cells are shed. Millions of cells are produced and shed each day. The epidermis contains no blood vessels.

The thick layer directly below the epidermis is called the *dermis*, or *true skin*. It is made up of connective tissue and contains blood vessels, nerve endings, hair follicles, and sweat and oil glands.

The subcutaneous tissue (or *hypodermis*), a thick, fat-containing tissue located below the dermis, serves to connect the skin to underlying muscles, bone, and organs.

Hair provides a protective function; for example, nasal hairs trap foreign particles to prevent them from being inhaled into the lungs. The hair follicle is a pouchlike depression in the skin from which the hair grows to extend above the skin surface. Oil glands (sebaceous glands) connect to the hair follicle through tiny ducts. Each sebaceous gland produces oil (sebum), which lubricates the hair and skin and inhibits bacterial growth.

The *sweat glands* (sudoriferous glands) are coiled, tube-like structures that are located mainly in the dermis. Each extends to the surface in the form of a tiny opening called a *pore*. Approximately 3000 pores can be found in the palm of a hand, and 2 million on the body surface. Sweat, a saline fluid, is produced by the sweat glands. As sweat evaporates on the body surface, it cools the body.

Skin color is determined by the amount of melanin in the epidermis of the skin. Skin color varies from pale yellow to black. A condition called *albinism* results when melanin cannot be formed by melanocytes. An albino can be recognized by the characteristic absence of pigment in the hair, eyes, and skin.

DISEASES AND CONDITIONS OF THE SKIN AND BODY CELLS

Cancer

Cancer (often abbreviated as *Ca*) is a disease in which unregulated new growth of abnormal cells occurs. It is normal for worn-out body cells to be replaced by new cell growth and also for new cells to form to repair tissue damage. Normal cell growth is regulated; in cancer, cell division is unregulated, and cells continue to reproduce until a mass known as a *tumor*, or

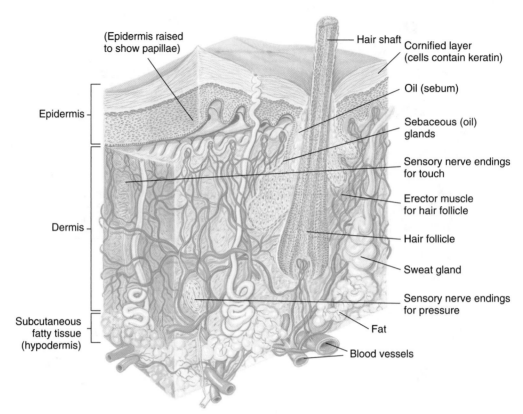

Figure labels:
- (Epidermis raised to show papillae)
- Hair shaft
- Cornified layer (cells contain keratin)
- Oil (sebum)
- Sebaceous (oil) glands
- Sensory nerve endings for touch
- Erector muscle for hair follicle
- Hair follicle
- Sweat gland
- Sensory nerve endings for pressure
- Fat
- Blood vessels
- Epidermis
- Dermis
- Subcutaneous fatty tissue (hypodermis)

Figure 22-6 The skin.

neoplasm, forms. Skin cancer arises from cell changes in the epidermis and is the most common form of human cancer. Exposure to broad-spectrum ultraviolet (UV) rays of the sun and artificial sources is thought to be an important factor in the development of skin cancer. Basal cell carcinoma and squamous cell carcinoma, two major types of skin cancers, both are very responsive to treatment and seldom metastasize (spread) to other body systems.

Cancerous tumors are malignant, which means they become progressively worse, whereas noncancerous tumors are benign or nonrecurrent. Malignant tumors grow in a disorganized fashion, interrupting body function and interfering with the food and blood supply to normal cells. Malignant cells may metastasize from one organ to another through the bloodstream or the lymphatic system. Malignant melanoma arises from the melanocytes (pigment-producing cells in the skin) and may metastasize to the brain, liver, lung, and other organs.

Cancer consists of many different diseases, and a single cause of abnormal cell division cannot be pinpointed. Genetic factors, steroidal estrogens, cigarette smoking, exposure to carcinogenic substances, and UV rays are believed to be among the causes of cancer.

Detection of cancer requires self-examination, x-ray imaging, blood tests, and microscopic tissue examination. Treatments for patients with cancer include surgery, chemotherapy, radiation, and gene therapy.

Cancer's Seven Warning Signals

The seven warning signals of cancer may be recalled easily by the mnemonic CAUTION.

- **C**hange in bowel or bladder habits
- **A** sore that does not heal
- **U**nusual bleeding of discharge
- **T**hickening or lump in the breast, testes, or elsewhere
- **I**ndigestion or difficulty in swallowing
- **O**bvious change in a wart or mole
- **N**agging cough or hoarsensess

Burns

All burns are dangerous if they are not treated properly, because infection can occur and because shock is possible in more serious burns as a result of fluid loss from the skin. Burns are classified according to degree of severity, which reflects the depth of the burn (full or partial thickness) (Fig. 22-7) and the extent of surface area involvement (Fig. 22-8).

1. *First-degree burns* damage the epidermis. Also called a *partial-thickness* burn, sunburn is an example of a first-degree burn in which redness, minor discomfort, and slight edema may be present.
2. *Second-degree burns* damage the epidermis and the dermis. Also called *partial-thickness burns*, second-degree burns account for symptoms such as redness, pain, edema, and blisters.
3. *Third-degree* burns destroy the epidermis, dermis, and subcutaneous tissue. They are also called *full-thickness burns.* No pain occurs because the skin's sensory receptors are destroyed. Third-degree burns heal only from the edges, and débridement (removal of dead skin) and skin grafts are necessary.

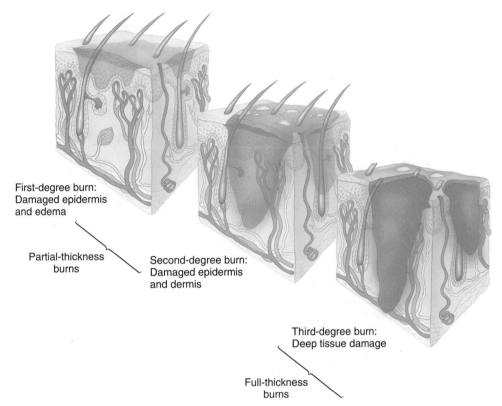

First-degree burn:
Damaged epidermis
and edema

Partial-thickness
burns

Second-degree burn:
Damaged epidermis
and dermis

Third-degree burn:
Deep tissue damage

Full-thickness
burns

Figure 22-7 First-degree burns damage the epidermis; second-degree burns damage the epidermis and the dermis; third-degree burns damage the epidermis, the dermis, and the subcutaneous tissue.

Abscesses

An *abscess* is a cavity that contains pus. Abscesses usually are caused by pathogenic microorganisms that invade the tissue through a break in the skin. As the microorganisms destroy the tissue, an increased blood supply is rushed to the area, causing inflammation in the surrounding tissue. Abscesses are formed by the body to wall off the pathogenic microorganisms and keep them from spreading throughout the body. It may be difficult to treat these infections, as antibiotics may not be able to permeate the wall of the abscess.

Lacerations and Abrasions

A *laceration* is a wound that is produced by tearing of body tissue. An *abrasion* is a scraping away of the skin. Keeping lacerations and abrasions clean is important because of the danger of infection. Suturing may be required to repair lacerations.

Gangrene

Gangrene, a serious medical condition, is the death of body tissue caused by lack of blood supply to an area of the body; often it is the result of infection or injury. Symptoms include fever, pain, darkening of the skin, and an unpleasant odor. Treatment, depending on the underlying cause, includes surgical débridement (removal with a sharp instrument) of necrotic tissue or amputation, administration of intravenous (IV) antibiotics, and the use of hyperbaric oxygen therapy to help kill the bacteria.

Infection

Infection is the invasion of the body by pathogenic microorganisms that reproduce and multiply, causing disease. Infections may be caused by streptococcal, staphylococcal, or *Pseudomonas* bacteria; by viruses; or by other organisms. Bacterial infections are treated with antibiotic therapy. Methicillin-resistant *Staphylococcus aureus* (MRSA) is one of several nosocomial (hospital- or health care setting–acquired) pathogens (see Chapter 14). Often the main mode of transmission of nosocomial infections in the clinical setting is through the hands of health care workers. These pathogens can be found on the skin, in the nose, and in blood and urine. Proper hand cleansing techniques should be reviewed with new employees by the infection control department of the clinical setting to avoid transmission of MRSA.

Decubitus Ulcer

Decubitus ulcer, also known as *bedsore* or *pressure sore*, is a vascular condition that arises in patients who sit or lie in one position for long periods of time. The weight of the body, typically over bony projections such as the hips, heels, and ankles, slows blood flow, causing ulcers to form, and infection may develop when microorganisms enter the affected area. The decubitus ulcer, similar to the burn, is categorized according to severity in terms of stages (stage I to stage IV). Beginning as a reddened, sensitive, unbroken patch of skin categorized as stage I, the pressure sore may progress to an open sore (ulcer) for which strict attention to

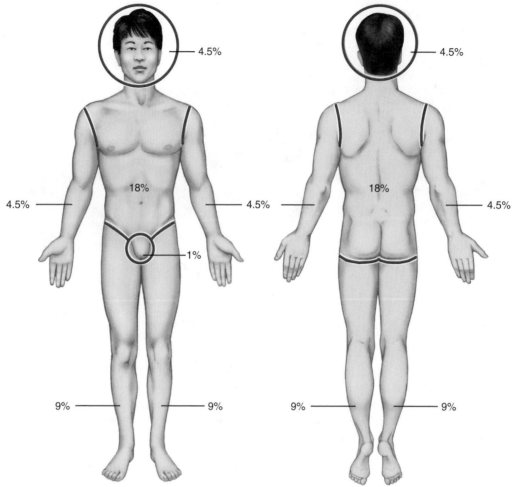

Figure 22-8 Surface area involvement of burns. The *rule of nines* is one method used to estimate the total body surface area (TBSA) burned in an adult. This method divides the TBSA into multiples of 9% (1% for the groin). The Lund-Browder chart is used for infants and children because the surface area of the head and neck is greater than for adults, and the limbs are smaller.

wound care is required. In stage IV the patient may experience full-thickness skin loss with damage to muscle, bone, or other body structures. Periodic body position changes and soft support cushions may help to prevent the onset of pressure sores.

⊖ REVIEW QUESTIONS

1. Describe the function and structure of body cells.

2. Identify and describe the function of four types of tissue.

3. Explain the structure of an organ and the structure of a system

4. List five body cavities and name a body organ contained in each cavity

5. List the four quadrants and nine regions of the abdominopelvic cavity.

6. Define the anatomical position.

7. Match each directional term in Column 1 with its correct meaning in Column 2.

Column 1
a. superior
b. inferior
c. lateral
d. medial
e. anterior
f. posterior
g. adduction
h. abduction
i. proximal
j. distal
k. deep
l. superficial

m. supine

n. prone
o. anteroposterior
p. posteroanterior

Column 2
1. in front of
2. pertaining to the middle
3. pertaining to away from
4. pertaining to the side
5. above
6. below
7. pertaining to toward
8. in back of
9. farther from the surface
10. nearer (point of reference)
11. closer to the surface
12. farther from (point of reference)
13. lying with face downward
14. lying on the back
15. from back to front
16. from front to back

8. List four functions of the skin.

9. What is the thin outermost layer of the skin called? What is the thick layer of skin directly below this layer called? What is the innermost layer of fat-containing tissue called?

10. Skin color is determined by the amount of _____ in the skin. Absence of this results in _____.

11. Name the glands that produce oil that lubricates the skin and hair.

12. _____ open to the surface of the skin in tiny openings called *pores*.

13. List the seven signs of cancer and describe first-, second-, and third-degree burns.

14. Match the terms in Column 1 with the phrases in Column 2.

Column 1	Column 2
a. burns	1. cavity that contains pus
b. abscess	2. classified according to degree of severity
c. laceration	3. invasion of the body by pathogenic microorganisms
d. gangrene	4. new growth of abnormal cells
e. infection	5. death of body tissue
f. cancer	6. wound produced by tearing
g. abrasion	7. pressure sore
h. decubitus ulcer	8. scraping away of skin

MEDICAL TERMINOLOGY RELATED TO BODY STRUCTURE, INTEGUMENTARY SYSTEM, AND ONCOLOGY

Objectives

On mastery of medical terminology for this unit, you will be able to:

1. Define, spell, and pronounce the medical terms listed in this unit.
2. Analyze the medical terms that are built from word parts.
3. Given the meaning of a medical condition, build the corresponding medical terms, using word parts.

Word Parts

Listed in the following table are the word parts you will be working with in this unit. You will need to memorize each one because you will continue to use them in this chapter and in your work environment. The exercises that follow these lists will assist you in this task. Practice pronouncing each word part aloud.

To review, a word root is the basic part of the word; a combining form is the word root plus a combining vowel (generally an *o*); a prefix is the modifying word part added to the beginning of a word; and a suffix is the modifying word part added to the end of a word root.

Word Roots/Combining Forms	Meaning
bi / o (bī′-yo)	life
cancer / o, carcin / o (kăn-sĕr-ō) (kar′-sĭn-ō),	cancer
cutane/ o (kyū-tā′-nē-ō),	skin
cyt / o (sī′-to)	cell
dermat / o (dĕr′-mĕ-tō)	skin
derm / o (dĕr′-mō)	skin
epitheli / o (ĕp-ĭ-thē′-lē-ō)	epithelium
hist /o (hĭs′-to)	tissue
lip / o (lĭp′-ō)	fat
onc / o (ŏn′-kō)	tumor
path / o (păth′-ō)	disease
sarc / o (sar′-cō)	connective tissue, flesh
trich / o (trĭk′-ō)	hair
ungu / o (ŭng′-ŭ-ō)	nail
viscer / o (vĭs′-ĕr-ō)	internal organs

Many of the suffixes presented in this course of study are made up of word roots and suffixes. For example, the suffix *-logy* (or *-ology*) is built from *log* (word root for "study") plus *-y* (suffix). For learning purposes, these will be studied as suffixes and analyzed as a single word part.

Prefixes	Meaning
sub-	under, below
trans- (trăns)	through, across, beyond

Suffixes	Meaning
-al, -ous	pertaining to
-genic (jĕn′-ĭk)	producing, originating, causing
-itis (ī′-tĭs)	inflammation
-oid (oyd)	resembling
-logist (lŏ′-jĭst)	one who specializes in the diagnosis and treatment of (doctor)
-logy (lŏ′ -jē)	study of
-oma (ō′-mah)	tumor
-opsy (ŏp′-sē)	to view

⊜ EXERCISE 1

Define each combining form listed.

1. viscer / o	9. sarc /o
2. dermat / o	10. epitheli / o
3. cyt / o	11. lip / o
4. hist / o	12. onc / o
5. derm / o	13. cutane / o
6. trich / o	14. cancer / o
7. path / o	15. ungu / o
8. carcin / o	16. bi / o

⊜ EXERCISE 2

Define each suffix and prefix listed.

1. -al	7. -genic
2. -logy	8. trans-
3. -logist	9. -ous
4. -oid	10. sub-
5. -itis	11. -opsy
6. -oma	

⊖ E X E R C I S E 3

Write the word parts for each definition. Indicate which word parts are suffixes by writing S in the space provided, indicate which word parts are word roots or combining forms by writing WR/CF in the space provided, and indicate which word parts are prefixes by writing P in the space provided.

Meaning	Word Part	Type of Word Part
Example: inflammation	-itis	S
1. cell		
2. skin		
a.		
b.		
c.		
3. specialist		
4. resembling		
5. internal organs		
6. tissues		
7. pertaining to		
a.		
b.		
8. study of		
9. through, across, beyond		
10. cancer		
a.		
b.		
11. under, below		
12. tumor		

MEDICAL TERMS RELATED TO BODY STRUCTURE AND SKIN

Listed here are the medical terms you need to know for this unit. Practice pronouncing these words aloud. Following the list are exercises that will assist you in learning these terms.

General Terms	Meaning
biopsy (bī´-yŏp-sē)	view of life (examination of tissue taken from a living patient)
carcinogenic (kar´-sĭn-ō-jēn´-ik)	producing cancer
cytoid (sī´-toyd)	resembling a cell
cytology (sī-tŏl´-o-jē)	study of cells
dermal (dēr´-mal)	pertaining to the skin (may also use the term *cutaneous*)
dermatoid (dēr´-măh-toyd)	resembling skin
dermatologist (dēr-măh-tŏl´-o-jĭst)	one who specializes in the diagnosis and treatment of skin (diseases)
dermatology (dēr-măh-tŏl´-o-je)	study of skin (branch of medicine that deals with diagnosis and treatment of skin disease)
dermoid (dĕrm´-ōid)	resembling skin
epithelial (ĕp-ĭ-thē´-lē-al)	pertaining to epithelium
histology (hĭs-tŏl´-o-jē)	study of tissues
oncologist (ŏn-kol´-o-jĭst)	one who specializes in the treament and diagnosis of tumors (cancer)

General Terms	Meaning
oncology (ŏn-kol´-o-jē)	study of tumors (cancer)
pathogenic (păth-ö-jĕn´-ĭk)	producing disease
pathologist (pă-thŏl´-o-jĭst)	one who specializes in the diagnosis and treatment of disease (body changes caused by disease)
pathology (pă-thŏl´-o-jē)	the study of disease
subcutaneous (sŭb-cŭ-tān´-ē-ŭs)	pertaining to under the skin
subungual (sŭb-ŭng´-ŭăl)	pertaining to under the nail
transdermal (trăns-dĕr´-mal), or transcutaneous	pertaining to (entering) through the skin
trichoid (trĭk´-oyd)	resembling hair
visceral (vĭs´-er-al)	pertaining to internal organs

Diagnostic Terms	Meaning
carcinoma (kăr-sĭ-nō´-mah)	cancerous tumor (malignant)
dermatitis (dĕr-mah-tī´-tĭs)	inflammation of the skin
epithelioma (ĕp-ĭ-thē-lē-ō´-mah)	tumor (composed of) epithelial cells
lipoma (li-pō´-mah)	tumor (containing) fat
sarcoma (sar-kō´-mah)	tumor (composed of) connective tissue (highly malignant)

⊖ E X E R C I S E 4

Analyze and define each term listed.

Example: pathologist
Analyze:
WR / CV / S
path / o / logist
Define: Specialist in the diagnosis and treatment of disease

1. cytology	14. epithelioma
2. trichoid	15. sarcoma
3. pathology	16. lipoma
4. pathogenic	17. pathologist
5. dermal	18. dermatoid/dermoid
6. cytoid	19. dermatology
7. visceral	20. transdermal
8. histology	21. oncology
9. dermatologist	22. subungual
10. dermatitis	23. subcutaneous
11. carcinogenic	24. biopsy
12. epithelial	25. oncologist
13. carcinoma	

⊖ E X E R C I S E 5

Build the medical terms that correspond with the definitions listed here. Remember that the beginning of the definition usually indicates the suffix that is needed to build the term.

1. resembling a cell
2. resembling hair
3. resembling skin (2 terms)

4. one who specializes in the diagnosis and treatment of disease (body changes caused by disease)
5. one who specializes in the diagnosis and treatment of skin (diseases)
6. pertaining to the skin (2 terms)
7. pertaining to the internal organs
8. study of tissues
9. study of disease
10. study of skin
11. producing disease
12. study of cells
13. inflammation of the skin
14. tumor containing fat
15. tumor composed of epithelial cells
16. pertaining to epithelium
17. producing cancer
18. a tumor composed of connective tissue
19. cancerous tumor
20. pertaining to through the skin
21. study of tumors (cancer)
22. pertaining to under the nail
23. pertaining to under the skin
24. view of life
25. one who specializes in the diagnosis and treatment of tumors (cancer)

EXERCISE 6

Write each of the 25 medical terms studied in this unit by having someone dictate all terms to you.

1.	10.	19.
2.	11.	20.
3.	12.	21.
4.	13.	22.
5.	14.	23.
6.	15.	24.
7.	16.	25.
8.	17.	
9.	18.	

ABBREVIATIONS

Abbreviation	Meaning
AP	anteroposterior
Bx	biopsy
Ca	cancer
Lat	lateral
LLQ	left lower quadrant
LUQ	left upper quadrant
PA	posteroanterior
RLQ	right lower quadrant
RUQ	right upper quadrant
SQ	subcutaneous

EXERCISE 7

Define the following abbreviations.

1. PA
2. RUQ
3. AP
4. RLQ
5. SQ
6. Lat
7. Ca
8. LLQ
9. LUQ
10. Bx

UNIT 3
The Musculoskeletal System

OUTLINE

UNIT OBJECTIVES

On completion of this unit, you will be able to:

1. Describe five functions of the skeletal system.
2. List four types of bones, and describe bone structure.
3. Name, specify numbers, and spell correctly the bones of the body.
4. Briefly describe 80 bones contained in the axial skeleton and 126 bones contained in the appendicular skeleton.
5. Explain the functions of joints and a ligaments.
6. Describe the four main functions of the muscular system.
7. Identify and discuss three types of muscles, and describe the function of tendons relating to skeletal muscle.
8. Discuss arthritis, a ruptured disk, osteoporosis, and Paget disease.
9. List six types of fractures, and describe the purpose and process of joint replacements.
10. Read the objectives related to medical terminology, and demonstrate ability to meet the objectives by correctly completing Exercises 1 through 13
11. Define the unit abbreviations.

THE SKELETAL SYSTEM

Organs of the Skeletal System

An adult skeleton has 206 bones.

Functions of the Skeletal System

- *Protection:* To protect the internal organs from injury
- *Support:* To provide a framework for the body
- *Movement:* To act with the muscles to produce body movement
- *Blood cell production:* To produce blood cells (hematopoiesis) in the red marrow of certain bones
- *Mineral storage:* To store calcium and phosphorus—minerals essential for cellular activities

Bone Structure

- There are four types of bones: long, short, flat, and irregular.
- Bones have their own system of blood vessels and nerves.
- Bones contain *red bone marrow* (produces RBCs, white blood cells, and platelets) and *yellow bone marrow* (consists mostly of adipose tissue, or fat).
- Bones are covered with a thin membrane called *periosteum*, which is necessary for growth and repair and is the attachment point for ligaments and tendons.

Axial Skeleton

The axial skeleton (80 bones) consists of skull, hyoid bone, vertebral column, and rib cage and is so named because the bones revolve around the vertical *axis* of the skeleton.

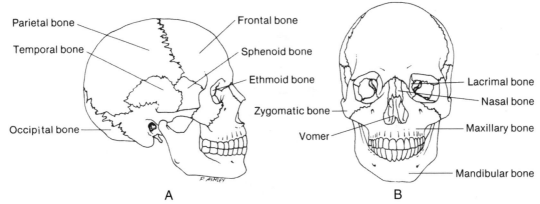

Figure 22-9 The bones of the skull. **A,** Cranial bones. **B,** Facial bones.

Bone Framework of the Head (Fig. 22-9)

Skull or Cranium (8 Bones)

- *Frontal bone (1):* Framework of the forehead and roof of the eye socket
- *Parietal bones (2):* Form the upper sides of the cranium
- *Temporal bones (2):* Form the lower sides of the cranium and contain parts of the ear
- *Ethmoid bone (1):* Forms part of the cranial floor and part of the nasal cavity
- *Sphenoid bone (1):* Bat-shaped bone that extends behind the eyes and forms part of the base of the skull
- *Occipital bone (1):* Composes the back and most of the base of the skull; connects with the parietal and temporal bones

Facial Bones (14 Bones)

- *Maxillary bones (2):* Upper jaw bones
- *Mandible bone (1):* Lower jaw bone; the only movable bone in the skull
- *Nasal bones (2):* Support the bridge of the nose
- *Lacrimal bones (2):* Corners of the eye sockets
- *Zygomatic bones (2):* Cheekbones
- *Vomer (1):* Lower portion of the nasal septum
- *Inferior nasal concha (2):* Lateral walls of the nasal cavity
- *Palatine (2):* Hard palate and part of nasal cavities and orbit walls

Other (7 Bones)

- *Hyoid bone (1):* U-shaped bone in the throat: anchors the tongue
- *Auditory ossicles—* in the middle ear: transmit sound, include:
  Malleus (2): Hammer
  Incus (2): Anvil
  Stapes (2): Stirrup

Vertebral Column (26 Vertebrae; Fig. 22-10)

- *Cervical (7):* The first seven vertebrae; form the neck
- *Thoracic (12):* The next 12 vertebrae; form the outward curve of the spine and join with 12 pairs of ribs
- *Lumbar (5):* The next five vertebrae, the largest and strongest; form the inward curvature of the spine
- *Sacrum (1):* The next five vertebrae; fuse together to form one sacrum in the adult
- *Coccyx (1):* The last three to five vertebrae; in the adult, these fuse together to form one coccyx

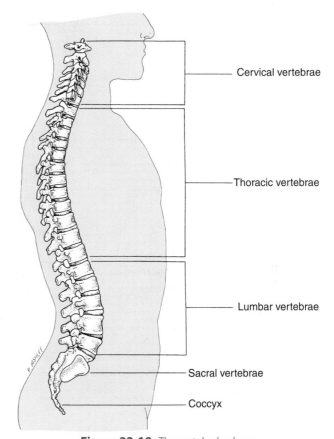

Figure 22-10 The vertebral column.

The vertebrae form the spinal column. Openings in the vertebrae provide a continuous space through which the spinal cord travels. The vertebrae are separated by disks (plates of cartilage). The central portion of the disk is filled with a pulpy elastic substance called *nucleus pulposus*. The disks allow for flexibility and absorb shock. The lamina is located on the posterior arch of the vertebra.

Rib Cage (24 Bones; Fig. 22-11)

All 24 ribs (12 pairs) are attached posteriorly to the thoracic vertebrae. The first seven pairs of ribs (*true ribs*) attach anteriorly to the sternum; the next three pairs converge and join the seventh rib anteriorly; the last two pairs remain free at the anterior ends. The last five pairs of ribs are called *false ribs*

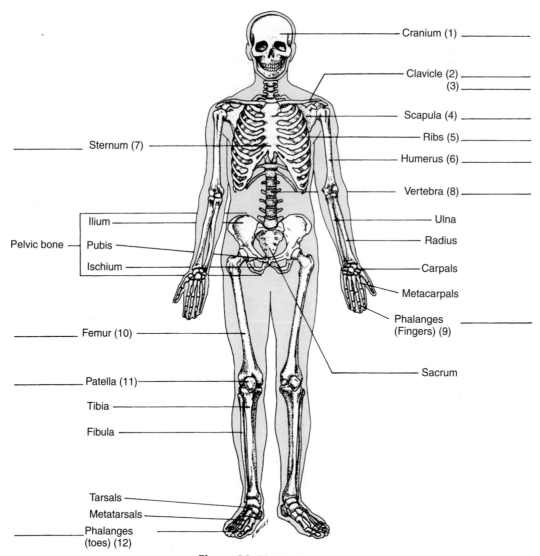

Figure 22-11 The skeleton.

because they do not attach directly to the sternum. The last two pairs are often referred to as *free* or *floating ribs*.

Sternum (1 Bone)

The sternum is the breastbone.

Appendicular Skeleton (126 Bones)

The appendicular skeleton consists of the limbs that have been appended to the axial skeleton.

Upper Extremities (64 Bones)

- *Clavicle (2):* Collar bone
- *Scapula (2):* Shoulder blade
- *Arm and hand bones (60):*
  - *Humerus (2):* Upper arm bone
  - *Ulna (2):* Smaller lower arm bone, small finger side
  - *Radius (2):* Larger lower arm bone, thumb side
  - *Carpals (16):* Wrist bones
  - *Metacarpals (10):* Bones of the hand
  - *Phalanges (28):* Three bones in each finger and two bones in each thumb

Lower Extremities (62 Bones)

In the child, the pelvic girdle consists of three pairs of separate bones: a superior element (the ilium) and two inferior elements (the ischium posteriorly and the pubis anteriorly). These bones fuse during adolescence and form the single pelvic bone on either side, characteristic of the adult.

- *Pelvic or hip bones (fused):*
  - *Ilium (2):* Upper hip bones
  - *Ischium (2):* Lower (sitting) hip bones
  - *Pubis (2):* Front hip bones
- *Leg and foot bones:*
  - *Femur (2):* Thigh bone; largest bone in the body
  - *Patella (2):* Kneecap
  - *Tibia (2):* Larger, inner lower leg bone (shin bone)
  - *Fibula (2):* Smaller, outer lower leg bone
  - *Tarsals (14):* Instep bones; form heel and back portion of foot
  - *Metatarsals (10):* Bones of the foot
  - *Phalanges (28):* Three bones in each toe, except for two in each big toe

Joints and Ligaments

A *joint* is that place in the skeleton where two or more bones meet. Joints allow for movement and hold bones together. Immovable joints, which are found only in the skull, are called *sutures.* In the newborn the sutures are not yet entirely closed; these fontanels or soft spots allow for "give" in the skull during the birth process. *Ligaments* are tough bands of tissue that connect one bone with another bone at a joint.

THE MUSCULAR SYSTEM

Organs of the Muscular System

Muscles: More than 600 muscles are included in the human body.

Muscular Functions

Muscles enable movement of body parts (including blood through blood vessels, food through the digestive system, and glandular secretions through ducts), maintain posture, stabilize joints, and generate heat. Supplies of oxygen and nerves to the muscle are necessary for adequate muscle function.

Types of Muscles

- *Skeletal muscle:* Skeletal muscles enable the body to move. These muscles are attached to the bones by tendons. Motion is produced by the contraction of muscles, and the muscles often work in pairs. Skeletal muscles are voluntary muscles in that they are controlled by the conscious portion of the brain.
- *Smooth muscle:* Smooth muscles generally make up the walls of hollow organs and serve to propel substances through body passageways and to adjust the pupil. Smooth muscles, which are involuntary muscles not under the control of the conscious part of the brain, may be found in the walls of blood vessels, in the eye, and in the digestive, urinary, and reproductive tracts.
- *Cardiac muscle:* Cardiac muscle, which is found only in the heart, is an involuntary muscle because it is not under the control of the conscious part of the brain, but it does respond to impulses from the autonomic nerves. It is especially conductive and contractile.

DISEASES AND CONDITIONS OF THE MUSCULOSKELETAL SYSTEM

Arthritis

More than 100 types of joint diseases are known; the two most common types are rheumatoid arthritis and osteoarthritis. Much is still unknown about the causes of arthritis; however, it has been observed that emotional upset can aggravate the disease.

Rheumatoid Arthritis

Rheumatoid arthritis, which is thought to be an autoimmune disease, usually occurs between the ages of 35 and 50 years, more commonly in women. The onset of symptoms, which include malaise, fever, weight loss, and stiffness of the joints, is gradual. The symptoms come and go. If the disease becomes chronic, degeneration of the joints, with permanent damage, occurs. Treatment consists of heat and drugs such as aspirin, nonsteroidal antiinflammatory drugs (NSAIDs), and corticosteroids, given to reduce inflammation and pain.

Osteoarthritis

Osteoarthritis, the most common form of arthritis, usually occurs in weight-bearing joints, such as the hips or knees, as chronic inflammation of the bone and joints caused by degenerative changes in the cartilage covering the surfaces of the joints. It occurs most often in older individuals. Treatment consists of drugs to reduce pain and inflammation and physical therapy to loosen the impaired joints.

Ruptured Disk

A *ruptured disk* also may be referred to as a *slipped* or *herniated disk* or as a *herniated nucleus pulposus (HNP)*. It is the abnormal protrusion of the soft, gelatinous core of an intervertebral disk (nucleus pulposus) into the neural canal that causes pressure on the spinal cord. Such herniation generally occurs in the lumbar spine (lower back). Treatment consists of bed rest, physical therapy, and analgesics. A laminectomy may be performed to remove a portion of the vertebra, creating more room for the protruding portion of the disk, or a diskectomy may be performed, in which the disk is removed and two or more vertebrae are fused together (Fig. 22-12).

Osteoporosis

Osteoporosis, an abnormal decrease in bone mass, is the leading cause of fractures because the bone tissue becomes porous, thin, and brittle. It is the most prevalent bone disease in the world. More than 20 million people in the United States have osteoporosis. Postmenopausal estrogen-deficient women are most likely to be affected. Age-related osteoporosis affects men and women equally. Osteoporosis is known as the "silent crippler," which results in a virtually symptomless process. Symptoms occur after the disease has progressed. The most common symptoms are pain and loss of height due to the bent-over position that the person assumes. The disease can cause up to an 8-inch loss in height. Fractures can occur in all parts of the skeletal system.

Osteoporosis is diagnosed by radiologic and laboratory studies performed to measure bone density and serum calcium levels. Because onset of the disease is virtually symptom free, the focus is on prevention to minimize bone loss. Preventive and therapeutic measures, aimed at improving bone density, include taking calcium supplements and vitamin D, performing weight-bearing exercise, undergoing hormone replacement therapy (if appropriate), and attending to correct posture. Bisphosphonates and calcitonin, drugs that slow down the dissolving process of the osteoclasts, are also useful in treating osteoporosis.

Paget Disease (Osteitis Deformans)

Paget disease, the second most common bone disease in the world, causes bones to become extremely weak. Affected individuals are generally older than 40 years of age. The bone may fracture with a very slight blow. If the vertebrae are involved, they may collapse. Bones are living substances that are involved

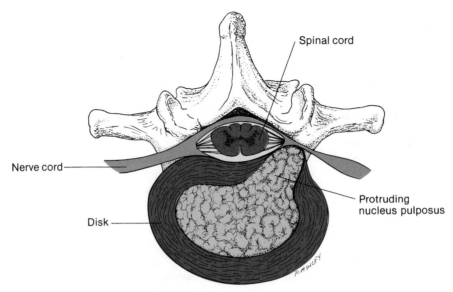

Figure 22-12 Ruptured disk.

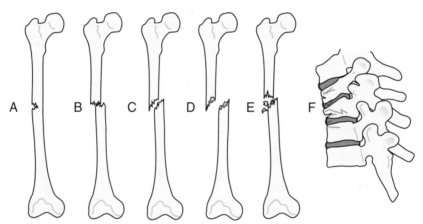

Figure 22-13 Types of fractures. **A,** Greenstick. **B,** Transverse. **C,** Oblique. **D,** Spiral. **E,** Comminuted. **F,** Compression.

in a constant process of dissolving and rebuilding. Osteoblasts are the cells that rebuild bone, and osteoclasts are the cells that dissolve bone. An imbalance of this dissolving and rebuilding process results in weak areas or lesions of the bone.

The symptoms of Paget disease depend on the bones that are affected. Lesions in long bones cause pain, bowing, and arthritic changes in the extremities. When the disease affects the skull, the patient may have headaches, ringing in the ears, hearing loss, and dizziness. If skull involvement affects the occipital region, pressure is placed on the cerebellum and may compress the spinal cord. Pressure on the spinal cord causes neurologic changes such as muscle weakness, loss of coordination, and ataxia.

Diagnosis is confirmed by abnormal radiologic studies characteristic of Paget disease and by elevated laboratory values for serum alkaline phosphatase, an enzyme produced by the osteoblasts during bone formation. Treatment for Paget disease includes use of a bisphosphonate or calcitonin to slow down the dissolving process of the osteoclasts.

Fractures

Fracture, the medical term for break (often abbreviated *Fx*), is an injury to a bone in which the bone is broken (Fig. 22-13).

A fracture is classified by the bone that is injured, such as fractured radius. Some types of fractures are listed here:

- *Closed (simple):* A broken bone with no open wound
- *Open (compound):* A broken bone with an open wound in the skin
- *Greenstick (incomplete):* A partially bent and partially broken bone; this is more commonly seen in children, in whom the bone is more pliable than in adults
- *Comminuted:* Splintered or crushed bone
- *Spiral:* A bone that has been twisted apart
- *Compression:* A fracture that occurs when the vertebrae collapse through trauma or pathology

An open or closed reduction is used to correct a displaced fracture to restore the fractured ends into normal alignment. In a closed reduction the bone is realigned through manipulation and/or traction without an incision, whereas an open reduction with internal fixation (ORIF) is performed after an incision has been made into the fracture site. Internal or external devices (plates, nails, screws, or rods) may be applied to maintain proper alignment of the bone during healing.

Joint Replacement

Joint replacement, a surgical procedure known as *arthroplasty,* is performed to replace an arthritic or damaged joint. An artificial joint, or *prosthesis,* is used to replace the patient's hip or knee joint. With total or partial arthroplasty, hip and knee joints and, less commonly, ankle, elbow, shoulder, wrist, and finger joints are replaced in cases of advanced osteoarthritis and improperly healed fracture, or to relieve a chronically painful or stiff joint.

⊖ REVIEW QUESTIONS

1. List five functions of the skeletal system.

2. What is the name of the thin membrane that covers bones.

3. List four types of bone, and describe bone structure.

4. Identify the 80 bones that are contained in the axial skeleton and the 126 bones that are contained in the appendicular skeleton.

5. Write the names of the bones that make up the cranium and the face. Indicate the number of each.

6. Name the bone in the throat that anchors the tongue.

7. Name the middle ear bones, and indicate the number of each.

8. List the five regions of the vertebral column, and indicate the number of vertebrae in each region.

9. Write the name of the bone to match the following definitions:
   a. shoulder
   b. collarbone
   c. upper arm bone
   d. lower arm bone, thumb side
   e. lower arm bone, finger side
   f. wrist bones
   g. bones of the hand
   h. finger bones

10. Write the names of three pairs of bones that are fused together to form the pelvis.

11. List the bones of the leg and foot.

12. Explain the function of joints and ligaments.

13. Describe four main functions of the muscular system.

14. Identify and discuss three types of muscles, and describe the function of tendons relating to skeletal muscles

15. Name and describe two types of arthritis.

16. Name two operations that may be performed for a ruptured disk.

17. What are cells that dissolve bone called, and what are cells that rebuild bone called?

18. What is an abnormal decrease in the amount of bone mass called?

19. In osteoporosis, what do preventive interventions include?

20. What symptoms are included when Paget disease affects the skull?

21. Define the following:

   a. closed fracture   d. comminuted fracture
   b. open fracture   e. greenstick fracture
   c. spiral fracture   f. compression fracture

22. What is another term for joint replacement, and what is the purpose of a joint replacement?

MEDICAL TERMINOLOGY RELATED TO THE MUSCULOSKELETAL SYSTEM—PREFIXES AND SUFFIXES

Objectives

On mastery of the medical terminology for this unit, you will be able to:

1. Define and spell the word parts and medical terms presented in this unit of study.
2. Analyze the medical terms built from word parts.
3. Given the meaning of a medical condition related to the musculoskeletal system, build with word parts the corresponding medical term.
4. Given descriptions of hospital situations in which the health unit coordinator (HUC) may encounter medical terminology, apply the correct medical terms to the situations.

Word Parts

In the following list are the word parts related to the skeletal system that you need to memorize. The exercises included in this unit will help you with this task. You will continue to use these word parts throughout the course and during employment. Practice pronouncing each word element aloud.

Skeletal System	Meaning
1. arthr / o (ar'-thrō)	joint
2. chondr / o (kŏn'-drō)	cartilage
3. clavic / o (klăv'-ĭ-kō)	clavicle (collarbone)
4. clavicul / o (klah-vĭk'-ū-lō)	clavicle (collarbone)
5. cost / o (kŏs'-tō)	rib
6. crani / o (krā'-nē-ō)	cranium (skull)
7. femor / o (fĕm'-or-ō)	femur (thigh bone)
8. humer / o (hūm'-er-ō)	humerus (upper arm bone)
9. lamin / o (lăm'-ĭ-nō)	lamina (bony arch of the vertebrae)

Skeletal System	Meaning
10. menisc / o (mĕ-nĭs′-kō)	meniscus (cartilage of the knee joint)
11. oste / o (ōs′-tē-ō)	bone
12. patell / o (pah-tĕl′-ō)	patella (kneecap)
13. phalang / o (fah-lăn′-jō)	phalange (finger or toe bone)
14. scapul / o (skăp′-ū-lō)	scapula (shoulder blade)
15. stern / o (ster′-nō)	sternum (breastbone)
16. vertebr / o (ver′-tĕ-brō)	vertebra (s), vertebrae (pl) (bones of the spine)

Muscular System	Meaning
muscul / o (mus′-kū-lō)	muscle
my / o (mĭ′-ō)	muscle
myos / o (mĭ′-ō-sō)	muscle

Other	Meaning
electr / o (ē-lĕk′-trō)	electricity, electrical activity
scoli / o (skō′-lē-ō)	crooked, curved (lateral)

EXERCISE 1

Write the combining forms for the skeletal system in the spaces provided on the diagram in Figure 22-11. The number preceding the combining form in the earlier list matches the number of the body part(s) in the diagram.

EXERCISE 2

Define each combining form listed.

1. arthr / o	11. scapul / o
2. oste / o	12. phalang / o
3. cost / o	13. vertebr / o
4. crani / o	14. clavic / o
5. femor / o	15. electr / o
6. my / o	16. lamin / o
7. humer / o	17. chondr / o
8. patell / o	18. menisc / o
9. stern / o	19. scoli / o
10. clavicul / o	

EXERCISE 3

Write the combining form for each part of the body listed.

1. finger bone	9. skull
2. joint	10. breastbone
3. bone	11. upper arm bone
4. thigh bone	12. rib
5. kneecap	13. muscle (3 forms)
6. shoulder blade	14. lamina
7. bones of the spine	15. cartilage
8. collarbone (2 forms)	16. meniscus

Recall from Units 1 and 2 that suffixes are letters that may be added to the end of a word root. The following list shows the suffixes that you need to know for this unit. Continue to use these throughout the chapter. The exercises will assist you in learning each suffix.

Suffix	Meaning
-algia (ăl′-ja)	pain
-ar, -ic	pertaining to (*Recall you have already learned -al, -ous*)
-centesis (sĕn-tē′-sĭs)	surgical puncture to aspirate fluid
-ectomy (ĕk′-to-mē)	surgical removal or excision
-gram	record, x-ray image, picture
-graph	instrument used to record
-graphy	process of recording, x-ray imaging, taking a picture
-osis (ō′-sĭs)	abnormal condition
-pathy (păthē)	disease of
-plasty (plăs′-tē)	surgical repair
-scope (skōp)	instrument used for visual examination
-scopy (skōp′-ē)	visual examination
-tomy (ŏt′-o-mē)	surgical incision, or to cut into
-trophy (trōf′-ē) (also may be used as a word root)	development, nourishment

EXERCISE 4

Write the suffix for each term listed.

1. surgical repair
2. pain
3. pertaining to (4 suffixes)
4. surgical incision
5. surgical removal
6. instrument used to record
7. process of recording
8. record, x-ray image, picture
9. development, nourishment
10. abnormal condition
11. instrument used for visual examination
12. visual examination
13. surgical puncture to aspirate fluid
14. disease of

EXERCISE 5

Write the definition for each suffix listed.

1. -algia	9. -ectomy
2. -graph	10. -ar
3. -gram	11. -osis
4. -graphy	12. -scopy
5. -tomy	13. -scope
6. -trophy	14. -centesis
7. -ic	15. -pathy
8. -plasty	

Recall from Unit 1 that prefixes are letters that may be added to the beginning of a word root to modify its meaning. Listed here are six prefixes that you need to memorize in this unit.

Prefix	Meaning
a-, an-	without or absence of (if used with a word root that begins with a vowel, use *an*; if used with a word root that begins with a consonant, use *a*)
dys- (dĭs)	difficult, painful, labored, abnormal
inter-	between

Prefix	Meaning
intra-	within
sub	below
supra-	above

 EXERCISE **6**

Write the prefix for each term listed.

1. within
2. painful
3. under
4. without
   (2 prefixes) a. b.
5. between
6. above

 EXERCISE **7**

Write the definition for each prefix listed. You may be asked to recall a prefix from previous study.

1. intra-
2. supra-
3. sub-
4. dys-
5. a-, an-
6. inter-

MEDICAL TERMS RELATED TO THE MUSCULOSKELETAL SYSTEM

In the following list are the medical terms for the musculoskeletal system that you need to know. Most are made up of the word roots, prefixes, and suffixes you have been working with; however, some words that relate to the musculoskeletal system are not made up of the word parts you have studied thus far. These are also included in the list. Following the list are exercises that will assist you in learning the meaning and spelling of each word. Practice pronouncing each word aloud.

General Terms	Meaning
atrophy (ăt′-rō-fē)	without development (a decrease in the size of a normally developed organ)
chondrogenic (kŏn-drō-jĕn′-ĭk)	producing cartilage
cranial (krā′-nē-al)	pertaining to the cranium
dystrophy (dĭs′-trō-fē)	abnormal development
femoral (fĕm′-ō-ral)	pertaining to the femur (or thigh bone)
humeral (hū′-mĕr-al)	pertaining to the humerus
intervertebral (ĭn-tĕr-vĕr′-tĕ-bral)	pertaining to between the vertebrae
intracranial (ĭn-trah-krā′-nē-al)	pertaining to within the cranium
orthopedics (or-thō-pē′-dĭks)	branch of medicine that deals with the diagnosis and treatment of disease, abnormalities, or fractures of the musculoskeletal system
orthopedist (or-thō-pē′-dist)	a doctor who specializes in orthopedics
osteoma (ŏs-tē-ō′-mah)	a tumor (composed of) bone
sternal (stĕr′-nal)	pertaining to the sternum

General Terms	Meaning
sternocostal (stĕr-nō-kŏs′-tal)	pertaining to the sternum and ribs
sternoid (stĕr′-noyd)	resembling the sternum
subcostal (sŭb-kŏs′-tal)	pertaining to below a rib or ribs
subscapular (sŭb-skăp′-ū-lar)	pertaining to below the scapula
suprascapular (soo-prah-skăp′-ū-lar)	pertaining to above the scapula
vertebrocostal (vĕr′-tĕ-brō-kŏs′-tal)	pertaining to the vertebrae and ribs

Surgical Terms	Meaning
arthroplasty (ar′-thrō-plăs′-tē)	surgical repair of a joint
arthrotomy (ar-thrŏt′-o-mē)	surgical incision of a joint
chondrectomy (kŏn-drĕk′-to-mē)	excision of a cartilage
clavicotomy (klăv-ĭ-kŏt′-o-mē)	surgical incision into the clavicle
costectomy (kŏs-tĕk′-to-mē)	excision of a rib
cranioplasty (krā′-nē-ō-plăs′-tē)	surgical repair of the cranium
craniotomy (krā-nē-ŏt′-o-mē)	surgical incision into the cranium
laminectomy (lăm-ĭ-nĕk′-to-mē)	surgical removal of lamina (often performed to relieve symptoms of a ruptured [slipped] disk)
meniscectomy (mĕn-ĭ-sĕk′-to-mē)	excision of the meniscus (of the knee joint)
patellectomy (păt-ĕ-lĕk′-to-mē)	excision of the patella
vertebrectomy (vĕr-tĕ-brĕk′-to-mē)	excision of a vertebra

Diagnostic Terms	Meaning
arthralgia (ar-thrăl′-ja)	pain in a joint
arthritis (ar-thrī′-tĭs)	inflammation of a joint
arthrosis (ar-thrŏ′-sĭs)	abnormal condition of a joint
chondritis (krŏn-drī′-tĭs)	inflammation of the cartilage
meniscitis (mĕn-ĭ-sī′-tĭs)	inflammation of the meniscus (of the knee joint)
muscular dystrophy (mŭs′-kū-lar) (dĭs′-trō-fē)	a number of muscle disorders characterized by a progressive, degenerative disease of the muscles
myoma (mī-ō′-mah)	a tumor (formed) of muscle (tissue)
myositis (mī-ō-sī′-tĭs)	inflammation of the muscles
scoliosis (skō-lē-ō′-sĭs)	abnormal condition of a (lateral) curve (of the spine)

Terms Related to Diagnostic Procedures	Meaning
arthrocentesis (ar-thrō-sĕn-tē′-sĭs)	surgical puncture to aspirate a joint
arthrogram (ar′-thrō-grăm)	x-ray image of a joint (contrast medium, dye, or air is used)
arthroscope (ar′-thrō-scōpe)	instrument used to visualize a joint (commonly the knee and shoulder)

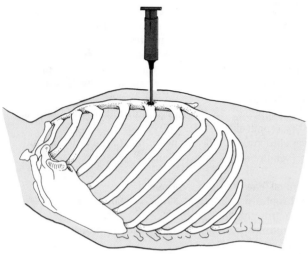

Figure 22-14 Sternal puncture. (From LaFleur M, Starr W: *Exploring medical language*, St Louis, 1985, Mosby, with permission.)

Terms Related to Diagnostic Procedures

	Meaning
arthroscopy (ar-thrŏs′-ko-pē)	visual examination of a joint (for diagnosing, identifying, and correcting problems)
electromyogram (ē-lĕk′-trō-mĭ′-ō-grăm) (EMG)	record of electrical activity of a muscle
electromyograph (ē-lĕk′-trō-mĭ′-ō-grăph)	instrument used to record the electrical activity of a muscle
electromyography (ē-lĕk′-trō-mī-ŏg′-rah-fē)	process of recording the electrical activity of muscle
sternal puncture (stĕr′-nal) (pŭngk′-chŭr)	insertion of a hollow needle into the sternum to obtain a sample of bone marrow to be studied in the laboratory (Fig. 22-14) (used for diagnosing blood disorders such as anemia and leukemia)

⊜ EXERCISE 8

Analyze and define each medical term listed.

1. electromyogram
2. myoma
3. sternoclavicular
4. cranial
5. vertebrocostal
6. arthritis
7. intervertebral
8. humeral
9. dystrophy
10. subscapular
11. arthrosis
12. electromyography
13. arthrogram
14. electromyograph
15. sternocostal
16. arthralgia
17. subcostal
18. femoral
19. clavicotomy
20. arthrotomy
21. intracranial
22. atrophy
23. arthroplasty
24. osteoma
25. costectomy
26. cranioplasty
27. patellectomy
28. vertebrectomy
29. craniotomy
30. suprascapular
31. myositis
32. chondrogenic
33. arthroscopy
34. chondritis
35. arthroscope
36. chondrectomy
37. laminectomy
38. sternal
39. meniscectomy
40. arthrocentesis
41. meniscitis

⊜ EXERCISE 9

Using word roots, prefixes, suffixes, and combining vowels as needed, build a medical term from each definition listed.

1. pertaining to the cranium
2. inflammation of muscle
3. pertaining to below the scapula
4. pertaining to the femur
5. surgical incision into a joint
6. excision of a cartilage
7. pain in a joint
8. inflammation in a joint
9. abnormal condition of a joint
10. pertaining to the humerus
11. without development
12. pertaining to the vertebrae and ribs
13. surgical incision into the cranium
14. surgical removal of a rib
15. pertaining to below the rib
16. x-ray image of a joint
17. surgical removal of a vertebra
18. record of the electrical activity of a muscle
19. surgical incision into the clavicle
20. process of recording electrical activity of a muscle
21. abnormal development
22. a tumor (formed) of muscle (tissue)
23. machine used to record electrical activity of a muscle
24. pertaining to the sternum and clavicle
25. pertaining to between the vertebrae
26. pertaining to within the cranium
27. pertaining to the sternum and rib
28. surgical removal of the patella
29. surgical repair of the cranium
30. a tumor composed of bone
31. surgical incision into the clavicle
32. producing cartilage
33. visual examination of a joint
34. instrument used for visual examination of a joint
35. inflammation of cartilage
36. excision of cartilage
37. surgical removal of the lamina
38. pertaining to the sternum
39. puncture and aspiration of a joint
40. excision of the meniscus
41. inflammation of the meniscus

⊜ EXERCISE 10

Define each medical term listed.

1. orthopedics
2. orthopedist
3. muscular dystrophy
4. sternal puncture

⊖ EXERCISE **11**

Spell each of the 45 medical terms studied in this unit by having someone dictate the terms to you.

1.	16.	31.
2.	17.	32.
3.	18.	33.
4.	19.	34.
5.	20.	35.
6.	21.	36.
7.	22.	37.
8.	23.	38.
9.	24.	39.
10.	25.	40.
11.	26.	41.
12.	27.	42.
13.	28.	43.
14.	29.	44.
15.	30.	45.

⊖ EXERCISE **12**

Answer the following questions.

1. What is the name of the nursing unit in the hospital that cares for patients with *fractures, abnormalities,* or *diseases of the bone?* What is the name of the doctor who specializes in this area of medicine?
2. A _____ tray is used by the doctor to obtain a *sample of bone marrow from the sternum.* The tray is named after the procedure.
3. The doctor ordered a procedure to determine the *electrical activity of a muscle.* What is this procedure called?
4. Following is a list of diagnostic phrases. In the space provided, write the name of the fractured bone.

   Example: fractured femur thigh bone

   a. fractured tibia

   b. fractured humerus

   c. fractured cervical 6 (C6)

   d. fractured ilium

   e. fractured clavicle

   f. fractured radius

5. A surgery schedule is a list of operations to be performed on a given day in the hospital. Following are the types of operations recorded on the surgery schedule. Indicate the terms that are incorrectly spelled by rewriting the term correctly.

   a. castectomy
   b. craniotomy
   c. lamonectomy
   d. clavictamy
   e. cranioplasty
   f. patelectomy
   g. ostoarthrotomy
   h. meniscectomy

6. The doctor ordered an x-ray procedure that requires the use of contrast medium to be performed on a joint. What is this procedure called? What is puncture and aspiration of a joint called?

ABBREVIATIONS

Abbreviation	Meaning
AKA	above the knee amputation
BKA	below the knee amputation
EMG	electromyogram
Fx	fracture
HNP	herniated nucleus pulposus
NSAID	nonsteroidal antiinflammatory drugs
ORIF	open reduction, internal fixation
THA	total hip arthroplasty
THR	total hip replacement

⊖ EXERCISE **13**

Define the following abbreviations.

1. AKA
2. BKA
3. Fx
4. ORIF
5. HNP
6. NSAID
7. EMG
8. THA
9. THR

UNIT 4
The Nervous System

UNIT OBJECTIVES

On completion of this unit, you will be able to:

1. Identify the two divisions of the nervous system, and identify the structures of each division.
2. Describe the overall functions of the nervous system.
3. Describe the structure and functions of the organs of the nervous system.
4. Describe the function of the meninges, and identify and describe the three layers of the meninges.
5. Discuss a cerebrovascular accident (CVA), a transient ischemic attack (TIA), Parkinson's disease, Alzheimer disease, amyotrophic lateral sclerosis (ALS), and epilepsy.
6. Read the objectives related to medical terminology, and demonstrate ability to meet the objectives by correctly completing Exercises 1 through 11.
7. Define the unit abbreviations.

THE NERVOUS SYSTEM

Organs of the Nervous System

- Nerves
- Brain
- Spinal cord

Divisions of the Nervous System

The nervous system is commonly divided into two parts:

1. The central nervous system (CNS) consists of the brain and spinal cord.
2. The peripheral nervous system (PNS) consists of the nerves of the body (12 pairs of cranial nerves and 31 pairs of spinal nerves). The autonomic (involuntary) and somatic (voluntary) nervous systems are subdivisions of the PNS. The autonomic nervous system is further divided into the sympathetic (fight or flight) and parasympathetic (tranquil: rest and digestion) nervous systems.

Functions of the Nervous System

All body parts and systems must work together to maintain a healthy body. The nervous system monitors, regulates, and controls the functions of body organs and body systems by using nerve impulses to transmit information from one part of the body to another (Fig. 22-15). The nervous system works in concert with the endocrine system to maintain homeostasis, a constant internal environment, by inhibiting or stimulating the release of hormones.

Nerves

A *nerve* is a cordlike structure that is located outside the CNS. It contains nerve cells called *neurons.* The neuron transmits nerve

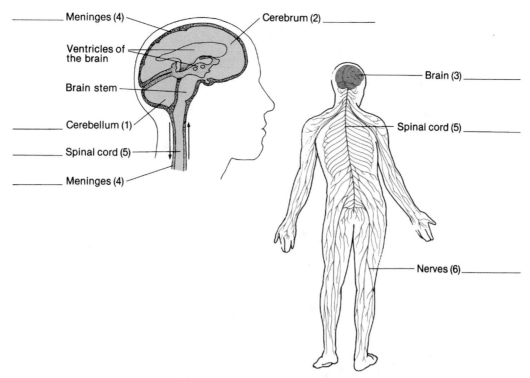

Figure 22-15 The nervous system.

impulses from one part of the body to another. Two types of neurons are as follows:

1. Sensory neurons, which transmit impulses to the brain and spinal cord
2. Motor neurons, which transmit impulses from the brain and spinal cord to the muscles or glands

Brain

The brain is located within the cranial cavity and is the main center for coordinating body activities. The brain is divided into three parts: the cerebrum, the cerebellum, and the brainstem. Each part of the brain is responsible for controlling certain body functions.

The *cerebrum* is the largest part of the brain. It is located in the upper portion of the cranium. The cerebrum is divided into right and left hemispheres, which are connected only at the lower middle portion. The cerebrum contains the sensory, motor, sight, and hearing centers. Memory, intellect, judgment, and emotional reactions also take place in the cerebrum.

Four spaces within the brain, called *ventricles,* produce a watery fluid known as *cerebrospinal fluid (CSF).* This cushion of fluid surrounds the brain and spinal cord. Its functions are to absorb shocks that may occur to the spinal cord or brain and to nourish and remove waste from the nervous tissue. The *cerebellum,* or "little brain," is situated below the posterior portion of the cerebrum. Its functions are to assist in the coordination of voluntary muscles and to maintain balance. The *brainstem* has three main parts: the midbrain, pons, and medulla oblongata. It contains the nerve fibers that form the connecting links between the different parts of the brain and the centers that control three vital functions: blood pressure (BP), respiration, and heartbeat.

Spinal Cord

The spinal cord extends from the brainstem and passes through the spinal cavity to between the first and second lumbar vertebrae (see Fig. 22-17, *A*). The spinal cord is the pathway for conducting *sensory impulses* up to the brain and *motor impulses* down from the brain. Injury to the spinal cord can result in paralysis, the loss of voluntary muscle function.

Meninges

The meninges are made up of three layers of connective tissue that completely surround and protect the spinal cord and brain. The outer tough layer is called the *dura mater.* The middle layer is the *arachnoid (mater),* a weblike structure. The inner thin, tender layer, the *pia mater,* carries blood vessels that provide nourishment to the nervous tissue. CSF flows through a space between the arachnoid and the pia mater called the *subarachnoid space* (see Fig. 22-17, *C*).

DISEASES AND CONDITIONS OF THE NERVOUS SYSTEM

Cerebrovascular Accident

Cerebrovascular accident (CVA), also called a *stroke,* is the interference of blood flow to the brain, which reduces the supply of oxygen and nutrients, causing damage to brain tissue. The major causes of CVA are embolism, thrombosis, and hemorrhage (Fig. 22-16). Strokes affect about 700,000 people each year, causing death in one quarter of them. Stroke is the third leading cause of death in the United States and the primary cause of disability.

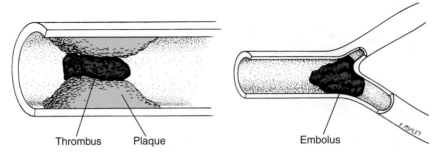

Thrombus   Plaque   Embolus

Figure 22-16 Thrombus (blood clot) or embolus (floating mass that blocks a vessel) in a cerebral artery can cause a cerebrovascular accident (CVA).

Damage to the brain tissue varies according to the artery affected. Paralysis is a result of the damage, and it may range from slight to complete hemiplegia (paralysis of one side of the body). CVA of the left hemisphere of the brain produces symptoms on the right side of the body, and CVA of the right side of the brain produces symptoms on the left side of the body. The more quickly the circulation returns, the better the chance for recovery.

⭐ HIGH PRIORITY

Cerebrovascular Accident (Stroke) Warning Signs and Treatment
Warning Signs
- Sudden numbness, weakness, or paralysis of the face, arm, or leg, especially on one side of the body
- Sudden confusion; problems with memory or perception
- Sudden loss of speech; difficulty speaking or understanding
- Sudden trouble seeing out of one or both eyes; blurred or double vision
- Sudden difficulty walking, dizziness, or loss of balance or coordination
- Sudden, severe headache with no known cause

Thrombolytic Treatment
Tissue plasminogen activator (tPA) is a thrombolytic agent (clot-busting drug) approved for use in certain patients who are having a heart attack or stroke caused by blood clots that block blood flow. This class of drugs may dissolve blood clots, which cause most heart attacks and ischemic strokes, if given within 3 hours of the onset of symptoms. Administered by hospital personnel through an intravenous line, tPA can reduce significantly the effects of a stroke caused by a clot, including permanent disability.

Transient Ischemic Attack

Transient ischemic attacks (TIAs) are recurrent episodes of decreased neurologic function that occur as double vision, slurred speech, weakness in the legs, and dizziness lasting from seconds to 24 hours, then clearing. TIAs are considered warning signs for strokes. TIAs are caused by small emboli that temporarily interrupt blood flow to the brain. Treatment includes administration of aspirin and anticoagulants to minimize

thrombosis in the hope of preventing a CVA. Preventive treatment may include a *carotid endarterectomy,* a surgical procedure that is performed to remove the thickened inner area of the carotid artery.

Parkinson Disease

Parkinson disease, also called *shaking palsy, parkinsonism,* and *paralysis agitans,* is one of the most common crippling diseases in the United States. Parkinson disease, a gradually progressive disorder of the CNS, occurs with degeneration of the dopamine-releasing neurons in the *substantia nigra,* an area of the brain. Dopamine, one of the chemical messengers (*neurotransmitters*) responsible for transmitting signals within the brain, initiates and controls movement and balance. The cause of Parkinson disease is most often unknown, but it is thought to result from genetic factors, viral infection, exposure to toxins, or cerebral arteriosclerosis. Symptoms include muscle rigidity, tremors, and a shifting gait. Deterioration is progressive. No cure is known; treatment is aimed at relieving symptoms and promoting function for as long as possible. Parkinson disease does not impair intellect. A recently developed device similar to a pacemaker is implanted in the brain and provides deep brain stimulation, which may offer some relief from tremors and involuntary movements.

Alzheimer Disease

Alzheimer disease, also called *presenile dementia,* is characterized by confusion, mental deterioration (dementia), restlessness, hallucinations, and the inability to carry out purposeful speech and movement. The patient may lose bowel and bladder control and refuse to eat. The disease is progressive and usually begins in later midlife. Because the precise cause of Alzheimer disease has not been identified, definitive treatment has not been established. Care of the patient generally includes maintaining proper hygiene, providing appropriate nutrition, preventing injury, and promoting purposeful activity. New medications and treatments continue to be developed to help the Alzheimer patient retain memory and to promote other mental functions for as long as possible.

Amyotrophic Lateral Sclerosis

Amyotrophic lateral sclerosis (ALS), often referred to as *"Lou Gehrig disease,"* is a progressive neurodegenerative disease that affects nerve cells in the brain and the spinal cord. The word *a-myo-trophic* comes from the Greek language. *A* means "no" or "negative." *Myo* refers to muscle, and *trophic* means "nourishment"—"No muscle nourishment." When a muscle has no nourishment, it "atrophies" or wastes away. *Lateral* identifies the areas in a person's spinal cord where portions of the nerve cells that signal and control the muscles are located. As this area degenerates, scarring or hardening *(sclerosis)* occurs in the region. When the motor neurons die, the ability of the brain to initiate and control muscle movement is lost. With voluntary muscle action progressively affected, patients in the later stages of the disease may become totally paralyzed.

Epilepsy

Epilepsy, a group of chronic disorders of the CNS, is the result of abnormal electrical (neuron) activity in the brain. It is common to hear epilepsy and seizure used synonymously; the difference is that epilepsy is the disease, and seizure is the result of the disease. Epilepsy usually occurs in childhood or after age 50. The disease can be classified as idiopathic (origin unknown) or acquired. Some of the known causes of acquired epilepsy are brain tumors, brain injury, and endocrine disorders. Seizures that result from fever, otitis media, or drug toxicity are usually isolated incidents and do not warrant the diagnosis of epilepsy.

Seizures are classified according to the origin of the abnormal brain signals. Involvement of the entire brain is known as *generalized seizure*, whereas a *partial seizure* is one in which abnormal electrical activity occurs in a particular region of the brain.

Seizure activity is divided into three stages. (1) During the *preictal* stage, the patient may experience abnormal somatic and psychic sensations, including strange sounds, tastes, and smells. These sensations are called an *aura*. (2) The second stage is called *interictal* and includes violent jerking of some parts of or the total body. The patient may experience a grand mal seizure characterized by incontinence of urine and stool, foaming or frothing from the mouth, changes in skin color, tongue biting, arching of the back, and turning of the head to one side. (3) The period immediately after the seizure is called the *postictal stage*. During this stage the patient may become confused and lethargic and may report headache and sore muscles. The petit mal seizure, another form of generalized seizure, is marked by a brief loss of consciousness along with unresponsive behaviors.

Diagnosis is confirmed by observation of the seizure activity, blood testing to rule out other ailments, and magnetic resonance imaging (MRI) or computed tomography (CT) scan of the brain to look for a lesion. An electroencephalogram (EEG) also may locate the site and possible cause of the disorder. Additional studies include EP (evoked potential), which is a group of tests that measure brain wave changes in response to various stimuli, and positron emission tomography (PET) scanning, a nuclear medicine test that more closely studies brain function and metabolism.

Treatment requires stabilization on anticonvulsant drugs (see Chapter 13 for a list of these drugs); 95% of the population responds to drug therapy. The other 5% is treated surgically to remove affected brain tissue. Patient education is included in the treatment regimen. Information about seizure triggers and how to avoid those triggers is an important part of patient education. A national association (National Association of Epilepsy Centers; www.naec-epilepsy.org) has been formed to help the patient deal with self-esteem issues and the stigma that is still attached to epilepsy. Because of stigmatization, many people who have epilepsy will not wear an identification bracelet and will not inform others of their illness.

 HIGH PRIORITY

Patients who are experiencing a seizure need to be protected from injury, especially head injury. Remove any furniture or other objects that the patient may strike. If possible, put a pillow under the patient's head. Call for help. *Do not try to restrain the movements of the patient.* Protect the patient's privacy. Ask those who are uninvolved with the care of patients to please leave the area.

REVIEW QUESTIONS

1. Identify the two divisions of the nervous system, and identify the structures of each division.

2. Describe the overall functions of the nervous system.

3. What is a nerve cell called? What are the two types of nerve cells?

4. Name three parts of the brain, and describe the functions of each.

5. Describe the location and function of the spinal cord.

6. The meninges are made up of three layers of tissue. What is the tough outer layer called? What is the middle layer called? What is the inner layer called?

7. Match the terms in Column 1 with the appropriate phrases in Column 2.

Column 1	Column 2
a. Parkinson disease	1. also called *shaking palsy*
b. Alzheimer disease	2. result of abnormal electrical (neuron) activity in the brain
c. transient ischemic attack	3. also called a stroke
d. cerebrovascular accident	4. also called Lou Gehrig disease
e. amyotrophic lateral sclerosis	5. symptoms include confusion and hallucinations
f. epilepsy	6. warning sign for strokes

8. Name the three stages of a seizure.

MEDICAL TERMINOLOGY RELATED TO THE NERVOUS SYSTEM AND PSYCHOLOGY

Objectives

On mastery of the medical terminology for this unit, you will be able to:

1. Spell and define the word parts and medical terms that relate to the nervous system.
2. Analyze the medical terms related to the nervous system that are built from word parts.
3. Given the meaning of a medical condition related to the nervous system, build with word parts the corresponding medical term.
4. Spell and use in sentence form the psychology terminology presented in this unit.
5. Given descriptions of hospital situations in which the HUC may encounter medical terminology, apply the correct medical terms to the situations.

Word Parts

The following list shows the word parts related to the nervous system that you need to memorize. The exercises included in this unit will help you with this task. You will continue to use these word parts throughout the course and during employment. Practice pronouncing each word element aloud.

Word Roots/Combining Forms	Meaning
1. cerebell / o (sĕr-ĕ-bĕl′-ō)	cerebellum (little brain)
2. cerebr/ o (sĕr′-ē-brō)	cerebrum (main portion of the brain)
3. dur / o (dū′-rō)	dura mater (outer meningeal layer)
4. encephal / o (ĕn-sĕf′-ah-lō)	brain
5. mening / o (mĕ-nĭng′-gō)	meninges (spinal cord covering)
6. myel / o (mī′-ĕl-ō)	spinal cord (also means *bone marrow*)
7. neur / o (nū′-rō)	nerve
8. phas / o (fāz′-ō)	speech
9. psych / o (sī′-kō)	mind

Other Word Root/ Combining Form	Meaning
poli / o (pō′-lē-ō)	gray matter
quadr/o (kwahd′-rō)	four

Prefixes	Meanings
hemi-	half
para-	beside, beyond, around

Suffixes	Meaning
-cele (sēl)	herniation or protrusion
-ia	abnormal condition of
-plegia (plē′-ja)	paralysis, stroke
-rrhagia (rah′-ja)	rapid flow of blood
-rrhaphy (rah′-fē)	to suture (surgical), repair
-rrhea (rē′-ah)	excessive discharge, flow

EXERCISE 1

Write in the spaces provided the combining forms for the parts of the nervous system shown on the diagram in Figure 22-15). The number preceding the combining form in the earlier list matches the number of the body part on the diagram.

EXERCISE 2

Define each combining form listed.

1. cerebr / o
2. encephal / o
3. neur / o
4. poli / o
5. mening / o
6. dur / o
7. myel / o
8. cerebell / o
9. phas / o
10. psych / o
11. quadr / o

EXERCISE 3

Write the combining forms for each term listed.

1. nerve
2. cerebrum
3. meninges
4. spinal cord
5. cerebellum
6. brain
7. dura mater
8. gray matter
9. speech
10. mind
11. four

EXERCISE 4

Write the suffix(es) that match each definition. (Note: This exercise includes suffixes from this unit and from previous units. Refer back as needed.)

1. tumor
2. surgical repair
3. pertaining to
4. to suture
5. excessive discharge
6. inflammation
7. specialist
8. record, x-ray image, picture
9. study of
10. rapid discharge
11. herniation
12. surgical removal
13. incision
14. pain
15. abnormal condition of

EXERCISE 5

Write the definition for each prefix and suffix listed. (Note: This exercise includes suffixes from this unit and from previous units. Refer back as needed.)

1. -gram
2. -itis
3. -logy
4. -rrhea
5. -rrhagia
6. -rrhaphy
7. -cele
8. -ar, -al
9. -ectomy
10. -plasty
11. -tomy
12. -algia
13. -osis
14. -ia
15. -plegia
16. hemi-
17. para-
18. -ic, -ous

MEDICAL TERMS RELATED TO THE NERVOUS SYSTEM

Listed here are medical terms related to the nervous system that you will need to know. Exercises following this list will assist you in learning these terms. Practice pronouncing these terms aloud.

General Terms	Meaning
aphasia (ah-fā′-zha)	abnormal condition characterized by no speech (loss of expression or understanding of speech or writing)
cerebrospinal (ser′-ē-brō-spī′-nal)	pertaining to the brain and spine
hemiplegia (hĕm-ĭ-plē′-ja)	paralysis of the right or left side of the body (usually caused by a stroke)
myelorrhagia (mī-ĕ-lō-rā′-ja)	rapid flow of blood into the spinal cord
neurologist (nū-rŏl′-o-jĭst)	one who specializes in the diagnosis and treatment of disorders of the nerves
neurology (nū-rŏl′-o-jē)	the study of nerves (the branch of medicine that deals with the diagnosis and treatment of disorders or diseases of the nervous system)
paraplegia (păr-ăh-plē′-ja)	paralysis of the legs and sometimes the lower part of the body, usually caused by injury to the spinal cord
quadriplegia (kwăd-rĕ-plē′-ja)	paralysis that affects all four limbs

Surgical Terms	Meaning
neuroplasty (nū′-rō-plăs′-tē)	surgical repair of a nerve
neurorrhaphy (nū-rŏr′-ah-fē)	suturing of a nerve

Diagnostic Terms	Meaning
cephalalgia (sĕf-ah-lăl′-ja)	pain in the head (headache)
cerebellitis (ser-ĕ-bĕl-ĭ′-tĭs)	inflammation of the cerebellum
cerebral palsy (ser′-ē-bral) (paul′-zē)	partial paralysis and lack of muscle coordination that results from a defect, injury, or disease of the brain that is present at birth or shortly thereafter
cerebrosis (ser-ĕ-brō′-sĭs)	abnormal condition of the cerebrum (of the brain)
cerebrovascular (ser′-ĕ-brō-văs′-kŭ-lăr) accident (CVA)	impaired blood supply to parts of the brain; also called a *stroke*
encephalitis (ĕn-sĕf-ah-lī′-tĭs)	inflammation of the brain
encephalocele (ĕn-sĕf′-ah-lō-sēl)	herniation of brain (tissue through a gap in the skull)
epilepsy (ĕp′-ĭ-lĕp-sē)	convulsive disorder of the nervous system characterized by chronic or recurrent seizures

Diagnostic Terms	Meaning
meningitis (mĕn-ĭn-jī′-tĭs)	inflammation of the meninges
meningomyelocele (mĕ-nĭng-gō-mī′-ĕ-lō-sĕl)	protrusion of the spinal cord and meninges (through the vertebral column)
multiple sclerosis (mŭl′-tĭ-pl) (sklĕ-rō′-sĭs) (MS)	a degenerative disease of the nerves that control the muscles, characterized by hardening patches along the brain and spinal cord
neuralgia (nū-răl′-ja)	pain in a nerve
neuritis (nū-rī′-tĭs)	inflammation of a nerve
neuroma (nū-rō′-mah)	a tumor made up of nerve (cells)
poliomyelitis (pō′-lē-ō-mī-ĕ-lī′-tĭs)	inflammation of the gray matter of the spinal cord (virally caused disease, commonly known as *polio*)
syncope (sĭng′-cō-pē)	fainting or "passing out," often because of a sudden decline of blood flow to the brain
subdural hematoma (sŭb-dū′-ral) (hēm-ah-tō′-mah)	blood tumor that pertains to the area below the dura mater (accumulation of blood in the subdural space)

Terms Related to Diagnostic Procedures	Meaning
CT scan (computed tomography)	use of radiologic imaging that produces images of bloodless "slices" of the body; CT scanning can detect hemorrhages, tumors, and brain abnormalities
electroencephalogram (ē-lĕk′-trō-ĕn-sĕf′-ăh-lō-grăm) (EEG)	record of the electrical activity of the brain
lumbar puncture (lŭm′-băr) (pŭngk′-chŭr) (LP)	removal of cerebrospinal fluid (CSF) for diagnostic and therapeutic purposes; a hollow needle is inserted into the subarachnoid space between the third and fourth lumbar vertebrae (Fig. 22-17)
magnetic resonance imaging (MRI)	noninvasive procedure for imaging tissues that cannot be seen via other radiologic techniques; the advantage of this diagnostic procedure is not only the avoidance of harmful radiation through its use of magnetic fields and radiofrequencies, but also the ability to detect small brain abnormalities; patients with pacemakers or any metallic foreign bodies generally cannot undergo this procedure
myelogram (mī′-ĕ-lō-grăm)	x-ray image of the spinal cord (injected dye is used as the contrast medium)

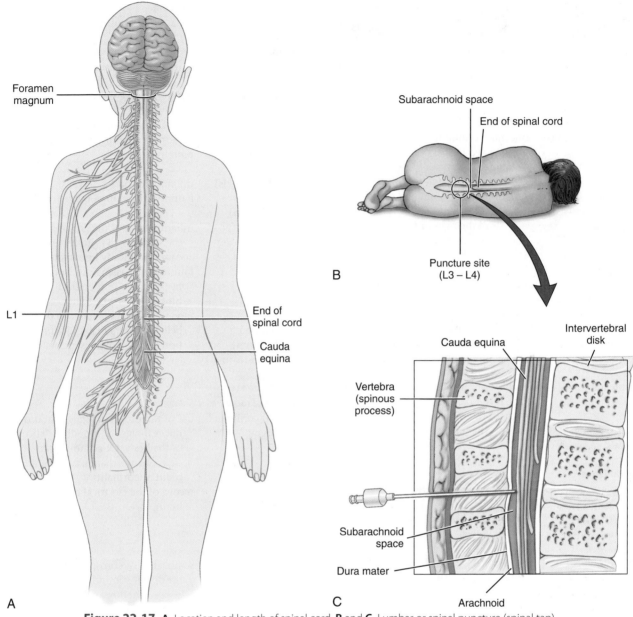

Figure 22-17 A, Location and length of spinal cord. **B** and **C,** Lumbar or spinal puncture (spinal tap).

⊜ E X E R C I S E **6**

Analyze and define each medical term listed.

1. neurology
2. cerebrospinal
3. neuralgia
4. poliomyelitis
5. neuroplasty
6. encephalitis
7. meningitis
8. neuropathy
9. neurologist
10. encephalocele
11. electroencephalogram
12. meningomyelocele
13. cerebellitis
14. cerebrosis
15. neuroma
16. myelorrhagia
17. myelogram
18. neuritis

⊜ E X E R C I S E **7**

Define each medical term listed.

1. multiple sclerosis
2. epilepsy
3. cerebral palsy
4. cerebrovascular accident
5. echoencephalography
6. hemiplegia
7. paraplegia
8. quadriplegia
9. lumbar puncture
10. subdural hematoma
11. CT scan
12. MRI
13. aphasia

⊜ EXERCISE 8

Using the word elements studied in this unit and in previous units, build a medical term from each of the definitions listed.

1. inflammation of a nerve
2. inflammation of the brain
3. inflammation of the meninges
4. surgical repair of a nerve
5. one who specializes in the diagnosis and treatment of nerves
6. disease of a nerve
7. tumor made of nerve cells
8. pain in a nerve
9. pertaining to the cerebrum and spine
10. herniation of the meninges and spinal cord (through the vertebral column)
11. inflammation of the cerebellum
12. herniation of the brain (through a gap in the skull)
13. rapid flow of blood into the spinal cord
14. record of the electrical activity of the brain
15. x-ray image of the spinal cord

⊜ EXERCISE 9

Spell each of the 33 medical terms studied in this unit by having someone dictate the terms to you.

1.	18.
2.	19.
3.	20.
4.	21.
5.	22.
6.	23.
7.	24.
8.	25.
9.	26.
10.	27.
11.	28.
12.	29.
13.	30.
14.	31.
15.	32.
16.	33.
17.	

TERMS RELATED TO PSYCHOLOGY

An extensive knowledge of psychology vocabulary is not necessary for general hospital employment; therefore we will discuss only those terms that you as a HUC may encounter in general medical and surgical areas of employment.

Psych / o is a combining form meaning "mind." The following words are developed from the word root *psych* and suffixes, most of which you have already studied.

Psychology Terms	Meaning
psychiatrist (sī-kī'-ah-trĭst)	a doctor who specializes in the mind
psychiatry (sī-kī'-ah-trē)	treatment of the mind (a branch of medicine that deals with the study, treatment, and prevention of mental illness)
psychologist (sī-kŏl'-ō-jĭst)	one who specializes in the diagnosis and treatment of the mind (a person trained to perform psychological analysis, therapy, or research, generally at a master's or doctoral [PhD] level of education)
psychology (sī-kŏl'-ō-jē)	study of the mind (behavior)
psychosis (sī-kō'-sĭs)	abnormal condition of the mind

Psychology Terms	Meaning
neur / o (nū'-rō)	the combining form that means "nerve"; it may be used to describe certain psychiatric disorders, as in the following terms
neurosis (nŭ-rō'-sĭs)	an emotional disorder considered less serious than a psychosis
neurotic (nŭ-rŏt'-ĭk)	having a neurosis
psychosomatic (sī-kō-sō-măt'-ĭk)	pertaining to the mind and body (relationship)

⊜ EXERCISE 10

Spell each of the eight psychology terms studied in this unit by having someone dictate the terms to you.

1.	5.
2.	6.
3.	7.
4.	8.

⊜ EXERCISE 11

Answer the following questions.

1. What is the name of the nursing unit in the hospital that cares for patients with disorders of the nervous system? What is the name of the doctor who specializes in this area of medicine?
2. The patient is admitted to the hospital with the admitting diagnosis of stroke or _____. What is the abbreviation for this term? The patient is paralyzed on the left side of her body. What does she have?
3. A child is diagnosed as having an inflammation of the meninges or _____. The doctor performs a procedure to obtain cerebrospinal fluid for diagnostic study. What is the procedure called? To perform this procedure, the doctor uses a special tray named after the procedure. What is this tray called?
4. Name four diagnostic procedures that end in the suffix *-graphy* that the doctor may order to gather information about the nervous system organs or about their functions.

ABBREVIATIONS

Abbreviation	Meaning
CNS	central nervous system
CSF	cerebrospinal fluid
CT	computed tomography
CVA	cerebrovascular accident (stroke)
EEG	electroencephalogram
EP	evoked potentials
LP	lumbar puncture
MRI	magnetic resonance imaging
MS	multiple sclerosis
PET	positron emission tomography
PNS	peripheral nervous system
TIA	transient ischemic attack

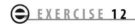 EXERCISE **12**

Define the following abbreviations.

1. CNS
2. CSF
3. CT
4. CVA
5. EEG
6. EP
7. LP
8. MS
9. PNS
10. PET
11. MRI
12. TIA

UNIT 5
The Eye and the Ear

OUTLINE

UNIT OBJECTIVES

On completion of this unit, you will be able to:

1. Describe the function and structure of the eye.
2. List five body structures that help protect the eye.
3. Identify and describe the parts and accessory structures of the eye, and briefly describe the function of each part.
4. Name and describe the functions of the two types of nerve cells located in the retina.
5. Describe the location and functions of the aqueous and vitreous humor.
6. List in order, beginning with the conjunctiva, the organs of the eye through which light rays travel to the retina.
7. Discuss cataract, glaucoma, retinal detachment, and macular degeneration.
8. Describe two functions of the ear.
9. List the parts of the outer ear, middle ear, and the inner ear.
10. Trace the travel of sound waves from the outside environment to the brain.
11. Describe and discuss two treatments for tinnitus.
12. Read the objectives related to medical terminology, and demonstrate ability to meet the objectives by correctly completing Exercises 1 through 8.
13. Define the unit abbreviations.

THE EYE

The eye (Fig. 22-18) is the organ of vision. The eye receives light waves that are focused on the retina and produces visual nerve impulses that are transmitted to the visual area of the brain by the optic nerve. The eye is divided into three layers: sclera, choroid, and retina.

The eye, a spherical, delicate structure, is protected by the skull bones and its accessory organs: eyelashes (close eyelids when disturbed), eyelids (protect and shade), lacrimal apparatus (glands secrete lubricating tears), and conjunctiva (protective membrane). The *conjunctiva* is a transparent membrane that lines the upper and lower eyelids and the anterior portion of the eye. It helps protect the eye from harmful bacteria.

The *sclera*, the outer protective layer of the eye, helps maintain the shape of the eyeball and is the site for muscle attachment. We can see the anterior portion of the sclera. It is often referred to as the *white of the eye*. The *cornea* is the transparent, avascular part of the sclera that lies over the iris of the eye and allows light rays to enter.

The middle layer of the eye is called the *choroid*. The choroid contains blood vessels that supply nutrients to the eye. The *iris* and the *ciliary muscle* make up the anterior middle portion of the choroid. The iris, the colored portion of the eye, has an opening in the center called the *pupil*. Muscles of the iris regulate the amount of light entering the eye through dilatation and contraction of the pupil.

> ### ★ HIGH PRIORITY
>
> The eye examination during the history and physical (H&P) may include the acronym *PERRLA*, meaning *pupils equal, round, reactive to light,* and *accommodation.*

The *lens*, located directly behind the pupil, focuses light rays on the retina. The ciliary muscle regulates the shape of the lens to make this possible through a process known as *accommodation.*

The inner layer of the eye is called the *retina*. Two different sets of nerve cells, or photoreceptor neurons, called *rods* and *cones*, are responsible for the adaptation to light. The cones are sensitive to bright light and are responsible for color vision. The rods, far more numerous than cones, adapt to provide both peripheral vision and vision in dim

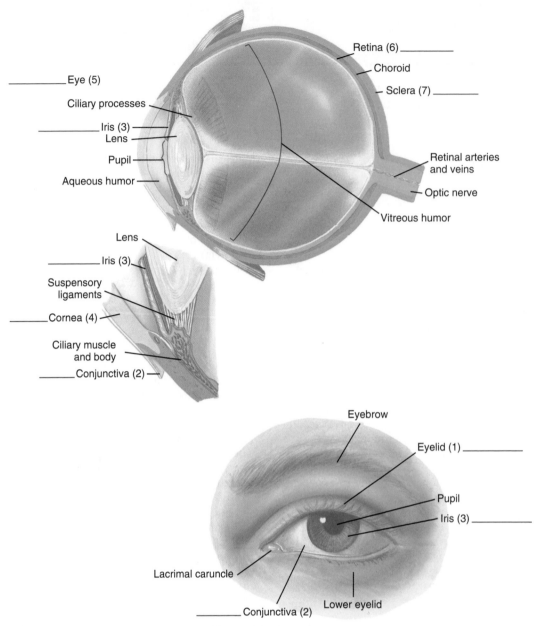

Retina (6) _____
Choroid
Sclera (7) _____

_____ Eye (5)
Ciliary processes
_____ Iris (3)
Lens
Pupil
Aqueous humor

Retinal arteries and veins
Optic nerve
Vitreous humor

Lens
_____ Iris (3)
Suspensory ligaments
_____ Cornea (4)
Ciliary muscle and body
_____ Conjunctiva (2)

Eyebrow
Eyelid (1) _____
Pupil
Iris (3) _____
Lacrimal caruncle
_____ Conjunctiva (2)
Lower eyelid

Figure 22-18 The eye.

light. The rods and cones transmit impulses to the optic nerve. The optic nerve carries these impulses to the vision center in the cerebrum, where they are registered as visual sensations.

The anterior and posterior cavities inside the eyeball are filled with fluid. The small anterior cavity in front of the lens is divided into an anterior and a posterior chamber. These chambers are filled with a watery substance called *aqueous humor*, which is constantly formed and drained. The large posterior cavity behind the lens is filled with a jelly-like substance called *vitreous humor*, which remains relatively constant. The functions of these fluids are to maintain the shape of the eyeball with proper intraocular pressure and to assist in bending the light rays to focus on the retina.

★ HIGH PRIORITY

Pathway of Light Rays
conjunctiva → cornea → aqueous humor → pupil → lens → vitreous humor → retina → optic nerve (converted to nerve impulses) → cerebrum

Diseases of the Eye
Cataracts

Cataracts are the gradually developed cloudiness of the lens of the eyes; they usually occur in both eyes. Most cataracts develop after a person is 50 years of age and are caused by degenerative changes. At first, vision is blurred; if not treated, cataracts eventually lead to loss of eyesight. Treatment consists of surgical removal of the lens followed by correction of the visual defects. Two types of surgery used to remove cataracts are extraction of the entire lens and *phacoemulsification,* which is the use of ultrasonic vibrations to break the lens into pieces, followed by *aspiration,* or sucking out of the pieces.

Correction of visual defects requires a lens implant. After removal of the cataract, a synthetic lens is inserted into the eye through a corneal incision. Corrective eyeglasses or contact lens also may be used to correct the visual defect caused by cataract extraction.

Glaucoma

Glaucoma is the abnormal increase in intraocular (within the eye) pressure. It is the most preventable cause of blindness and yet is the cause of 15% of all cases of blindness in the United States. Pressure is caused by overproduction of aqueous humor or obstruction of its outflow, which causes damage to the retina that results in blindness.

Two forms of glaucoma exist: chronic and acute. Chronic glaucoma affects vision gradually and may not be diagnosed until after some loss of vision has occurred. The acute form causes severe pain and sudden dimming of vision.

Treatment varies, but glaucoma often is treated with drugs that help to reduce intraocular pressure. The patient has to understand that the medication must be taken for the rest of his or her life.

Retinal Detachment

Retinal detachment is the separation of the retina from the choroid in the back of the eye, which allows vitreous humor to leak between the choroid and the retina. Retinal detachment may be caused by trauma but is often the result of aging. *Photocoagulation, cryosurgery,* and *scleral buckling* are the surgical procedures that are used for treatment.

Macular Degeneration

Macular degeneration is the loss of vision in the center of the visual field as a result of damage to the retina. It is more common in adults over the age of 50 (age-related macular degeneration [AMD]). No medical or surgical treatment is currently available, but some vitamin supplements high in antioxidants may slow the progression of the disease.

THE EAR

Two functions of the ear include hearing and equilibrium (sense of balance). The ear is divided into three main parts: the outer ear, the middle ear, and the inner ear (Fig. 22-19).

The Outer Ear

The outer ear is made up of two parts: the pinna, or auricle, and the auditory canal. The *pinna* is the appendage we see on each side of the head. The *auditory canal* is the tube that leads from the outer ear to the middle ear through which sound waves pass.

The Middle Ear

The *tympanic membrane* (eardrum) separates the outer ear from the middle ear. Located just inside the eardrum are three small bones, or *ossicles,* called the *malleus,* the *incus,* and the *stapes.* These three small bones form a chain across the middle ear from the tympanic membrane (eardrum) to the oval window. They transfer vibrations of the eardrum to the inner ear. The middle ear also contains the *eustachian tube,* which leads from the middle ear to the pharynx (throat). The eustachian tube serves to equalize pressure on both sides of the tympanic membrane. Disease-causing bacteria, especially in children, may travel from the throat to the middle ear through the eustachian tube, resulting in middle ear infection.

The Inner Ear (or Labyrinth)

The *oval window* separates the middle ear from the inner ear. The structure next to the oval window in the inner ear is the *cochlea,* an organ that is shaped like a snail, with receptors for hearing. It contains special fluids that carry sound vibrations. The inner ear also contains the *semicircular canals.* The cerebellum interprets impulses from the semicircular canals to maintain balance and equilibrium.

> ### ⭐ HIGH PRIORITY
>
> **Pathway of Sound Waves through the Ear**
> pinna → auditory canal → tympanic membrane → ossicles (malleus, incus, stapes) → oval window → cochlea → auditory nerve (converted to nerve impulses) → cerebrum

Diseases and Disorders of the Ear
Tinnitus

Tinnitus, a symptom in most disorders of the ear, is described as a ringing, buzzing, or roaring noise in the ears. In some patients this noise can be heard by others with the use of a stethoscope (objective tinnitus) and may be caused by muscle spasm or an abnormality in blood vessels. Common causes of tinnitus include chronic infection, head injury, prolonged exposure to loud environmental noise, hypertension, and cardiovascular disease. Another common cause of tinnitus is intake of drugs that are ototoxic. Ringing in the ears is a very common adverse effect of aspirin.

Persistent and severe noises in the ear can interfere with the person's ability to carry on normal activities such as resting and sleeping. Medical treatment begins with an audiologic and vascular examination that is performed to try to determine the underlying cause of the tinnitus. Many cases have been unresponsive to all conventional methods of treatment. One frequent approach to treatment is to try to mask ear noises by providing soft background music. Biofeedback has been marginally effective in cases caused by stress or hysteria. Because the condition is so prevalent, two national associations have been established (American Tinnitus Association—www.ata.org; or American Speech-Language-Hearing Association—www.asha.org). One of the primary goals of the associations is management and study of the condition.

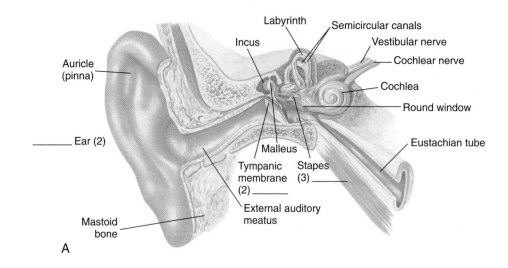

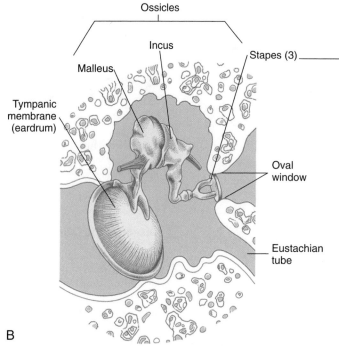

Figure 22-19 A, The ear. **B,** Enlarged view of inner ear.

REVIEW QUESTIONS

1. Describe the function and structure of the eye.

2. What are five body structures that help protect the eye in various ways?

3. Match the terms in Column 1 with the definitions in Column 2.

Column 1
a. choroid

b. pupil

c. stapes

d. retina

e. auditory nerve

f. cornea

g. cochlea

h. iris

i. sclera
j. lens
k. optic nerve

Column 2
1. anterior transparent part of the sclera

2. the colored portion of the eye

3. located directly behind the pupil

4. outer protective layer of the eye

5. the opening in the center of the iris

6. inner layer of the eye

7. transmits impulses from the retina to the brain

8. middle layer of the eye

4. Name and describe the functions of the two types of nerve cells located in the retina.

5. Describe the location and function of the aqueous and vitreous humor.

6. List in order, beginning with the conjunctiva, the organs of the eye through which light rays travel to the retina.

7. Describe the clinical presentation of cataracts.

8. What will the physician's eye pressure examination for glaucoma reveal?

9. What will an examination reveal in which retinal detachment is the diagnosis?

10. What are three surgical procedures used to treat retinal detachment?

11. Define macular degeneration, and identify a treatment used to slow down the progress of the disease.

12. Describe two functions of the ear.

13. List the parts of the outer ear, the middle ear, and the inner ear.

14. Trace the travel of sound waves from the outside environment to the brain.

15. List six factors that cause tinnitus.

16. List two treatments for tinnitus.

MEDICAL TERMINOLOGY RELATED TO THE EYE AND THE EAR

Objectives

On mastery of the medical terminology for this unit, you will be able to:

1. Spell and define the word parts and medical terms for the eye and the ear.
2. Given the meaning of a medical condition related to the eye or the ear, build the corresponding medical term with word parts.
3. Analyze the medical terms that are built from word parts that relate to the eye and ear.
4. Given a description of hospital situations in which the HUC may encounter medical terminology, apply the correct medical terms to the situations.

Word Parts

Listed here are the combining forms for this unit. Memorize each combining form. Practice pronouncing each word part aloud.

Word Roots/Combining Forms	Meaning
Eye	
1. blephar / o (blĕf'-ah-rō)	eyelid
2. conjunctiv / o (kŏn-jŭnk'-tĭv-ō)	conjunctiva (membrane covering the eye and lining of the eyelid)
3. irid / o (ĭ'-rĭd-ō)	iris (colored portion of the eye)
4. kerat / o (kĕr'-ah-tō)	cornea (clear anterior covering of the eye; also means "hard")
5. ophthalm / o (ŏf-thal'-mō)	eye
6. retin / o (rĕt'-ĭn-ō)	retina (inner layer of eye)
7. scler / o (skleù'-rō)	sclera (white covering of the eye)
Ear	
1. myring / o (mĭ-rĭng'-gō)	tympanic membrane (eardrum)
2. ot / o (ō'-tō)	ear
3. staped / o (stā-pē'-dō)	stapes (in middle ear)

⊜ EXERCISE 1

1. Write the combining forms for the eye in the spaces provided on the diagram in Figure 22-18. The number that precedes the combining form in the earlier list matches the number of the body part on the diagram.
2. Write the combining forms for the ear in the spaces provided on the diagram in Figure 22-19. The number preceding the combining form in the earlier list matches the number of the body part on the diagram.

⊜ EXERCISE 2

Define each combining form listed.

1. retin / o	6. ot / o
2. kerat / o	7. myring / o
3. scler / o	8. blephar / o
4. ophthalm / o	9. irid / o
5. conjunctiv / o	10. staped / o

⊜ EXERCISE 3

Write the word roots for each part of the body listed.

1. eye	6. sclera
2. eyelid	7. conjunctiva
3. retina	8. iris
4. ear	9. cornea
5. eardrum	10. stapes

MEDICAL TERMS RELATED TO THE EYE AND THE EAR

The following list consists of medical terms related to the eye and the ear that you will need to know. Exercises following this list will assist you in learning these terms. Practice pronouncing these terms aloud.

General Terms	Meaning
ophthalmologist (ŏf-thal-mŏl′-o-jĭst)	one who specializes in the diagnosis and treatment of the eye (doctor)
ophthalmology (ŏf-thăl-mŏl′-o-jē)	study of the eye (and its diseases and disorders)
optometrist (ŏp-tŏm′-e-trĭst)	a professional person trained to examine the eyes and prescribe glasses
otorhinolaryngologist	specialist of ear, nose, and throat
otorrhea (ō-tō-rē′-ah)	discharge from the ear

Surgical Terms	Meaning
blepharoplasty (blĕf′-ah-rō-plăs′-tē)	surgical repair of the eyelid
blepharorrhaphy (blĕf′-ah-rōr′-ah-fē)	suturing of an eyelid
cataract extraction (kăt′-ah-răkt) (ĕk-străk′-shŭn)	removal of the clouded lens of the eye
corneal (kor′-nē-al) transplant	transplantation of a donor cornea into the eye of the recipient
enucleation (ē-nū-klē-ā′-shŭn)	removal of an organ; often used to indicate surgical removal of the eyeball
iridectomy (īr-ĭ-dĕk′-to-mē)	excision of (a part of) the iris
iridosclerotomy (īr-ĭ-dō-sklē-rŏt′-o-mē)	incision into the iris and the sclera
keratectomy (kĕr-ah-tĕk′-to-mē)	procedure whereby an excimer laser is used to correct myopia; includes removal of part of the cornea (PRK, photorefractive keratectomy)

General Terms	Meaning
keratoplasty (kĕr-ah-to-plăs′-tē)	procedure in which the laser is used to correct myopia; involves reshaping corneal tissue below the surface (LASIK [laser-assisted in situ keratomileusis])
keratotomy (kĕr-ah-tot′-ō-mē)	incision into the cornea (RK, radial keratotomy, is an operation in which a series of incisions, in spokelike fashion, are made in the cornea; done to correct myopia [nearsightedness]); photorefractive keratectomy (PRK) is a related procedure
LASIK (lā′- sĭk)	LASIK (laser assisted in situ keratomileusis) is a procedure done to correct myopia, hyperopia, and astigmatism; flaps are created in the cornea instead of incisions

General Terms	Meaning
myringoplasty (mĭ-rĭng′-gō-plăs′-tē)	surgical repair of the tympanic membrane
myringotomy (mĭ-rĭng-gŏt′-o-mē)	incision of the tympanic membrane
ophthalmectomy (ŏf-thal-mĕk′-to-mē)	excision of the eye
scleroplasty (sklŭ-rō-plăs′-tē)	surgical repair of the sclera
sclerotomy (skĕ-rŏt′-o-mē)	incision into the sclera
stapedectomy (stā-pē-dĕk′-to-mē)	excision of the stapes

Diagnostic Terms	Meaning
cataract (kăt′-ah-răkt)	cloudiness of the lens of the eye
conjunctivitis (kŏn-jŭnk-tī-vī′-tĭs)	inflammation of the conjunctiva (pinkeye)
glaucoma (glaw-kō′-mah)	an eye disease caused by increased pressure within the eye
keratocele (kĕr′-ah-tō-sĕl)	herniation (of a layer) of the cornea
keratoconjunctivitis (kĕr′-ah-tō-kŏn-jŭnk-tĭ-vī′-tĭs)	inflammation of the cornea and the conjunctiva
otitis media (ō-tī′-tĭs) (mē-dē-ah) (OM)	inflammation of the middle ear
retinal detachment (rĕt′-ĭn-al) (dē-tăch′-mĕnt)	complete or partial separation of the retina from the choroid
strabismus (străh-bĭz′-mŭs)	weakness of the muscle of the eye that causes the eye to look in different directions (medical term for crossed eyes)

Terms Related to Diagnostic Procedures	Meaning
ophthalmoscope (ŏf-thal′-mō-skōp)	instrument used for visual examination of the eye
otoscope (ō′-tō-skōp)	instrument used for visual examination of the ear

⊜ EXERCISE 4

Analyze and define each medical term listed.

1. ophthalmoscope
2. ophthalmologist
3. ophthalmectomy
4. otorrhea
5. otoscope
6. iridosclerotomy
7. iridectomy
8. blepharoplasty
9. blepharorrhaphy
10. keratoconjunctivitis
11. keratocele
12. conjunctivitis
13. myringotomy
14. myringoplasty
15. keratotomy
16. otorhinolaryngologist

⊜ EXERCISE 5

Build a medical term from each definition listed.

1. inflammation of the middle ear
2. instrument used for visual examination of the eye

3. suturing of the eyelid
4. discharge from the ear
5. incision into the iris and the sclera
6. surgical repair of the sclera
7. excision of part of the iris
8. herniation of the cornea
9. instrument used for visual examination of the ear
10. excision of the eye
11. incision of the sclera
12. surgical repair of the eyelid
13. incision into the tympanic membrane
14. surgical repair of the tympanic membrane
15. inflammation of the cornea and the conjunctiva
16. inflammation of the conjunctiva
17. incision into the cornea
18. ear, nose, and throat specialist

⊖ EXERCISE **6**

Define each medical term listed.

1. cataract
2. cataract extraction
3. retinal detachment
4. enucleation of the eye
5. strabismus
6. glaucoma
7. optometrist
8. corneal transplant

⊖ EXERCISE **7**

Spell each of the 28 medical terms studied in this unit by having someone dictate the terms to you.

1.
2.
3.
4.
5.
6.
7.
8.
9.
10.
11.
12.
13.
14.
15.
16.
17.
18.
19.
20.
21.
22.
23.
24.
25.
26.
27.
28.

⊖ EXERCISE **8**

Answer the following questions.

1. Instruments used to examine the eye and the ear visually are usually part of the equipment stored at the nurses' station in the hospital. What is the instrument used to examine the eye? What is the instrument used to examine the ear?
2. Children often develop inflammation of the middle ear, called _____. Children who have had repeated middle ear infections may have a buildup of fluid in the middle ear. The doctor may surgically treat this condition by making an incision into the eardrum, known as _____, and inserting tiny tubes.
3. The patient is admitted to the hospital with a diagnosis of cloudiness of the lens of the right eye, or _____. She is scheduled for surgical removal of the diseased lens. What is the operation called?
4. Two medical words are used to describe surgical removal of the eyeball. What are they?
5. What is the medical term for crossed eyes?

ABBREVIATIONS

Abbreviation	Meaning
ENT	Ear, nose and throat specialist (called an *otorhinolaryngologist*)
OD	oculus dexter (right eye)
OM	otitis media (middle ear infection)
OS	oculus sinister (left eye)
OU	oculus uterque (both eyes)
PERRLA	pupils equal, round, reactive to light, and accommodation
PRK	photorefractive keratectomy
RK	radial keratotomy

⊖ EXERCISE **9**

Define the following abbreviations.

1. PERRLA
2. OM
3. PRK
4. RK
5. OD
6. OS
7. OU
8. ENT

UNIT 6
The Cardiovascular and Lymphatic Systems

OUTLINE

UNIT OBJECTIVES

On completion of this unit, you will be able to:

1. List the organs and describe three functions of the circulatory system.
2. Identify the pericardium, and list three layers and four chambers of the heart.
3. Name types of blood vessels, and briefly describe the function of each.
4. Trace the flow of blood through the blood vessels of the body and the circulation of blood through the heart.
5. Describe what systolic and diastolic blood pressure represent.
6. Describe the three main functions of blood, and briefly describe the composition of blood and the functions of the three types of blood cells.
7. List the two primary functions of the lymphatic system.
8. Name and describe the functions of the organs of the lymphatic system.
9. Discuss coronary artery disease, congestive heart failure, anemia, varicose veins, abdominal aortic aneurysm, and acquired immunodeficiency syndrome.
10. Read the objectives related to medical terminology, and demonstrate ability to meet the objectives by correctly completing Exercises 1 through 7.
11. Define the unit abbreviations.

THE CARDIOVASCULAR SYSTEM

Organs of the Circulatory System

- Heart
- Blood vessels
- Blood

Functions of the Circulatory System

- *Transportation* of nutrients, oxygen, and hormones to cells, and removal of wastes
- *Protection* by white blood cells and antibodies to defend the body against foreign invaders
- *Regulation* of body temperature, fluids, and water volume of cells

All living cells, which are metabolically active structures, need constant nourishment and oxygen for life and for continuous removal of their waste products. The circulatory system provides the vital transportation service that carries nourishment (oxygen, nutrients, and hormones) to the cells of the body and carries away the waste (nitrogenous wastes, carbon dioxide, and heat). Blood is the tissue that is most frequently examined by clinicians to determine the state of health.

The heart pumps blood to the lungs and the body cells through a network of tubing called *blood vessels*. Blood is the

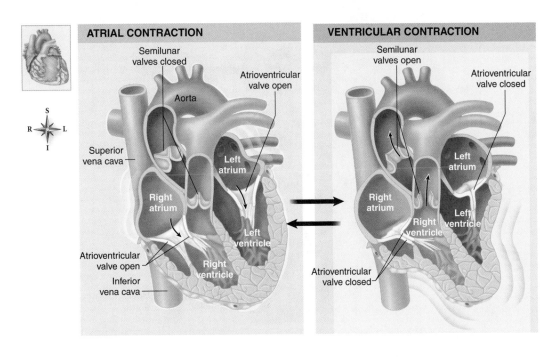

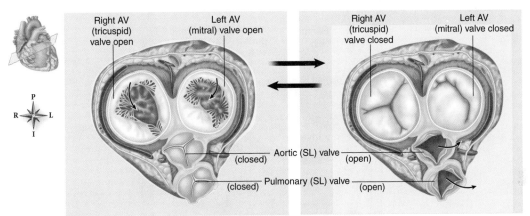

Figure 22-20 The heart. (From Patton KT, Thibodeau GA: *The human body in health & disease,* ed 6, St. Louis, 2014, Mosby.)

carrying agent for food, oxygen, waste, and other materials needed for or produced by cell function.

THE HEART

The heart is located in the mediastinum, the cavity between the lungs that is situated behind the sternum. It is a four-chambered organ the size of a fist, and it weighs less than a pound. The heart performs the action of pumping the blood through the blood vessels to all parts of the body, circulating it in a one-way movement. The heart is surrounded by the *pericardium*, a loose-fitting double-layered sac. Serous membranes of the pericardium secrete a small amount of fluid to prevent irritation as the heart contracts.

Structure of the Heart

The heart wall is made up of three layers. The outer layer of the heart wall, the *epicardium*, is the visceral layer of the pericardium. The thickest, muscular middle layer is called the *myocardium*. The *endocardium*, the inner lining of the heart, also forms the heart valves.

The heart is divided into four cavities or chambers (Fig. 22-20), through which blood entering the heart travels. Each chamber has a valve (or one-way door) that prevents the blood from flowing backward into the chamber. The *septum* is a partition that divides the heart into a right and a left side. Each side is divided by halves into two upper chambers—the *right atrium* and the *left atrium*—and two lower chambers—the *right ventricle* and the *left ventricle*. The left atrium is separated from the left ventricle by the *bicuspid*, or *mitral*, *valve*. On the right side, the right atrium is separated from the right ventricle by the *tricuspid*, or *atrioventricular (AV), valve*. The *semilunar valves* (pulmonary and aortic) are located between the right ventricle and the pulmonary artery and between the left ventricle and the aorta.

Conduction System of the Heart

Regular and coordinated cardiac muscle contraction is conducted by electrical impulses that originate within the heart

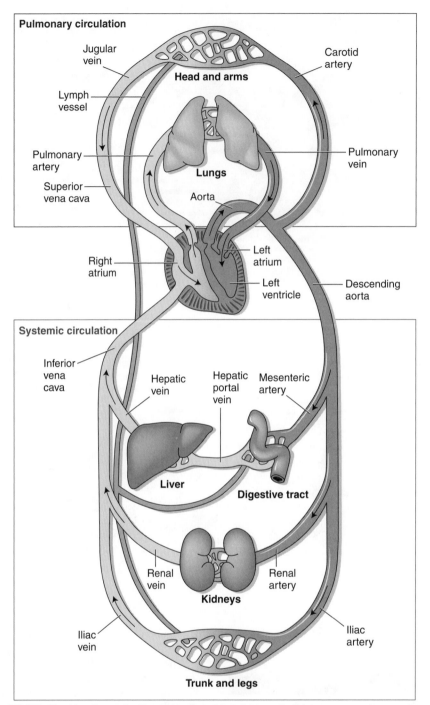

Figure 22-21 The blood vessels. (From Warekois RS, Robinson R: *Phlebotomy: worktext and procedures manual,* ed 2, St Louis, 2007, Saunders.)

muscle; it is regulated by the CNS as well as by hormones. A normal heartbeat begins with an impulse from the sinoatrial (SA) node to the AV node, through the bundle branches, and finally through the Purkinje fibers to effect a complete heart contraction. The electrical impulses that generate the rhythm are measured by the electrocardiogram (ECG [or EKG]). (See Fig. 16-3, for an ECG.)

BLOOD VESSELS

Blood vessels are the tubular structures through which blood flows to and from the heart to the body parts (Fig. 22-21).

Three major types of blood vessels are present: arteries, capillaries, and veins.

Arteries, except for the pulmonary artery, carry blood away from the heart. The pulmonary artery is the only artery in the body that carries blood with low levels of oxygen and a high concentration of carbon dioxide from the heart to the lungs. All other arteries carry blood that is high in oxygen concentration from the heart to the body cells. *Arterial walls* are the thickest because they must withstand the pumping force of the heart. Within the walls are smooth muscles, whose contraction and relaxation affect BP. Arteries branch into *arterioles,* tiny arteries that connect the arteries to capillaries. The aorta, the largest artery of the body, measures approximately 1 inch in diameter. It carries blood away from the left ventricle of the heart.

Veins are the vessels that carry blood from the capillary beds back to the heart. Veins , except for the pulmonary vein, carry carbon dioxide and other waste products. The pulmonary vein carries blood that is high in oxygen concentration from the lungs to the heart. Vein walls are thinner than arterial walls, and they contain tiny valves that help to prevent the backward flow of blood and to keep it moving in one direction. *Venules* are tiny veins that connect the capillaries with the veins. The *superior vena cava* and the *inferior vena cava* are large veins through which the blood returns from the body to the right atrium.

Capillaries are microscopic, thin-walled blood vessels. The exchange of substances takes place between the blood and the body cells while the blood is in the capillaries. The cells take in nutrients and oxygen from the blood and give off waste and carbon dioxide to the blood. Blood carries the waste to the organ that removes it from the body. Capillaries provide the links between arteries and veins.

Flow of Blood through the Blood Vessels of the Body

Blood leaves the heart through the aorta. It travels first through the arteries and then through the arterioles to the capillaries, where the exchange of gases, nutrients, and waste takes place. The blood returns from the capillaries by first entering the venules and then flowing through the veins, finally entering the right atrium of the heart through the superior and inferior venae cavae. The superior vena cava returns blood to the heart from the upper part of the body, and the inferior vena cava returns blood to the heart from the lower part of the body.

Circulation of Blood through the Heart

Blood that carries the waste product carbon dioxide returns from circulating through the body and enters the right atrium of the heart through the superior vena cava and the inferior vena cava. Blood travels through the tricuspid valve to the right ventricle. The right ventricle pumps the blood through the *pulmonary arteries* to the lungs. (The pulmonary artery is the only artery that transports waste-carrying blood.) The blood, while in the lungs, gets rid of the carbon dioxide and takes on oxygen. This exchange changes the appearance of the blood from a bluish-red color to a bright red color. Oxygenated blood returns to the left atrium through the *pulmonary veins.*

The pulmonary vein is the only vein in the body that carries oxygenated blood. The blood passes through the bicuspid valve to the left ventricle. The left ventricle pumps the blood through the aorta and out to the body parts. Refer to Figure 22-20; the arrows indicate the passage of blood through the heart.

★ **HIGH PRIORITY**

Pathway: blood saturated with carbon dioxide (CO_2) returns to the right side of the heart via the inferior and superior venae cavae → right atrium → tricuspid valve → right ventricle → pulmonary valve → pulmonary artery → to the lungs → (exchange of CO_2 and oxygen [O_2] takes place in the lungs) from the lungs saturated with O_2 → pulmonary veins → left atrium → bicuspid valve (mitral valve) → left ventricle → aortic valve → aorta

---

Blood Pressure

BP, measured in milliliters of mercury (mm Hg) (e.g., 120/70), records the forces created by circulating blood against the walls of the arteries, veins, and chambers of the heart. The upper number—systolic BP—represents the pressure in the aorta and other large arteries during ventricular contraction. The lower number—diastolic BP—represents the pressure during relaxation of the heart.

BLOOD

Blood is the carrying agent of the transportation system. It is a warm, sticky fluid that ranges in color from dark bluish-red to bright red, according to the amount of oxygen it is carrying. An adult has approximately 5.7 L (6 qt) of blood.

Function of Blood

The blood has three main functions: transportation, fighting of infection, and regulation.

Transportation

The blood carries oxygen from the lungs and nutrients from the digestive tract to the body cells. It carries waste products from the cells, carbon dioxide to the lungs, and other waste (urea) to the kidneys. The blood also transports hormones and other chemicals.

Fighting Infection

Certain blood cells help the body to fight disease-causing organisms. White blood cells, or leukocytes, acting as the main line of defense against infection, respond when they encounter microbes or toxins. Certain leukocytes (e.g., B lymphocytes) produce proteins called *antibodies* (or immunoglobulins), which neutralize these foreign substances.

Regulation

The blood distributes hormones and other chemicals as needed, maintains body temperature through dilatation and constriction of blood vessels in the skin, and maintains the homeostatic balance of fluids necessary for survival.

Blood Composition

Blood is made up of plasma and cells.

Plasma

Plasma is the clear, fluid portion of the blood in which blood cells are suspended. Plasma consists of approximately 90% water and contains more than 100 other constituents, such as glucose, fibrinogen, and protein. It makes up approximately 50% of the total amount of the blood. Plasma transports nutrients, waste material, hormones, and so forth, to and from the body cells. Fibrinogen in the plasma assists in the blood-clotting process.

Blood Cells, or Formed Elements

Three types of *blood cells* have been identified; each carries out certain functions.

- *Erythrocytes* (RBCs) are produced by the red bone marrow. Red bone marrow is found in the flat bones of the body, such as the sternum and the pelvic bones. A *sternal puncture* is a procedure that is performed to obtain bone marrow from the sternum. The bone marrow is then studied to determine its ability to produce RBCs. The function of RBCs is to carry oxygen (carbon dioxide is dissolved in the plasma). *Hemoglobin* is the oxygen-carrying protein of the erythrocyte that gives blood its color. The average RBC count is 4.5 to 5 million/mm³ of blood. Erythrocytes exist for approximately 4 months. It is estimated that each erythrocyte travels approximately 700 miles during its lifetime.

- *Leukocytes* (white blood cells) are colorless cells that are produced by the spleen, bone marrow, and lymph nodes. Their chief function is to fight against pathogenic microorganisms (disease-causing bacteria). The normal white blood cell (WBC) count is 5000 to 9000/mm³ of blood. An elevated blood count may indicate the presence of infection in the body. Leukocytes last a very short time—approximately 14 hours or less.
- *Platelets* (thrombocytes) also are formed in the red bone marrow. Their prime function is to aid in the clotting of blood. A normal platelet count is about 250,000/mm³ of blood. Platelets exist for a short time in the bloodstream and are replaced approximately every 4 days.

★ HIGH PRIORITY

Because leukocytes fight incompatible blood cells, it is absolutely essential that patients be typed and cross-matched before receiving blood. Before scientists learned to group blood into types that could be safely given from one person to another, many deaths resulted from incompatible blood transfusions. The blood types are O, A, B, and AB.

★ HIGH PRIORITY

Rh blood groups, a complex system of erythrocyte surface antigens, were first identified in rhesus monkeys in 1940. The presence of even one antigen on the red blood cell makes a person Rh positive. Rh incompatibility is generally not a problem during the first pregnancy because the mother does not produce anti–Rh-positive antibodies until after birth. Rh incompatibility may cause problems in subsequent pregnancies, necessitating treatment of mother and baby to correct the disorder. Rh-negative women who carry Rh-positive babies in subsequent pregnancies will form anti–Rh antibodies unless they are treated with RhoGAM (Rh0[D] immune globulin) before or shortly after birth.

LYMPHATIC SYSTEM

The lymphatic system consists of the spleen, thymus gland, lymph nodes, a fluid called *lymph,* and the lymphatic vessels.

The two principal functions of the lymphatic system involve the maintenance of fluid balance and immunity. Lymphatic vessels collect excessive tissue fluids and return them to the blood circulation.

Spleen

The *spleen,* the largest lymphatic organ, is located in the upper left abdomen and is protected by the lower ribs. Two important functions of the spleen are to destroy old RBCs, bacteria, and germs and to store blood for emergency use. The spleen produces RBCs in the fetus.

Thymus Gland

The *thymus gland,* one of the primary lymphatic organs, plays an important role in the development of the body's defenses against infection by promoting the maturation of cells that provide immune responses (T lymphocytes).

DISEASES AND DISORDERS OF THE CIRCULATORY SYSTEM

Coronary Artery Disease

Coronary artery disease (CAD) usually is caused by blockage or narrowing of the arteries which develop when plaque accumulates on the arterial walls, a condition called *atherosclerosis. Angina pectoris* is a condition characterized by chest pain that is caused by lack of oxygen to the myocardium as a result of atherosclerosis of the coronary arteries. Atherosclerosis can block the artery completely, creating a condition called *coronary occlusion,* or a *thrombus* (blood clot) can develop on segments of the artery that contain plaque, causing a partial or complete blockage. This condition is referred to as *coronary thrombosis.* Both conditions may lead to *myocardial infarction (MI)* (heart attack) because they reduce the flow of blood to the heart, which denies the myocardium the oxygen and nutrients it needs. A symptom of an MI is sudden onset of chest pain, sometimes radiating to the arms. The severity of the heart attack depends on which artery is blocked and to what extent it is blocked.

Coronary artery bypass graft surgery (CABG) may be performed in patients with CAD to improve the blood supply to the myocardium. This type of surgery consists of using a vein from the leg that is grafted to the aorta and the clogged coronary artery to form an alternative route for the flow of blood. A minimally invasive bypass (mid-CAB) may now be done endoscopically and is an alternative intervention for patients who are not good candidates for surgery.

Angioplasty, surgical repair of a blood vessel, refers to various techniques such as the use of surgery, lasers, or tiny balloons at the tip of a catheter to repair or replace damaged blood vessels. *Percutaneous transluminal coronary angioplasty (PTCA)* is a cardiac procedure in which fatty plaques in the blood vessels are flattened against vessel walls by passage of a balloon within a catheter through the affected blood vessels. A coronary stent, a wire mesh tube, is commonly placed in the cleared artery to maintain its patency. *Laser angioplasty* makes use of light amplification through stimulated emission of radiation (laser beam) through a fiberoptic probe to open blocked arteries. Less commonly, the plaque may be removed by a cutting device such as a rotoblade.

Congestive Heart Failure

Congestive heart failure (CHF) occurs when the heart is unable to pump the required amount of blood, resulting in accumulation of blood in the lungs and the liver. CHF develops gradually. Symptoms include fatigue, dyspnea (shortness of breath), and peripheral edema. Diagnostic testing includes chest x-ray examination, ECG, echocardiogram, angiogram, and blood tests. Treatment consists of dietary changes (i.e., restricted sodium, fats, cholesterol, fluids) and administration of medications such as angiotensin-converting enzyme (ACE) inhibitors, β-blockers, digoxin, and diuretics. Surgical options that may be used to correct the underlying cardiac problem include coronary bypass surgery, valve repair or replacement, cardiac resynchronization therapy, ventricular remodeling, and heart transplantation.

Anemia

Anemia is a disorder that is characterized by an abnormally low level of hemoglobin in the blood, or inadequate numbers of RBCs. It may result from decreased RBC production, from increased RBC destruction, or from blood loss. Treatment varies according to the cause. The anemic person becomes easily fatigued. Pallor also may indicate anemia. Sternal puncture to obtain bone marrow for study and blood tests are used to diagnose anemia.

Varicose Veins

Varicose veins are swollen, distended, and knotted veins that usually are found among the superficial veins of the leg. One-way valves in the veins assist in moving the blood upward to the heart. Standing or sitting for prolonged periods causes the valves to dilate from the weight of pooled blood and can result in loss of elasticity of the valves. Other causes of varicose veins include pregnancy, obesity, illness, injury, and heredity. Elevation of the leg and the use of elastic stockings reduce blood pooling in the great saphenous vein, the largest superficial vein. Minimally invasive surgery, in which the affected veins are pulled out, called *ambulatory phlebectomy*, may be required in more severe cases. Hemorrhoids are internal or external varicose veins in the rectal area.

Abdominal Aortic Aneurysm

Abdominal aortic aneurysm (AAA) results from the weakening of the wall of the aorta as it passes through the abdomen. If the aneurysm dissects, it may rupture and cause death. If it is stable, it may be monitored with regular abdominal ultrasound studies. Surgical intervention is usually required, or the aneurysm may be repaired endoscopically through use of a catheter and an endoluminal graft.

Acquired Immunodeficiency Syndrome

In *acquired immunodeficiency syndrome (AIDS)*, which manifests as the destruction of patients' immune systems, carriers are highly susceptible to infection. AIDS is caused by the human immunodeficiency virus (HIV), which infects certain WBCs of the body's immune system and gradually destroys the body's ability to fight infection. Many infected persons develop previously rare types of pneumonia (*Pneumocystis jiroveci* pneumonia) and a form of skin cancer (Kaposi sarcoma).

HIV has been isolated from semen and blood and is transmitted via direct or intimate contact involving the mucous membranes or breaks in the skin, across the placenta from mother to fetus, or before or during birth. The sharing of hypodermic needles among IV drug users, blood transfusions, and needle sticks are other ways by which infection is spread. The virus cannot penetrate intact skin. AIDS had become one of the deadliest epidemic diseases of modern times and will remain a major global health concern until more definitive treatment can be provided. In the United States, recently developed medications are available and have increased the life expectancy and quality of life for many chronically ill patients for whom the disease may be managed.

⊖ REVIEW QUESTIONS

1. List three functions of the cardiovascular system.

2. Label the following diagram of the heart, including the blood vessels through which the blood enters and leaves the heart. Include the following parts:

endocardium	aorta
myocardium	superior vena cava
pericardium	inferior vena cava
bicuspid valve	right atrium
tricuspid valve	left atrium
pulmonary artery	right ventricle
pulmonary vein	left ventricle

3. Using arrows, trace on the same diagram the circulation of blood from the superior and inferior venae cavae to the aorta.

4. Blood travels through a network of tubes called *blood vessels*. Name, in sequence, the types of blood vessels through which the blood travels when it leaves the heart until reentry, and describe the function of each.

5. Describe what systolic and diastolic blood pressure represent.

6. The fluid portion of the blood is called what? What are its functions?

7. List three types of blood cells (formed elements), and briefly describe the function of each.

8. Name the four blood types.

9. List the two primary functions of the organs of the lymphatic system.

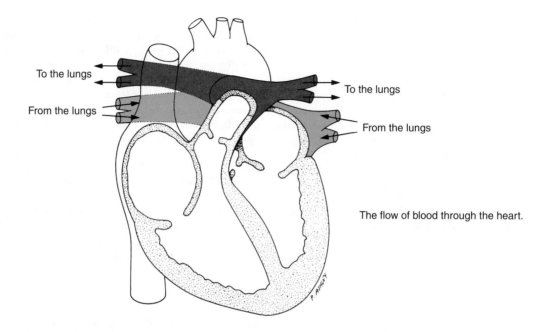

The flow of blood through the heart.

10. Match the terms in Column 1 with the phrases in Column 2.

Column 1
a. anemia
b. CHF
c. CAD
d. coronary thrombosis
e. myocardial infarction
f. CABG
g. angina pectoris
h. ambulatory phlebectomy
i. AIDS
j. abdominal aortic aneurysm

Column 2
1. pain caused by lack of oxygen to the myocardium
2. the heart is unable to efficiently pump blood
3. narrowing of arteries because of plaque
4. below normal level of hemoglobin
5. causes occlusion of an artery
6. surgery for varicose veins
7. damage to the heart muscle
8. results from the weakening of the wall of the aorta as it passes through the abdomen
9. surgery that restores blood flow to the heart
10. caused by HIV

MEDICAL TERMINOLOGY RELATED TO THE CIRCULATORY SYSTEM

Objectives
On mastery of the medical terminology for this unit, you will be able to:

1. Spell and define the word parts and the medical terms for the circulatory system.
2. Given the meaning of a medical condition related to the circulatory system, build with word parts the corresponding medical term.
3. Analyze the medical terms that are built from word parts that relate to the circulatory system.
4. Given a list of word parts, identify them as word roots, suffixes, or prefixes.

5. Given descriptions of hospital situations in which the HUC may encounter medical terminology, apply the correct medical terms to the situations.

Word Parts
The following list contains the word parts related to the circulatory system that you need to memorize. The exercises included in this unit will help you with this task. You will continue to use these word parts throughout this course and during your employment. Practice pronouncing each word part aloud.

Word Roots/Forms	Combining Meaning
angi / o (ăn′-jē-ō)	blood vessel
aort / o (ā-ŏr′-tō)	aorta
arteri / o (ar-tē′-rē-ō)	artery
cardi / o (kar′-dē-ō)	heart
hem / o (hē′-mō); hemat / o (hĕm′-ah-tō)	blood
phleb / o (flĕb′-ō); ven / o (vē′-nō)	vein
splen / o (splē′-nō)	spleen
thromb / o (thrŏm′-bō)	clot

Color Word Roots/Combining Forms	Meaning
cyan / o (sī′-ah-nō)	blue
erythr / o (ĕ-rĭth′-rō)	red
leuk / o (loo′-kō)	white

Prefixes	Meaning
brady- (brā′-dee)	slow
endo- (ĕn′-dō)	inside
hyper- (hī′-per)	above normal
hypo- (hī′-pō)	below normal
peri- (pĕr′-ē)	surrounding (outer)
tachy- (tăk′-kē)	fast, rapid

Suffixes	Meaning
-emia (ē′-mē-ah) (also may be used as a word root)	condition of the blood
-megaly (mĕg′-ah-lē)	enlargement

Suffixes	Meaning
-pexy (pĕk′-sē)	surgical fixation (suspension)
-sclerosis (sklĕ-rō′-sĭs)	hardening (also may be used as a word root)
-stenosis (stĕ-nō′-sĭs)	narrowing (also may be used as a word root)

⊖ EXERCISE 1

Identify each word part listed here by writing P for prefix, S for suffix, or WR/CF for word root in the space provided. Then define each word part in the space provided. Word parts studied in previous units are also included in this exercise.

Word Part	Type	Meaning
Example: pexy	S	surgical fixation
1. hypo		
2. a, an		
3. hem		
4. spleen		
5. cyt		
6. stenosis		
7. endo		
8. leuk		
9. erythr		
10. angi		
11. cardi		
12. arteri		
13. peri		
14. inter		
15. intra		
16. sclerosis		
17. emia		
18. megaly		
19. phleb		
20. aort		
21. thromb		
22. hyper		
23. tachy		
24. brady		

⊖ EXERCISE 2

Write the word parts for the meanings listed. Identify each word part that you write in the answer column. Use P for prefix, S for suffix, and WR for word root or combining form. For review purposes, word parts from previous units are included in this exercise.

Meaning	Type	Word Parts
1. aorta		
2. enlargement		
3. hardening		
4. between		
5. artery		
6. blood vessel		
7. white		
8. narrowing		
9. spleen		
10. without		
11. surgical fixation		
12. inside		
13. blood		
14. cell		
15. below normal		
16. redī		
17. heartī		
18. surrounding (outer)		
19. blood condition		
20. veinī		
21. clotī		
22. fast, rapid		
23. slow		

MEDICAL TERMS RELATED TO THE CIRCULATORY SYSTEM

The following list is made up of medical terms for the circulatory system that you will need to know. Exercises following this list will assist you in learning these terms. Practice the pronunciation of these terms out loud.

General Terms	Meaning
aortic (ā-or′-tĭk)	pertaining to the aorta
arrhythmia (ah-rĭth′-mē-ah)	variation from a normal rhythm, especially of the heartbeat (also called *dysrhythmia*)
bradycardia (brā-dy-cār′-dĭă)	condition of slow heart (rate)
cardiac arrest (kar′-dē-ăk) (ah-rĕst′)	sudden and often unexpected stoppage of the heartbeat
cardiologist (kar-dē-ŏl′-o-jĭst)	one who specializes in the diagnosis and treatment of the heart (doctor)
cardiology (kar-dē-ŏl′-o-jē)	the study of the heart (and its functions and diseases)
cardiomegaly (kar′-dē-ō-mĕg′-ah-lē)	enlargement of the heart
cardiovascular (kar′-dē-ō-văs′-kū-lar)	pertaining to the heart and blood vessels
coronary (kŏr′-ō-nā-rē) blood vessels	a term used to describe blood vessels that supply blood to the heart
endocardial (ĕn-dō-kar′-dē-al)	pertaining to within the heart
erythrocyte (ĕ-rĭth′-rō-sīt)	red blood cell (RBC)
hemorrhage (hĕm′-ō-rĭj)	the rapid flow of blood (from a blood vessel)
hypertension (hī-per-tĕn′-shŭn) (HTN)	high blood pressure
hypotension (hī-pō-tĕn′-shŭn)	low blood pressure
intravenous (ĭn-trah-vē′-nŭs)	within a vein
leukocyte (loo′-kō-sīt)	white blood cell (WBC)
phlebotomy (flĕ-bŏt′-ō-mē)	incision into the vein (to withdraw blood)
splenomegaly (splĕ-nō-mĕg′-ah-lē)	enlargement of the spleen
tachycardia (tăk-ĕ-kar′-dē-ah)	condition of rapid heart (rate)
thrombosis (thrōm-bō′-sĭs)	abnormal formation of a blood clot

Surgical Terms	Meaning
angioplasty (ăn′-jē-ō-plăs′-tē)	surgical repair of a blood vessel (Fig. 22-22)
angiorrhaphy (ăn-jĕ-ōr′-ah-fĕ)	suturing of a blood vessel
hemorrhoidectomy (hĕm-ō-roi-dĕk′-tō-mē)	excision of hemorrhoids
splenectomy (splĕ-nĕk′-tō-mē)	excision of the spleen
splenopexy (splĕ-nō-pĕk-sē)	surgical fixation of the spleen

Diagnostic Terms	Meaning
anemia (ah-nē′-mē-ah)	condition of blood without (deficiency in the number of erythrocytes [RBCs])
aneurysm (ăn′-ū-rĭzm)	dilatation of a weak area of the arterial wall
arteriosclerosis (ar-tē′-rē-ō-sclĕ-rō′-sĭs)	abnormal condition of hardening of the arteries
arteriostenosis (ar-tē′-rē-ō-stĕ-nō′-sĭs)	abnormal condition of narrowing of an artery
congestive heart failure (CHF)	inability of the heart to pump sufficient amounts of blood to the body parts
coronary occlusion (kŏr′-ŏ-nā-rē) (ō-kloo′-zhŭn)	the closing off of a coronary artery, which usually results in damage to the heart muscle; commonly referred to as a *heart attack*
coronary thrombosis (kŏr′-ŏ-nā-rē) (thrŏm-bō′-sĭs)	the blocking of a coronary artery by a blood clot; commonly referred to as a *heart attack*
edema (ĕ-dē′-mah)	an abnormal accumulation of fluid in the intercellular spaces of the body
embolism (ĕm′-bō-lĭzm)	a floating mass that blocks a vessel
endocarditis (ĕn-dō-kar-dī′-tĭs)	inflammation of the inner (lining) of the heart
hematology (hē-mah-tŏl′-o-jē)	study of the blood (also, a diagnostic division within a hospital laboratory that performs diagnostic tests on blood components)
hematoma (hē-mah-tō′-mah)	a tumor-like mass formed from blood (in the tissues)
hemophilia (hē-mō-fĭl′-ē-ah)	a congenital disorder characterized by excessive bleeding
hemorrhoid (hĕm′-ōrr-oyd)	enlarged veins in the rectal area
leukemia (loo-kē′-mē-ah)	a type of cancer characterized by rapid abnormal production of white blood cells
myocardial infarction (mī-ō-kar′-dē-al) (ĭn-fark′-shŭn) (MI)	damage to the heart muscle caused by insufficient blood supply to the area; a condition the layperson refers to as a *heart attack*
pericarditis (pĕr-ĭ-kar-dī′-tĭs)	inflammation of the outer (sac) of the heart (or pericardium)

Diagnostic Terms	Meaning
thrombophlebitis (thrŏm′-bō-flĕ-bī′-tĭs)	inflammation of a vein (as the result of a clot)
ventricular fibrillation (VFib)	life-threatening uncoordinated contractions of the ventricles; immediate application of an electrical shock with a defibrillator is necessary treatment

Terms Related to Diagnostic Procedures	Meaning
angiogram (ăn′-jē-ō-grăm)	an x-ray image of a blood vessel (using dye as a contrast medium)
aortogram (ā-ōr′-tō-grăm)	an x-ray image of the aorta (using dye as a contrast medium)
arteriogram (ar-tē′-rē-ō-grăm)	an x-ray image of an artery (using dye as a contrast medium)
cardiac catheterization (kar-dē-ăk) (kăth′-ĕ-ter-ĭ-zā′-shŭn) may also be referred to as angiography (ăn′-jē-ŏg′-rah-fĕ)	a diagnostic procedure used to visualize the heart to determine the presence of heart disease or heart defects; a long catheter is threaded from a blood vessel to the heart cavities and vessels; contrast medium (dye) is injected into the blood vessels for the purpose of taking real-time x-ray images (fluoroscopy)
electrocardiogram (ē-lĕk′-trō-kar′-dē-ō-grăm) (EKG/ECG)	a record of the electrical activity of the heart
electrocardiograph (ē-lĕk′-trō-kar′-dē-ō-grăf)	an instrument used to record electrical activity of the heart
electrocardiography (ē-lĕk′-trō-kar-dē-ōg′-rah-fĕ)	the process of recording the electrical activity of the heart
extracorporeal membrane oxygenation (ECMO)	method in which a machine similar to a heart-lung machine provides cardiac and respiratory support (oxygenation and circulation); the procedure to place the patient on ECMO is performed by a surgeon
hematocrit (hē-măt′-ō-krĭt)	hematocrit, which means "to separate blood," is a laboratory test that measures the volume percentage of RBCs in whole blood
hemoglobin (hē′-mō-glō′-bĭn)	the oxygen-carrying protein of the RBCs

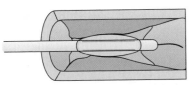

Balloon catheter positioned
in stenotic area

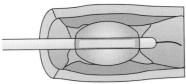

Inflated balloon presses
plaque against arterial wall

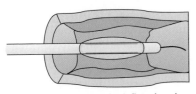

Balloon is deflated and
blood flow reestablished

A

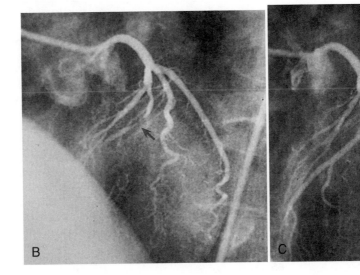

B

C

Figure 22-22 A, Percutaneous transluminal coronary angioplasty (PTCA). **B,** Coronary artery before PTCA. Arrow indicates a stenotic area, estimated at 95% minimum blood flow distal to the lesion. **C,** Coronary arteriogram after PTCA in the same patient. Blood flow is estimated to be 100%.

EXERCISE 3

Analyze and define each medical term listed.

1. aortic
2. splenomegaly
3. hemorrhage
4. thrombosis
5. leukocyte
6. erythrocyte
7. cardiologist
8. cardiomegaly
9. phlebotomy
10. angiorrhaphy
11. splenectomy
12. splenopexy
13. endocarditis
14. arteriosclerosis
15. arteriostenosis
16. thrombophlebitis
17. hematoma
18. hematology
19. leukemia
20. anemia
21. electrocardiogram
22. electrocardiograph
23. electrocardiography
24. angiogram
25. arteriogram
26. aortogram
27. pericarditis
28. tachycardia
29. bradycardia
30. angioplasty

EXERCISE 4

Using the word elements you have studied in this unit and in previous units, build a medical term from each definition listed.

1. x-ray image of the aorta
2. x-ray image of an artery
3. x-ray image of a blood vessel
4. a record of the electrical activity of the heart
5. inflammation of the inner lining of the heart
6. hardening of the arteries
7. inflammation of a vein owing to blood clot formation
8. study of the blood
9. study of the heart
10. one who specializes in the diagnosis and treatment of the heart
11. enlarged heart
12. incision into a vein
13. excision of the spleen
14. surgical fixation of the spleen
15. rapid discharge of blood
16. white blood cell
17. red blood cell
18. inflammation of the outer (sac) of the heart

EXERCISE 5

Define each medical term listed.

1. hematocrit
2. hemoglobin
3. cardiac arrest
4. cardiovascular
5. hemorrhoidectomy
6. myocardial infarction
7. hemorrhoid
8. intravenous
9. cardiac catheterization
10. aneurysm
11. embolism
12. hypertension
13. hypotension
14. congestive heart failure
15. coronary blood vessels
16. edema
17. arrhythmia
18. tachycardia

⊖ EXERCISE 6

Spell each of the 53 medical terms studied in this unit by having someone dictate the terms to you.

1. _____   28. _____
2. _____   29. _____
3. _____   30. _____
4. _____   31. _____
5. _____   32. _____
6. _____   33. _____
7. _____   34. _____
8. _____   35. _____
9. _____   36. _____
10. _____   37. _____
11. _____   38. _____
12. _____   39. _____
13. _____   40. _____
14. _____   41. _____
15. _____   42. _____
16. _____   43. _____
17. _____   44. _____
18. _____   45. _____
19. _____   46. _____
20. _____   47. _____
21. _____   48. _____
22. _____   49. _____
23. _____   50. _____
24. _____   51. _____
25. _____   52. _____
26. _____   53. _____
27. _____

⊖ EXERCISE 7

1. Name the division within the laboratory that performs diagnostic tests on blood components. Name two tests performed in this laboratory division whose results yield RBC information.
2. The coronary care unit (CCU) in the hospital is an intensive care unit that is set up to care for patients who have had heart attacks. Name the three possible admitting diagnoses of these patients.
3. Following is a list of medical terms. Circle the terms that may be found on the surgical schedule. Underline the part of the word that makes it a surgical procedure.

   cardiology   hemorrhoidectomy
   electroencephalogram hypertension
   endocarditis   splenectomy

4. A doctor who performs surgery on the heart or blood vessels may be called a _____ surgeon.
5. A patient is having symptoms that suggest the presence of a disease or a complication involving the circulatory system. The attending doctor is a good practitioner. He wishes the patient to see a heart specialist. He will contact a _____.
6. Each hospital has a team of people to call for emergency conditions such as sudden stoppage of the heart or _____. This team may be called the _____ team.

7. A doctor orders a diagnostic procedure to record the electrical activity of the heart, called a(n) _____. The technician brings a(n) _____ (machine) to the patient's bedside to perform this test.
8. A patient is scheduled for a diagnostic test that uses dye as a contrast medium to visualize parts of the heart. A long catheter is threaded from a blood vessel to the heart. What is the name of this test? May also be referred to as an _____.
9. Below are listed three types of blood cells. Look under "Doctors' Orders for Hematology Studies." Write the name of the laboratory test used to study each cell listed:
   a. leukocyte
   b. erythrocyte
   c. platelet
10. What is the clear, fluid portion of the blood that may be ordered by the doctor to be administered intravenously to the patient?

ABBREVIATIONS

Abbreviation	Meaning
AAA	abdominal aortic aneurysm
ASHD	atherosclerotic heart disease
BP	blood pressure
CABG	coronary artery bypass graft
CAD	coronary artery disease
CHF	congestive heart failure
DVT	deep vein thrombosis
ECG	electrocardiogram
EchoCG	echocardiogram
ECMO	extracorporeal membrane oxygenation
EKG	electrocardiogram
HIV	human immunodeficiency virus
HTN	hypertension (high blood pressure)
MI	myocardial infarction
PTCA	percutaneous transluminal coronary angioplasty
PVD	peripheral vascular disease
RBC	red blood cell (erythrocyte)
Vfib	ventricular fibrillation
WBC	white blood cell (leukocyte)

⊖ EXERCISE 8

Define the following abbreviations.

1. BP   11. Vfib
2. ASHD   12. MI
3. CABG   13. PTCA
4. CAD   14. PVD
5. CHF   15. RBC
6. ECG   16. WBC
7. EchoCG   17. DVT
8. EKG   18. ECMO
9. HIV   19. AAA
10. HTN

UNIT 7
The Digestive System

UNIT OBJECTIVES

On completion of this unit, you will be able to:

1. List seven organs of the digestive tract and five accessory organs.
2. Define four functions of the digestive system.
3. Discuss the process that begins in the mouth, and identify the accessory organs that aid in the process.
4. Name and discuss the purpose of the five sphincters of the digestive tract.
5. Identify the term for the involuntary wavelike movements that move food through the digestive tract.
6. Describe the function of the stomach in continuing the chemical breakdown of food until it is liquefied (chyme), and explain the time it takes for the stomach to completely empty.
7. Identify the 20-foot long organ in which, after secretions of enzymes and bile, digestion is completed and absorption takes place.
8. Describe two functions of the large intestine.
9. Trace the passage of food through the digestive tract.
10. Discuss the functions of the liver, gallbladder, and pancreas and explain how each contributes to the digestive process.
11. Describe gastritis and peptic ulcer disease, diverticular disease, cholelithiasis (gallstones) and choledocholithiasis, and pyloric stenosis.
12. Read the objectives related to medical terminology, and demonstrate ability to meet the objectives by correctly completing Exercises 1 through 8.
13. Define the unit abbreviations.

ORGANS OF THE DIGESTIVE SYSTEM

Digestive Tract

- Mouth
- Pharynx
- Digestive sphincter muscles
- Esophagus
- Stomach
- Small intestine
- Large intestine

Accessory Organs
- Salivary glands
- Teeth and tongue
- Liver
- Gallbladder
- Pancreas

The accessory organs play a vital role in the digestive process. Although food does not pass through the salivary glands, liver, gallbladder, or pancreas, these organs provide secretions necessary for the chemical digestion of food.

Functions of the Digestive System

- *Ingestion:* Taking nutrients into the digestive tract through the mouth
- *Digestion:* The mechanical and chemical breakdown of food for use by body cells
- *Absorption:* The transfer of digested food from the small intestine to the bloodstream
- *Elimination:* The removal of solid waste from the body

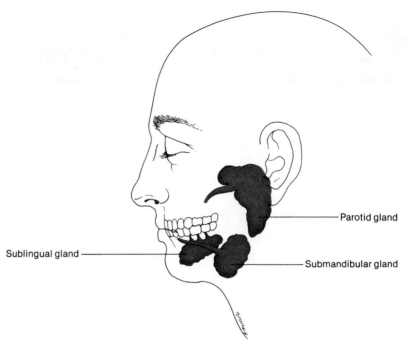

Figure 22-23 The salivary glands.

Food passes through a long tubular structure called the *digestive tract* (also called the *alimentary canal* and the *gastrointestinal [GI] tract*), which extends from the mouth to the rectum. Along the way, food is prepared for absorption by the organs of the digestive tract and the accessory organs. Waste material—that material that is not transferred to the bloodstream during absorption—is eliminated from the body. Ingestion, digestion, absorption, and elimination are the main functions of the digestive system.

THE DIGESTIVE TRACT

Mouth

In the mouth, the chewing of food, or *mastication*, starts the mechanical breakdown of food necessary for *metabolism*, the utilization of digested food by body cells. The tongue helps guide the food to the teeth, where mechanical digestion begins. The salivary glands (Fig. 22-23) produce saliva that contains the enzyme amylase. This enzyme starts the chemical breakdown of carbohydrates (starches and sugars). The three pairs of salivary glands are as follows:

1. *Parotid:* The largest, located near the ear
2. *Submandibular:* Located near the lower jaw
3. *Sublingual:* The smallest, located under the tongue

Each salivary gland has a duct (canal) that opens into the mouth to allow for the flow of saliva.

Pharynx

The *pharynx* (throat) allows for the passage of food from the mouth to the esophagus and is about 5 inches (12.5 cm) long. The pharynx is shared with the respiratory tract because it is also used for the passage of air. The epiglottis,

a flexible flap of cartilage, prevents food from entering the respiratory system.

Digestive Sphincter Muscles

Sphincters, circular muscles that close or open a natural body opening, regulate the passage of substances. The arrangement of the circular fibers creates a central opening when relaxed and closure when they are contracted. Five sphincter muscles are located along the digestive tract. These digestive sphincters are called *upper esophageal, lower esophageal (cardiac), pyloric, ileocecal,* and *anal* sphincters.

Esophagus

The *esophagus* is a muscular tube that extends from the pharynx to the stomach. It passes through the thoracic cavity, behind the heart, to the abdominal cavity. The esophagus is approximately 9 inches (22.5 cm) long. Its function is simply the passage of food, which is propelled along by involuntary wavelike movements; this action is called *peristalsis.* The movement of food into and out of the esophagus is regulated by an upper esophageal sphincter and the lower esophageal (cardiac) sphincter, located between the esophagus and the stomach.

Stomach

The stomach is located in the upper left portion of the abdomen, below the diaphragm. It is a container for food during part of the digestive process. Gastric glands located in the mucous membrane lining of the stomach secrete enzymes (lipase and pepsin) and hydrochloric acid. These secretions continue the chemical breakdown of food. The smooth muscles of the stomach are circular, diagonal, and longitudinal. This muscular construction of the stomach makes the organ very strong (Fig. 22-24). The function of the stomach is to secrete the enzymes

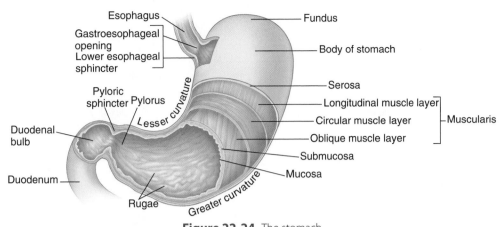

Figure 22-24 The stomach.

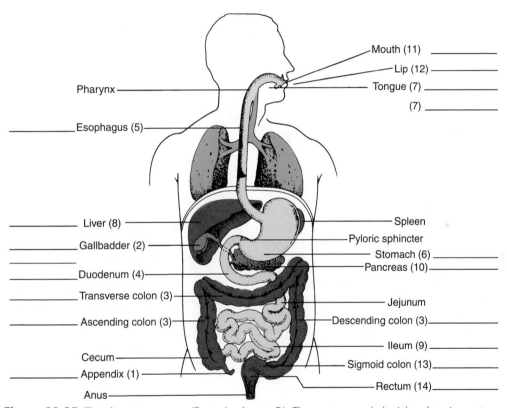

Figure 22-25 The digestive system. (From Applegate EJ: *The anatomy and physiology learning system,* Philadelphia, 1995, WB Saunders, with permission.)

and mix and churn the food to a liquid consistency. This process of mixing and churning continues the mechanical breakdown of food. When the food is liquefied, it is referred to as *chyme.*

After about 30 minutes, the food begins to leave the stomach at 30-minute intervals. It passes through the pyloric sphincter muscle into the duodenum, which is the first part of the small intestine. It takes 2 to 4 hours for the stomach to empty completely.

Small Intestine

The small intestine, so called because it is smaller in diameter than the large intestine, is approximately 20 feet long. It extends from the stomach to the large intestine (Fig. 22-25). The first

part of the small intestine is called the *duodenum.* Two accessory organs, the *pancreas* and the *gallbladder,* secrete into the duodenum through tiny tubes called *ducts.* The pancreas secretes many enzymes necessary for digestion. The gallbladder secretes bile that has been produced by the liver and stored in the gallbladder. The *jejunum,* followed by the *ileum,* forms the remainder of the small intestine. (The *ilium,* one of the pelvic bones studied in the musculoskeletal system, has the same pronunciation as *ileum.* Correct spelling of the word to communicate the proper meaning is absolutely essential.) The mucosal cells located in the lining of the small intestine secrete enzymes that continue the chemical breakdown of food. These enzymes include sucrase, maltase, lipase, peptidase, and lactase. Digestion is completed in the small intestine, and absorption takes place here.

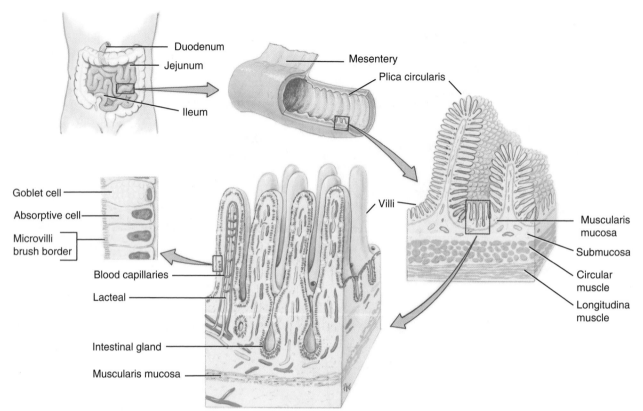

Figure 22-26 Intestinal villi. (From Applegate EJ: *The anatomy and physiology learning system,* Philadelphia, 1995, WB Saunders, with permission.)

Absorption is the passage of the end products of digestion from the small intestine into the bloodstream. The passage of nutrients from the small intestine to the bloodstream is facilitated through the capillary walls of the villi, which have a surface area of approximately 100 square feet. The *villi,* which are tiny, finger-like projections that line the walls of the small intestine (Fig. 22-26), increase the surface area of the small intestine to make it the main site of digestion and absorption. The blood carries the nutrients to all body cells, where they are used according to need. The process of cell utilization of nutrients is called *metabolism.*

The food substance (waste) that is not absorbed continues to move by peristalsis through the ileocecal sphincter into the large intestine.

Large Intestine

The large intestine is approximately 5 feet long. Peristalsis continues into the large intestine. The large intestine extends from the ileum to the *anus,* the opening at the end of the rectum to the outside. The large intestine is divided into the following parts, listed in sequence extending from the ileum: the *cecum;* the *colon,* which is divided into four parts—the ascending colon, the transverse colon, the descending colon, and the sigmoid colon; and the *rectum.* The function of the large intestine is the absorption of water and the elimination of solid waste products of digestion from the body.

The appendix is a small blind tube attached to the cecum. It has no function.

★ **HIGH PRIORITY**

Pathway: food ingestion → mouth → esophagus → cardiac sphincter → stomach → pyloric sphincter → small intestine (duodenum, jejunum, ileum) → nutrients absorption by the blood and carried to all cells for metabolic waste → ileocecal sphincter → large intestine (cecum, ascending colon, transverse colon, descending colon, sigmoid colon, rectum) → anal sphincter → elimination

Accessory Organs: Liver, Gallbladder, and Pancreas

The liver, the largest gland in the body, is located in the upper right portion of the abdominal cavity. Although it has many important functions, only one is discussed here: the production of bile. The liver secretes bile, which aids in the digestion of fats. Bile is stored in the gallbladder, a small sac located under the liver. The gallbladder concentrates the bile by reabsorbing water. When food (especially food that contains fat) enters the duodenum from the stomach, the gallbladder is stimulated to contract and release bile into the duodenum.

The pancreas is located behind the stomach. Part of its function is to secrete the enzymes lipase, protease, amylase, and bicarbonate into the duodenum. These enzymes continue the digestion process by chemically breaking down food particles. The islets of Langerhans are contained in the pancreas. They secrete two hormones—glucagon and insulin—that are released directly into the bloodstream. Insulin is necessary for the metabolism of carbohydrates in the body, and it decreases blood glucose levels. Glucagon, also instrumental in digestion, increases blood glucose.

DISEASES AND CONDITIONS OF THE DIGESTIVE SYSTEM

Gastritis and Peptic Ulcer Disease

Gastritis describes a group of conditions with one thing in common, inflammation of the lining of the stomach. Gastritis may occur suddenly (acute gastritis) or it can occur slowly over time (chronic gastritis). Symptoms may include a burning ache or pain (indigestion) in your upper abdomen that may become either worse or better with eating, nausea, vomiting, and/or a feeling of fullness in upper abdomen after eating. Usually gastritis isn't serious and improves quickly by avoiding alcohol and eating any foods such as those that are spicy, aciic, fried, or fatty. If the condition worsens and goes untreated, gastritis can lead to ulcers.

A peptic ulcer is a lesion, or sore, of the mucous membrane of the stomach (gastric ulcer) or duodenum (duodenal ulcer) (Fig. 22-27). A combination of factors causes peptic ulcer disease (PUD); these factors include excessive secretion of gastric enzymes, hydrochloric acid, *Helicobacter pylori*, heredity, and the use of certain drugs, especially NSAIDs.

Symptoms include pain 1 to 3 hours after eating, which is usually relieved by eating or taking antacids. Also, a gnawing sensation in the epigastric region is experienced. If untreated, bleeding, hemorrhage, or perforation may occur. Perforation allows the contents of the stomach or the small intestine to escape into the peritoneal cavity. The GI series, gastroscopy, and gastric analysis are used for diagnosing peptic ulcers. Because symptoms of peptic ulcer are similar to symptoms of stomach or duodenal cancer, early diagnosis is important. Early treatment includes diet control, medication, and, if present, eradication of *H. pylori* bacteria with antibiotics. Surgery may be indicated when scarring, recurrent bleeding, or perforation occurs.

Diverticular Disease

Diverticular disease is caused by the formation of small pouches, called *diverticula*, on the wall of the large intestine, generally the colon (Fig. 22-28). Two forms of diverticular disease may occur: diverticulosis and diverticulitis. In diverticulosis, diverticula are present but for most people cause no symptoms. In diverticulitis, diverticula are inflamed or infected and may cause obstruction, infection, or hemorrhage. There is evidence that diverticular disease is related to the consumption of a low-fiber diet.

Symptoms include cramping in the abdomen and muscle spasms. Medical treatment includes eating a high-fiber or restricted diet and taking antibiotics to treat infection. Severe cases may require surgical removal of the involved segment of the intestine and a temporary colostomy (surgical opening between the colon and the body surface).

Cholelithiasis and Choledocholithiasis

Cholelithiasis (or *gallstones*), a condition that affects 20% of the population older than 40 years of age, is more common in women than in men (Fig. 22-29). The stones form because

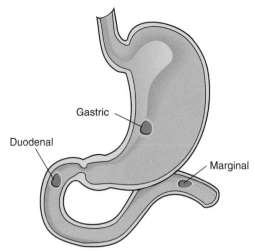

Figure 22-27 Types of ulcers.

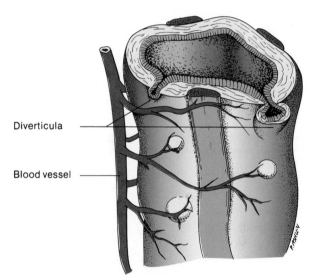

Figure 22-28 Diverticula.

of changes in bile content. Gallstones can lodge in the common bile duct, which leads to the duodenum. This condition is called *choledocholithiasis*. Pain is caused by buildup of pressure in the gallbladder.

Symptoms of a typical gallbladder attack include acute abdominal pain after eating a fatty meal. Sometimes the pain is so severe that the patient may seek emergency treatment. Other symptoms involve digestive disturbances, such as belching and flatulence. MRI, CT scan, cholecystogram, or abdominal ultrasound may be used for diagnosing gallstones. Treatment includes laparoscopic cholecystectomy and choledocholithotomy.

Pyloric Stenosis

Pyloric stenosis is an obstruction that is caused by narrowing of the pyloric sphincter muscle. The condition may be congenital or acquired. In adults the condition most often is caused by peptic ulceration or tumors that may be cancerous. Symptoms include vomiting that becomes progressively more frequent and forceful. Infants with pyloric stenosis may be diagnosed at first with failure to thrive. Adults experience a gradual weight loss.

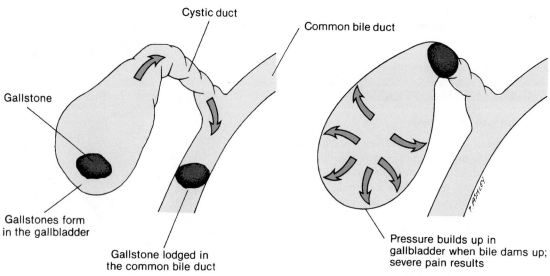

Cystic duct

Common bile duct

Gallstone

Gallstones form
in the gallbladder

Gallstone lodged in
the common bile duct

Pressure builds up in
gallbladder when bile dams up;
severe pain results

Figure 22-29 Gallstones.

Diagnosis is confirmed by an upper GI examination in which barium is used as a contrast medium. Treatment is usually surgical. In infants, a formula that is thickened with cereal may be sufficient to stretch out the sphincter muscle if stenosis is not severe.

REVIEW QUESTIONS

1. List seven organs of the digestive tract and five accessory organs.

   a. ingestion   c. absorption
   b. digestion   d. elimination

2. Define the following four functions of the digestive system:

3. Discuss the process that begins in the mouth, and identify the accessory organ that produces a substance that aids in the process in the mouth.

4. Name and discuss the purpose of the five sphincters of the digestive tract.

5. Identify the term for the involuntary wavelike movements that move food through the esophagus.

6. Describe the function of the stomach in continuing the chemical breakdown of food until it is liquefied (chyme), and explain the time it takes for the stomach to completely empty.

7. Identify the 20-foot-long organ in which, after bile is secreted from the gallbladder, digestion is completed and absorption takes place.

8. Describe two functions of the large intestine

9. Beginning with the mouth, list in order the organs through which food passes during ingestion, digestion,

and elimination. Include the names of the parts of the small intestine, large intestine, and sphincter muscles.

10. Match the terms in Column 1 with the definitions in Column 2.

Column 1	Column 2
a. diverticulitis	1. lesion of the mucous membrane of the stomach
b. cholelithiasis	2. inflamed diverticula
c. cholecystectomy	3. stones in the gallbladder
d. diverticulosis	4. stone in the common bile duct
e. peptic ulcer	5. diverticula with no symptoms
f. choledocholithiasis	

MEDICAL TERMINOLOGY RELATED TO THE DIGESTIVE SYSTEM

Objectives
On mastery of the medical terminology for this unit, you will be able to:

1. Spell and define the word parts and medical terms related to the digestive system.
2. Given the meaning of a medical condition related to the digestive tract, build with word parts the corresponding medical term.
3. Given a list of medical terms, identify those that are surgical procedures and those that are diagnostic studies.
4. Compare the three -*tomy* suffixes.
5. Analyze and define medical terms built from word parts that relate to the digestive system.
6. Given a description of hospital situations in which the HUC may encounter medical terminology, apply the correct medical terms to the situations.

Word Parts

The following list contains the word parts related to the digestive system that you need to memorize. The exercises included

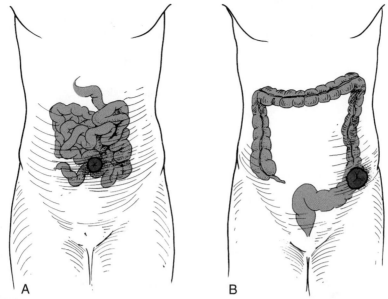

Figure 22-30 A, Ileostomy. **B,** Colostomy. (From LaFleur M: *Exploring medical language,* ed 5, St Louis, 2002, Mosby.)

in this unit will help you with this task. You will continue to use these word parts throughout this course and during your employment. Practice pronouncing each part aloud.

Word Roots/Combining Forms	Meaning
1. abdomin / o (ăb-dŏm′-ī-nō)	abdomen
2. appendic / o (ăp-ĕn-dĕk′-ō)	appendix
3. cheil / o (kī′-lō)	lip
4. chol / o (kō′-lō) or chol / e (kō′-lē)	bile, gall
5. col / o (kō′-lō)	colon
6. colon / o (kō′-lŏ- nō)	colon
7. cyst / o (sĭs′-tō)	bladder (urinary unless otherwise used)
8. duoden / o (doo-ō-dē′-nō)	duodenum
9. enter / o (ĕn′-ter-ō)	intestine
10. esophag / o (ĕ-sŏf′-ah-gō)	esophagus
11. gastr / o (găs′-trō)	stomach
12. gloss / o (glŏss′-ō); lingu / o (lĭng′-gwō)	tongue
13. hepat / o (hĕp′-a-tō)	liver
14. herni / o (her′-nē-ō)	protrusion of a body part
15. ile / o (ĭl′-ĕ-ō)	ileum
16. lapar / o (lăp′-ah-rō)	abdomen
17. lith / o (lĭth′-ō)	stone or calculus
18. pancreat / o (păn′-krē-ă-tō)	pancreas
19. proct / o (prŏk′-tō)	rectum
20. sigmoid / o (sĭg′-moy-dō)	sigmoid colon (part of the colon)
21. stomat / o (stō′-mah-tō)	mouth

Suffixes	Meaning
-iasis (ī′-ah-sĭs)	condition of
-ostomy (ŏs′-to-mē)	creation of an artificial opening into

-tomy Suffixes

You are already familiar with two *-tomy* suffixes that are used to describe surgical procedures. These include *-tomy,* which means an incision into a part of the body, and *-ectomy,* which means surgical removal of a part of the body. The third *-tomy* suffix you will study in this unit is *-stomy,* which describes a surgical procedure that is performed to create an artificial opening into a part of the body. For example, in the medical term *colostomy* (col / o is the combining form for colon), a portion of the colon is attached to the surface of the abdomen, which creates an artificial opening between the colon and the abdominal surface (Fig. 22-30). This artificial opening is used for the passage of stools.

⊜ EXERCISE **1**

Write the combining forms for the digestive system in the spaces provided on the diagram in Figure 22-25). The number preceding the combining form in the preceding list matches the number of the body part in the diagram.

⊜ EXERCISE **2**

Define the word parts listed. Indicate the word parts that are suffixes by writing S after each in the space provided.

Word Parts	Definition	Suffix?
1. stomat		
2. gloss		
3. gastr		
4. proct		
5. pancreat		
6. enter		
7. hepat		
8. cheil		
9. esophag		
10. iasis		
11. chol		
12. cyst		

Word Parts	Definition	Suffix?
13. duoden		
14. col		
15. ile		
16. abdomin		
17. appendic		
18. lapar		
19. lith		
20. stomy		
21. herni		
22. sigmoid		

⊜ EXERCISE 3

Define the three -tomy suffixes. Build a medical term using each suffix, and write the meaning of each term you have built.

1. -tomy   **2.** -ectomy   **3.** -stomy

MEDICAL TERMS RELATED TO THE DIGESTIVE SYSTEM

Following is a list of medical terms related to the digestive system that you will need to know. Exercises following this list will assist you in learning these terms. Practice pronouncing each term aloud.

General Terms	Meaning
abdominal (ăb-dŏm′-ĭn-al)	pertaining to the abdomen
diarrhea (dī-ah-rē′-ah)	frequent discharge of watery stool
duodenal (doo-ō-dē′-nal)	pertaining to the duodenum
dysentery (dĭs′-ĕn-tĕr-ē)	condition of bad or painful intestines accompanied by diarrhea
glossoplegia (glŏss-ō-plē′-ja)	paralysis of the tongue
hepatoma (hĕp-ah-tō′-mah)	a tumor of the liver
hepatomegaly (hĕp′-ah-tō-mĕg′-ah-lē)	enlargement of the liver
hernia (her′-nē-ah)	an abnormal protrusion of a body part through the containing structure
jaundice (jawn′-dĭs)	yellowness of the skin and eyes; a symptom of hepatitis
pancreatic (păn-krē-ăt′-ĭk)	pertaining to the pancreas
proctorrhea (prŏk-tō-rē′-ah)	excessive discharge from the rectum
stomatogastric (stō′-mah-tō-găs′-trĭk)	pertaining to the mouth and stomach
sublingual (sŭb-lĭng′-gwal)	pertaining to under the tongue
ulcer (ŭl′-ser)	a sore of the skin or mucous membrane

Surgical Terms	Meaning
abdominal herniorrhaphy (ăb-dŏm′-ĭn-al) (her-nē-ōr′-ah-fē)	suturing of a weak spot or opening in the abdominal wall to prevent protrusion of organs

Surgical Terms	Meaning
appendectomy (ăp-ĕn-dĕk′-to-mē)	excision of the appendix
cheiloplasty (kī′-lō-plăs′-tē)	surgical repair of the lip
cholecystectomy (kō-lē-sĭs-tĕk′-to-mē) *Note: e* is used as the combining vowel between the word roots *chol* and *cyst*.	excision of the gallbladder
colectomy (kō-lĕk′-to-mē)	excision of the colon
colostomy (kō-lŏs′-to-mē)	creation of an artificial opening into the colon; a portion of the colon is attached to the surface of the abdomen for the passage of stools
esophagoenterostomy (ē-sŏf′-ah-gō-ĕn-ter-ŏs′-to-mē)	creation of an artificial opening between the esophagus and the intestine
gastrectomy (găs-trĕk′-to-mē); pyloroplasty (pī-lōr′-ō-plăs′-tē); and vagotomy (vā-gŏt′-o-mē)	surgical procedures performed for treatment of ulcers; gastrectomy is the removal of the stomach; pyloroplasty is the plastic repair of the pyloric sphincter, located at the lower end of the stomach; vagotomy is an incision into the vagus nerve, performed to reduce the quantity of gastric juices in the stomach
gastric bypass—malabsorptive	surgical procedure for obesity in which a small pouch is created at the top of the stomach to restrict food intake
gastrostomy (găs-trŏs′-to-mē)	creation of an artificial opening into the stomach (for feeding purposes)
glossorrhaphy (glŏ-sŏr′-ah-fē)	suturing of the tongue
herniorrhaphy (her-nē-ōr′-ah-fē)	surgical repair of a hernia (suturing of the containing structure, for example, the abdominal wall)
ileostomy (ĭl-ē-ŏs′-to-mē)	creation of an artificial opening into the ileum; a portion of the ileum is attached to the surface of the abdomen for passage of stools
laparoscopy (lăp-ah-rŏs′-ko-pē)	visual examination of the abdomen (with instruments introduced through incisions, often done in order to perform minimally invasive surgery)
laparotomy (lăp-ah-rŏt′-o-mē)	incision into the abdominal wall

Diagnostic Terms	Meaning
appendicitis (ah-pĕn-dĭ-sī′-tĭs)	inflammation of the appendix
cholecystitis (kō-lē-sĭs-tī′-tĭs)	inflammation of the gallbladder

Diagnostic Terms	Meaning
cholelithiasis (kō-lē-lǐ-thī′-ah-sǐs) *Note: e is used as the combining vowel between the word roots chol and lith.*	a condition of gallstones
Crohn (krōn) disease	chronic inflammatory disease that can affect any part of the bowel, most often the lower small intestine
diverticulitis (dī-ver-tǐk-ū-lī′-tǐs)	inflammation of the diverticula (small pouches in the intestinal wall)
duodenal ulcer (dū-ō-dē′-nal) (ǔl′-sěr)	ulcer (sore open area) in the duodenum
gastric ulcer (găs′-trǐk) (ǔl′-ser)	ulcer pertaining to the stomach
gastritis (găs-trī′-tǐs)	inflammation of the stomach
hepatitis (hěp-ah-tī′-tǐs)	inflammation of the liver
ileitis (ǐl-ē-ī′-tǐs)	inflammation of the ileum
infectious hepatitis (ǐn-fěk′-shǔs) (hěp-ah-tī′-tǐs)	inflammation of the liver (caused by a virus)
pancreatitis (păn-krē-ah-tī′-tǐs)	inflammation of the pancreas
stomatitis (stǒ-mah-tī′-tǐs)	inflammation of the mouth
ulcerative colitis (ǔl′-sě-ră-tǐv) (kō-lī′-tǐs)	inflammation of the colon with the formation of ulcers

Terms Related to Diagnostic Procedures / **Meaning**

abdominocentesis (ăb-dǒm′-ǐ-nō-sěn-tē′-sǐs)	aspiration of fluid from the abdominal cavity
barium enema (bă′-rē-ǔm) (ěn′-ē-mah) (BE)	x-ray examination of the colon (fasting x-ray); barium is used as the contrast medium
cholangiogram (kō-lăn′-jē-ǒ-grăm)	x-ray image of the bile ducts (fasting x-ray), usually done after a cholecystectomy; dye is the contrast medium
cholecystogram (kō-lē-sǐs′-to-grăm)	x-ray image of the gallbladder (most commonly done intraoperatively); contrast medium is used
colonoscope (kō-lǒn′-ō-skōp)	instrument used for visual examination of the colon

Terms Related to Diagnostic Procedures / **Meaning**

colonoscopy (kō-lǒn-ǒs′-ko-pē)	visual examination of the colon
esophagogastroduodenoscopy (ě-sǒf′-ah-gō-gas-trō-doo-odd-ěn-ǒs′-ko-pē) (EGD)	visual examination of the esophagus, stomach, and duodenum
esophagoscope (ě-sǒf′-ah-gō-skōp)	instrument used for visual examination of the esophagus
esophagoscopy (ě-sǒf′-ah-gǒs′-ko-pē)	visual examination of the esophagus

Terms Related to Diagnostic Procedures / **Meaning**

gastroscope (găs′-trō-skōp)	instrument used for visual examination of the stomach
gastroscopy (găs-trǒs′-ko-pē)	visual examination of the stomach
proctoscope (prǒk′-tō-skōp)	instrument used for visual examination of the rectum
proctoscopy (prǒk-tǒs′-ko-pē)	visual examination of the rectum
sigmoidoscopy (sǐg-mol-dǒs′-ko-pē)	visual examination of the sigmoid colon
upper gastrointestinal (găs′-trō-ǐn-těs′-tǐ-nal) (UGI)	x-ray examination of the esophagus and the stomach (fasting x-ray); barium is used as the contrast medium; UGI with small-bowel follow-through is an x-ray examination of the stomach and small intestines

⊖ EXERCISE 4

Analyze and define the terms listed.

1. glossoplegia
2. appendectomy
3. cholecystectomy
4. gastrostomy
5. hepatomegaly
6. ileostomy
7. pyloroplasty
8. proctorrhea
9. cholecystitis
10. gastritis
11. sublingual
12. ileitis
13. cholecystogram
14. sigmoidoscopy
15. gastrectomy
16. gastroscopy
17. gastroscope
18. colitis
19. hepatitis
20. colostomy
21. herniorrhaphy
22. colonoscope
23. colonoscopy
24. esophagogastroduodenoscopy

⊖ EXERCISE 5

Using the word parts studied in this unit and in previous units, build medical terms from the definitions listed. Also, identify which are surgical procedures by writing S in the space provided, and which are diagnostic studies by writing D in the space provided. Underline the word part that indicates that the word is a surgical procedure or a diagnostic study. (Note: Some words in the list will not fall into either of these categories.)

Examples:	gastr<u>ectomy</u>	S
	gastro<u>scopy</u>	D

1. inflammation of the mouth
2. inflammation of the gallbladder
3. a condition of gallstones
4. x-ray image of the gallbladder
5. excision of the gallbladder
6. inflammation of the pancreas
7. instrument used for visual examination of the rectum
8. visual examination of the rectum
9. aspiration of fluid from the abdominal cavity

★ **HIGH PRIORITY**

Scope It Out

Modern medical advances and surgical innovation have paved the way for a growing number of minimally invasive surgeries. In procedures that range from appendectomy and blepharoplasty (cosmetic repair of eyelids) to cardiac and foot surgery, the thin, flexible tube with a small video camera and a light on the end is able to penetrate organs, joints, and cavities; to diagnose and correct various conditions; and to record the episode at the same time. Local or general anesthesia may be used during the procedure. Frequently, conscious sedation is administered, with a combination of sedatives and pain relievers that achieve an altered state of consciousness. Most endoscopies are performed on an outpatient basis.

Expanding use of the fiberoptic endoscope beyond the digestive system is responsible for smaller incisions, shorter recovery time, and lower medical costs. Nearly all specialties are making use of endoscopy as a more efficient means of providing diagnostic and therapeutic interventions.

The endoscope, an instrument used for visual examination within a hollow organ or body cavity, is introduced through a small incision. Through a separate small incision, tiny folding surgical instruments (e.g., forceps, scissors, brushes, snares, baskets for tissue excision) are introduced and manipulated within the tissue.

- *Arthroscopy:* Examination of joints for diagnosis and treatment.
- *Bronchoscopy:* Examination of the trachea and lung bronchial trees to diagnose abscesses, bronchitis, carcinoma, tumors, tuberculosis, alveolitis, infection, and inflammation.
- *Capsule endoscopy:* Remote examination of the inside of the entire digestive system by using a small capsule device with a camera that is swallowed by the patient.
- *Colonoscopy:* Examination of the inside of the colon and large intestine to detect polyps, tumors, ulceration, inflammation, colitis diverticula, and Crohn disease, and for discovery and removal of foreign bodies.
- *Colposcopy:* Direct visualization of the vagina and cervix to detect cancer, inflammation, and other conditions.
- *Cystoscopy:* Examination of the bladder, urethra, urinary tract, ureteral orifices, and prostate (men) performed with insertion of the endoscope through the urethra.
- *Endoscopic biopsy:* Removal of tissue specimens for pathologic examination and analysis.

- *Endoscopic laser foraminoplasty:* With the use of an endoscope and a laser to create an opening through the foramen (itself an opening) into the epidural space, the endoscopic surgeon can visualize the nerves in the spinal column to repair ruptured or herniated disks.
- *Endoscopic retrograde cholangiopancreatography (ERCP):* Makes use of the endoscope for radiographic examination with contrast medium introduced through a catheter. The endoscopist visualizes the liver's biliary tree, the gallbladder, the pancreatic duct, and other nearby anatomy to check for stones, obstructions, and disease. Fluoroscopic x-ray images are taken to show any abnormality or blockage. If disease is detected, it sometimes can be treated at the same time, or biopsy can be performed to test for cancer or other pathologic conditions. ERCP may reveal biliary cirrhosis, cancer of the bile ducts, pancreatic cysts, pseudocysts, pancreatic tumors, chronic pancreatitis, and gallbladder stones.
- *Esophagogastroduodenoscopy (EGD):* Visual examination of the upper gastrointestinal (GI) tract (also referred to as *gastroscopy*) to diagnose hemorrhage, hiatal hernia, inflammation of the esophagus, and gastric ulcers.
- *Gastroscopy:* Examination of the lining of the esophagus, stomach, and duodenum. Gastroscopy often is used to diagnose ulcers and other sources of bleeding and to guide the biopsy of suspected GI cancers.
- *Hysteroscopy:* Visual examination of the uterus.
- *Laparoscopy:* Visual examination of the abdominal cavity: stomach, liver, and other abdominal organs, including the female reproductive organs (e.g., fallopian tubes, uterus, ovaries).
  - Laparoscopic adrenalectomy
  - Laparoscopic appendectomy
  - Laparoscopic cholecystectomy
  - Laparoscopic choledochoscopy and choledocholithotomy
  - Laparoscopic tubal ligation
- *Laryngoscopy:* Visual examination of the larynx (voice box).
- *Proctoscopy, proctosigmoidoscopy, sigmoidoscopy:* Visual examination of the rectum and sigmoid colon.
- *Thoracoscopy:* Visual examination of the thorax (chest: pleura [sac that covers the lungs], pleural spaces, mediastinum, and pericardium).

10. creation of an artificial opening into the colon
11. creation of an artificial opening into the ileum
12. visual examination of the esophagus
13. instrument used for visual examination of the stomach
14. creation of an artificial opening between the esophagus and the intestines

15. inflammation of the stomach
16. suturing of the tongue
17. surgical repair of the lip
18. excision of the colon
19. paralysis of the tongue
20. pertaining to the mouth and stomach
21. pertaining to under the tongue
22. discharge from the rectum
23. enlargement of the liver
24. tumor of the liver

25. pertaining to the pancreas
26. inflammation of the appendix
27. surgical removal of the appendix
28. visual examination of the colon
29. instrument used for visual examination of the colon
30. visual examination of the esophagus, stomach, and duodenum

EXERCISE 6

Define the following medical terms.

1. dysentery
2. upper gastrointestinal (UGI)
3. barium enema
4. cholecystogram
5. jaundice
6. ulcerative colitis
7. gastric ulcer
8. Crohn disease

EXERCISE 7

Spell each of the 59 medical terms studied in this unit by having someone dictate the terms to you.

1.	31.
2.	32.
3.	33.
4.	34.
5.	35.
6.	36.
7.	37.
8.	38.
9.	39.
10.	40.
11.	41.
12.	42.
13.	43.
14.	44.
15.	45.
16.	46.
17.	47.
18.	48.
19.	49.
20.	50.
21.	51.
22.	52.
23.	53.
24.	54.
25.	55.
26.	56.
27.	57.
28.	58.
29.	59.
30.	

EXERCISE 8

Answer the following questions.

1. A surgical procedure to make an artificial opening from the small intestine to the abdomen is listed on the surgery schedule. Circle the correct surgical term for this procedure, and explain your choice:
   a. iliostomy
   b. ileostomy
   c. ileotomy
2. A patient enters the hospital with a diagnosis of gallstones. In medical terms, what will be the admitting diagnosis? The doctor orders a diagnostic study to visualize the gallbladder to determine the presence of disease or gallstones. The order is for a _____. The result of the diagnostic study indicates surgery for removal of the gallbladder. What is the medical term for this operation?
3. The doctor orders a medication to be administered under the patient's tongue. What is the word written on the doctors' order sheet to indicate this?
4. List three visual examinations of the digestive tract that the doctor may order, and name the instrument used for each examination.
5. A patient enters the hospital for surigical procedures for the treatment of ulcers. The doctor plans to remove the stomach, repair the pyloric sphincter, and make an incision into the vagus nerve. What are the medical terms used to describe the surgery?
6. The following surgical procedures are listed on the surgical schedule, and you are preparing consent forms for them. Circle the terms that are spelled incorrectly, and correctly spell the misspelled terms.
   a. laportotomy
   b. appendectomy
   c. herniorraphy
   d. collectomy
   e. gastrostomy

ABBREVIATIONS

Abbreviation	Meaning
BE	barium enema
EGD	esophagogastroduodenoscopy
GE	gastroenterology, gastroenterologist
GERD	gastroesophageal reflux disease
GI	gastrointestinal
PUD	peptic ulcer disease
UGI	upper gastrointestinal

EXERCISE 9

Define the following abbreviations.

1. BE
2. GI
3. GE
4. GERD
5. EGD
6. PUD
7. UGI

UNIT 8
The Respiratory System

OUTLINE

UNIT OBJECTIVES

On completion of this unit, you will be able to:

1. Describe the overall function of the respiratory system, and identify the organs included in the upper and lower respiratory systems.
2. Compare internal respiration with external respiration.
3. Name and discuss the function of each organ of the respiratory system.
4. Describe the pathway of air from the outside to the capillary blood in the lungs.
5. Discuss pneumothorax, hemothorax, pulmonary embolism, chronic obstructive pulmonary disease (COPD), and acute respiratory distress syndrome (ARDS).
6. Read the objectives related to medical terminology, and demonstrate ability to meet the objectives by correctly completing Exercises 1 through 8.
7. Define the unit abbreviations.

THE RESPIRATORY SYSTEM

Organs of the Respiratory System

- Nose
- Pharynx
- Larynx
- Trachea
- Bronchi
- Lungs

Division of the Respiratory System

The *upper respiratory system* refers to the nose, nasal cavities, sinuses, pharynx, and larynx. The *lower respiratory system* refers to the trachea, bronchi, alveoli, and lungs (Fig. 22-31).

Function of the Respiratory System

The function of the respiratory system is to exchange gases. Oxygen is taken into the body and carbon dioxide is removed. This process is referred to as *respiration*. The respiratory system also helps to regulate the acid-base balance and enables the production of vocal sounds.

Respiration

External respiration, or breathing, is the exchange of gases between the lungs and the blood. Oxygen is inhaled into the lungs and passes through the capillary wall into the blood to be carried to the blood cells. Carbon dioxide passes out of the capillary blood to the lungs to be exhaled to the outside environment.

An exchange of gases also takes place within the body between the blood in the capillaries and individual body cells. This is called *internal respiration.* Body cells take on oxygen from the blood and at the same time give off carbon dioxide to the blood to be transported back to the lungs, where it is exhaled from the body.

The Nose

Air enters the respiratory system through the nose. The nose is divided into a right and a left nostril by a partition called the

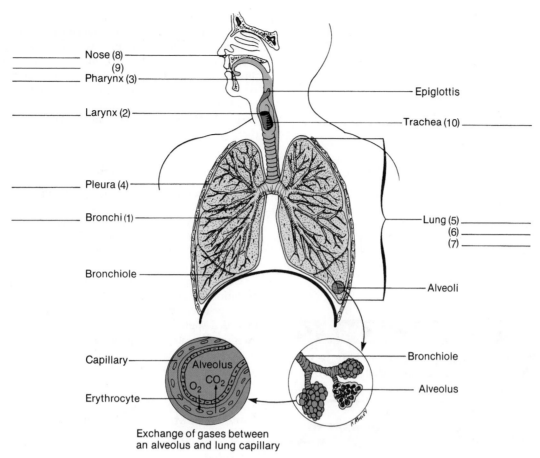

Nose (8)
(9)
Pharynx (3)
Larynx (2)
Pleura (4)
Bronchi (1)
Bronchiole
Capillary
Alveolus
CO_2
O_2
Erythrocyte

Epiglottis
Trachea (10)
Lung (5)
(6)
(7)
Alveoli
Bronchiole
Alveolus

Exchange of gases between
an alveolus and lung capillary

Figure 22-31 The respiratory system.

nasal septum. The nose prepares the air for the body by (1) warming and moistening the air, (2) removing pathogenic microorganisms, and (3) removing foreign particles, such as dust, from the air. Tiny, hairlike growths in the nose called *cilia* trap and move foreign particles toward the outside and away from delicate lung tissue. Particles too large to be handled by the *cilia* produce a sneeze or a cough, which forcibly expels the foreign particles.

The Pharynx

Both air and food travel through the *pharynx* (throat). Food passes from the pharynx to the esophagus, and air passes from the pharynx into the larynx, which is located anterior to the esophagus.

The Larynx

The *larynx* (voice box) is a tubular structure located below the pharynx. As was mentioned earlier, the pharynx is a passageway for both food and air. A flap of cartilage, called the *epiglottis,* automatically covers the larynx during the act of swallowing to prevent the passage of food from the pharynx into the larynx. The larynx contains the *vocal cords.* As air is exhaled past the vocal cords, the vibration of the cords produces sound.

The Trachea

The *trachea* (windpipe), a vertical tube 4 to 5 inches (10 to 12.5 cm) long, extends from the larynx to the bronchi. A series of C-shaped cartilage rings prevents the trachea from collapsing. The function of the trachea is the passage of air.

Bronchi

Behind the heart, close to the center of the chest, the trachea branches into two tubes: one leading to the right lung and the other leading to the left lung. These tubes are called *bronchi* (singular: *bronchus*). The function of the bronchi is the passage of air.

The Lungs

The lungs are cone-shaped organs located in the thoracic cavity. The right lung is the larger of the two and is divided into three lobes. The left lung is divided into two lobes. After the bronchus enters the lung, it divides into smaller tubes and continues to subdivide into even smaller tubes called *bronchioles.* At the end of each bronchiole is a grape-like cluster of air sacs called *alveoli* (singular: *alveolus*). The walls of the alveoli are single celled, which allows for an exchange of gases to take place between the alveoli and the capillaries. The *pleura* is a double sac that surrounds each lung and lines the walls of the thoracic cavity. The *visceral pleura* lines the outer surface of the lungs, whereas the *parietal pleura* covers the chest wall. The small amount of fluid within the sacs allows the lungs to expand and contract without friction.

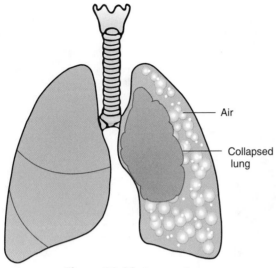

Figure 22-32 Pneumothorax.

 HIGH PRIORITY

Pathway: air → nose → pharynx → larynx → trachea → bronchi → bronchioles → alveoli, where the exchange of carbon dioxide and oxygen takes place

CONDITIONS OF THE RESPIRATORY SYSTEM

Pneumothorax and Hemothorax

Pneumothorax

Pneumothorax is the collection of air or gas in the pleural cavity, resulting in a collapsed lung, or *atelectasis* (Fig. 22-32). It may be caused by a chest wound, or it may be a spontaneous collapse resulting from lung disease. The pleural cavity is airtight, with negative pressure. As air enters the pleural cavity, it creates pressure against the lung, causing it to collapse.

Symptoms include sudden sharp chest pain, shortness of breath, cyanosis, and stopping of normal chest movements on the affected side. Treatment ranges from observation and supplemental oxygen for an uncomplicated pneumothorax to a thoracentesis to remove the air or gas from the cavity and a thoracotomy with insertion of chest tubes. The tubes are connected to an underwater drainage system with suction and remain in place until air is no longer expelled from the pleural space.

Hemothorax

A *hemothorax* is the collection of blood in the pleural cavity; it usually is caused by chest trauma. Symptoms include chest pain, shortness of breath, respiratory failure, tachycardia, and anxiety. Treatment includes stabilizing the patient, stopping the bleeding, inserting a chest tube to evacuate blood and air from the pleural space, and reexpanding the lung.

Pulmonary Embolism

Pulmonary embolism (PE) is the most common complication in hospitalized patients. It strikes 6 million adults each year, causing 100,000 deaths. Pulmonary embolism is usually caused by a blood clot that has been dislodged from a leg or pelvic vein—*deep vein thrombosis* (DVT)—and blocks a pulmonary artery. Symptoms include cough, dyspnea (difficulty in breathing), chest pain, cyanosis (blue tinge to the skin), tachycardia, and shock. It is difficult to distinguish between pneumonia and MI. Chest x-ray examination, pulmonary arteriography, arterial blood gases, and lung perfusion scans coupled with a lung ventilation scan are used to diagnose PE. Treatment includes thrombolytic, anticoagulant, and oxygen therapy.

Chronic Obstructive Pulmonary Disease

Chronic obstructive pulmonary disease (COPD) is the persistent obstruction of bronchial air flow. This chronic condition of the respiratory system is the second leading cause of hospital admissions in this country. COPD is actually a group of respiratory diseases, of which bronchitis, asthma, and emphysema are the most common.

COPD is attributed to cigarette smoking, environmental pollution, occupational hazards, and chronic infection. Symptoms include shortness of breath, chronic cough, wheezing, increased sputum production, and fatigability on even mild exertion. Symptoms are progressive, and lung damage is irreversible. No cure is known. Treatment focuses on maintaining remaining lung function and relieving symptoms as much as possible.

Acute Respiratory Distress Syndrome

Acute (or adult) respiratory distress syndrome (ARDS) is respiratory failure, usually in the adult patient, that occurs as a result of disease or injury. Symptoms include pulmonary edema (swelling in the lungs), dyspnea (difficulty breathing), tachypnea (rapid respiratory rate), and hypoxemia (decreased oxygen levels in the blood) with cyanosis. The patient with ARDS usually requires intensive medical intervention (in an intensive care unit [ICU]), and the mortality rate is approximately 50% to 60%.

REVIEW QUESTIONS

1. Describe the overall function of the respiratory system, and identify the organs in the upper and lower respiratory systems.

2. In external respiration, the blood in the capillaries takes on _____ and gives off _____ to the lungs.

3. In internal respiration, the body cells take on _____ from the blood in the capillaries and at the same time give off _____ to the blood in the capillaries to be transported to the lungs.

4. Name and discuss the functions of each of the organs in the respiratory system.

5. List in sequence the organs through which the air from the outside travels to the blood in the capillaries of the lung.

6. Where are the vocal cords are located?

7. Answer the following questions.
   a. What is blood in the pleural cavity called?
   b. What is a collection of air or gas in the pleural cavity called?
   c. What is a collapsed lung known as?
   d. What is a thrombus that blocks a pulmonary artery?

8. In what condition are the symptoms progressive and the lung damage irreversible?

9. List four factors that cause COPD.

10. A patient with pulmonary edema (swelling in the lungs), dyspnea (difficult breathing), tachypnea (rapid respiratory rate), and hypoxemia (decreased oxygen levels in the blood with cyanosis) would be diagnosed with _____.

MEDICAL TERMINOLOGY RELATED TO THE RESPIRATORY SYSTEM

Objectives
On mastery of the medical terminology for this unit, you will be able to:

1. Spell and define the terms related to the respiratory tract.
2. Given the meaning of a medical condition related to the respiratory system, build with word parts the corresponding medical term.
3. Analyze and define medical terms that are built from word parts that relate to the respiratory system.
4. State the meaning of the abbreviations used in this unit.
5. Given a description of a hospital situation in which the HUC may encounter medical terminology, apply the correct medical term to the situation described.

Word Parts

The following list contains word parts for the respiratory system that you need to memorize. The exercises included in this unit will help you with this task. You will continue to use these word parts throughout the course and during your employment. Practice pronouncing each word part aloud.

Combining Forms	Meaning
1. bronch / o (brŏn′-kō)	bronchus (s.); bronchi (pl.)
2. laryng / o (lah-rĭng′-gō)	larynx (voice box)
3. pharyng / o (fah-rĭng′-gō)	pharynx (throat)
4. pleur / o (ploo′-rō)	pleura
5. pneum / o (nū′-mō)	lung (also means air)
6. pneumon / o (nū-mŏn′-ō)	lung
7. pulmon / o (pŭl′-mŏ-nō)	lung
8. rhin / o (rī′-nō)	nose
9. thorac / o (thŏ′-rah-kō)	thorax (chest)
10. tonsill / o (tŏn′-sĭl-ō)	tonsil
(*Note:* The word root for tonsil has a double *l*.)	
11. trache / o (trā′-kē-ō)	trachea (windpipe)

Prefix

dys- (dĭs)	difficult, labored, painful, abnormal

Suffix

-pnea (nē′-ah)	respiration, breathing

 E X E R C I S E 1

Write the combining forms for the respiratory system in the spaces provided on the diagram in Figure 22-31. The number preceding the combining form in the earlier list matches the number of the body part on the diagram.

 E X E R C I S E 2

Write the combining forms (and suffix) for each term listed.

1. lung		6. bronchus	
2. pharynx		7. pleura	
3. larynx		8. nose	
4. trachea		9. breathing	
5. tonsil		10. chest	

MEDICAL TERMS RELATED TO THE RESPIRATORY SYSTEM

The following list is made up of medical terms for the respiratory system that you will need to know. Exercises following this list will assist you in learning these terms. Practice the pronunciation of these terms aloud.

General Terms	Meaning
adenoids (ăd′-ĕn-oyds)	tissue in the nasopharynx
apnea (ăp′-nē-ah)	without breathing (temporary stoppage of breathing)
bronchotracheal (brŏn-kō-trā′-kē-al)	pertaining to the bronchi and trachea
dyspnea (dĭsp-nē′-ah)	difficulty in breathing
endotracheal (ĕn-dō-trā′-kē-al) (ET)	pertaining to within the trachea
pharyngocele (fah-rĭng′-gō-sēl)	(an abnormal) protrusion in the pharynx
pharyngoplegia (fah-rĭng′-gō-plē′-ja)	paralysis of the pharynx
pulmonary (pŭl′-mŏ-nĕr-ē)	pertaining to the lungs
thoracentesis (thō-rah-sĕn-tē′-sĭs)	surgical puncture and drainage of fluid from the chest cavity (for diagnostic or therapeutic purposes)
thoracic (thō-răs′-ĭk)	pertaining to the chest
thoracocentesis (thō′-rah-kō-sĕn-tē′-sĭs)	surgical puncture and drainage of fluid from the chest cavity (for diagnostic or therapeutic purposes [the same as thoracentesis])
tracheoesophageal (trā′-kē-ō-ĕ-sŏf′-ah-jē′-al)	pertaining to the trachea and esophagus

Surgical Terms	Meaning
adenoidectomy (ăd′-ĕ-noy-dĕk′-to-mē)	surgical removal of the adenoids
laryngectomy (lar-ĭn-jĕk′-to-mē)	excision of the larynx
lobectomy (lō-bĕk′-to-mē)	excision of a lobe (of a lung—also may refer to the brain or liver)
pleuropexy (ploo′-rō-pĕk′-sē)	surgical fixation of the pleura
pneumonectomy (nū-mŏ-nĕk′-to-mē)	excision of the lung (may be total or partial removal of a lung)
rhinoplasty (rhī-nō-plăs′-tē)	surgical repair of the nose
thoracotomy (thō-rah-kŏt′-o-mē)	incision into the chest cavity
tonsillectomy (tŏn-sĭl-lĕk′-to-mē)	surgical removal of the tonsils
tracheostomy (trā-kē-ŏs′-to-mē)	artificial opening into the trachea (through the neck)

Diagnostic Terms	Meaning
adenoiditis (ăd′-ĕ-noy-dī′-tĭs)	inflammation of the adenoids
asthma (ăz′-mah)	chronic disease characterized by periodic attacks of dyspnea, wheezing, and coughing
bronchitis (brŏn-kī′-tĭs)	inflammation of the bronchi
chronic obstructive pulmonary disease (COPD)	chronic obstruction of the airway that results from emphysema, asthma, or chronic bronchitis
emphysema (ĕm-fĭ-sē′-mah)	degenerative disease characterized by destructive changes in the walls of the alveoli, resulting in loss of elasticity to the lungs
laryngitis (lar-ĭn-jī′-tĭs)	inflammation of the larynx
pharyngitis (fah-rĕn-jī′-tĭs)	inflammation of the pharynx
pleuritis (ploo-rī′-tĭs); pleurisy (ploo′-rĕ-sē)	inflammation of the pleura
pneumonia (nū-mō′-nē-ah)	abnormal condition of the lung
pneumonitis (nū-mō-nī′-tĭs)	inflammation or infection of the lung
pneumothorax (noo-mō-thor′-ăks)	air in the pleural cavity causes the lung to collapse
rhinopharyngitis (rī′-nō-făr-ĭn-jī′-tĭs)	inflammation of the nose and throat
rhinorrhagia (rī-nō-rā′-ja)	bleeding from the nose, also called *epistaxis*
tonsillitis (tŏn-sĭ-lī′-tĭs)	inflammation of the tonsils
upper respiratory infection (rĕs′-pi-rah-tō-rē) (URI)	infection of nose, sinuses, pharynx, larynx, and bronchi

Terms Related to Diagnostic Procedures	Meaning
bronchogram (brŏn′-kō-grăm)	x-ray image of the bronchi and lung (with the use of a contrast medium)
bronchoscope (brŏn′-kō-skōp)	instrument used to visually examine the bronchi
bronchoscopy (brŏn-kŏs′-ko-pē)	visual examination of the bronchi
laryngoscope (lăr-răng′-gō-skōp)	instrument used for visual examination of the larynx

⊜ EXERCISE 3

Analyze and define each medical term listed.

1. dyspnea
2. pharyngocele
3. apnea
4. bronchotracheal
5. tracheoesophageal
6. endotracheal
7. pharyngoplegia
8. rhinopharyngitis
9. rhinorrhagia
10. bronchoscope
11. bronchoscopy

⊜ EXERCISE 4

Using the word parts studied in this unit and in previous units, build a medical term from each definition listed.

1. inflammation of the bronchi
2. inflammation of the larynx
3. artificial opening into the trachea
4. excision of a lung
5. excision of a lobe (of the lung)
6. surgical fixation of the pleura
7. surgical repair of the nose
8. incision into the chest cavity
9. surgical puncture and drainage of the chest cavity
10. inflammation of the tonsils
11. inflammation of the adenoids

⊜ EXERCISE 5

Complete the spelling of each medical term listed.

Medical Term	Meaning
1. pn _ _ _ o_thor _ _	air in the pleural cavity that causes the lungs to collapse
2. em _ _ _ se _ _	disease of the alveoli of the lung
3. _ _ _ umon _ _	an inflammation or infection of the lung
4. pleuro _ _ _ _	surgical fixation of the pleura
5. phar _ _ _ itis	inflammation of the pharynx

EXERCISE 6

Define each medical term listed.

1. adenoids
2. lobectomy
3. emphysema
4. pneumonia
5. upper respiratory infection
6. apnea
7. dyspnea
8. pharyngocele
9. laryngectomy
10. pneumothorax
11. rhinorrhagia
12. bronchogram
13. laryngoscope
14. asthma
15. chronic obstructive pulmonary disease
16. tuberculosis

EXERCISE 7

Spell each of the 42 terms studied in this unit by having someone dictate the terms to you.

1.	22.
2.	23.
3.	24.
4.	25.
5.	26.
6.	27.
7.	28.
8.	29.
9.	30.
10.	31.
11.	32.
12.	33.
13.	34.
14.	35.
15.	36.
16.	37.
17.	38.
18.	39.
19.	40.
20.	41.
21.	42.

EXERCISE 8

Answer the following questions.

1. A patient was admitted to the hospital with the diagnosis of hemothorax. The doctor is planning to perform a procedure on the patient to remove fluid from the chest cavity by surgical puncture. What is this procedure called?

2. A patient suddenly stops breathing. During this emergency the doctor may perform the following procedure to ensure the opening of the air passageway. The doctor uses a _____ (an instrument for visual examination of the larynx) to insert a(n) _____

(pertaining to within the trachea) tube. These two items of equipment may be used during an emergency. You may be asked to locate these items for the nursing staff or doctor. On assignment to a nursing unit, locate and be able to identify this equipment.

3. The patient is having difficulty breathing, or _____. The doctor performs a procedure called _____ (artificial opening into the trachea) to facilitate breathing. A tube is inserted into the trachea to prevent it from collapsing. It has the same name as the procedure. It is called a(n) _____ tube. A tray that has the same name as the procedure, called a(n) _____, is used by the nursing staff to care for the patient. A patient with a tracheostomy may have difficulty talking; therefore the HUC should not use the intercom to communicate with this patient.

4. A patient is scheduled for a visual examination of the bronchus, called a _____. What is the instrument the doctor uses to perform the examination?

5. The patient is admitted to the hospital with a(n) _____ (a collapsed lung). The patient is having difficulty breathing; what is the medical term for this? The doctor treats this condition by making a surgical incision into the chest wall, called a(n) _____, for the purpose of inserting tubes. A tray that has the same name as the procedure, a(n) _____ tray, is obtained from the central service department for the doctor's use.

6. T&A is the abbreviation for excision of the tonsils, called _____, and excision of the adenoids, called _____.

ABBREVIATIONS

Abbreviation	Meaning
ARDS	acute respiratory distress syndrome
COPD	chronic obstructive pulmonary disease
ET	endotracheal
NP	nasopharyngeal
PE	pulmonary embolism
RSV	respiratory syncytial virus
SARS	severe acute respiratory syndrome (viral)
TB	tuberculosis (mycobacterial)
URI	upper respiratory infection

EXERCISE 9

Define the following abbreviations.

1. ARDS
2. COPD
3. ET
4. NP
5. PE
6. RSV
7. SARS
8. TB
9. URI

UNIT 9
The Urinary System and the Male Reproductive System

OUTLINE

UNIT OBJECTIVES

On completion of this unit, you will be able to:

1. Describe the overall functions of the urinary system.
2. Name the organs of the urinary system, and describe the function of each organ.
3. Name the components of urine.
4. Describe the overall functions of the male reproductive system.
5. Name the organs of the male reproductive system, and describe the function of each organ.
6. State the location and describe the function of the seminal vesicle glands and the prostate gland.
7. Describe the passageway of sperm from the testes to the outside of the body.
8. Discuss pyelonephritis, renal calculi, and tumors of the prostate gland.
9. Read the objectives related to medical terminology, and demonstrate ability to meet the objectives by correctly completing Exercises 1 through 7.
10. Define the unit abbreviations.

THE URINARY SYSTEM

Organs of the Urinary System

- Kidneys (2)
- Ureters (2)
- Bladder (1)
- Urethra (1)

Functions of the Urinary System

The functions of the urinary system are to monitor and regulate extracellular fluids and to remove waste products from the blood and excrete them from the body. Although toxic substances also are eliminated through the skin, lungs, and intestines, the urinary system is a major contributor to homeostasis in the body because it maintains the proper balance of water, electrolytes, and pH of body fluids. The urinary system also may be referred to as the *excretory system*.

The Kidneys

The kidneys are two fist-sized, bean-shaped organs located in the lumbar region on either side of the spine, posterior to the abdominal cavity. The primary functions of the kidneys are to remove waste from the blood, to balance the water and electrolytes in the body by removing and retaining water, and to assist in RBC production by releasing erythropoietin (eh-rith'-ro-poy'-eh-tin). Nephrons, the basic functional unit of the kidney, begin to remove waste and water as the blood flows into the kidney through the renal artery. Each kidney contains about one million nephrons. At the entrance of each nephron is a cluster of capillaries called the *glomerulus* (plural: *glomeruli*), where the process of filtering the blood begins. The antidiuretic hormone (ADH) released by the posterior pituitary gland (neurohypophysis) stimulates the production of urine that contains soluble waste. When danger of dehydration is present, the posterior pituitary gland decreases the amount of ADH that is released. The nephrons continue to remove waste, but the fluid portion of urine decreases. Voided urine is more concentrated

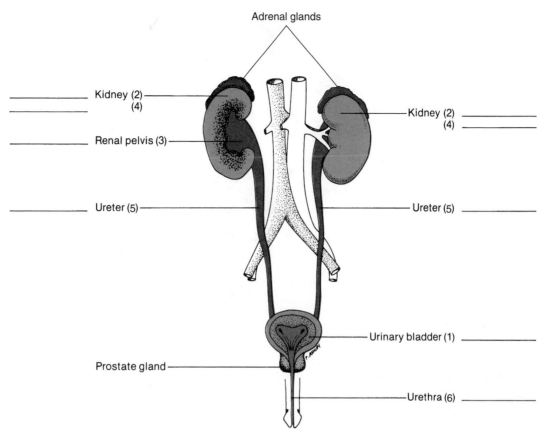

Figure 22-33 The male urinary system.

and occurs in smaller amounts. This process maintains the fluid balance in the body. Diuretics commonly prescribed for edema, hypertension, and CHF are chemicals that serve to increase the rate of urinary output. After urine is produced, it drains into a space in the kidney called the *renal pelvis*. From the renal pelvis, urine is transported to the bladder via the ureters.

The Ureters

The ureters are tubes that provide the drainage system for urine from the renal pelvis of each kidney to the bladder (Fig. 22-33). They are small in diameter and are approximately 10 to 12 inches (25 to 30 cm) long. They extend from the renal pelvis of the kidney and enter the posterior portion of the bladder.

The ureters have muscular walls that contract to keep urine moving toward the bladder. A backup of urine into the kidney is prevented by a flap fold of mucous membrane at the entrance of the ureters into the bladder.

The Urinary Bladder

The urinary bladder is a hollow muscular bag located in the pelvic cavity. The bladder is a temporary reservoir for the urine it receives from the ureters. The need to urinate, or void, is stimulated by distention of the bladder as it fills with urine.

The Urethra

The urethra is the tube through which urine passes from the bladder to the outside of the body. The female urethra is approximately 1 to 2 inches (3.75 cm) long, and the male urethra, which is also a part of the male reproductive system (also carries seminal fluid at the time of ejaculation), is approximately 8 inches (20 cm) long.

Urine

Urine is a straw-colored fluid that is made up of approximately 95% water and 5% waste material (urea, uric acid, creatinine, and ammonia). The amount of urine produced daily by the kidneys is about 1500 mL.

 HIGH PRIORITY

Production and Pathway of Urine
blood flows via the renal artery into the nephrons of the kidneys, where filtering of the blood takes place and urine is produced → renal pelvis → ureter → bladder → urethra → outside

THE MALE REPRODUCTIVE SYSTEM

Organs of the Male Reproductive System (Fig. 22-34)

- Testes
- Scrotum
- Vas deferens
- Urethra
- Seminal vesicles
- Prostate
- Penis

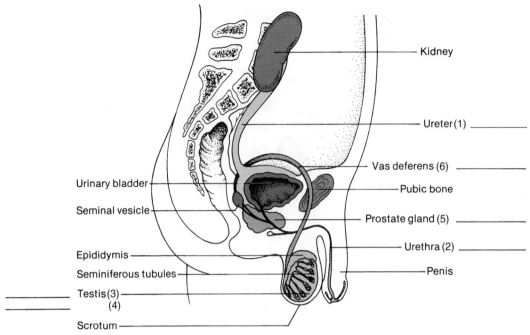

Figure 22-34 The male reproductive system.

Functions of the Male Reproductive System

The functions of the male reproductive system are to produce and eject the male reproductive cell (sperm, or spermatozoa) and to secrete the hormone testosterone.

The Testes

The testes (singular: testis), or testicles, are a pair of egg-shaped organs located outside the body, suspended in a sac called the *scrotum*. They are the main sex glands of the male, and because they produce the male reproductive cells, they are also called gonads. The function of the testes is to produce sperm (sex cells) and testosterone (hormone). Testosterone is responsible for the development of male secondary sex characteristics, such as beard and deep voice, and for the function of certain reproductive organs.

Production of Sperm

Sperm is produced in coiled tubes, located inside the testes, called *seminiferous tubules*. The sperm passes on to a tiny 20-foot tube called the *epididymis*, which is located in the scrotum. Sperm is stored in the epididymis for a short time, during which it matures and becomes motile (able to move by itself). It then travels through a pair of tubes about 2 feet long called the *vas deferens*. The vas deferens carries sperm to the urethra. The urethra connects with both the bladder and the vas deferens and passes through the penis to the outside. It is a passageway for both semen and urine. The seminal vesicles are glands located near the bladder that open into the vas deferens just before it joins with the urethra. The seminal vesicles produce a secretion that nourishes the sperm. This secretion makes up much of the volume of semen (sperm plus secretions). The junction of the vas deferens and the urethra is surrounded by a gland called the *prostate gland*.

The Prostate Gland

The prostate gland secretes a fluid that aids in the motility of sperm. The prostate gland also aids in ejaculation (expulsion of semen from the male urethra). Each ejaculation contains an average of 200 million sperm. Erection (stiffening) of the penis, produced by an increased blood supply to the spongelike tissue of the penis, allows for the deposit of sperm in the female vagina during ejaculation. A fold of skin called the *prepuce*, or *foreskin*, covers the tip of the penis; this often is removed shortly after birth through the surgical procedure of circumcision.

★ **HIGH PRIORITY**

Passageway of Sperm
from the seminiferous tubules (production) → epididymis (sperm matures and becomes motile) → vas deferens (passageway) → seminal vesicles (add nourishing secretions) → prostate (add motility secretions) → urethra (passageway) → to the outside

DISEASES AND CONDITIONS OF THE URINARY SYSTEM AND THE MALE REPRODUCTIVE SYSTEM

Pyelonephritis

Pyelonephritis is an infection of the renal pelvis and the kidney that is caused by bacterial invasion of the urinary tract. Typically, infection spreads from the bladder to the urethra to the kidneys. The three stages of the disease process include pyelitis—inflammation of the renal pelvis; pyelonephritis—inflammation of the renal pelvis and kidney; and pyonephrosis—collection of pus in the renal pelvis. As the disease progresses, the name changes. Symptoms include dysuria (pain or burning during urination), nocturia (excessive urination at night), and hematuria (blood in the urine). Urinalysis and culture and sensitivity of bacterial specimens from the urine are used to diagnose the condition. Treatment includes antibiotic therapy.

Labels in figure:
- Kidney
- Ureter (1) _____
- Vas deferens (6) _____
- Pubic bone
- Prostate gland (5) _____
- Urethra (2) _____
- Penis
- Urinary bladder
- Seminal vesicle
- Epididymis
- Seminiferous tubules
- _____ Testis (3)
- _____ (4)
- Scrotum

Renal Calculi

Renal calculi, or kidney stones, usually form in the renal pelvis, where they may remain, or they may enter the ureter and cause obstruction. Back pain or renal colic, resulting from the obstruction, is usually the key symptom. Kidney, ureter, and bladder x-ray imaging (KUB); intravenous pyelography (IVP); and kidney ultrasonography are used in diagnosing renal calculi. Treatment is to promote normal passage of the stone. Extracorporeal shock wave lithotripsy (ESWL), the crushing of kidney stones by laser beams, is replacing the need for surgery. Endoscopy also is used to remove small calculi from the lower part of the ureters. If indicated, a stone may be removed through a small incision in the skin (percutaneous nephrolithotomy).

Tumors of the Prostate Gland

Tumors of the prostate gland may be malignant (cancer of the prostate) or benign (benign prostatic hyperplasia). Often the growth is not diagnosed until it is large enough to obstruct urinary outflow. Treatment of choice is surgical removal of the tumor. A radical, or perineal, prostatectomy is the excision of the entire gland and its capsule through an incision in the perineum. Suprapubic prostatectomy is removal of the prostate gland through an incision in the abdomen and the bladder. Retropubic prostatectomy is surgical removal of the prostate gland through an incision in the abdomen, but the bladder is not excised. Transurethral prostatic resection is removal of a portion of the prostate gland through the urethra. No surgical incision is required.

REVIEW QUESTIONS

1. Describe the overall function of the urinary system.

2. Name the organs of the urinary system, and describe the function of each organ.

3. Identify the basic units of the kidneys.

4. Urine is made up of approximately 95% _____ and 5% _____.

5. Describe the overall function of the male reproductive system.

6. Name the organs of the male reproductive system, and describe the function of each.

7. Trace the travel of the sperm from the testicles to the outside of the body. Indicate which glands add secretions to the sperm along the passageway.

8. Match the terms in Column 1 with the phrases in Column 2.

Column 1	Column 2
a. nephrotripsy	1. kidney stone
b. pyelonephritis	2. growth that may obstruct urinary outflow
c. renal calculi	3. infection of the renal pelvis and kidney
d. hydrolithotripsy	4. crushing of a kidney stone

Column 1	Column 2
e. benign prostatic hyperplasia	
f. perineal prostatectomy	
g. lithotripsy	

MEDICAL TERMINOLOGY RELATED TO THE URINARY SYSTEM AND THE MALE REPRODUCTIVE SYSTEM

On mastery of the medical terminology for this unit, you will be able to:

1. Correctly spell and define the terms related to the urinary system and the male reproductive system.
2. Given the meaning of a medical condition related to the urinary system and the male reproductive system, build with word parts the correct corresponding medical term.
3. Analyze and define medical terms built from word parts that relate to the urinary system and the male reproductive system.
4. Write the meaning of each abbreviation used in this unit.
5. Given a description of a hospital situation in which the HUC may encounter medical terminology, apply the correct medical terms to the situations described.

Word Parts

The following list contains the word parts for the urinary system and the male reproductive system that you need to memorize. The exercises included in this unit will help you with this task. You will continue to use these word parts throughout the course and during employment. Practice pronouncing each word part aloud.

Urinary System

Word Roots/Combining Forms	Meaning
1. cyst / o (sĭs′-tō)	bladder, sac
2. nephr / o (nĕf′-rō)	kidney
3. pyel / o (pī′-ĕ-lō)	renal pelvis
4. ren / o (rē′-nō)	kidney
5. ur / o (ū′-rō)	urine, urinary tract
6. ureter / o (ū-rē′-ter-ō)	ureter
7. urethr / o (ū-rē′-thrō)	urethra
8. urin / o (ū′-rĭ-nō)	urine (urinary tract, urination)

Male Reproductive System

Word Roots/Combining Forms	Meaning
9. orchi / o (or′-kē-ō)	testicle, testis
10. orchid / o (or′-kĭ-dō)	testicle, testis
11. prostat / o (prŏs′-tăt-ō)	prostate
12. vas / o (văs′-ō)	vessel, duct

EXERCISE 1

a. Write the combining forms for the urinary system in the spaces provided on the diagram in Figure 22-33. The number preceding the combining form in the earlier list matches the number of the body part on the diagram.

b. Write the combining forms for the male reproductive system in the spaces provided on the diagram in Figure 22-34. The number preceding the combining form in the earlier list matches the number of the body part on the diagram.

⊖ E X E R C I S E 2

Write the combining forms for each term listed.

1. urine, urinary tract
2. renal pelvis
3. kidney
4. ureter
5. bladder
6. testicle
7. vessel, duct
8. urethra
9. prostate

MEDICAL TERMS RELATED TO THE URINARY SYSTEM AND THE MALE REPRODUCTIVE SYSTEM

The following list is made up of medical terms for the urinary system and the male reproductive system that you will need to know. Exercises following this list will assist you in learning these terms. Practice pronouncing each term aloud.

General Terms	Meaning
hematuria (hēm-ah-tū′-rē-ah)	blood in the urine
scrotum (scrō′-tŭm)	the skin-covered sac that contains the testes and their accessory organs
urethral (ū-rē′-thral)	pertaining to the urethra
urinary (ū′-rĭ-nĕr-ē)	pertaining to urine
urinary catheterization (kăth′-ĕ-ter-ĭ-zā′-shŭn)	insertion of a sterile tube through the urethra into the bladder to remove urine
urination (ū-rĭ-nā′-shŭn)	passage of urine from the body; also called *micturition*
urologist (ū-rŏl′-o-jĭst)	one who specializes in the diagnosis and treatment of (diseases) of the urinary tract (doctor)
urology (ū-rŏl′-o-jē)	study of the urinary tract (the branch of medicine that deals with the diagnosis and treatment of diseases of the male and female urinary tract and of the male reproductive organs)
void (voyd)	to pass urine or feces from the body (generally used with reference to passing urine from the bladder to the outside of the body)

Surgical Terms	Meaning
circumcision (sur′-kŭm-sĭzh′-ŭn)	surgical removal of the foreskin of the penis
nephrectomy (nĕ-frĕk′-to-mē)	excision of the kidney
nephrolithotomy (nĕf′-rō-lĭ-thŏt′-o-mē)	incision into the kidney (to remove a stone)

Surgical Terms	Meaning
nephropexy (nĕf′-rō-pĕk-sē)	surgical fixation of a kidney
orchiectomy (ōr-kē-ĕk′-to-mē)	excision of (one or both) testes
prostatectomy (prŏs-tah-tĕk′-to-mē)	surgical removal of the prostate gland
transurethral resection (trăns-ū-rē′-thral) (rē-sĕk′-shŭn) of the prostate gland (TURP)	removal of a portion of the prostate through the urethra by resecting the abnormal tissue in successive pieces
ureterolithotomy (ū-rē′-ter-ō-lĭ-thŏt′-o-mē)	incision into the ureter (to remove a stone)
urethroplasty (ū-rē′-thrō-plăs′-tē)	surgical repair of the urethra
urethrorrhaphy (ū-rē-thrōr′-ah-fē)	suturing of a urethral tear
vasectomy (vah-sĕk′-to-mē)	excision of a duct (vas deferens or a portion of the vas deferens; produces sterility in the male)

Diagnostic Terms	Meaning
cystitis (sĭs-tī′-tĭs)	inflammation of the bladder
cystocele (sĭs′-tō-sēl)	herniation of the urinary bladder
hydrocele (hī′-drō-sēl)	scrotal swelling caused by the collection of fluid in the membrane covering the testes
nephritis (nĕ-frī′-tĭs)	inflammation of the kidney
nephrolithiasis (nĕf′-rō-lĭ-thī′-ah-sĭs)	a kidney stone
pyelonephritis (pī′-ĕ-lō-nĕ-frī′-tĭs)	inflammation of the renal pelvis and kidney
renal calculus (rē′-nal) (kăl′-cū-lŭs)	a kidney stone
uremia (ū-rē′-mē-ah)	urine in the blood (caused by inability of the kidneys to filter out waste products from the blood)
ureteralgia (ū-rē-ter-al′-ja)	pain in the ureter

Terms Related to Diagnostic Procedures	Meaning
blood urea nitrogen (BUN)	laboratory test performed on a blood sample to determine kidney function
creatinine (Cr)	laboratory test usually performed with the BUN to determine kidney function
cystogram (sĭs′-tō-grăm)	x-ray image of the (urinary) bladder; dye is used as a contrast medium
cystoscopy (sĭs-tŏs′-ko-pē)	visual examination of the bladder; usually performed in the operating room so the patient may be anesthetized
intravenous pyelogram (ĭn-trah-vē′-nŭs) (pī′-ĕ-lō-grăm) (IVP)	x-ray image of the kidney, especially the renal pelvis and ureters; contrast medium is used; also called *intravenous urogram* (IVU)

Terms Related to Diagnostic Procedures	Meaning
kidneys, ureters, and bladder (KUB)	x-ray image of the kidneys, ureters, and bladder
urinalysis (ū-rǐ-năl′-ǐ-sǐs) (UA)	a laboratory test to analyze several constituents of urine to assist in the diagnosis of disease

EXERCISE 3

Analyze and define each medical term listed.

1. uremia
2. urologist
3. nephrolithotomy
4. prostatectomy
5. nephritis
6. urology
7. orchiectomy
8. nephrolithiasis
9. cystocele
10. cystoscopy
11. nephrectomy
12. nephropexy
13. pyelonephritis
14. ureteralgia
15. urethral
16. ureterolithotomy
17. cystitis
18. urethroplasty
19. urethrorrhaphy

EXERCISE 4

Using the word parts studied so far, build a medical term from each definition listed.

1. visual examination of the urinary bladder
2. inflammation of the kidney
3. excision of the kidney
4. a doctor who specializes in urology
5. blood in the urine
6. urine in the blood
7. suturing of a urethral tear
8. excision of a duct (vas deferens or a portion of it)
9. excision of the prostate gland
10. pain in the ureter
11. herniation of the bladder
12. x-ray image of the bladder
13. inflammation of the kidney and the renal pelvis
14. incision into the kidney to remove a stone
15. surgical repair of the urethra
16. surgical fixation of a kidney
17. branch of medicine that deals with the male and female urinary systems and the male reproductive system
18. excision of the testes

EXERCISE 5

Define each medical term listed.

1. urinalysis
2. renal calculus
3. hydrocele
4. transurethral resection
5. circumcision
6. urinary
7. urination

EXERCISE 6

Spell each of the 36 medical terms studied in this unit by having someone dictate the terms to you.

1.
2.
3.
4.
5.
6.
7.
8.
9.
10.
11.
12.
13.
14.
15.
16.
17.
18.
19.
20.
21.
22.
23.
24.
25.
26.
27.
28.
29.
30.
31.
32.
33.
34.
35.
36.

EXERCISE 7

Answer the following questions.

1. A patient is unable to void. The doctor writes an order to pass a sterile tube through the urethra into the bladder to remove the urine. What is this procedure called? The doctor wants a sample of this urine sent to the lab to be analyzed, a procedure called a(n) _____.
2. A patient is admitted to the hospital with a diagnosis of inflammation of the bladder, or _____.
3. A doctor orders an image of the kidneys, ureters, and urinary bladder. What is the abbreviation for this x-ray procedure? The doctor also orders a blood test to determine kidney function. What is this test called, and what is the abbreviation for this test?
4. A doctor writes an order on the patient's chart for a consultation with a doctor who specializes in the treatment of diseases of the urinary tract and male reproductive system. What is this specialist is called?
5. A patient is scheduled for the operating room for a procedure to visualize the urinary bladder. What is the procedure called? Why may the patient be scheduled for this procedure in the operating room?

ABBREVIATIONS

Abbreviation	Meaning
ADH	antidiuretic hormone
BPH	benign prostatic hyperplasia
BPM	benign prostatomegaly
BUN	blood urea nitrogen
Cr	creatinine

Abbreviation	Meaning
IVP	intravenous pyelogram (x-ray image produced with use of contrast medium)
IVU	intravenous urogram (x-ray image produced with use of contrast medium)
KUB	kidneys, ureters, and bladder (x-ray study of the abdomen)
TURP	transurethral resection of the prostate
UA	urinalysis
UTI	urinary tract infection

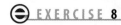 EXERCISE **8**

Define the following abbreviations.

1. ADH
2. BPH
3. BPM
4. BUN
5. Cr
6. IVP

7. IVU
8. KUB
9. UTI
10. UA
11. TURP

UNIT 10
The Female Reproductive System

OUTLINE

UNIT OBJECTIVES

On completion of this unit, you will be able to:

1. Describe the primary functions and identify the organs of the female reproductive system.
2. Discuss the structure of the uterus, and describe its role in pregnancy and in menstruation.
3. Describe the function of the ovaries, and name and describe the functions of two hormones produced by the ovaries.
4. Describe the functions of the fallopian tubes and vagina.
5. Identify the term that describes the pelvic floor of both the male and the female—most frequently refers to the area between the vaginal opening and the anus of the female.
6. Describe the function of the mammary glands.
7. Name and describe the function of the external reproductive structures.
8. Discuss endometriosis, pelvic inflammatory disease, and ectopic pregnancy.
9. Read the objectives related to medical terminology, and demonstrate ability to meet the objectives by correctly completing Exercises 1 through 10.
10. Define the unit abbreviations.

THE FEMALE REPRODUCTIVE SYSTEM

Organs of the Female Reproductive System (Fig. 22-35)

- Uterus (1)
- Ovaries (2)
- Fallopian tubes (2)
- Vagina (1)
- External genitalia
- Mammary and Bartholin glands

The reproductive organs do not mature and begin to perform reproductive functions until about the age of 11. The maturing of the reproductive organs is called *puberty.*

Functions of the Female Reproductive System

The functions of the female reproductive system are to produce the female reproductive cell (ovum), to produce hormones, and to provide for conception and pregnancy.

The Uterus

The uterus is a thick, muscular, pear-shaped organ that is located in the pelvic cavity between the rectum and the urinary bladder. Three layers make up the uterus: the outer perimetrium, the middle myometrium, and the inner endometrium. In pregnancy the uterus functions to contain and nourish the unborn child. Rhythmic myometrial contractions during labor assist in the birthing process. The uterus also plays a role in menstruation as the endometrium disintegrates and sloughs off if a fertilized egg is not implanted. The upper rounded region of the uterus is called the *fundus.* The wide, central portion of the uterus is the body, and the lower, narrow end that extends into the vagina is called the *cervix.*

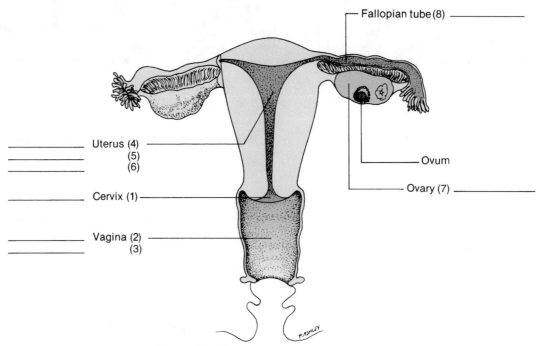

Figure 22-35 The female reproductive system.

The Ovaries

The ovaries, a pair of small oval organs located within the pelvic cavity, produce the female reproductive cell called the *ovum* (plural: *ova*). Because they produce the reproductive cells, they are also called gonads. At birth the female has nearly 1 million ova in the ovaries, of which approximately 300,000 remain during the reproductive lifetime. At puberty the ovaries, in response to follicle-stimulating hormone (FSH), release a mature ovum about every 28 days. This process is called *ovulation*, and it occurs about halfway through the menstrual cycle.

The ovaries, also called *female endocrine glands*, produce two hormones—estrogen and progesterone. Estrogen is responsible for the development of the female reproductive organs and the development of female secondary sex characteristics, such as breasts and pubic hair. The hormone progesterone plays a part in the menstrual cycle by helping to maintain the lining of the uterus for conception and in pregnancy.

The Fallopian Tubes

A pair of tubes, each approximately 5 inches (12.5 cm) long, called the *fallopian tubes* provide a passageway for the ovum from the ovaries to the uterus. The fallopian tubes are not connected to the ovaries; however, after ovulation the ovum is swept into one of the fallopian tubes, which are connected to the uterus. Fertilization, the union of the sperm and the ovum, usually takes place within the fallopian tube. It takes approximately 5 days for the ovum to pass through the fallopian tube to the uterus.

The Vagina

The vagina is a muscular tube about 3 inches long that connects the uterus to the outside of the body (Fig. 22-36). The outside opening of the vagina is located between the rectum (posterior) and the urethra (anterior) of the pelvic floor. The vagina receives the penis during sexual intercourse and is the lower part of the birth canal through which the newborn baby passes from the uterus to the outside of the body. Bartholin glands (or greater vestibular glands), mucus-producing glands at the external opening of the vagina, secrete lubricating substances.

The Perineum

The pelvic floor of both the male and the female is called the *perineum.* However, this term is used most frequently to refer to the area between the vaginal opening and the anus of the female.

Mammary Glands

The mammary glands, specialized organs of milk production, are located within the breasts. Each adult mammary gland contains 15 to 20 glandular lobes. During pregnancy, estrogen and progesterone stimulate development of the mammary glands. The hormone prolactin (PRL) initiates milk production after birth.

External Reproductive Structures

The *vulva* (a collective term for the external genitalia) consists of the labia majora and the labia minora, the two folds of adipose tissue surrounding the vagina, as well as the vestibule, the recess formed by the labia minora. The clitoris, a small erectile structure, is located anterior to the urethra.

DISEASES AND CONDITIONS OF THE FEMALE REPRODUCTIVE SYSTEM

Endometriosis

Endometriosis is a condition in which endometrial tissue (lining of the uterus) is found outside of the uterus, especially in

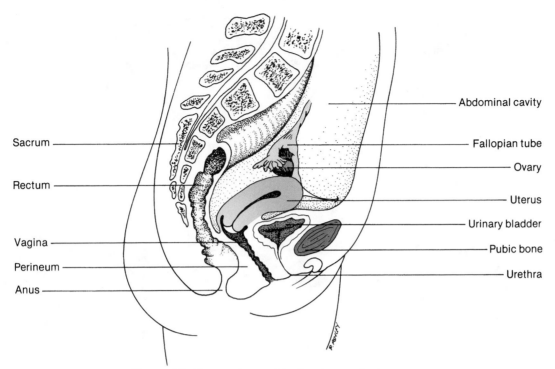

Figure 22-36 Lateral view of the female reproductive system.

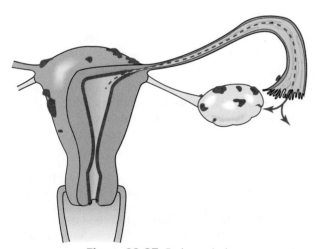

Figure 22-37 Endometriosis.

the pelvic area, but it can appear anywhere in the body (Fig. 22-37). The misplaced endometrial tissue undergoes changes, including bleeding, during menstruation. Symptoms include dysmenorrhea (painful menstruation), which causes constant pain in the vagina and the lower abdomen. The cause is unknown.

Treatment varies according to the severity of the disease and according to the age and childbearing desires of the patient. Hormonal treatment may be recommended for milder forms of endometriosis. Endometrial ablation may be performed to suppress ovarian function and to halt the growth of endometrial tissue. Conservative surgery may involve removal of cysts or lysis (freeing) of adhesions. For severe cases and for women who do not wish to bear children, a total hysterectomy and bilateral salpingo-oophorectomy is recommended (Fig. 22-38).

Pelvic Inflammatory Disease

Pelvic inflammatory disease (PID) is any infection of the female pelvic organs; most often it is caused by bacterial infection. Early diagnosis and treatment prevent damage to the reproductive organs. If untreated, PID can lead to infertility and to other severe medical complications. Symptoms include vaginal discharge, abdominal pain, and fever. Treatment includes antibiotic therapy.

Ectopic Pregnancy

In an ectopic (tubal) pregnancy, the fertilized ovum is implanted outside of the uterus; more than 90% implant in the fallopian tubes. The fetus may grow large enough to rupture the tube, creating a life-threatening situation. Symptoms of a ruptured fallopian tube include severe abdominal pain on one side and vaginal bleeding. Treatment is surgical repair or removal of the fallopian tube and removal of the products of conception.

⊖ REVIEW QUESTIONS

1. Describe the primary functions of the female reproductive system.

2. List the organs of the female reproductive system, and describe the function of each.

3. What are the names of two hormones produced by the ovaries? What is the hormone responsible for secondary sex characteristics and that aids in the development of the female reproductive organs?

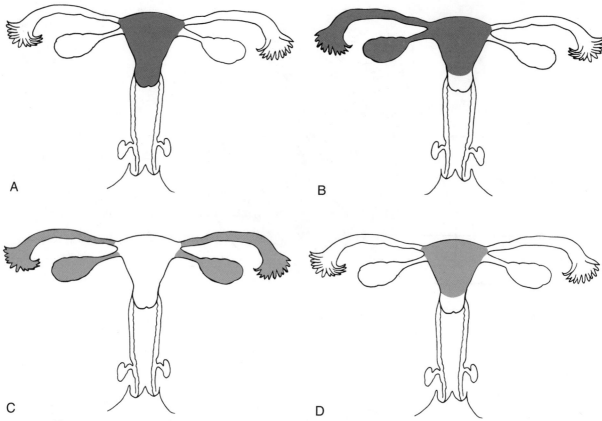

Figure 22-38 A, Total hysterectomy. **B,** Hysterosalpingo-oophorectomy. **C,** Bilateral salpingo-oophorectomy. **D,** Subtotal hysterectomy.

4. Identify the term that describes the pelvic floor of both the male and female and most frequently refers to the area between the vaginal opening and the anus of the female.

5. What is the term for an infection of the female pelvic organs that if left untreated can lead to infertility?

6. What is a pregnancy that occurs outside the uterus called?

7. What is the name of a condition in which endometrial tissue is found outside the uterus?

MEDICAL TERMINOLOGY RELATED TO THE FEMALE REPRODUCTIVE SYSTEM

Objectives

On mastery of the medical terminology for this unit, you will be able to:

1. Spell and define the terms related to the female reproductive system.
2. Given the meaning of a medical condition related to the female reproductive system, build with word parts the correct corresponding medical terms.
3. Analyze and define medical terms that are built from word parts related to the female reproductive system.
4. Define terms related to pregnancy, childbirth, and the newborn.

5. Given a description of a hospital situation in which the HUC may encounter medical terminology, apply the correct medical term to the situation described.

Word Parts

The following list contains the word parts for the female reproductive system that you need to learn. The exercises included in this unit will help you with this task. You will continue to use these word parts throughout the course and during employment. Practice pronouncing each word part aloud.

Word Roots/Combining Forms

	Meaning
1. cervic / o (ser'-vĭ-ko)	cervix (the necklike portion of the uterus)
2. colp / o (kŏl'-pō)	vagina
3. gynec / o (gī'-nĕ-kō, jīn'-ĕ-kō)	woman
4. hyster / o (hĭs'-ter-ō)	uterus (womb)
5. mamm / o (măm'-mō)	breast
6. mast / o (măs'-tō)	breast
7. men / o (mĕn'-ō)	menstruation
8. metr / o (meù'-trō)	uterus (womb)
9. oophor / o (ō-ŏf'-ō-rō)	ovary

Word Roots/Combining Forms	Meaning
10. perine / o (pĕr-ĭ-nē′-ō)	perineum (the pelvic floor); in the female, the area between the vaginal opening and the anus, and in the male, the region between the scrotum and the anus
11. salping / o (săl-pĭng′-gō)	fallopian or uterine tube
12. uter / o (ū′-tĕr-ō)	uterus (womb)
13. vagin / o (văj′-ĭ-nō)	vagina

⊜ E X E R C I S E **1**

Write the combining forms for the female reproductive system in the spaces provided on the diagram in Figure 22-35. The number preceding the combining form in the earlier list matches the number of the body part on the diagram.

⊜ E X E R C I S E **2**

Write the combining forms for each of the following.

1. menstruation	6. ovary
2. woman	7. uterus
3. vagina	8. cervix
4. perineum	9. breast
5. fallopian or uterine tube	

MEDICAL TERMS RELATED TO THE FEMALE REPRODUCTIVE SYSTEM

The following list contains the medical terms for the female reproductive system that you need to memorize. The exercises included in this unit will help you with this task. You will continue to use these medical terms throughout the course and during your employment. Practice pronouncing each term aloud.

General Terms

General Terms	Meaning
gynecologist (gī-nĕ-kŏl′-o-jĭst, jīn-ĕ-kŏl′-o-jĭst)	specialist in the diagnosis and treatment of women (doctor)
gynecology (gī-nĕ-kŏl′-o-jē, jīn-ĕ-kŏl′-o-jē)	study of women (the branch of medicine that deals with diseases and disorders of the female reproductive system)
menopause (mĕn′-ō-pawz)	the period during which the menstrual cycle slows down and eventually stops
menstrual (mĕn′-stroo-ăl)	pertaining to menstruation
menstruation (mĕn-stroo-ā′-shŭn)	discharge of blood and tissue from the uterus, normally occurring every 28 days
ovum (ō′-vŭm) (s.); ova (ō′-vă) (pl.)	female reproductive cell; may be referred to as the female reproductive egg
ureterovaginal (ū-rē′-ter-ō-văj′-ĭ-nal)	pertaining to the ureter and the vagina
uterine (ū′-ter-ĭn)	pertaining to the uterus
vaginal (văj′-ĭ-nal)	pertaining to the vagina
vaginoperineal (văj-ĭ-nō-pĕr-ĭ-nē′-al)	pertaining to the vagina and the perineum

Surgical Terms

Surgical Terms	Meaning
cervicectomy (sĕr-vĭ-sĕk′-to-mē)	excision of the cervix
colporrhaphy (kōl-por′-ah-fē)	suturing of the vagina
dilation and curettage (dī-la′-shŭn) (kū-rĕ-tăhzh′) (D&C)	surgical procedure to dilate the cervix and scrape the inner walls of the uterus (endometrium) for diagnostic and therapeutic purposes
endometrial ablation (en-dō-mē′-trē-al ab-lā′-shun)	use of laser to destroy endometrium in abnormal uterine bleeding
hysterectomy (hĭs-tĕ-rĕk′-to-mē)	surgical removal of the uterus
hysterosalpingo-oophorectomy (hĭs′-ter-ō-săl-pĭng′-gō-ō-ŏf-ō-rĕk′-o-mē)	excision of the uterus, fallopian tubes, and ovaries
mammoplasty (măm′-ō-plăs′-tē)	surgical repair of the breast(s) to enlarge (augmentation) or reduce (reduction) in size, or to reconstruct after surgical removal of a tumor
mastectomy (măs-tĕk′-to-mē)	surgical removal of a breast
oophorectomy (ō-ŏf-ō-rĕk′-to-mē)	excision of an ovary; if both ovaries are removed, it is referred to as a bilateral oophorectomy
perineoplasty (pĕr-ĭ-nē′-ō-plăs′-tē)	surgical repair of the perineum
salpingo-oophorectomy (săl-pĭng′-gō-ō-ŏf-o-rĕk′-to-mē)	excision of a fallopian tube and an ovary
salpingopexy (săl-pĭng′-gō-pĕk-sē)	surgical fixation of a fallopian tube

Diagnostic Terms

Diagnostic Terms	Meaning
amenorrhea (ā-mĕn-ō-rē′-ah)	without menstrual discharge
cervicitis (ser-vĭ-sī′-tĭs)	inflammation of the cervix
dysmenorrhea (dĭs-mĕn-ō-rē′-ah)	painful menstrual discharge
menometrorrhagia (mĕn-ō-mĕt-rō-rā′-ja)	rapid flow of blood from the uterus at menstruation (and between menstrual periods)
metrorrhagia (mĕ-trō-rā′-ja)	rapid flow of blood from the uterus (bleeding at irregular intervals other than that associated with menstruation)
metrorrhea (mĕ-trō-rē′-ah)	(abnormal) uterine discharge
oophoritis (ō-ŏf-ō-rī′-tĭs)	inflammation of an ovary
salpingitis (săl-pĭn-jī′-tĭs)	inflammation of a fallopian tube
salpingocele (săl-pĭng′-gō-sēl)	herniation of the fallopian tube

Terms Related to Diagnostic Procedures

Procedures	Meaning
cervical Pap smear	a laboratory test used to detect cancerous cells; commonly performed to detect cancer of the cervix and the uterus
colposcope (kŏl′-pō-skōp)	an instrument used for visual examination of the vagina (and cervix)
colposcopy (kŏl-pŏs′-kō-pē)	visual examination of the vagina (and cervix)
hysterosalpingogram (hĭs′-ter-ō-săl-pĭng′-gō-grăm)	x-ray image of the uterus and fallopian tubes
mammogram (măm′-ō-grăm)	x-ray image of the breast
vaginal speculum (spĕk′-ū-lŭm)	instrument used for expanding the vagina to allow for visual examination of the vagina and cervix

⊜ EXERCISE 3

Analyze and define the following medical terms.

1. gynecology
2. colporrhaphy
3. oophorectomy
4. oophoritis
5. salpingo-oophorectomy
6. salpingopexy
7. hysterectomy
8. dysmenorrhea
9. colposcope
10. mammoplasty
11. amenorrhea
12. mammogram
13. hysterosalpingogram
14. colposcopy

⊜ EXERCISE 4

Using the word parts you have studied, build a medical term from each definition listed.

1. excision of the ovary
2. study of women (branch of medicine that deals with diseases of the reproductive organs of women)
3. surgical fixation of a fallopian tube
4. inflammation of an ovary
5. an instrument used for visual examination of the vagina
6. (abnormal) uterine discharge
7. excision of the cervix
8. excision of the uterus, ovaries, and fallopian tubes
9. herniation of a fallopian tube
10. pertaining to the ureter and vagina
11. inflammation of the cervix
12. excision of the uterus
13. suture of the vagina
14. surgical repair of the perineum
15. pertaining to the vagina
16. surgical removal of a breast
17. excision of a fallopian tube and ovary
18. painful menstruation

19. x-ray image of the uterus and fallopian tubes
20. without menstrual discharge
21. x-ray image of the breast
22. surgical repair of the breast
23. visual examination of the vagina (and cervix)

⊜ EXERCISE 5

Define the following medical terms.

1. gynecologist
2. uterine
3. vaginal speculum
4. menometrorrhagia
5. dilation and curettage
6. ovum

⊜ EXERCISE 6

A surgery schedule lists all the operations to be performed in the hospital on a given day. Information on a surgery schedule includes the patient's name, the operation, and the surgeon. In the following sample, identify the terms spelled incorrectly in the operations listed. Spell the term correctly in the space provided.

Patient Name	Surgery	Doctor
a. Ms. Wallace	dilation and curettage	Dr. Lewis
b. Ms. Kelly	histero-solpingo oopherec-tomy	Dr. Robinowitz
c. Ms. Thomas	periniplasty	Dr. Cohen
d. Ms. Clark	colporhaphy	Dr. Jacobson
e. Ms. Cohen	salpangpexy	Dr. Sheets

⊜ EXERCISE 7

Spell each of the 38 medical terms studied in this unit by having someone dictate the terms to you.

1.	20.
2.	21.
3.	22.
4.	23.
5.	24.
6.	25.
7.	26.
8.	27.
9.	28.
10.	29.
11.	30.
12.	31.
13.	32.
14.	33.
15.	34.
16.	35.
17.	36.
18.	37.
19.	38.

TERMS RELATED TO OBSTETRICS

Following is a list of terms commonly used in the field of obstetrics and their definitions.

Obstetric Terms	Meaning
abortion (ah-bor′-shŭn)	termination of pregnancy before the fetus is capable of survival outside the uterus; may be spontaneous or therapeutic abortion
amniotic (ăm-nē-ŏt′-ĭk) fluid	fluid that surrounds the fetus
cesarean (sē-să′-rē-ăn) section (C/S)	incision into the uterus through the abdominal wall to deliver the fetus
congenital (kŏn-jĕn′-ĭ-tal)	term to describe a condition that exists at birth
ectopic (ĕk-tŏp′-ĭk) pregnancy	the fertilized ovum is implanted outside the uterus
fetus (fē′-tŭs)	the unborn child in the uterus from the third month of development to birth
natal (nā′-tal)	pertaining to birth
neonatal (nē′-ō-nā′-tal)	pertaining to the first 4 weeks after birth
obstetrician (ŏb-stĕ-trĭsh′-ăn)	a doctor who practices obstetrics
obstetrics (ŏb-stĕt′-rĭks) (OB)	branch of medicine that deals with pregnancy and childbirth
placenta (plah-sĕn′-tah) (afterbirth)	a spongy structure developed during pregnancy through which the unborn child is nourished
postnatal (pōst-nā′-tal)	pertaining to after birth
prenatal (prē-nā′-tal)	pertaining to before birth

⊜ EXERCISE 8

Match the word in Column 1 with its meaning in Column 2.

Column 1	Column 2
a. congenital	**1.** occurring before birth
b. abortion	**2.** present at birth
c. fetus	**3.** early termination of pregnancy
d. postnatal	**4.** unborn child
e. natal	**5.** a branch of medicine
f. prenatal	**6.** pregnancy outside the uterus
g. obstetrics	**7.** occurring after birth
h. ectopic pregnancy	**8.** birth

⊜ EXERCISE 9

Define each term listed.

1. obstetrician
2. placenta
3. amniotic fluid
4. cesarean section

⊜ EXERCISE 10

Answer the following questions.

1. In a large hospital, there is usually a nursing unit for patients who are hospitalized for surgery of the female reproductive tract. What is this unit called? A separate nursing unit is used for delivery and care of the newborn and for care of the mothers. What is this unit called?
2. The doctor plans to perform a pelvic examination of a female patient. What is the name of the instrument she or he uses to expand the vagina? During the pelvic examination, the doctor plans to remove some cells from the cervix to be studied for the presence of cancer. The cells are sent to the laboratory for a _____ test.

ABBREVIATIONS

Abbreviation	Meaning
BSO	bilateral salpingo-oophorectomy
C/S or C-section	cesarean section
D&C	dilation and curettage
EDD	estimated date of delivery
FSH	follicle-stimulating hormone
OB	obstetrics, obstetric
PID	pelvic inflammatory disease
PP	postpartum (after having given birth)
TPAL	term-premature-abortions (terminations)-living

⊜ EXERCISE 11

Define the following abbreviations.

1. C/S
2. D&C
3. FSH
4. OB
5. PID
6. PP
7. TPAL
8. EDD
9. BSO

UNIT 11
The Endocrine System

OUTLINE

UNIT OBJECTIVES

On completion of this unit, you will be able to:

1. Describe the overall function of the endocrine system.
2. Compare endocrine glands with exocrine glands.
3. Name the glands of the endocrine system, and describe the hormones produced by each gland and the function of each of the hormones.
4. Discuss diabetes mellitus and Graves disease.
5. Read the objectives related to medical terminology, and demonstrate ability to meet the objectives by correctly completing Exercises 1 through 6.
6. Define the unit abbreviations.

THE ENDOCRINE SYSTEM

Primary Organs of the Endocrine System
(Fig. 22-39)

- Hypothalamus
- Pituitary
- Thyroid gland
- Parathyroid gland
- Pancreas (islets of Langerhans)
- Adrenal glands
- Ovaries (female) and testes (male)

Functions of the Endocrine System

The functions of the endocrine system are much the same as those of the nervous system—communication, integration, and control; however, endocrine functions are carried out in a much different manner. Both systems use chemicals (hormones and neurotransmitters), but neurotransmitters act immediately and are short-lived, and the effects of endocrine system hormones are farther reaching and longer lasting. The organs of the endocrine system are the endocrine glands, which produce controlling substances called *hormones*. Endocrine, or ductless, glands do not have tubes to carry their secretions to other parts of the body; endocrine secretions go directly into the bloodstream, which carries them to other parts of the body. In contrast to the endocrine glands, the exocrine glands of the body have tubes that carry their secretions from the producing gland to other parts or organs of the body. For example, the saliva produced by the parotid gland (an exocrine gland) flows from the parotid gland through a tube into the mouth. Some nonendocrine organs such as the heart, lungs, kidneys, liver, and placenta also produce and release hormones.

The Pituitary Gland

The pituitary gland, often referred to as the master gland, has a master of its own! Although the pituitary gland produces hormones that stimulate the functions of other endocrine glands, it is the hypothalamus of the brain that directly regulates the secretory activity of the pituitary gland. The pituitary gland, which is attached to the hypothalamus, is a pea-sized gland located in the cranial cavity at the base of the brain. The pituitary gland is divided into two lobes: the anterior and the posterior.

The anterior lobe, or adenohypophysis, produces the following five hormones:

- *Adrenocorticotropic hormone (ACTH):* Stimulates the action of part of the adrenal gland.

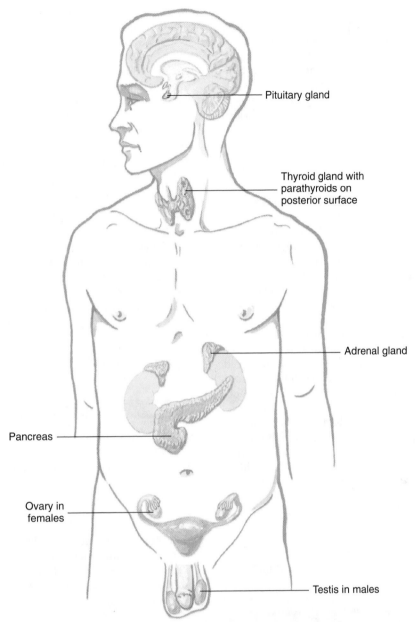

Figure 22-39 Primary organs of the endocrine system.

- *Thyroid-stimulating hormone (TSH):* Stimulates the action of the thyroid gland.
- *Growth hormone (GH):* Promotes body growth.
- *Prolactin (PRL):* Stimulates and sustains milk production in lactating females. PRL has no known effect in males.
- *Gonadotropins:* Stimulate growth and maintenance of the gonads (ovaries [female] and testes [male]). FSH stimulates follicles in the ovaries (female) and seminiferous tubes (male), and luteinizing hormone (LH) stimulates ovulation (female) and production of the male sex cell (spermatogenesis).

The posterior lobe, or neurohypophysis, produces two hormones:

- *Antidiuretic hormone (ADH):* Stimulates reabsorption of water by the kidney.

- *Oxytocin:* Stimulates uterine contractions while a woman is in labor.

The Thyroid Gland

The thyroid gland, which is shaped like a butterfly, is located in the lower neck on the front and sides of the trachea. It produces the hormone thyroxine, which maintains metabolism of body cells. Iodine is necessary in the body for the production of thyroxine by the thyroid gland, which is critical for normal growth and development.

The Parathyroid Glands

The parathyroid glands are four small bodies that are located posterior to the thyroid gland. They produce parathyroid hormone, which regulates the amount of calcium in the blood.

The Pancreas

The pancreas functions as both an exocrine gland and an endocrine gland. The endocrine component, the islets of Langerhans, consists of microscopic bunches of cells scattered throughout the pancreas (refer to Unit 7 of this chapter). These cells secrete the hormones insulin and glucagon, which are necessary for the metabolism of carbohydrates in the body. Glucagon works with insulin to regulate blood glucose levels.

The Adrenal Glands

The adrenal glands, situated on top of each kidney, are divided into two parts: the adrenal cortex (outer part) and the adrenal medulla (inner part). The adrenal cortex produces three steroid hormones: mineralocorticoids, glucocorticoids, and androgens. Mineralocorticoids regulate electrolyte balance, which is essential to normal body function and to life itself. Cortisol and cortisone are two glucocorticoids that influence protein, sugar, and fat metabolism. Cortisone, because of its antiinflammatory effects, is used therapeutically for the treatment of patients with various ailments. During physical or emotional stress, cortisol secretions increase to assist with the body's response. Androgens are hormones that are responsible for the masculinizing effect in males. Testosterone produced by the testes has the same masculinizing effect and is discussed further in Unit 9, The Urinary System and the Male Reproductive System.

The adrenal medulla produces two hormones—epinephrine (or adrenaline) and norepinephrine—that help the body respond to emergency or stressful situations by increasing the function of vital organs (heartbeat and respiration), raising BP, and providing extra nourishment for the voluntary muscles so they can perform extra work.

The Sex Glands

The ovaries of the female and the testes of the male are endocrine glands. Ovaries are described in Unit 10, and the testes are discussed in Unit 9.

DISEASES OF THE ENDOCRINE SYSTEM

Diabetes Mellitus (Type 1 or Type 2)

Diabetes mellitus, one of the most common endocrine disorders, results in the inability of the body to store and use carbohydrates in the usual manner. Contributing factors are the inability of the islets of Langerhans to produce enough insulin, an increase in the rate at which the body uses insulin, an increase in the rate of insulin storage in the body, and a drop in the efficiency of the use of insulin. In type 1 the beta cells of the pancreatic islets are destroyed and the patient must take regular injections of insulin. In type 2 the body is unable to respond normally to its insulin. Patients tend to be overweight—a factor that is believed to be responsible for the characteristic insulin resistance. Individuals with type 2 diabetes control their blood sugar level with diet, exercise, oral hypoglycemics, and insulin injections.

Symptoms of diabetes mellitus include polyuria, an increase in urine output; polyphagia, an increase in appetite; polydipsia, an increase in thirst; glycosuria, an elevation of sugar in the urine; and hyperglycemia, an elevation of sugar in the blood.

Diagnostic studies include urinalysis, fasting blood sugar, and hemoglobin A_{1c}. Treatment depends on the severity of the disease. Mild diabetes can be controlled by a diet that usually contains limited quantities of sugar, carbohydrates, and fats. Some patients may need to take oral hypoglycemics while adhering to their diet modifications. Moderate to severe diabetes may require insulin therapy. Too much glucose in the blood may cause a condition called *diabetic coma*, whereas too much insulin in the blood may cause a condition called *insulin shock*.

Graves Disease

Graves disease, a form of hyperthyroidism, causes overproduction of thyroxine, an increase in the size of the thyroid gland (goiter), and many changes in the other systems. Accompanying symptoms include intolerance to heat, nervousness, loss of weight, and goiter. The cause of Graves disease is unknown, but it is five times more common in women than in men. It usually occurs between the ages of 20 and 40 years. T_3 and T_4 uptake tests and a thyroid scan may be used to diagnose Graves disease. Treatment includes antithyroid drugs, radioactive iodine, and subtotal thyroidectomy.

⊜ REVIEW QUESTIONS

1. What is the overall function of the endocrine system?

2. What is necessary in the body for the production of thyroxine?

3. Compare endocrine glands with exocrine glands.

4. Indicate the hormones produced by each endocrine gland by writing the letter of the hormone listed in Column 1 by the name of the endocrine gland listed in Column 2. You may wish to write more than one number in each space.

Column 1	Column 2
a. parathyroid hormone	1. anterior pituitary gland
b. GH	2. adrenal cortex gland
c. TSH	3. thyroid gland
d. FSH	4. posterior pituitary gland
e. oxytocin	5. parathyroid gland
f. ACTH	6. islets of Langerhans
g. cortisone	7. adrenal medulla gland
h. epinephrine	
i. insulin	
j. PRL	
k. thyroxine	
l. ADH	

5. Insulin is secreted by the _____ located throughout the _____.

6. What is the function of insulin in the body?

7. List the symptoms of diabetes mellitus.

8. Graves disease is a form of _____.

MEDICAL TERMINOLOGY RELATED TO THE ENDOCRINE SYSTEM

Objectives

On mastery of the medical terminology for this unit, you will be able to:

1. Spell and define the terms related to the endocrine system.
2. Given the meaning of a medical condition related to the endocrine system, build with word parts the correct corresponding medical term.
3. Given a description of a hospital situation in which the HUC may encounter medical terminology, apply the correct medical term to the situation described.

Word Parts

The following list contains the word parts for the endocrine system that you need to memorize. The exercises included in this unit will help you with this task. You will continue to use these word parts throughout the course and during employment. Practice pronouncing each word part aloud.

Word Roots/Combining Forms	Meaning
aden / o (ăd′-ĕ-nō)	gland
adren / o (ah-drē′-nō)	adrenal
adrenal / o (ah-drē′-nal-ō)	adrenal
parathyroid / o (păr-ah-thī′-roy-dō)	parathyroid
thyr / o (thī′-rō)	thyroid
thyroid / o (thī′-roy-dō)	thyroid

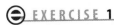 E X E R C I S E **1**

Write the combining forms for each medical term listed.

1. gland
2. thyroid
3. adrenal
4. parathyroid

MEDICAL TERMS RELATED TO THE ENDOCRINE SYSTEM

The following list is made up of medical terms for the endocrine system that you will need to know. Exercises following this list will assist you in learning these terms. Practice pronouncing each term aloud.

General Terms	Meaning
adenitis (ăd-ĕ-nī′-tĭs)	inflammation of a gland
adenoid (ăd′-ĕ-noyd)	resembling a gland (adenoids: glandular tissue located in the nasopharynx)
adenoma (ăd-ĕ-nō′-mah)	a tumor of glandular tissue
adenosis (ăd-ĕ-nō′-sĭs)	abnormal condition of a gland

General Terms	Meaning
adrenal (ah-drē′-nal)	adrenal gland located near the kidney
adrenalitis (ah-drē-năl-ī′-tĭs)	inflammation of the adrenal gland
endocrinologist	specialist who treats glandular diseases
gland (gland)	a secretory organ that produces hormones or other substances
hormones	chemical messengers produced by the endocrine system
secretion (sē-krē′-shŭn)	a substance produced by a gland

Surgical Terms	Meaning
parathyroidectomy (păr-ah-th-ī-roy-děk′-to-mē)	excision of the parathyroid gland
thyroidectomy (th-ī-roy-děk′-to-mē)	surgical removal of the thyroid gland

Diagnostic Terms	Meaning
Addison (ăd′-i-sŭn) disease	disease caused by lack of production of hormones by the adrenal gland
Cushing (koosh′-ĭng) disease	a disorder caused by overproduction of certain hormones by the adrenal cortex
diabetes insipidus (dī-ah-bē′-tĭs) (ĭn-sĭp′-ĭ-dĭs)	disease caused by inadequate antidiuretic hormone production by the posterior lobe of the pituitary gland
diabetes mellitus (dī-ah-bē′-tĭs) (mĭl-ī′-tĭs) (DM)	disease that results in the inability of the body to store and use carbohydrates in the usual manner; may be caused by inadequate production of insulin by the islets of Langerhans
hyperthyroidism (hī-per-thī′-roy-dĭzm)	excessive production of thyroxine and often an enlarged thyroid gland (goiter); also called *Graves disease* or *exophthalmic goiter*
hypothyroidism (hī-pō-thī′-roy-dĭzm)	condition of underproduction of thyroxine by the thyroid gland

Terms Related to Diagnostic Procedures	Meaning
blood glucose monitoring	method of monitoring the patient's glucose level by using a finger stick to obtain blood; performed by nursing staff
fasting blood sugar (FBS)	laboratory test to determine the amount of glucose in the blood after patient has fasted for 8 to 10 hours; may be used to diagnose and/or monitor diabetes mellitus

Terms Related to Diagnostic Procedures | **Meaning**

hemoglobin A_{1c} (HbA1c) | laboratory test performed to assess more precisely the control of diabetes; test result shows the percentage of glycated (or glycosylated) hemoglobin in the blood; excess glucose in the bloodstream, which usually occurs when diabetes is poorly controlled, binds (or glycates) with hemoglobin molecules in the RBCs (also called glycohemoglobin [glycoHb])

protein-bound iodine | laboratory test performed on a sample of blood to determine thyroid activity

T_3, T_4, and T_7 uptake | studies performed on a blood sample to determine the function of the thyroid gland

thyroid scan | diagnostic study performed in the nuclear medicine department for thyroid gland function

EXERCISE 2

Using the word parts studied in this unit and in previous units, build a medical term from each definition listed.

1. inflammation of a gland
2. surgical removal of the thyroid gland
3. surgical removal of the parathyroid gland
4. resembling a gland
5. tumor of glandular tissue
6. abnormal condition of a gland
7. inflammation of the adrenal gland

EXERCISE 3

The following are conditions caused by oversecretion or undersecretion of endocrine glands. Write the name of the gland involved with the condition.

1. diabetes mellitus
2. hyperthyroidism
3. Addison disease
4. hypothyroidism
5. Cushing disease
6. diabetes insipidus

EXERCISE 4

Complete the following words.

1. dia _ _ t _ _ ins _ p _ d _ _
2. Ad _ _ _ on dis _ _ se
3. Cu _ _ ing dis _ _ se
4. h _ poth _ _ oid _ _ m
5. sec _ _ ti _ ns

EXERCISE 5

Spell each of the 23 terms studied in this unit by having someone dictate the terms to you.

1.   9.   17.
2.   10.   18.
3.   11.   19.
4.   12.   20.
5.   13.   21.
6.   14.   22.
7.   15.   23.
8.   16.

EXERCISE 6

Answer the following questions.

1. A patient is admitted to the hospital with a possible diagnosis of _____, caused by an inadequate amount of insulin in the body. Insulin is produced by the _____. The doctor may order any of these three laboratory tests: _____, _____, or _____, to assist in diagnosing the patient's condition. The doctor also orders _____ to be performed by the nursing staff to determine the patient's glucose level.

2. If a patient has an insufficiency of a certain hormone in the body, the doctor may order a hormonal medication to be given to the patient to make up for the deficiency. The following is a list of hormonal medications. Indicate which endocrine gland should secrete each hormone.

   a. ACTH
   b. cortisone
   c. insulin
   d. epinephrine
   e. Premarin (estrogen)
   f. testosterone
   g. thyroid preparation

3. The patient is admitted to the hospital with a diagnosis of a thyroid condition. List three tests the doctor may order to gather information about the patient's thyroid function.

ABBREVIATIONS

Abbreviation	Meaning
ACTH	adrenocorticotropic hormone
DKA	diabetic ketoacidosis
DM	diabetes mellitus
FSH	follicle-stimulating hormone
HbA1c	hemoglobin A_{1c}, or glycosylated hemoglobin
LH	luteinizing hormone
PRL	prolactin
PTH	parathyroid hormone
TSH	thyroid-stimulating hormone

EXERCISE 7

Define the following abbreviations.

1. ACTH
2. DM
3. FSH
4. HbA_{1c}
5. LH
6. PRL
7. PTH
8. TSH

Websites of Interest

The Merck Manual of Diagnosis and Therapy: www.merckmanuals.com/professional/index.html

American Heart Association: www.heart.org

National Institute of Diabetes and Digestive and Kidney Diseases: www.niddk.nih.gov

National Institute of Mental Health: www.nimh.nih.gov

Epilepsy Foundation: www.epilepsyfoundation.org

American Lung Association: www.lung.org

American Cancer Society: www.cancer.org

National Kidney Foundation: www.kidney.org

Abbreviations

The following is a list of alphabetized abbreviations that are used frequently in doctors' orders. Most of the abbreviations related to specific departments, such as laboratory and diagnostic imaging, are not included here. For those, please refer to the chapters that discuss those departments.

Abbreviation	Meaning
c̄	with
p̄	after
/	per, by run
@	at
<	less than
>	greater than
Δ	change
↑ or >	increase, above, or elevate
↓ or <	decrease, below, or lower
°	degree or hour
ā	before
A&O	alert and oriented
A1C	glycosylated hemoglobin (chemistry)
AA	active assisted
AAA	abdominal aortic aneurysm
Ab	antibody
abd	abdomen; abdominal
ABGs	arterial blood gases
ABI	ankle brachial index
ABR	absolute bed rest
ac	before meals
ACTH	adrenocorticotropic hormone (chemistry)
ad lib	as desired
ADA	American Diabetic Association
ADD	Attention Deficit Disorder
ADE	adverse drug event
ADH	antidiuretic hormone (chemistry)
ADLs	activities of daily living
ADS	adult distress syndrome
ADT log book	book used to record all admissions, discharges, and transfers on a nursing unit
ADT log sheet	form used to record admissions, discharges, and transfers on a nursing unit on a daily basis
AFB	acid-fast bacillus (microbiology)
Ag	antigen
AHA	American Heart Association; American Hospital Association
AIDS	acquired immunodeficiency syndrome
AKA	above-the-knee amputation

Abbreviation	Meaning
ALP or alk phos	alkaline phosphatase (chemistry)
AMA	against medical advice
amb	ambulate
ANA	American Nurses Association; antinuclear antibody (serology)
ANCC	American Nurses Credentialing Center
AP	anteroposterior
app	application—An app is a piece of software. It can run on the Internet, on a computer, or on a phone or other electronic device.
appt	appointment
APS	Adult Protective Services
ARC	AIDS-related complex
ARDS	acute respiratory distress syndrome
ARRA	American Recovery and Reinvestment Act (of 2009)
as tol	as tolerated
ASA	acetylsalicylic acid, aspirin
ASAP	as soon as possible
ASHD	atherosclerotic heart disease
ASI	arterial stiffness index
asst	assistance
Ax	axilla or axillary
B/L	bilateral (both sides)
BAER	brain stem auditory evoked response; also called *auditory brainstem evoked potential* (ABEP)
BC	blood culture (microbiology)
BCOC or LOC	bowel care of choice, laxative of choice
BE	barium enema
BIBA	brought in by ambulance
bid	two times per day
bili	bilirubin
BiPAP	bilevel positive airway pressure
BiW	twice a week
BKA	below-the-knee amputation
BLE	both or bilateral lower extremities
BMI	body mass index
BMP	basic metabolic panel (chemistry)
BNP	brain natriuretic protein (chemistry)
BP	blood pressure
BPH	benign prostatic hyperplasia
BPM	benign prostatomegaly
BR	bed rest
BRP	bathroom privileges
BS	bedside

Abbreviation	Meaning	Abbreviation	Meaning
BSC	bedside commode	COO	chief operating officer
BSO	bilateral salpingo-oophorectomy	COPD	chronic obstructive pulmonary disease
BUE	both or bilateral upper extremities	CP	cold pack
BUN	blood urea nitrogen (chemistry)	CPAP	continuous positive airway pressure
Bx	biopsy (cytology)	CPK or CK	creatine phosphokinase *or* creatine kinase (chemistry)
C&S	culture and sensitivity (microbiology)		
C/O	complains of	CPM	continuous passive motion
C/S or C-section	cesarean section	CPOE	computer physician order entry
C. diff	*Clostridium difficile* (microbiology and serology)	CPR	cardiopulmonary resuscitation
		CPS	Child Protective Services
Ca	cancer	CPT	chest percussion therapy
Ca or Ca⁺	calcium (chemistry)	Cr	creatinine
CABG	coronary artery bypass graft	CRKP	carbapenem-resistant *Klebsiella pneumoniae* (microbiology and serology)
CAD	coronary artery disease		
cal	calorie		
cath	catheterize		
CBC	complete blood (cell) count (hematology)	CRP	C-reactive protein (chemistry); critical response performance
CBG	capillary blood gases	CSF	cerebrospinal fluid (chemistry, hematology, microbiology)
CBI	continuous bladder irrigation		
CBNT	continuous bronchodilator nebulizer therapy	CT	computed tomography
		Cult	culture (microbiology)
CBR	complete bed rest	CVA	cerebrovascular accident (stroke)
cc	cubic centimeters	CVC	central venous catheter
(same as "mL" and may not be allowed in some facilities, as may be confused with "u" if poorly written)		CVP	central venous pressure
		Cx	culture (microbiology)
		CXR	chest x-ray examination
		D&C	dilation and curettage
		D/C *or* DC	discontinue or discharge
		D/LR	dextrose in lactated Ringer's
		$D_{10}W$	10% dextrose in water
CC, creat cl, or cr cl	creatinine clearance (chemistry)	D_5W	5% dextrose in water
		DAT	diet as tolerated
CCM	certified case manager	DBP	diastolic blood pressure
CDC	Centers for Disease Control and Prevention	diff	differential (hematology)
		disch	discharge
CDSS	clinical decision support system	DKA	diabetic ketoacidosis
CE	covered entity	DM	diabetes mellitus
CEA	carcinoembryonic antigen (chemistry)	DME	durable medical equipment
		DMS	document management system
CEO	chief executive officer	DNR/DNI	do not resuscitate/do not intubate
CFO	chief financial officer	DO	doctor of osteopathy
CHF	congestive heart failure	DOA	dead on arrival
CHO	carbohydrate	DPI	dry powder inhaler
chol	cholesterol	DRG	diagnosis-related group
CHUC	certified health unit coordinator	drsg	dressing
CI	clinical indications	DSA	digital subtraction angiography
cl	clear	DSU	day surgery unit
Cl	chloride (chemistry)	DVT	deep vein thrombosis
cm	centimeter	DW	distilled water
CMP	comprehensive metabolic panel (chemistry)	Dx	diagnosis
		EBV	Epstein-Barr virus (serology)
CMS	circulation, motion, sensation	ECF	extended care facility
CMT	cardiac monitor technician	ECG, EKG	electrocardiogram
CMV	cytomegalovirus (microbiology, serology)	EchoCG	echocardiogram
		ECMO	extracorporeal membrane oxygenation
CNA	certified nursing assistant		
CNS	central nervous system	ED or ER	emergency department, emergency room
CO_2	carbon dioxide (chemistry)		
con't	continue, continuous	EDD	estimated date of delivery

Abbreviation	Meaning
EEG	electroencephalogram
EGD	esophagogastroduodenoscopy
eICU	electronic intensive care unit
EKG	electrocardiogram
EMG	electromyogram
EMR or EHR	electronic medical (health) record
ENG	electronystagmography (electrooculography)
ENT	ear, nose, and throat specialist (otorhinolaryngologist)
EP	evoked potential
EPC	electronic pain control
EPHI	electronic protected health information
EPS	electrophysiologic study
ERCP	endoscopic retrograde cholangiopancreatography
ES	electrical stimulation
ESR or sedrate	erythrocyte sedimentation rate (hematology)
ET	endotracheal
ETS	elevated toilet seat
F/U	follow-up
FBS	fasting blood sugar (chemistry)
Fe	iron (chemistry)
FF	force fluids
FPG	fasting plasma glucose (chemistry)
FS	full strength; frozen section (cytology)
FSH	follicle-stimulating hormone
FWW	front-wheel walker
Fx	fracture
G, gm, or g	gram
GB	gallbladder
GE	gastroenterologist; gastroenterology
GERD	gastroesophageal reflux disease
GI	gastrointestinal
GPS	Global Positioning System
gr	grain
GTT or OGTT	glucose tolerance test; oral glucose tolerance test (chemistry)
gtt(s)	drop(s)
H&H	hemoglobin and hematocrit (hematology)
H&P	history and physical
H/O	history of
H_2O_2	hydrogen peroxide
h, hr, hrs	hour, hours
HA	heated aerosol
HA or H/A	headache
HbA_{1c}	hemoglobin A1C, or glycosylated hemoglobin
HBOT	hyperbaric O_2 therapy
HBsAg	hepatitis B surface antigen (serology)
HBV	hepatitis B virus
hCG	human chorionic gonadotropin (test for pregnancy [chemistry])
Hct	hematocrit (hematology)
HCV	hepatitis C virus

Abbreviation	Meaning
HD	hemodialysis
HDL	high-density lipoprotein (chemistry)
Hgb	hemoglobin (hematology)
HIMS	health information management services; health information management system
HIMSS	Healthcare Information and Management Systems Society
HIPAA	Health Insurance Portability and Accountability Act
HITECH	Health Information Technology for Economic and Clinical Health Act
HIV	human immunodeficiency virus
$HIVB_{24}Ag$	human immunodeficiency virus antigen screen (serology)
HL or hep lock	heparin lock; also called a *saline lock*
HMO	health maintenance organization
HNP	herniated nucleus pulposus
HO	house officer
HOB	head of bed
HP	hot packs
hs	hour of sleep
HSV	herpes simplex virus (serology)
HTN	hypertension (high blood pressure)
HUC	health unit coordinator
Hx	history
I&O	intake and output
ICD	implantable cardioverter-defibrillator; International Statistical Classification of Diseases and Related Health Problems
ICG	impedance cardiography
ID labels	identification labels
IgG, IgM	immunoglobulin G, immunoglobulin M (serology)
IIHI	individually identifiable health information
IM	intramuscular
IPG	impedance plethysmogram
IPPB	intermittent positive-pressure breathing
irrig	irrigate
IS	incentive spirometry
ISOM	isometric
IV	intravenous
IVDU	intravenous drug user
IVF	intravenous fluids
IVP	intravenous push
IVP	intravenous pyelogram (x-ray study using contrast medium)
IVPB	intravenous or IV piggyback
IVU	intravenous urogram (x-ray using contrast medium); synonymous with IVP
K or K^+	potassium
KCl	potassium chloride
KO	keep open

Abbreviation	Meaning
KUB (also called a flat plate of abdomen)	kidneys, ureters, and bladder (x-ray of the abdomen)
L	liter
L&S	liver and spleen
L/min	liters per minute
lat	lateral chest
Lat	lateral
Lbs or #	pounds
LDL	low-density lipoprotein (chemistry)
LE	lower extremities
LH	luteinizing hormone
liq	liquid
LIS	low intermittent suction
LLE	left lower extremity
LLL	left lower lobe
LLQ	left lower quadrant
LOC	leave on chart (when it follows ECG, LOC ECG or EKG)
LP	lumbar puncture (also called spinal tap)
LPN	licensed practical nurse
LR	lactated Ringer's
LS	lumbosacral
lt or ⓛ	left
LTC	long-term care
LUE	left upper extremities
LUL	left upper lobe
LUQ	left upper quadrant
lytes	electrolytes (chemistry)
MAR	medication administration record
mcg	microgram
MD	medical doctor
MDA	medical doctor of anesthesia
MDI	metered-dose inhaler
mEq	milliequivalent
mets	metastasis
mg	milligram
Mg or Mg⁺	magnesium (chemistry)
MI	myocardial infarction
min, m	minute
mL or ml (same as cc, which may not be allowed in some facilities, as it may be confused with "u" if poorly written)	milliliter (same as cubic centimeter)
MN	midnight
MR	may repeat
MRA	magnetic resonance angiography
MRI	magnetic resonance imaging
MRSA	methicillin-resistant *Staphylococcus aureus* (microbiology)
MS	multiple sclerosis
MSSU	medical short-stay unit
N/V	nausea and vomiting
Na	sodium (chemistry)

Abbreviation	Meaning
Na or Na⁺	sodium
NAS	no added salt
NC or NP	nasal cannula or nasal prongs
NCS	nerve conduction studies
ND or NMD	doctor of naturopathic medicine or naturopathic medical doctor
nec	necessary
NG	nasogastric
NINP	no information, no publication
NKA	no known allergies
NKDA	no known drug allergies
NKFA	no known food allergies
NKMA	no known medication allergies
noc	night
NP	nasopharyngeal; nasopharynx; nurse practitioner
NPO	nothing by mouth
NS	normal saline
NSA	no salt added (same as NAS)
NSAID	nonsteroidal antiinflammatory drug
NTG	nitroglycerin
NVS or neuro ✓s	neurologic vital signs or checks
NWB	non–weight-bearing
O&P	ova and parasites (parasitology)
O₂	oxygen
OB	obstetrics, obstetric
OBS	observation
OD	oculus dexter (right eye)
OM	otitis media (middle ear infection)
OOB	out of bed
OPS	outpatient surgery (ambulatory surgery)
OR	operating room
ORE	oil-retention enema
ORIF	open reduction, internal fixation
OS	oculus sinister (left eye)
OSA	obstructive sleep apnea
OSHA	Occupational Safety and Health Administration
OT	occupational therapy or occupational therapist
OTC	over-the-counter
OU	oculus uterque (both eyes)
oz	ounce
P	pulse
PA	physician assistant; posteroanterior
PACS	picture archiving and communication system
PACU	postanesthesia care unit
PAP	prostatic acid phosphatase (serology)
pc	after meals
PC	packed cells (blood bank); personal computer
PCA	patient-controlled analgesia
PCN	penicillin
PCP	primary care physician
PCR	polymerase chain reaction (serology)

Abbreviation	Meaning	Abbreviation	Meaning
PCTS	Patient Care Technology Systems	q day	every day or daily
PCV	packed-cell volume (hematology; same as hematocrit)	q other day	every other day
		QEEG	quantitative electroencephalography
PCXR	portable chest x-ray study	qh or q h	every hour or every (fill in number) hours
PD	peritoneal dialysis		
PDA	personal data assistant	qid	four times a day
PDPV	postural drainage, percussion, and vibration	R	rectal
		RA	room air
PE	pulmonary embolism	RACE	*Rescue* individuals in danger.
PEG	percutaneous endoscopic gastrostomy		*Alarm:* Sound the alarm.
			Confine the fire by closing all doors and windows.
PEP	positive expiratory pressure		
PERRLA	pupils equal, round, reactive to light and accommodation		*Extinguish* the fire with the nearest suitable fire extinguisher.
PET	positron emission tomography	RBC	red blood cell (erythrocyte); red blood cell count (hematology)
PFT	pulmonary function test		
PHI	protected health information	RBS or BS	random blood sugar or blood sugar (chemistry)
PICC	peripherally inserted central catheter		
		RD	registered dietitian
PID	pelvic inflammatory disease	RDW	red cell distribution width (hematology)
PKU	phenylketonuria (chemistry)		
PNS	peripheral nervous system	reg	regular
PO	per os (by mouth)	retics	reticulocytes (hematology)
PO_4 or phos	phosphate or phosphorus (chemistry)	RIS	radiology information system
		RK	radial keratotomy
POCT or PCT	point-of-care testing (performed on the nursing unit)	RLE	right lower extremities
		RLL	right lower lobe
postop	after surgery	RLQ	right lower quadrant
PP	postpartum (after having given birth); postprandial (chemistry)	RML	right middle lobe
		RN	registered nurse
PPE	personal protective equipment	ROM	range of motion
PPO	preferred provider organization	Rout	routine
PR or R	per rectum	RPR	rapid plasma reagin (serology)
preop	before surgery	RR	respiratory rate
PRK	photorefractive keratectomy	RSV	respiratory syncytial virus (microbiology)
PRL	prolactin		
prn	pro re nata (as needed)	RT	respiratory therapist
PROM	passive range of motion	rt, ®	right
PSA	patient support associate; prostatic specific antigen (serology)	RUE	right upper extremity
		RUL	right upper lobe
pt	patient	RUQ	right upper quadrant
PT	physical therapy or physical therapist	Rx	take (e.g., treatment, medication) prescription
PT/INR	prothrombin time/international normalized ratio (coagulation–hematology)	S&A	sugar and acetone (urinalysis)
		SAD or SDS	save-a-day surgery, same-day surgery (patient admitted on the day of surgery)
PTA	physical therapy assistant		
PTC or PTHC	percutaneous transhepatic cholangiography		
PTCA	percutaneous transluminal coronary angioplasty	Sao or O_2 sats	oxygen saturation (on pulse oximetry, not ABGs)
		SARS	severe acute respiratory syndrome (viral)
PTH	parathyroid hormone		
PTT or APTT	partial thromboplastin time *or* activated partial thromboplastin time (coagulation—hematology)	SBFT	small bowel follow-through
		SBP	systolic blood pressure
		SCD	sequential compression device
PUD	peptic ulcer disease; peripheral vascular disease	SEP	somatosensory evoked potential
		SHUC	student health unit coordinator
PVR or RV	postvoid residual urine volume, residual volume	SIDS	sudden infant death syndrome
		SNAT	suspected nonaccidental trauma
q	every	SNF	skilled nursing facility

Abbreviation	Meaning	Abbreviation	Meaning
SOB	shortness of breath	TPR	temperature, pulse, respiration
sol'n	solution	trans	transfer
SPECT or SPET	single-photon emission computer tomography	trig or TG	triglycerides (chemistry)
		TSH	thyroid-stimulating hormone (chemistry)
SQ, sq, sub-q	subcutaneous		
SSE	soap suds enema	TT	tilt table
SSU	short-stay unit	TTOT	transtracheal oxygen therapy
st	straight retention	TTT	tilt table test
stat	urgent; rush (may be written in uppercase or lowercase)	TURP	transurethral resection of the prostate
(from Latin word *statim* meaning "immediately")		TWE	tap water enema
		Tx	traction
STM	soft tissue massage	U/O	urine output
STO	specimen to be obtained (i.e., by nurse)	UA or U/A	urinalysis
		UC	urine culture
subling, sl	sublingual (under tongue)	UD	unit dose
supp	suppository	UGI	upper gastrointestinal
SVN	small volume nebulizer	URI	upper respiratory infection
syr	syrup	US	ultrasound
T&S	type and screen (blood bank)	USN	ultrasonic nebulizer
T&X-match or T&C	type and crossmatch (blood bank)	UTI	urinary tract infection
T_3, T_4, T_7	thyroid tests (chemistry)	$\dot{V}/\dot{Q}$	ventilation/perfusion (quotient)
TB	tuberculosis (mycobacterial)	VAD	vascular access device
TCDB	turn, cough, and deep breathe	VEP	visual evoked potential
TEE	transesophageal echocardiography	Vfib	ventricular fibrillation
temp or T	temperature	VRE	vancomycin-resistant *Enterococcus* (microbiology)
TENS	transcutaneous electrical nerve stimulation		
		VS	vital signs
THA or THR	total hip arthroplasty or replacement	WA or W/A	while awake
		WBAT	weight bearing as tolerated
TIA	transient ischemic attack	WBC	white blood cell (leukocyte); white blood cell count (hematology)
TIBC	total iron-binding capacity (chemistry)		
tid	three times a day	WHO	World Health Organization
tinct or tr	tincture	wk	week
TJC	The Joint Commission (formerly the Joint Commission on Accreditation of Healthcare Organizations [JCAHO])	WNL	within normal limits
		WOW	workstation on wheels
		WP	whirlpool
		wt	weight
TKO	to keep open	www	World Wide Web
TKA or TKR	total knee replacement or arthroplasty	x	times
TPAL	term-premature-abortions (terminations)-living	XDR-TB	extensively drug-resistant tuberculosis (microbiology)

APPENDIX B

Word Parts

Each word element present in Chapter 22 is noted in **bold text** along with its meaning and the unit of Chapter 22 in which it is found. Additional word parts that you may encounter in your medical work are provided in normal text, and instead of a unit number, a sample medical term incorporating the word part is provided.

Word Element	Meaning	Unit Number (or Sample Medical Term)
a	without	3
abdomin / o	abdomen	7
aden / o	gland	11
adren / o	adrenal	11
adrenal / o	adrenal	11
-al	pertaining to	2
-algia	pain	3
an-	without	3
angi / o	blood vessel	6
aort / o	aorta	6
appendic / o	appendix	7
-ar	pertaining to	3
arteri / o	artery	6
arthr / o	joint	3
bi / o	life	2
blephar / o	eyelid	5
brady-	slow	6
bronch / o	bronchus	8
cancer / o	cancer	2
carcin / o	cancer	2
cardi / o	heart	1, 6
-cele	herniation, protrusion	4
-centesis	surgical puncture to aspirate fluid	3
cerebell / o	cerebellum	4
cerebr / o	cerebrum	4
cervic / o	cervix	10
cheil / o	lip	7
cholangi / o	bile duct	*cholangioma*
chol / e, chol / o	bile, gall	7
choledoch / o	common bile duct	*choledocholithiasis*
chondr / o	cartilage	3
clavic / o	clavicle	3
clavicul / o	clavicle	3
col / o	colon	7
colon / o	colon	7
colp / o	vagina	10
conjunctiv / o	conjunctiva	5

Word Element	Meaning	Unit Number (or Sample Medical Term)
cost / o	rib	3
crani / o	cranium	3
cutane / o	skin	2
cyan / o	blue	6
cyst / o	bladder, sac	7, 9
cyt / o	cell	1, 2
derm / o	skin	2
dermat / o	skin	2
duoden / o	duodenum	7
dur/o	dura mater (outer meningeal layer)	4
dys-	difficult, labored, painful, abnormal	3, 8
-ectomy	excision, surgical removal	1, 3
electr / o	electricity, electrical activity	1, 3
-emia	condition of the blood	6
encephal / o	brain	4
endo-	within	6
enter / o	intestine	7
epi-	upon	1
epitheli / o	epithelium	2
erythr / o	red	6
esophag / o	esophagus	7
femor / o	femur	3
gastr / o	stomach	1, 7
-genic	producing, originating, causing	2
gloss / o	tongue	7
-gram	record, x-ray image	1, 3
-graph	instrument used to record	3
-graphy	process of recording, x-ray imaging	3
gynec / o	woman	10
hem / o	blood	6
hemat / o	blood	6
hepat / o	liver	1, 7
herni / o	protrusion of a body part	7
hist / o	tissue	2
humer / o	humerus	3

Word Element	Meaning	Unit Number (or Sample Medical Term)	Word Element	Meaning	Unit Number (or Sample Medical Term)
hyper-	above normal	6	-pathy	disease	*neuropathy*
hypo-	below normal	6	peri-	surrounding (outer)	6
hyster / o	uterus	10	perine / o	perineum	10
-ia	abnormal condition of	4	-pexy	surgical fixation	6
-iasis	condition of	7	phalang / o	phalange	3
-ic	pertaining to	1, 3	pharyng / o	pharynx	8
ile / o	ileum	7	phas / o	speech	4
inter-	between	*intervertebral*	phleb / o	vein	6
intra-	within	1, 3	-plasty	surgical repair	3
irid / o	iris	5	-plegia	paralysis, stroke	4
-itis	inflammation	1, 2	pleur / o	pleura	8
kerat / o	cornea	5	-pnea	respiration, breathing	8
lamin / o	lamina	3	pneum / o	air, lung	8
lapar / o	abdomen	7	pneumon / o	lung	8
laryng / o	larynx	8	poli / o	gray matter	4
leuk / o	white	6	proct / o	rectum	7
lingu / o	tongue	7	prostat / o	prostate	9
lip / o	fat	2	psych / o	mind	4
lith / o	stone, calculus	7	pulmon / o	lung	8
-logist	one who specializes in the diagnosis and treatment of	2	pyel / o	renal pelvis	9
			ren / o	kidney	9
			retin / o	retina	5
-logy	study of	1, 2	rhin / o	nose	8
mamm / o	breast	10	-rrhagia	rapid flow of blood	4
mast / o	breast	10			
-megaly	enlargement	6	-rrhaphy	surgical repair	4
men / o	menstruation	10	-rrhea	excessive discharge, flow	4
mening / o	meninges	4			
menisc / o	meniscus	3	salping / o	fallopian or uterine tube	10
metr / o	uterus	10			
muscul/o	muscle	3	sarc / o	connective tissue, flesh	2
my / o	muscle	3			
myel / o	spinal cord, bone marrow	4	-sarcoma	malignant tumor	*rhabdomyosarcoma*
myos/o	muscle	3	scapul / o	scapula	3
myring / o	tympanic membrane	5	scler / o	sclera, hard	5
			-sclerosis	hardening	6
nephr / o	kidney	1, 9	scoli/o	crooked, curved (lateral)	3
neur / o	nerve	4			
-oid	resembling	2	-scope	instrument used for visual examination	3
-oma	tumor	2			
onc / o	cancer	2			
oophor / o	ovary	10	-scopy	visual examination	3
ophthalm / o	eye	5			
-opsy	to view	*biopsy*	sigmoid / o	sigmoid colon	7
orchi / o	testicle, testis	9	splen / o	spleen	6
orchid / o	testicle, testis	9	staped / o	stapes	5
-osis	abnormal condition	3	-stenosis	narrowing	6
			stern / o	sternum	3
oste / o	bone	3	stomat / o	mouth	7
ot / o	ear	5	-stomy	creation of an artificial opening	7
-ous	pertaining to	2			
pancreat / o	pancreas	7			
parathyroid / o	parathyroid	11	sub-	under, below	1, 2
patell / o	patella	3	supra-	above	*suprascapular*
path / o	disease	2	tachy-	fast, rapid	6

Word Element	Meaning	Unit Number (or Sample Medical Term)	Word Element	Meaning	Unit Number (or Sample Medical Term)
thorac / o	chest	8	ungu / o	nail	2
thromb / o	clot	6	ur / o	urine, urinary tract	9
thyr / o	thyroid	11			
thyroid / o	thyroid	11	ureter / o	ureter	9
-tomy	surgical incision or to cut into	3	urethr / o	urethra	9
			urin / o	urine	9
tonsill / o	tonsil	8	uter / o	uterus	10
trache / o	trachea	8	vagin / o	vagina	10
trans-	through, across, beyond	1, 2	vas / o	vessel, duct	9
			vertebr / o	vertebra	3
trich / o	hair	2	viscer / o	internal organs	2
-trophy	development, nourishment	3			

Answers

CHAPTER 1

Exercise 1

1. CHUC
2. EMR, EHR
3. SHUC
4. pt
5. HUC
6. CDSS
7. CPOE
8. HIMSS
9. www

Exercise 2

1. certified health unit coordinator
2. electronic medical record, electronic health record
3. student health unit coordinator
4. clinical decision support system
5. health unit coordinator
6. patient
7. computer physician order entry
8. Health Information Management Systems Society
9. World Wide Web

Review Questions

1. a. tasks performed at the bedside or in direct contact with the patient
   b. tasks performed away from the bedside
   c. use of certified EMR technology in ways that can be measured significantly in quality and in quantity
   d. the process of testifying to or endorsing that a person has met certain standards
   e. a process used to communicate the doctors' orders to the nursing staff and other hospital departments; computers or handwritten requisitions are used
   f. A computer program that allows one to search for and view (or hear) various kinds of information on the Web, such as websites, videos, and audio files.
   g. a website that collects and organizes content from all over the Web
   h. a company that provides Internet connections and services to individuals and organizations for a monthly fee
   i. the electronic transmission of prescription information from the prescriber's computer (hospital or doctor's office) to a pharmacy computer
   j. the use of different search engines on the Web to locate information
   k. keywords that when entered after "http://www" on the Web will take the user to a specified location, referred to as a *website*

l. an interactive decision support system (DSS); computer software designed to assist physicians at the point of order entry

2. a. clinical
   b. nonclinical
   c. nonclinical
   d. nonclinical
   e. clinical
   f. nonclinical
   g. nonclinical
   h. clinical
   i. nonclinical

3.
   - World War II—shortage of registered nurses
   - advanced technology—the workload of the doctor increased, many tasks shifted to the nursing staff
   - hospitals larger and more complex
   - more specialists ordering newly available tests and treatments
   - Federally sponsored health programs required more detailed record keeping, and nonclinical demands of every hospitalized patient increased proportionately

4. a. on-the-job training
   b. formal education
   c. formation of a national association
   d. certification or licensure

5. a. professional representation
   b. forum for sharing ideas and challenges—assistance in being prepared and proactive regarding changes that are taking place in health care and the HUC profession
   c. national networking
   d. national directory
   e. opportunity to develop leadership skills

6.
   - increased credibility
   - gaining a broader perspective of health unit coordinating (not just one specialty)—be prepared and proactive regarding changes that are taking place in the health unit coordinator profession
   - increased mobility, geographically and vertically
   - peer and public recognition and respect
   - improved self-image

7. August 23

8. a. *nursing personnel*—any three of the following:
   - communicate all new doctors' orders or messages to the patient's nurse
   - maintain the patient's paper chart or manage the electronic record
   - communicate information involving new patient arrivals and requests for patient transfers

- perform the nonclinical tasks required for admission, discharge, and transfer of a patient
- prepare the patient's chart for surgery (if a paper chart is in use)
- prepare necessary consent forms for patient surgeries or procedures
- handle all telephone communication for the nursing unit
- maintain nursing unit supplies

Additional responsibilities may include the following:

- create time schedules for nursing unit staff
- monitor and maintain documentation required by The Joint Commission (TJC) on licenses and certifications and in-services for nursing unit staff

b. *doctors*—any three of the following:

- assist in finding patients' charts
- assist as necessary with physician order entry if EMR is used
- transcribe the doctors' orders (if paper charts are used)
- scan reports or documents into the patient's electronic record
- procure requested equipment for patient examinations
- place calls to and receive calls from doctors' offices
- obtain information for the physician regarding whether previously ordered procedures have been completed

c. *hospital departments*—any three of the following:

- order, schedule, and coordinate diagnostic procedures and treatments when required
- relay messages and information to appropriate departments as required
- request services from maintenance and other service departments
- work closely with the admitting department to admit, transfer, and discharge patients
- order supplies for the nursing unit ranging from food to paper products and patient care supplies

d. *patients*—any three of the following:

- instruct new patients on how to use the call light, turn on the television, and operate bed controls
- relay patient requests to nursing personnel when answering the intercom located in each patient's room
- greet and listen to concerns or requests of patients who come to the nursing station

The HUC usually has little bedside contact with patients.

e. *hospital visitors*—any three of the following:

- assist visitors looking for a patient by locating the patient on the computer
- provide information about the location of bathrooms, visitors' lounge, cafeteria, and so on
- inform visitors about the rules of visitation, and explain any special precautions that may be required during their visit to a patient's room
- receive telephone calls from relatives or friends who are inquiring about the patient's condition
- listen to (document) and handle visitor concerns

9. a. The use of EMR and CPOE with e-prescribing in hospitals as well as in doctor's offices can significantly improve patient care by reducing the risk of human error in interpreting doctor's handwriting. Also, the ability to access all of the patient information, organized in one place, at the click of a mouse eliminates the duplication of tests, reduces delays in treatment, and can help doctors collaborate more effectively, as patients often see a variety of specialists.

b. The CDSS will provide prompts that warn against the possibility of a drug interaction, an incorrect dose, or a patient allergy. The system also may provide reminders to the physician, such as a reminder to order aspirin for a patient who is going home after undergoing heart surgery.

10. Any of the following examples:

- alerts doctor of a patient allergy at point of ordering a medication to which the patient is allergic
- alerts doctor of drug interactions at point of ordering a medication that would be a problem because of another medication the patient is taking
- alerts doctor of an incorrect dosage at point of ordering a medication

11. a.

- Complete a Health Unit Coordinator program.
- Complete communication and management classes related to health care.
- Complete classes in advanced computer skills (typing and keyboarding, Microsoft Office including Word, Excel, PowerPoint, Access, and Outlook).
- Become a member of the National Association of Health Unit Coordinators.
- Become certified by taking the National Health Unit Coordinator certification test.

b.

- Attend job related in-services that are offered through the hospital.
- Take classes that are available at local community colleges. (Most hospitals have a continuing education program.)
- Stay active in the National Association of Health Unit Coordinators.
- Receive and read the NAHUC newsletter and attend conferences.
- Keep certification current by taking the certification test or by obtaining continuing education units.
- Be curious—research new procedures or information on the Web.

12. a. telemetry technician

b. case management assistant or secretary

c. CNA

In a few hospitals, HUCs are also trained to perform electrocardiography and/or phlebotomy.

13. a. Clinical Research Associate

b. Health Information Manager

CHAPTER 2

Exercise 1

1. AHA
2. app
3. CCM
4. CEO
5. CFO
6. COO
7. DRG
8. ECF

9. HIMS
10. HMO
11. ICD
12. LTC
13. PPO
14. SNF
15. TJC
16. WHO

Exercise 2

1. American Hospital Association
2. application
3. certified case manager
4. chief executive officer
5. chief financial officer
6. chief operating officer
7. diagnosis-related group
8. extended care facility
9. health information management system
10. health maintenance organization
11. International Statistical Classification of Diseases and Related Health Problems
12. long-term care
13. preferred provider organization
14. skilled nursing facility
15. The Joint Commission
16. World Health Organization

Review Questions

1. a. classification system used to determine payments from Medicare by assigning a standard flat rate to major diagnostic categories. This flat rate is paid to hospitals regardless of the full cost of the services provided.
   b. insurance coverage that is responsible for paying claims first and protects against medical expenses up to the policy's limit, regardless of whatever other insurance the purchaser holds
   c. a person who is extremely poor—lacking necessities of life, such as food and clothing; impoverished
   d. insurance coverage used to supplement existing policies or to cover any gaps in insurance coverage—billed after primary insurance has paid
   e. the combined use of telecommunications and computer technologies to improve the efficiency and effectiveness of health care services by eliminating the traditional constraints of place and time
   f. a local, PC-based large-vocabulary voice-recognition engine that generates reports, often using macros and templates to make the process more efficient and reduce recognition errors
   g. recognition that a health care organization has met an official standard
   h. payment method whereby the provider of care receives a set dollar amount per patient, regardless of services rendered
   i. a temporary coverage gap in Medicare that occurs after the beneficiary and his or her Medicare Part D Drug Plan have spent a set amount of money in total prescription drug expenses. The beneficiary pays 100% of drug costs while in the donut hole until another set amount is reached, then the beneficiary receives catastrophic coverage.
   j. equipment and services provided to patient in his or her home to ensure comfort and care
   k. supportive care for terminally ill patients and their families
   l. not for profit (nonprofit)
   m. coverage a Medicare beneficiary has after reaching a certain amount of "out of pocket" monies paid for his or her medications during the temporary coverage gap. The beneficiary will pay a coinsurance amount (such as 5% of the drug cost) or a copayment ($2.15 or $5.35 for each prescription) for the rest of the calendar year.
   n. unskilled care given for the primary purpose of meeting personal needs, such as bathing and dressing
   o. for profit
   p. a secure Web-based system that allows a patient to register for an appointment, schedule an appointment, request prescription refills, send and receive secure patient-physician messages, view lab results, or pay bills electronically

2. Any five of the following:
   - more than 50 million people uninsured in 2010
   - a disparity in care provided to insured people as compared with the uninsured or underinsured, many of whom belong to racial and ethnic minorities
   - the staggering cost of advanced technology
   - increasing insurance costs and out-of-pocket costs that continue to soar
   - Many doctors and health care facilities are refusing to treat Medicare patients or limiting the number of Medicare patients they treat owing to slow and low pay.
   - The Medicaid health insurance program for low-income people announced $112.8 million in cuts.
   - Medical errors are one of the nation's leading causes of death and injury.

3. Any four of the following:
   - A new health insurance marketplace will be created in 2014.
   - The exchanges will guarantee that all people have a choice for high-quality, affordable health insurance even if a job loss, job switch, move, or illness occurs.
   - A preexisting condition insurance plan will provide new coverage options to individuals who have been uninsured for at least 6 months.
   - In 2014 patients will no longer be discriminated against based on a preexisting condition.
   - Insurance companies will be prohibited from imposing lifetime dollar limits on essential benefits.
   - Young adults will be allowed to stay on their parent's plan until they turn 26 years old.
   - All new plans must cover certain preventive services such as mammograms and colonoscopies without charging a deductible, copay, or coinsurance.
   - There will be a requirement for health plans to begin adopting and implementing rules for the secure, confidential, electronic exchange of health information (EMR).
   - The law establishes a hospital Value-Based Purchasing (VBP) program in original Medicare; this offers financial incentives to hospitals to improve the quality of care.

- Hospital performance is required to be publicly reported, beginning with measures relating to heart attacks, heart failure, pneumonia, surgical care, health care–associated infections, and patients' perception of care.
- Most individuals who can afford it will be required to obtain basic health insurance coverage or pay a fee to help offset the costs of caring for uninsured Americans.

4. It is important to stay current with any additional changes made, as the changes may have an impact on health care providers as well as everyone receiving health care.

5. A national electronic medical record system will allow the federal government to track the course and impact of a pandemic in real time and would provide local, state, and federal governments with the necessary data to direct therapies, medical personnel, and supplies during an emergency.

6. There is a balancing act between ease of access for prompt medical care and the maintenance of confidentiality. Health care providers must make sure their EMR system is HIPAA compliant and that the EMR systems installed take care of all the privacy and information security issues.

7. *Client server–based EMR*—The software is hosted on the hospital internal server, and the licenses are purchased outright. *Cloud- or Web-based EMR*—The facility uses an Internet site to host data and programs instead of keeping them on an internal computer.

8. VistA

9. HIPAA-compliant mobile EMR—An EHR service that allows doctors to access critical patient records and office information from their iPhones. The iSALUS new mobile EMR-EHR application enables physicians to securely access real-time patient information such as progress notes, medical images, and contact and insurance information. It also provides doctors and practice managers with access to office items such as schedules, rounds, task lists, dictations, patient charges, and office communications.

   Patient portal applications might allow patients to register and complete forms online, allow patients to request prescription refills online, order eyeglasses and contacts, access medical records, pay bills, review lab results, and schedule necessary medical appointments.

10. Three categories of telemedicine:
    a. acquiring medical data such as medical images and biosignals (e.g., ECG tracings) and then transmitting this data to a doctor or medical specialist at a remote site
    b. remote monitoring—enables medical professionals to monitor a patient remotely through use of various technologic devices
    c. interactive real-time interactions between patient and provider—provided through telephone conversations, online communication, and home visits

    Three major advances aided by surgical robots:
    a. computer assisted surgery—commonly used in orthopedic surgeries
    b. telesurgical systems—enhances the surgery by providing three-dimensional visualization deep within hard-to-reach places such as the heart, as well as enhancing wrist dexterity and control of tiny instruments

    c. shared control systems—monitor the surgeon, providing stability and support during the procedure; the human does the bulk of the work. Before getting started, the surgeons program the robots to recognize safe, close, boundary, and forbidden territories within the human body. Safe regions are the main focus of the surgery. When the forbidden zone is reached, the robotic system actually locks up to prevent any further injury. Shared-control systems might work best for brain surgeries; the surgeon provides the action, but the robot arm steadies the hand.

11. *Indemnity insurance:*
    - provides individuals freedom and flexibility in choosing doctor and medical treatments
    - premiums are higher, and there are deductibles and other out-of-pocket expenses
    - most plans come with an annual coinsurance maximum; once it has been met, the insurance company will pay 100% of the medical costs for the rest of the calendar year
    - does not pay for preventative care
    - covers accidents and illnesses

    Managed care:
    - has a lower deductible and smaller copayment than an indemnity plan
    - limited choices when it comes to doctors or hospitals
    - physicians must be authorized by the managed care provider
    - permission must be obtained from the primary doctor to see a specialized doctor
    - Managed care systems most often are associated with health maintenance organizations (HMOs) that have management responsibility for providing comprehensive health care services on a prepayment basis (capitation) to voluntarily enrolled persons within a designated population.

    Worker's compensation:
    - The employer pays a premium to an insurance carrier for worker's compensation coverage.
    - The policy pays the medical bills and a significant portion of the lost wages when an on-the-job accident or illness results in injury or disability.
    - The injured worker must fill out a claim form and send it to the insurance carrier.
    - The injured worker receives no bill, pays no deductible, and is covered 100% for medical expenses related to that injury or illness.

12. Medicaid is a federal and state program that provides medical assistance for the indigent.

13. Medicare Part A—hospital insurance—helps cover inpatient care in hospitals and helps cover skilled nursing facility, hospice, and home health care

    Medicare Part B—medical insurance—helps cover doctors' services, hospital outpatient care, and home health care and helps cover some preventive services to help maintain health and to keep certain illnesses from getting worse

    Medicare Part D—prescription drug coverage—a prescription drug option run by Medicare-approved private insurance companies that helps cover the cost of prescription drugs until a preset amount of money has been reached; then the Medicare beneficiary is in a temporary donut hole.

14. nursing homes or health care centers, extended care facilities (ECFs), physical medicine and rehabilitation facilities, hospice
15. Hospice provides palliative and supportive care for terminally ill patients and their families. Emphasis is placed on control of symptoms and preparation for and support before and after death.
16. a. the care and treatment of the sick
    b. education of physicians and other health care personnel
    c. research
    d. prevention of disease
    e. local health center
17. a. type of service offered
    b. ownership of the hospital
    c. the type of accreditation the hospital has been given
18. a. Magnet status is an award given by the ANCC to hospitals that satisfy a set of criteria designed to measure the strength and quality of their nursing.
    b. Hospital benefits include:
       • enhanced nursing care
       • increased staff morale
       • appeal to high-quality physicians
       • reinforced positive collaborative relationships
       • creation of a "Magnet culture"
       • improved patient quality outcomes
       • enhanced nursing recruitment
       • retention
       • competitive advantage
19. a. American Hospital Association (AHA)
    b. The Joint Commission (TJC)
20. Governing board—responsibilities include establishing policy, providing adequate financing, and overseeing personnel standards.
21. a. Chief executive officer (CEO)
    b. responsibilities include planning for the implementation of policies set forth by the governing board. (The chief operating officer (COO) is responsible for the day-to-day operations of the hospital and reports directly to the CEO. The chief financial officer (CFO) is responsible for the fiscal aspects of the hospital administration and reports directly to the CEO).
22. a. managing patient accounts
    b. admission of patients
    c. diagnostic procedures on specimens from the body
    d. x-ray, nuclear medicine, and ultrasound studies
    e. treatment of cancer growths
    f. distribution of medications
    g. rehabilitation of patients
    h. treatment related to respiratory function
    i. preparation of food and meals
    j. diagnostic procedures performed with the use of endoscopes
    k. diagnostics studies related to the digestive system
    l. tests related to heart and blood vessels
    m. studies of the nervous system
    n. managing patient charts or electronic medical records
    o. storage and distribution of supplies and equipment used for patient care
    p. assistance to patients and families
    q. housekeeping duties
    r. protection of the hospital, patient, visitors, and employees

s. installation and repair of electronics including computers, printers, and software
    t. keeps equipment in working order
    u. recruitment, employee payroll, exit interviews
23. Any of three of the following:
    • surf the Web for local job openings
    • check newspaper classifieds
    • school job placement, career counselors, instructors
    • health care hotlines
    • employment agencies
    • library resources
    • health care facility websites and bulletin boards
    • networking with professionals in the field
    • networking with NAHUC members

CHAPTER 3

Exercise 1

1. ANA
2. ANCC
3. CNA
4. DO
5. DSU
6. ENT
7. eICU
8. ED, ER
9. HO
10. LPN
11. MDA
12. MD
13. ND, NMD
14. NP
15. OR
16. PCP
17. PSA
18. PA
19. PACU
20. RN
21. SAD (surgery), SDSurgery

Exercise 2

1. American Nurses Association
2. American Nurses Credentialing Center
3. certified nursing assistant
4. doctor of osteopathy
5. day surgery unit
6. electronic intensive care unit
7. emergency department, emergency room
8. ear, nose, and throat doctor (otorhinolaryngologist)
9. house officer
10. licensed practical nurse
11. medical doctor
12. medical doctor of anesthesia
13. doctor of naturopathy, naturopathic medical doctor
14. nurse practitioner
15. operating room
16. physician's assistant
17. postanesthesia care unit
18. primary care physician
19. patient support associate
20. registered nurse
21. save-a-day (surgery), same-day surgery

Review Questions

1. a. level of care patients would require on the basis of their medical condition; used to evaluate staffing needs
   b. level of health care, generally provided in hospitals or emergency departments, for sudden, serious illnesses or trauma
   c. long-lasting; describes an illness or medical condition that lasts for a long period and sometimes causes a long-term change in the body
   d. term applied to a physician who admits and is responsible for a hospital patient
   e. patient to receive medical or surgical care whose doctor has written an admission order
   f. specializes in the care of critically ill patients, usually in an intensive care unit (ICU)
   g. any act by a nurse that implements the nursing care plan or clinical pathway or any specific objective of that plan or pathway
   h. a patient receiving medical or surgical care while registered as an outpatient and whose doctor has not written an admission order; the patient's doctor may order the patient to stay overnight for observation without writing an admitting order
   i. meeting of a patient's doctor or resident, primary nurse, case manager or social worker, and other health care professionals for the purpose of planning the patient's care
   j. a general practitioner or internist, chosen by an individual to serve as his or her health care professional (sometimes referred to as a "gatekeeper")
   k. a graduate of a medical school who is gaining experience in a hospital
   l. a health unit coordinator, a nurse, or a group of health care workers who are on call for all units in the hospital to provide assistance as needed

2. a. neonatologist
   b. psychiatrist
   c. otolaryngologist
   d. pathologist
   e. anesthesiologist
   f. endocrinologist
   g. allergist
   h. hospitalist
   i. geriatrist
   j. internist
   k. pediatrician
   l. gynecologist
   m. cardiologist
   n. dermatologist
   o. pulmonologist

3. a. radiologist
   b. neurologist
   c. oncologist
   d. emergency room doctor
   e. ophthalmologist
   f. radiation oncologist
   g. urologist
   h. proctologist
   i. surgeon
   j. orthopedist
   k. obstetrician
   l. physiatrist

m. intensivist
n. interventional radiologist

4. a. telemetry
   b. behavioral health
   c. surgical
   d. cardiovascular
   e. urology
   f. pediatrics
   g. rehab
   h. oncology
   i. orthopedics
   j. GYN
   k. medical
   l. neurology
   m. L&D
   n. obstetrics

5. a. physician's assistant (PA)
   b. nurse practitioner (NP)

6. Any two of the following:
   • Chiropractic medicine—complementary and alternative health care profession with the purpose of diagnosing and treating mechanical disorders of the spine and musculoskeletal system
   • Acupuncture—originated in China—based on a belief that all living things have a vital energy, called *qi*
   • Homeopathy—a natural medicine that treats the whole person with natural medicines
   • Native American healing—the practices and healing beliefs of hundreds of indigenous tribes of North America; a combination of religion, spirituality, herbal medicine, and rituals
   • Naturopathic medicine—based on the belief that the human body has an innate healing ability

7. The nursing service department is basically responsible for ensuring the physical and emotional care of the hospitalized patient. Other responsibilities include patient assessment and recording, planning and implementing patient care plans, and patient teaching. Implementation of the electronic medical record (EMR) requires the nurse to enter documentation directly into the patient's record at the bedside via computer.

8. a. The *director of nursing* (also called the *vice president of nursing*) is responsible for the overall administration of nursing service. Setting nursing practice standards and staffing are two examples of the responsibilities of the director of nursing.
   b. The *nurse manager* (also called *clinical manager, patient care manager,* or *unit manager*) is responsible for the patients and nursing personnel on the unit for 24 hours a day. Managerial responsibilities include the planning and coordinating of high-quality nursing care for patients hospitalized on the unit. Selecting, supervising, scheduling, and evaluating personnel employed on the unit are other managerial responsibilities of the nurse manager.

9. a. specialist referral services
   b. interactive telemedicine services
   c. remote patient monitoring
   d. medical education
   e. consumer medical and health information

10. Allows intensivists and critical care nurses to care and monitor ICU 24/7. Video conferencing allows tele-ICU physicians and nurses to see and communicate directly

with patients, families and on-site clinicians from a central control station. The system also provides automated alerts that can identify trends in the patient's condition before an on-site caregiver might notice. The advanced ICU intensivist-led program helps hospitals improve patient outcomes and support continuous quality improvement.

11. Any three of the following:
    - nurse or clinical manager: assists the director of nursing in carrying out administrative responsibilities and is usually in charge of one or more nursing units
    - assistant nurse manager: assists the nurse manager in coordinating the activities of the nursing units
    - registered nurse: may give direct patient care or supervise patient care given by others
    - licensed practical nurse: gives direct patient care; functions under the direction of the RN
    - certified nursing assistant: a health care provider who performs basic nursing tasks such as bathing and feeding patients

12. a. preoperative area—area in the hospital where patients are prepared for surgery
    b. intraoperative care—operating room; area in the hospital where surgery is performed
    c. postoperative (postanesthesia care)—area in the hospital where patients are cared for immediately after surgery until they have recovered from the effects of the anesthesia

13. Critically ill patients are admitted to an intensive care unit (ICU) to receive constant specialized acute nursing care. As the condition of a critically ill patient improves (not enough to go to a floor unit), the patient is transferred to the intermediate care (IMC) or stepdown unit for less intensive nursing care.

14. a. Emergency department—care of patients who need emergency treatment
    b. Hospice inpatient—care of terminally ill patients in need of more care than can be managed at home, or whose symptoms require more intensive management than a family caregiver can provide
    c. Chronic pain management—treatment of individuals in chronic pain

15. A patient who is to receive medical or surgical care and has been preapproved by his or her insurance company is considered an inpatient when a doctor formally writes an admission order.

16. The team patient care model is made up of the charge nurse who oversees the nursing unit, two or three team leaders (RNs), and three or four team members who work under the supervision of each team leader. Members of the team may be RNs, LPNs, and/or CNAs.

   In total patient care, the RN assigned to a patient is responsible for planning, organizing, and performing all care, including providing personal hygiene, medications and treatments, emotional support, and education required for a group of patients during an assigned shift.

17. Clinical pathways, also called *critical paths*, are used as a method of outlining a patient's path of treatment for a specific diagnosis, procedure, or symptom.

   Goals for developing and using clinical pathways include the following: (1) identify patient and family needs, (2) determine realistic patient outcomes and time frames required to achieve those outcomes, (3) reduce length of stay and inappropriate use of resources, and (4) clarify the appropriate care setting, providers, and timelines of intervention.

18. The assignment sheet indicates the nursing staff assigned to each patient on that nursing unit. The form also may include lunch times and break times for nursing personnel.

19. Holistic nursing care is the modern nursing practice that expresses the philosophy of comprehensive patient care (total patient care) and considers the physical, emotional, social, economic, and spiritual needs of the patient, his or her response to illness, and the effect of the illness on ability to meet self-care needs.

20. a. facilitates continuous quality improvement
    b. improves patient care
    c. decreases errors
    d. provides "total patient care"
    e. maximizes resources
    f. increases professional satisfaction for health care givers

CHAPTER 4

Exercise 1

1. CRP
2. DMS
3. GPS
4. PC
5. PCTS
6. PDA
7. WOW

Exercise 2

1. critical response performance
2. document management system
3. Global Positioning System
4. personal computer
5. Patient Care Technology Systems
6. personal data assistant
7. workstation on wheels

Review Questions

1. a. methods for uniquely recognizing humans based on one or more intrinsic physical or behavioral traits
   b. a mobile computer that can be taken to a patient's bedside, allowing nurses and other health care providers the ability to access and enter information into patient records
   c. an alphabetic listing of names, telephone numbers, and directory telephone numbers of physicians on staff (most hospitals have made this available on computer)
   d. a nonmobile personal computer (PC) intended to be used at the same dedicated location day after day for use by one computer operator at any given moment
   e. a computer system (or set of computer programs) used to track and store electronic documents and/or images of paper documents
   f. a paper order form (requisition) that is used to process information when the computer is not available for use
   g. a mechanical device for transporting food or supplies from one hospital floor to another

h. a message usually involving a laboratory value of such variance with normal as to be life-threatening unless some intervention is done by the physician, and for which there are interventions possible

i. a portable computer; some laptops are actually in a tablet form (tablets are essentially just laptops with a touchscreen and possibly a pen for input)

j. a handheld mobile device that functions as a personal information manager (also called a *personal digital assistant* or *palmtop computer*)

k. used to make up for nursing and staff shortages; robots used to dispense medication, make deliveries, visit patients, and help doctors reach patients across distance

l. computer that may be removed from its base, or a portable computer that can be taken into patient rooms, with a stylus used to enter information directly into a patient's electronic record, as in a notebook

m. provides network services to other computers on a network

n. a brand of laptop designed to withstand vibration, drops, spills, extreme temperature, and other rough handling used in many hospitals

o. a relatively powerful kind of desktop with a faster processor, more memory, and other advanced features compared with a more basic desktop.

2. a. Answer the telephone promptly and professionally, preferably prior to the third ring. If engaged in a conversation at the nurses' station, excuse yourself to answer the telephone.

b. Identify yourself properly by stating location, name, and status. For example: "4 East, Stacey, Health Unit Coordinator."

c. Speak into the telephone—be sure the mouthpiece is not under your chin, making it difficult for the caller to hear.

d. Give the caller your undivided attention—it is difficult to focus on the telephone conversation while attempting to do something else.

e. Speak clearly and distinctly—do not eat food or chew gum while talking on the telephone.

f. Always be courteous—say "Please" and "Thank you."

g. When you do not know the answer, state that you will locate someone who can help the caller.

h. If necessary to step away or answer another call, place the caller on hold *after asking permission to do so and waiting for an answer.* For example: "May I put you on hold, Mr. Phillips, while I find Jenny to speak to you?"

3. Place caller on hold:

a. when it is necessary to locate information or a person

b. when it is necessary to answer other telephone lines

c. when it is necessary to leave telephone for any reason to protect patient confidentiality (caller will not hear conversations)

Transfer a caller when:

a. the caller reached the wrong department or wrong extension

b. the caller has questions that only another person or department can answer

4. a. who the message is for

b. the caller's name

c. date and time of the call

d. purpose of the call

e. phone number to call if a return call is expected

f. your name

5. Most messages received on the nursing unit need to be communicated immediately to avoid delays in patient care. It is important to gain the trust and confidence of medical staff and nursing team members; putting messages in writing may be the first important step toward gaining that confidence while guaranteeing accuracy during the communication process.

6. a. The person taking the message should read back the critical value to the person providing the message.

b. The name of the person providing the message and the person taking the message should be documented.

7. Have the information or the patient's chart handy so that facts will be available when questions are asked; write down the main facts that need to be discussed and the telephone number to be called; alert the person requesting the call be made when the call is being placed.

8. a. voice message on telephone, voice pocket pager, or wireless device

- Speak slowly and distinctly so the person listening to the message can hear and understand what is being communicated.
- If leaving a message, include the name of the patient and/or the doctor; give the first and last names, and spell the last name.
- If the message includes a telephone number or laboratory values, speak slowly and repeat the numbers twice, allowing time for the listener to record the information.
- Always leave your name and telephone number, and repeat both twice (at the beginning of the message and at the end of the message) so the listener can call for clarification if necessary.

b. text message on telephone or pocket pager

- keep texts brief and to the point
- do not use abbreviations that may not be understood

9. a. alphabetized directory of department numbers and key personnel; hospitals using the individual pocket pager also may publish a directory of pocket pager numbers

b. names of the doctors (in alphabetic order) with an indication of who has admitting or visiting privileges, medical specialties, office telephone numbers, and answering service telephone numbers

10. a. pneumatic tube system

b. telelift system

c. dumbwaiter

11. a. dispense medication

b. make deliveries

c. visit patients

12. Any three of the following wireless communication systems:

- Vocera communication system
- Polycom SpectraLink
- Ascom 914T Pocket Receiver
- locator tracking and communication system

13. Any of the following capabilities and benefits:

- Hospital workers are able to quickly reach area law enforcement as well as one another for help.
- The nurses' stations are quieter and less hectic as calls are made directly to caregivers.

- Can be integrated with third-party applications such as nurse call systems and in-building PBX systems. The nurse call system integration allows nurses to respond faster to patient needs.
- Patients and families have the ability to contact the nurse directly from both inside and outside the hospital.
- When paged, the health care professionals do not have to waste time finding a phone, so they do not have to leave whatever they are doing at the moment. Now they can take the call directly without leaving the bedside, even in the intensive care unit.
- Easy to use with naturally spoken commands; hands-free conversations
- No need to memorize telephone or extension numbers
- Saves money by lowering or eliminating phone and pager costs

14. part of a disaster or emergency preparedness plan—the ability to communicate critical information to tens, hundreds, or thousands of individuals, anywhere, anytime, and on any device

15. Any of the following:
    - a multiple injury car, train, or airplane accident
    - a bombing
    - an earthquake
    - an infectious disease outbreak

16. Any of the following:
    - locates key equipment (such as crash carts, IV pumps, and wheelchairs) and maintains inventory—provides immediate, real-time information on the location and condition of equipment
    - tracks patients and personnel
    - provides the status of bed availability and the nearest skilled staff resources needed to care for patients (to improve workflow and track exposure to infection)
    - improves efficiency of transport and order turnaround times to departments such as pharmacy, laboratory, or radiology
    - provides the information needed to effectively move patients to appropriate levels of care, or discharge them, in a timely, safe, and cost-effective way.
    - performs condition monitoring as in temperature-controlling equipment (refrigerators, freezers, warmers)—tags are used in pharmacies, blood banks, laboratories, operating rooms, and nursing units where proper temperature conditions are critical
    - monitors the temperature of warming blankets in the operating room and on nursing units

17. a. Ultra-Scan fingerprint technology
    b. Fujitsu PalmSecure (vascular biometrics)
    c. iris recognition systems

18. Any of the following:
    - reduces risk of wrong body part being operated on
    - reduces risk of medication given to wrong patient
    - reduces errors caused by getting a patient's chart confused with another patient's chart
    - reduces problem of sending a baby home with the wrong mother; can be eliminated if the baby's and mother's physical characteristics can be matched with certainty
    - improves issues of potential patient fraud
    - lowers the risk of writing in the wrong medical record
    - has reduced registration time for patients by about 10 seconds each

19. a. Most hospitals have bins located on each nursing unit that are emptied periodically and taken to an area where the contents are shredded in the shredder; blank documents with any patient information (label) on them have to be shredded.
    b. Whiteboards, usually in the nurses' station area, on which to record census information including unit room numbers, admitting doctors' names, and the name of the nurse assigned to each patient
    c. The HUC may be given the responsibility of maintaining the nursing unit bulletin board; includes posting material in an attractive manner and keeping posted material current.
    d. A device used to transmit images of paper documents and pictures to be entered into the patient's electronic record
    e. Used for instant two-way voice conversation without the need to remember a phone number or use a handset
    f. Used to communicate between the nurses' station and patient rooms on the nursing unit
    g. Transport tubes used for carrying supplies, requisitions, or some lab specimens from one hospital unit or department to another
    h. Used to print patient labels from information entered into the computer; located near the health unit coordinator's area
    i. Worn by nursing personnel, including health unit coordinators, so their location may be detected on the interactive console display when necessary
    j. When activated by entering a series of numbers into a telephone, delivers a digital or voice message to the carrier of the pager
    k. Transmits copies of written material over a telephone wire from one site to another
    l. Used for making copies of written or typed materials—the fax machine also can be used to make a minimal number of copies

20. It may result in confidential patient information being sent to the wrong location and could cause one to lose his or her job.

21. a. desk top
    b. laptop or notebook
    c. hand held
    d. server or application server

22. a. do not use for personal messages
    b. do not use to send inappropriate material such as jokes
    c. respond to the necessary person or department only; refrain from sending to "all" or using "reply to all" unless necessary

23. E-mail and social networks are not to be used for personal communication, can be easily tracked, and could cause one to lose his or her job.

24. Icons appear on the computer screen next to the patient's name on the census sheet when there is a HUC task that must be performed. E-mail may also be used to indicate tasks that need to be completed.

25. a. printed reports
    b. handwritten doctor's progress notes
    c. electrocardiograms (ECGs)

26. When paper charts are used, the HUC's main focus is transcribing doctors' orders; when the EMR is used, the HUC's role is more administrative.

CHAPTER 5

Exercise 1

1. a
2. b
3. b
4. c
5. d
6. d
7. d
8. c
9. a
10. b

Exercise 2

1. AS
2. AG
3. NA
4. NA
5. AS
6. AG
7. AS
8. AG
9. AG
10. AS
11. AG
12. NA
13. AS
14. AG
15. AG
16. NA
17. AS
18. AS

Exercise 3

Answers will vary. Following are examples of responses for each behavior:

1. Assertive: "It really embarrassed me when you asked if I know what I'm supposed to do in front of my co-workers. Of course I know what needs to be done—I had a very busy day and just didn't have time to do everything."
   Nonassertive: Be upset and say nothing.
   Aggressive: "This is a 24-hour facility; what I don't get done, you can do!"

2. Assertive: "I understand that you would prefer someone who is accustomed to working in pediatrics. I may need a little assistance and will do my best to get the job done." *(Fogging)*
   - Nonassertive: "I'm sorry; I know I'm not qualified to work in pediatrics."
   - Aggressive: "You're lucky to have me; if you don't want me to be here, I'll leave."

3. Assertive: "You're right, I did miss that order; I'll order it right now." *(Negative assertion)*
   Nonassertive: "I'm sorry; I'm so stupid! What should I do now?"
   Aggressive: "Well, maybe if you gave me a little more help, I wouldn't be missing orders!"

4. Assertive: "Only relatives may visit the patient, on the instructions of the physician." Repeat as necessary. *(Broken record)*

- Nonassertive: "I don't think you're supposed to visit, but maybe just this once we could sneak you in."
- Aggressive: "You are not allowed to visit; I don't care who you are!"

5. Assertive: "I was not aware that you felt this way. What about my work is sloppy?" *(Negative inquiry)*
   - Nonassertive: "I've always been sloppy. It's just the way I am. I'm sorry."
   - Aggressive: "I'm a lot neater than most of the other people around here!"

6. Assertive: "I know it must seem that nothing is done right here; however, most things are done very well. I'll scan the report into the patient's record now."
   - Nonassertive: "I'm sorry; I should have scanned it as soon as you asked me too. I am so forgetful sometimes."
   - Aggressive: "You don't understand how hectic it is around here. You doctors always think everyone else is incompetent!"

Review Questions

1. a. the process of transmitting feelings, images, and ideas from the mind of one person to the mind of another person by the use of speech, signals, writing, or behavior
   b. translating mental images, feelings, and ideas into verbal and nonverbal symbols to communicate them to the receiver
   c. the process of translating verbal and nonverbal symbols received from the sender to determine the message
   d. a disagreement or clash between ideas, values, principles, or people
   e. a person who facilitates oral communication between or among parties who are conversing in different languages
   f. attempts at influencing or controlling others' actions or behaviors to one's own advantage
   g. repeating a message back to the sender in your own words to clarify meaning
   h. a type of aggressive behavior characterized by an indirect expression of negative feelings, resentment, and aggression in an unassertive way (as through sullenness, obstructionism, stubbornness, and unwillingness to communicate)
   i. a set of values, beliefs, and traditions that are held by a specific social group
   j. factors such as age, gender, race, religion, and socioeconomic status
   k. dealing with conflict in such a way that the solution is satisfactory to all parties
   l. subgroup within a culture; people with a distinct identity but who have specific ethnic, occupational, or physical characteristics found in a larger culture

2. a. diversity
   b. ageism
   c. elitism
   d. empathy
   e. stereotyping
   f. ethnocentrism

3. Answers will vary. Following are examples of patient needs.
   a. physiologic—The patient is "NPO" for tests.
   b. safety and security—The patient is concerned about his job and how long he will be unable to work.

c. love and belonging —The patient's family has not visited or called for 2 days.

d. esteem—The patient is a quiet, shy gentleman, and a nurse calls him "sweetie" and "honey."

4. a. sender
   b. message
   c. receiver
   d. feedback

5. a. A poor choice of words or an inconsistency between verbal and nonverbal messages may result in unsuccessful communication.
   b. Inconsistency in the verbal and nonverbal symbols received from the sender

6. Answers will vary.

7. a. poor choice of words
   b. contradiction of verbal and nonverbal language used

8. a. poor listening skills
   b. poor feedback skills

9. Any three of the following:
   - clothing
   - hair
   - jewelry
   - body art
   - cosmetics
   - automobile
   - house
   - perfume or cologne

10. Any three of the following:
    - posture
    - ambulation
    - touching
    - personal distance
    - eye contact
    - breathing
    - hand gestures
    - facial expressions

11. a. 55%
    b. 38%
    c. 7%

12. a. unsuccessful decoding: The nurse was not aware of the patient's cultural background (see Table 5-1).
    b. unsuccessful encoding: Joe was disrespectful in using the term *honey* and also used medical terms that Mrs. Fredrick did not understand. Mrs. Fredrick, by crying, was expressing both her esteem and safety and security needs.
    c. unsuccessful decoding: Sue was distracted and failed to listen for the page.
    d. unsuccessful decoding: Cindi was stereotyping Mr. Potter on the basis of his status and personal hygiene.

13. a. *ignoring:* making no effort to listen
    b. *pretend listening:* giving the appearance that you are listening
    c. *selective listening:* hearing only the parts that interest you
    d. *attentive listening* (also called active listening): paying attention and focusing on what the speaker says and comparing it with your own experience
    e. *empathic listening:* listening and responding with both the heart and the mind to truly understand, realizing that all persons have the right to feel as they do

14. a. Stop talking.
    b. Teach yourself to concentrate.
    c. Take time to listen.
    d. Listen with your eyes.
    e. Listen to what is being said—not only to how it is being said.
    f. Suspend judgment.
    g. Do not interrupt the speaker.
    h. Remove distractions.
    i. Listen for both feeling and content (seek to understand).

15. a. Use paraphrasing (repeat the message to the sender in your own words).
    b. Repeat the last word or words of the message (to allow the speaker to more fully develop the thought).
    c. Use specific rather than general feedback.
    d. Use constructive feedback rather than destructive feedback.
    e. Do not deny senders' feelings.

16. Care that involves understanding and being sensitive to a patient's cultural background; also called *cultural competence*. It is essential for health care workers to understand and evaluate their own values, beliefs, and customs before working with and caring for people of varying cultures in health care. Many conflicts occur in the health care delivery system because of cultural misunderstandings (e.g., verbal and nonverbal language, lack of courtesy, objectivity).

17. a. Understand and evaluate your own values, beliefs, and customs before working with and caring for people of varying cultures.
    b. Take the time to learn about the cultural backgrounds of patients, which may involve incorporating their beliefs and practices into their care.
    c. Do not judge other people by the standards of your own values and beliefs.
    d. Avoid stereotyping or making assumptions about a patient or a co-worker that are based on race or ethnicity.
    e. Treat all people with respect as unique individuals regardless of their gender, age, economic status, religion, sexual status, education, occupation, physical makeup or limitations, or command of the English language.

18. a. nonassertive
    b. aggressive
    c. assertive

19. a. a skill that allows you to say no over and over again without raising your voice or getting irritated or angry
    b. a skill that allows you to accept manipulative criticism and anxiety-producing statements by offering no resistance and by using a noncommittal reply
    c. a skill that allows you to accept your errors and faults without becoming defensive or resorting to anger
    d. a skill that allows you to actively prompt criticism so you can use the information or, if manipulative, exhaust it

20. a. Always identify yourself by nursing unit, name, and status.
    b. Avoid putting the person on hold.
    c. Listen to what the caller is saying.
    d. Write down what the caller is saying.
    e. Acknowledge the anger.
    f. Do not allow the caller to become abusive.

21. a. Provide the student and the student's instructor or the new employee a copy of dates and times that the student or new employee is to be on the nursing unit to complete the clinical experience.
    b. Obtain a list of objectives (provided by the hospital or the school).
    c. Take the student or new employee on a tour of the nursing unit and hospital so that he or she is aware of where restrooms, cafeteria, and hospital departments are located.
    d. Set a positive example.
    e. If the student or new employee does not call before being late or absent, notify the instructor or nurse manager.
    f. Notify the student, nursing unit, new employee, and nurse manager if you are going to be tardy, absent, or transferred to another unit (preferably an hour before start of shift).
    g. Stay with the student or new employee to monitor his or progress and check off objectives as completed, with competence defined as instructed in the clinical or orientation packet.
    h. Provide feedback to the student or new employee, and provide suggestions for improvement.
    i. Notify the student's instructor or new employee's nurse manager if the student or new employee is not attired according to hospital or school dress code, is not performing in an appropriate, professional manner, or is having difficulty completing objectives.
    j. Notify the student's instructor or new employee's nurse manager if there are any questions or concerns.
    k. Notify the student's instructor or new employee's nurse manager immediately if there are serious concerns.
    l. Complete an evaluation form regarding the student clinical experience.
22. a. Be sure you know when and where you are to complete your clinical experience, and know the name of your preceptor.
    b. If you are a student, provide your preceptor with a list of objectives and the instructor's telephone and or pager numbers.
    c. The student or new employee should notify the nursing unit, the preceptor, and the instructor or nurse manager an hour before the start of shift (except in the case of an emergency) if he or she is going to be tardy or absent.
    d. The student must notify the instructor if he or she will leave the hospital before the end of the shift.
    e. It is the student's responsibility to notify the instructor if the preceptor is going to be late, absent, or transferred to another unit.
    f. The student or new employee should arrive dressed appropriately and prepared to learn and work each day and should be accountable for his or her learning.
    g. The student must be flexible and refrain from saying, "That's not the way we were taught in class," or "That's not the way we did it at Previous Community Hospital."
    h. The student or new employee should communicate openly with the preceptor, instructor, or nurse manager regarding any problems with his or her clinical performance.
    i. The student or new employee should have the list of objectives or evaluation forms completed and signed off by the preceptor 2 days before the last day of clinical.
    j. The student or new employee should complete an evaluation form regarding his or her clinical experience or orientation.
23. a. obtaining information
    b. providing information
    c. developing trust
    d. showing understanding
    e. relieving stress
24. With the implementation of the electronic medical record, the HUC role is expanding. The HUC is often the "go-to" person in assisting doctors, nurses, and ancillary personnel in entering and retrieving information regarding the patient's electronic medical record. The HUC has a larger role in listening to visitors, patients, and nursing unit personnel complaints and problem solving.

CHAPTER 6

Exercise 1

1. APS
2. ARRA
3. CPS
4. NINP
5. SNAT
6. HIPAA
7. HITECH
8. PHI
9. CE
10. CPR
11. EPHI
12. IIHI

Exercise 2

1. Adult Protective Services
2. American Recovery and Reinvestment Act
3. Child Protective Services
4. no information, no publication
5. suspected nonaccidental trauma
6. Health Insurance Portability and Accountability Act
7. Health Information Technology for Economic and Clinical Health Act
8. protected health information
9. covered entities
10. cardiopulmonary resuscitation
11. electronic protected health information
12. individually identifiable health information

Exercise 3

Personal answers required; answers will vary.

Review Questions

1. a. attitude
   b. autonomy
   c. workplace behavior
   d. accountability
   e. ethics
   f. fidelity
   g. code of ethics
   h. confidence

i. confidentiality

j. respect

k. philosophy

2 a. expert witness

b. liability

c. damages

d. defendant

e. statute of limitations

f. deposition

g. negligence

h. plaintiff

i. statute

3. a. philosophy and standards of the organization

b. leadership style of supervisors

c. meaningfulness or importance of the work

d. how challenging the work is

e. relationship with co-workers

f. one's personal characteristics such as abilities, interests, aptitudes, values, and expectations

g. external factors such as the person's family life, health, and recreational habits

4. a. Personal values describe the beliefs of an individual or culture, evolve from circumstances with the external world, and can change over time.

b. Answers will vary. *Example:* A patient is admitted with complications of alcoholism. The health unit coordinator's religion prohibits drinking.

5. Any six of the following:

- dependability
- accountability
- consideration
- cheerfulness
- empathy
- trustworthiness
- respectfulness
- courtesy
- tactfulness
- conscientiousness
- honesty
- cooperation
- attitude

6. *Privacy Rule:* Establishes regulations for the use and disclosure of protected health information (PHI) and gives patients' rights over their health information, including rights to examine and obtain a copy of their health records, and to request corrections

Security Rule: To protect the confidentiality, integrity, and availability of individually identifiable health information (IIHI) that is created, received, transmitted, used, or maintained by a covered entity

7. a. provides over $30 billion for health care infrastructure and the adoption and meaningful use of health information technology

b. widens the scope of privacy and security protections available under HIPAA; applies the same HIPAA privacy and security requirements (and penalties) for covered entities to business associates; increases the potential legal liability for noncompliance; and provides for more enforcement

8. Any six of the following:

- names
- all geographic subdivisions smaller than a state, including street address, city, county, precinct and ZIP code

- all elements of dates (except year) for dates directly related to an individual, including birth date, admission date, discharge date, date of death; and all ages over 89 and all elements of dates (including year)
- phone numbers
- fax numbers
- electronic mail addresses
- Social Security numbers
- medical record numbers
- health plan beneficiary numbers
- account numbers
- certificate and license numbers
- vehicle identifiers and serial numbers, including license plate numbers
- device identifiers and serial numbers;
- Web Universal Resource Locators (URLs)
- Internet Protocol (IP) address numbers
- biometric identifiers, including fingerprints and voiceprints
- full-face photographic images and any comparable images
- any other unique identifying number, characteristic, or code (this does not mean the unique code assigned by the investigator to code the data

9. a. Right to receive Notice of Privacy Practices and notice of the uses and disclosures of protected health information that may be made by the covered entity.

b. Right to request restrictions on use and disclosure of protected health information (PHI). The health care provider is not required to agree to a restriction.

c. Right to receive confidential communication. The health care provider must accommodate reasonable requests from individuals to receive communications of PHI by alternative means or at alternative locations and cannot require a reason for the request.

d. Right to not be listed in hospital directory when admitted to hospital.

e. Right to access, inspect, and copy PHI. The health care provider can deny request under certain conditions, and the requesting individual may appeal a denial of his or her right to access PHI.

f. Right to amend PHI. The health care provider can deny request and must provide a timely denial in plain language and include the basis for the denial.

g. Right to receive an accounting of disclosures of PHI—required by law.

10. a. to avoid verbally repeating confidential information

b. to manage the patient's electronic record in a manner that ensures confidentiality of its contents or to control the patient's paper chart

11. Answers will vary. Examples:

a. Response: "I cannot discuss this information, especially not in the cafeteria."

b. Walk over to the two members, say "Excuse me," and change the subject; after the wife is out of hearing distance, explain that their discussion could be overheard.

c. Direct the visitor away from the conversation, and ask if you can help him or her.

d. Ask the reporter to hold so that he or she may be transferred to the nurse in charge.

e. Deny any knowledge of the patient; if he becomes insistent or rude, ask him to hold while being transferred to the nurse in charge.

f. Explain that patient information cannot be discussed, and change the subject

g. Ask the woman if there is something she needs—this would also alert the nurse.

12. Professional appearance will earn the trust, respect, and confidence of one's employer, co-workers, patients, and others. A professional appearance also demonstrates self-confidence and sends a message that one has self-respect and respects his or her position.

13. *Preclinical or employment screenings and requirements:*
a. drug testing
b. fingerprinting and background check
c. immunizations
d. signed HIPAA confidentiality statement
The Joint Commission requirements:
a. Certification in CPR (cardiopulmonary resuscitation) training
b. Fire and safety in-service
c. Infectious disease in-service
d. HIPAA in-service

14. a. If a smell of alcohol (a drug) is detected on a student's or employee's breath, or if inappropriate behavior is observed.
b. If the student or employee refuses the drug test or tests positive for drug use, she or he will be sent home and most likely will be terminated from the HUC program or employment.

15. a.
- Respect people in close proximity (speak more softly, turn cell phone off when appropriate to do so, and pay attention to your surroundings).
- When in a public place, keep conversations brief. Remember that you are a professional.
- When out to dinner, spend time with who you are with, not with a phone.
- Follow rules for cell phone use in hospitals, schools, and airplanes and while pumping gas.
- Do not drive while using a cell phone.

b.
- When the elevator button light is lit, it is not necessary to continue to push the button; this may be causing the door to close on someone on another floor who is trying to enter or exit the elevator.
- When the elevator does arrive, stand aside and allow people to exit before you try to enter.
- When you are riding on an elevator and are going to a higher floor in the building, stand to the side or in the back, so others may exit on their floors.
- Patients who are being transported on stretchers and personnel who are pushing hospital equipment have priority for using elevators.

16. a. Guidelines regarding attendance, punctuality, and breaks are usually provided by the employer in an employment packet during orientation.
b. It is essential that nursing unit personnel work as a team and that each member of the team be reliable and act in a responsible, professional manner. When a student is completing his or her clinical experience on a nursing unit, this should be viewed as an extended

evaluation or appraisal period. A student's preceptor and the other nursing unit personnel will be continually appraising the student's knowledge, attendance, punctuality, and professionalism.

17. a. verbally expressed anger and frustration
b. body language, such as threatening gestures
c. signs of drug or alcohol use
d. presence of a weapon
e. the presence of someone who has a restraining order that prohibits him or her from being there

18. The HUC should not approach the threatening person but should present a calm attitude and should call security immediately.

19. a. Advise the person to stop; tell him or her that you do not like or welcome this behavior.
b. Document the comments and behavior of the person.
c. File a complaint with the supervisor or with management.

20. a. to provide feedback
b. to make compensation decisions (concerning salary increases)

21. Keeping a written record of accomplishments, classes taken, and in-services attended during the evaluation period would be mutually beneficial to the individual (HUC) being evaluated as well as the evaluator (nurse manager). Often employee evaluations are based only on the most recent work history, so keeping a record or diary will produce a more accurate work history.

22. a. The purpose of a résumé is to get an interview; it is hoped that the interview will result in your getting a job. The résumé is a marketing tool intended to create interest in one's abilities and potential.
b. Type using a simple font such as Times New Roman, 12 point (avoid using fancy type such as outline, shadow, script, or other styles that are difficult to read). Use standard 8½ × 11–inch paper in white, ivory, or gray (avoid flashy colors).
Keep a 1-inch margin on all four sides.
Limit résumé to one page, if possible.
Use single space within sections.
Use double space between sections.
Bold, underline, or capitalize section headings to make them stand out.
Use everyday language; be specific. Give examples.
Do a spelling and grammar check.
Produce high-quality photocopies.
c.
- Name, address, telephone number, e-mail address, website address
- Objective. Be specific about the job wanted. Example: "To obtain a HUC position within a health care facility to apply my organizational skills and medical knowledge."
- Education. New graduates without a lot of work experience should list their educational information first. List most recent education first; add grade point average (GPA) if higher than 3.0.
- List NAHUC (National Association of Health Unit Coordinators) certification, if applicable.
- Work experience. Briefly describe work experience, including specific duties performed). List most recent work experience first. Be accurate with dates of employment.

- Other information. May include special skills or competencies, such as being bilingual or leadership experience in volunteer organizations. Your instructor can advise you on other information to add to your résumé.
- "References furnished on request." Ask people if they are willing to serve as references before giving their names to a potential employer. Do not include reference information on your résumé.

23. *In-person interview:*
- Arrive on time (at least one-half hour early).
- Stand until you are asked to sit down.
- Make eye contact with interviewer.
- Give a firm handshake.
- Use body language to show interest—smile, nod, and give nonverbal feedback to the interviewer.

Telephone interview:
- Be ready to answer phone or to call in—employers usually call candidates, but employers may ask a candidate to call them to test how serious they are.
- Stand during the telephone interview; this allows one's voice to project and sound more confident.
- Choose a location and time so that there will be no distractions.
- Relax and speak clearly and slowly—do not sound rushed or anxious (the HUC position requires excellent telephone skills).

Both in-person and telephone interviews:
- Think in advance of work situations and how you would handle them.
- Role-play—rehearse responses to difficult or uncomfortable issues that may come up.
- Project a positive attitude and confidence.
- Listen attentively to questions.
- Keep answers brief and to the point.
- Never criticize a former employer.
- Be prepared to give a positive summary of your education, work history, and interests.
- Be aware of the job description for the position for which you are applying.
- Ask questions. Avoid yes or no answers. Avoid long silences.
- Ask about the next step in the process.
- Thank the interviewer.
- Write a thank-you letter to anyone you have spoken to.
- Follow up with a telephone call if you do not hear back from the interviewer in 3 days.

24. a. respect
    b. autonomy
    c. veracity
    d. beneficence
    e. non-maleficence
    f. role fidelity
    g. confidentiality
25. a. the Constitution
    b. statutes
    c. common law
26. a. Professional negligence of a health care professional; failure to meet a professional standard of care, resulting in harm to another—for example, failure to provide "good and accepted medical care."
    b. The standard of practice is established by expert witness testimony—Evidence of the standard of care may also be found in textbooks, standards from NAHUC, policy and procedure manuals, or standards of The Joint Commission.
27. a. Know your job description.
    b. Keep current with the employer's current policies and procedures.
    c. Keep current in your practice.
    d. Do not assume anything.
    e. Do not perform nursing tasks, even as favors.
    f. Be aware of relationships with patients.
28. Answers will vary.

CHAPTER 7

Exercise 1
1. ADT log book
2. ADT sheet
3. CQI

Exercise 2
1. admission, discharge, transfer log book
2. admission, discharge, transfer log sheet
3. continuous quality improvement

Exercise 3
Answers will vary.

Review Questions
1. a. scientific field that is concerned with human factors in the design and operation of machines and the physical environment
   b. saying or doing the first thing that comes to mind and allowing negative emotions to take over in response to another person or event (a negative choice)
   c. a positive approach to a person or event that puts distance between you and the event (a positive choice)
2. a. a list of patients including room and bed numbers and other relevant information that may be printed from a computer menu
   b. a notepad kept by the telephone and used to write down messages that need to be relayed and tasks that need to be completed
   c. a computerized or written record of the quantity of each item that the nursing unit currently needs to last until the next supply order date (separate lists are found inside cabinet doors, in supply drawers, and on the code or crash cart)
   d. a sheet of paper used by all nursing unit personnel to jot down items that need reordering
   e. form used on a nursing unit that includes a list of patients' names and room and bed numbers, with blank spaces next to each name; may be used by the HUC to record patient activities (may also be called a patient information sheet or a patient activity sheet)
   f. form used to record daily admissions, discharges, and transfers for quick reference and to assist in tracking empty beds
3. a. management of nursing unit supplies and equipment
   b. management of activities at the nurses' station
   c. management related to the performance of tasks
   d. management of time
   e. management of stress

4. a. purchasing
   central service
   nutritional care
   pharmacy
   laundry or linen
   b. the HUC and/or a unit aide determining the supplies needed and ordering them from the supplying department; the supplying department maintains a list, takes daily inventory, and restocks supplies
5. a. purchasing
   b. nutritional care
   c. pharmacy
   d. laundry or linen
   e. central service
6. a. IT department
   b. IT department
   c. maintenance or temperature control
   d. IT department
   e. maintenance or plumbing
   f. IT department
   g. maintenance
7. The code or crash cart is usually stored on each nursing unit or in an area between nursing units. Other emergency equipment includes fire extinguishers and fire doors.
8. an intravenous infusion pump
9. a. Patient safety hinges on a complete and correct exchange of information.
   b. Any of the following:
      • scheduled diagnostic procedures
      • surgeries
      • planned discharges
      • transfers
      • do not resuscitate (DNR), or no code information
      • NINP (no information, no publication)
      • no visitors allowed
      • no phone calls to the patient's room
      • patient is in respiratory isolation
      • patient is out on a temporary pass
      • the nurse who is assigned to the patient
      • the resident or attending physician who is assigned to the patient
10. a. The time and destination are recorded next to the patient's name on the census worksheet when the patient leaves the nursing unit for surgery, a diagnostic study, to visit the cafeteria with a relative, or for any other reason. When the patient returns to the nursing unit, a line is drawn through this recording.
    b. Keeping track of and locating misplaced charts are essential for ensuring efficient use of time by doctors, nurses, and other professionals.
11. a. After an order is written to obtain a patient's medical records from another health care facility or doctor's office, the HUC prepares a medical record release form for the patient to sign. After the form has been signed, the HUC notifies the facility or doctor's office of the request, obtains the appropriate fax number, and provides the return fax number as needed; the release form is then sent, and the requested records or reports are faxed to the nursing unit. When EMRs are in use, the signed release and faxed documents are scanned into the patient's EMR, and hard copies of the release and faxed documents are placed in a receptacle to be sent to health information management. If paper charts are in use, the HUC places the signed release form and the faxed documents into the patient's chart.
    b.
      • Label the document with the appropriate patient's ID label.
      • Scan the records using the nursing unit scanner as required or requested in a timely manner.
      • The records will then be certified by an HIMS specialist and will be entered into the patient's EMR.
      • Stamp the original documents as "scanned," and write the date, the time, and your initials.
      • Place the original documents in a box or bin to be delivered to HIMS.
    c.
      • When possible, file at the same time each day.
      • Separate the records according to the patients' names.
      • Always check the patient's name within the chart with the name on the record before filing it.
      • Be especially alert when two patients on the unit have the same name.
      • Place the record behind the correct chart divider.
      • Initial each record before filing.
      • Never discard any patient's records.
12. a. The HUC records all admissions, discharges, and transfers on the ADT sheet each day for quick reference regarding nursing unit activity for that day, and to determine the number of empty beds on the unit.
    b. When a patient is admitted to the nursing unit, the HUC places the patient's label in the admission, discharge, and transfer (ADT) log book and writes the date and time of admission next to the label. If a patient is transferred to another unit within the hospital, the date and time of transfer and the destination are written next to the patient's label in the ADT book. If the patient is discharged to another facility or to home, the date, time, and name of the facility to which the patient is going (if not to home) are written next to the patient label.
    c. Patient labels (at least five sheets) are stored in each patient's chart when paper charts are used, and newly discharged patient labels are often kept in a "patient label book" in case additional charges or credits have to be made to the discharged patient's account. When EMR has been implemented, inpatient (at least five sheets) and newly discharged patient labels are stored in a patient label book.
13. nurse's progress records
    CSD cards (not used when CSD items are scanned into patient's EMR)
    recopying MARs if required
14. a. Listen carefully and attentively to what the person is saying.
    b. Ask pertinent, objective questions, and gather as many facts as possible.
    c. Respond to the complaint appropriately.
    d. Refrain from eating or chewing gum when communicating with visitors.
    e. Try to avoid answering the phone, but if it must be answered, ask the person on the phone to hold; then return to handling the complaint.

f. Document the complaint and your responses after the conversation has ended, and relay the information to the patient's nurse as soon as possible.

g. Demonstrate empathy.

15. a. When EMR is used, the HUC can view diagnostic test results by choosing a patient and then choosing "summary," which will display the patient's diagnostic test results.

b. When EMR is not used, most diagnostic test results may be retrieved from the computer by selecting "Laboratory results" or "Diagnostic imaging results" and then selecting the patient's name. The results will be displayed on the computer screen and may be printed. In some hospitals, recorded diagnostic test results may be obtained by telephone by calling a specified number.

16. a. A patient in a medical crisis—calling a code is the highest priority.

b. The ringing telephone would be the second highest priority.

c. The doctor would understand that the code and telephone would be the higher priorities.

Tending to the tube that arrived in the pneumatic tube system could be done as soon as you have called the code, answered the telephone, and informed the doctor that the medical records would be obtained as soon as possible. Then the order for the surgery permit (preparing the consent for the patient's nurse to have signed) and the two discharge orders would be processed (whatever that would involve [e.g., printing out information for a new Rx, notifying admitting and/or family]).

17. a. Ask for assistance when needed.

b. Monitor electronic medical records or paper charts for new orders frequently.

c. Complete one task before beginning another.

d. Follow the 10 steps of transcription (outlined in Chapter 9).

e. Plan for rush periods.

f. Plan a daily schedule for routine.

g. Group activities.

h. Know the job and perform it well.

i. Take breaks as assigned.

j. Delegate tasks to volunteers.

k. Avoid unnecessary conversation.

l. Use a memory sheet.

18. a. Perennial stress. Example: Answers will vary—traffic, difficult relationships, and so on.

b. Crisis stress. Example: Answers will vary—death, divorce, serious illness, and so on.

19. a. Effective time management is the first step in managing stress.

b. Follow the time management techniques.

c. Realize that nurses, doctors, and other health care workers may be working under a lot of stress, so do not take their expressions of frustration personally.

d. Say "no" tactfully when asked to do additional work if there truly is not time.

e. Keep a sense of humor. Humor is a great stress reliever as long as it is timely and appropriate.

20. a. Acute. Example: Answers will vary—fractures, low back strain injuries.

b. Cumulative. Example: Answers will vary—carpal tunnel syndrome, tendonitis, or low back pain.

21. Any four of the following:

- The computer monitor should be located where it will reduce awkward head and neck postures; position the monitor so that you must look slightly downward to look at the middle of the screen. The preferred viewing distance is 18 to 24 inches (see Fig. 7-7).
- Chairs should be adjusted so that one can sit straight yet in a relaxed position, with a backrest supporting the small of the back and feet flat on the floor.
- Adjust chair back to a slightly backward position and extend legs out slightly, so there are no sharp angles that result in pressure on hip or knee joints.
- Wrists should be straight while typing, with forearms level and elbows close to the body—reduce bending of the wrists by moving the entire arm.
- Use a computer wrist pad.
- Eliminate situations that would require constant bending over to complete tasks.
- Shift weight in the chair frequently.
- Use proper body mechanics when lifting—do not bend over with legs straight or twist while lifting, and avoid trying to lift above shoulder level.
- Take frequent mini-stretches of the neck (lower head in each direction for a 5-second count).
- Stand, walk, and stretch back and legs at least every hour.

22. a. Any of the following:

- The label printer should be in close proximity to the work space.
- Frequently used forms should be stored within reaching distance.
- Charts (if paper charts are being used) should be located in an area where they can be easily reached.
- The telephone should be within easy reach.
- The fax machine should be in close proximity to the work space.
- The unit scanner should be in close proximity to the work space.
- The unit shredder or receptacle for paper to be shredded should be in close proximity.
- Any unit reference books and manuals should be kept within reaching distance.

b. Any six of the following:

- *Physicians' Desk Reference* (PDR)
- hospital formulary
- institutional policy and procedures manual
- disaster manual
- laboratory manual
- diagnostic imaging manual
- If not computerized, indexes of frequently used hospital extension numbers, in-hospitaloffice numbers, and pager numbers are kept on the nursing unit and are kept up-to-date by the HUC.
- A communication book may be used to preserve organizational information between shifts.

23. Not monitoring the patient's EMR or paper chart for orders or tasks could delay diagnostic tests and the

patient's diagnosis, thereby delaying treatment. Delaying treatment could place the patient in danger.

24. Improvement in products and services—Continuous quality improvement (CQI) results in products and services of better quality. Competition to provide the best product and service in the most efficient manner has increased worldwide.

25. a. Identify and analyze the problem.
   b. Identify alternative plans for resolving the problem.
   c. Choose the best plan.
   d. Put the best plan into practice.
   e. Evaluate the plan after it has been in place for a given time.

26. a. Listen to Mrs. Mendez with understanding and empathy; tell her that you will ask her husband's nurse to come talk to her. After the conversation, document what Mrs. Mendez said and your responses. Locate Mr. Mendez's nurse and relate all of the information that you have documented.
   b. Advise the visitor of the doctor's order, and if she persists in wanting to visit Mr. Blair, ask the patient's nurse to speak to her.
   c. Go into the room and ask that only two visitors be in the room at one time, or suggest (if possible) that they all go out to the waiting room or to the cafeteria.
   d. Ask the other HUCs who regularly work on the nursing unit and the nurse manager if it could be moved to a more convenient place. The nurse manager may suggest bringing it up at the health unit coordinator meeting for discussion.
   e. Suggest that you would be glad to help in any other way, but you are not trained or legally covered by your job description to assist patients in going to the restroom.

CHAPTER 8

Exercise 1

1. Hx
2. NKA
3. ID labels
4. H&P
5. MAR
6. NKMA
7. NKDA
8. NKFA

Exercise 2

1. identification labels
2. no known food allergies
3. medication administration record
4. no known allergies
5. no known drug allergies
6. history and physical
7. history
8. no known medication allergies

Review Questions

1. a. placing extra chart forms in patients' paper charts so they will be available when needed
   b. patient's current paper chart after portions have been removed when the chart became so full that it was unmanageable
   c. labels that contain individual patient information for identifying patient records or other personal items
   d. a method of alerting staff when two or more patients with the same or similarly spelled last names are located on a nursing unit
   e. labels affixed to the front cover of a patient's paper chart that indicate a patient's allergies
   f. a patient's paper record from previous admissions stored in the health information management department that may be retrieved for review when a patient is admitted to the emergency room, nursing unit, or outpatient department; older microfilmed records also may be requested by the patient's doctor
   g. a locked workstation that is located on the wall outside a patient's room; it stores the patient's paper chart or a laptop computer, and when unlocked, it forms a shelf to write on
   h. a preassembled packet of standard chart forms to be used on admission of a patient to the nursing unit

2. a. means of communication
   b. documentation and planning of patient care
   c. research
   d. education
   e. legal record or document
   f. history of patient illnesses, care, treatment, and outcomes

3. a. All entries into the EMR must be accurate.
   b. Handwritten progress notes, electrocardiograms, consents, anesthesia records, and outside records and reports must be scanned into the EMR.
   c. Errors made in care or treatment must be documented and cannot be falsified.
   d. All entries into the EMR must include the date and time (military or traditional) of the entry.
   e. Abbreviations may be used in keeping with the health care facility's list of "approved abbreviations."

4. a. All paper chart form entries must be made in ink.
   b. Written entries on paper chart forms must be legible and accurate.
   c. Recorded entries on the paper chart may not be obliterated or erased.
   d. All written entries on paper chart forms must include the date and time (military or traditional) of the entry.
   e. Abbreviations may be used in keeping with the health care facility's list of "approved abbreviations."

5. a. face sheet or information form—contains information about the patient, such as name, address, telephone number, name of employer, admission diagnosis, health care insurance policy information, and next of kin
   b. admission or service agreement form—provides legal permission to the hospital or doctor to treat the patient and also serves as a financial agreement
   c. patient rights—copies must be given to each patient or legal guardian of the patient on admission; vary in wording among hospitals, but all are based on following the basic ethical principles
   d. advance directive checklist—documents that a patient was informed of his or her choice to declare health care decisions

6. a. the form on which the doctor requests care and treatment procedures for the patient

b. usually precedes or leads into the nurse's notes—contains a short nursing history regarding the patient's daily living activities, present illness, and medications the patient is taking plus patient's vital signs, height, weight, and any allergies to food or medications

c. a form on which the physician records the patient's progress during the patient's hospitalization

d. used to outline the patient's care and treatment and to record the treatment, progress, and activities of the patient

e. form listing all medications administered to the patient along with the date, drug, dosage, route, and time and frequency of administration of the medication

f. used by the physician to summarize the treatment and diagnosis the patient received while hospitalized; includes discharge information

g. used to prepare the patient for discharge from the health care facility—the nurse usually records information about the patient's health status at the time of discharge and provides instructions

7. The H&P contains the medical history and the present symptomatic history of the patient. A review of all body systems or physical assessment of the patient is also recorded.

8. a. Forms that are additional to the standard chart forms according to specific care and treatment provided
   b. Any of the following forms:
   - clinical pathway record form
   - anticoagulant therapy record
   - diabetic record
   - consultation form
   - operating room records
   - therapy records
   - parenteral fluid or infusion record

9. Accuracy and timeliness in the recording of vital signs information is a must, because the doctor may use this information to prescribe treatment for the patient.

10. a. *A minor error on the graphic portion of the record*—Write "mistaken entry" or "error" in ink on the incorrect connecting line, and record your first initial, your last name, and your status above the error; then graph the correct value.
   b. *A numbered entry*, such as the respiration value—Draw a line through the entry in ink, and write in ink "mistaken entry" or "error," your first initial, your last name, and your status near it. As closely as possible, insert the correct numbers.
   c. *A series of errors* on the graphic record—The entire record must be recopied to show the correct data. Prepare a new graphic record, and label with the patient's ID label. Transfer in ink all the information onto the new graphic record, including the correction of errors. Draw a diagonal line through the old graphic record in ink, and record in ink on the line "mistaken entry" or "error." Place the old record behind the recopied record because it must remain as a permanent part of the chart, and in ink write "recopied," followed by your name, your status, and the date on the new graphic record, then place it behind the correct divider in the patient's chart.

11. a. A number of conditions require the patient or a responsible party to sign a special form granting permission for surgery or other invasive procedures to be performed on the patient.
   b.
   - Affix the patient's ID label to the consent form.
   - Write in black ink the first and last names of the doctor who is to perform the surgery or invasive medical procedure.
   - Write in black ink the surgery or invasive medical procedure to be performed, exactly as the physician wrote it on the physician's order sheet except that abbreviations must be spelled out.
   - Spell correctly, and write all information legibly.
   - Do not record the date and time. The person who obtains the patient's signature will enter the date and time.

12. Forms that constitute the patient's paper chart are usually kept together in a three-ring binder, and binders are stored in a chart rack in which each slot on the rack holds one patient chart. Charts are identified with patient identification labels.

13. a. 1500
    b. 0715
    c. 1230
    d. 0115

14. a. 10:20 am
    b. 7:40 pm
    c. 11:19 am
    d. 9:30 pm

15. a. release of side rails
    b. consent to receive blood transfusion
    c. refusal to permit blood transfusion
    d. consent form for human immunodeficiency virus (HIV) testing

16. a. Monitor the patient's EMR consistently, and complete HUC tasks as required and in a timely manner.
    b. Assist nurses, doctors, and ancillary personnel as necessary in entering information and orders into the computer.
    c. Report any necessary repairs regarding nursing unit computers and/or printers to the hospital information systems department.
    d. Scan documents as required such as handwritten progress notes, electrocardiograms, outside medical records, consent forms, operating room records, and reports in a timely manner.
    e. Place and maintain patient ID labels in a patient label book.
    f. Place patient face sheets into the face sheet binder, which may be the same as the label book, to provide to physicians as requested.
    g. Always log out of the EMR when not in use to protect patient confidentiality.

17. a. Place all charts in proper sequence (usually according to room number) in the chart rack when they are not in use.
    b. Place new chart forms in each patient's chart before the immediate need arises; label each chart form with the patient's ID label before placing it in the chart.
    c. Place diagnostic reports in the correct patient's chart behind the correct divider.

d. Review the patient's charts frequently for new orders.

e. Properly label the patient's chart so it can easily be located at all times.

f. Check each chart to be sure that all forms are labeled with the correct patient's name.

g. Check the chart frequently for patient information forms or face sheets.

h. Assist physicians or other professionals in locating the patient's chart.

18. a. The paper chart of a patient who remains in the health care facility for a long time becomes very full and eventually becomes unmanageable. When this occurs, the HUC may "thin" or "split" the chart. A doctor's order is not required to thin a patient's chart. In thinning the chart, some categories of chart forms may be removed and placed in an envelope for safekeeping on the unit.

- Remove older nurse's notes, medication forms, and other forms that are no longer needed in the chart binder. (Check the hospital policy and procedures manual to verify forms that may and may not be removed.)
- Place the removed forms in an envelope.
- Place the patient's ID label on the outside of the envelope.
- Write "thinned chart" and record the date with your first initial and last name (of the person thinning the chart) on the outside of the envelope.
- Place a label stating that the chart was thinned, along with the date, first initial, and last name (of the person thinning the chart) on the front of the patient's chart.
- If the patient is transferred to another unit, transfer the thinned-out forms with the patient's chart.
- When the patient is discharged, send all thinned-out forms with the patient's paper chart to the health information management department.

b. Placing new chart forms in each patient's chart before the immediate need arises. Label each chart form with the patient's ID label before placing it in the chart. New chart forms are placed on top of old chart forms for easy access. The new forms may be folded in half to show that the old form has not been completely used.

c. Availability of patient medical records is necessary to ensure continuity of care when a patient is discharged to another facility. When EMR is used, the patient's EMR is available on computer to other health care facilities, or the records may be printed from the computer. The patient will be required to sign a release form for the records to be available or copied. When paper charts are used, the records will need to be reproduced on a copy machine, the patient's doctor must write an order specifying the specific chart forms to be copied, and the patient will be required to sign a release form. Depending on hospital policy, the HUC may have the responsibility of copying the paper chart forms, or the patient's chart may be sent to the health information management services department to be copied. After the forms have been reproduced on the copier, the original forms are replaced in the patient's chart, and the copied records are sent to the receiving facility.

19. a. Draw (in black ink) one single line through the error; record the words "mistaken entry" or "error" along with the date, the time, and the first initial, last name, and status of the person correcting the error in a blank area near (directly above or next to) the error.

b. Patient chart forms that are affixed with the wrong or incorrect ID label may be shredded if no notations have been made on them. Draw an X with a black ink pen through the incorrect label and write "mistaken entry" with the date, the time, and the first initial, last name, and status of the person correcting labeling error above the incorrect label. Affix the correct patient ID label on the form next to the incorrect label (do not place the correct label over the incorrect label). It is also permissible to handprint the patient information in black ink next to the incorrect label that has an X drawn through it.

CHAPTER 9

Review Questions

1. a. the process of requisitioning diagnostic procedures, treatments, or supplies from hospital departments other than nursing

b. the process of recording and updating doctors' orders on the Kardex form (many hospitals have eliminated the paper Kardex form in favor of entering all patient orders into the computer)

c. a paper form used to order diagnostic procedures, treatments, or supplies from hospital departments other than nursing when the computer is down (also called a *downtime requisition*)

d. a method used by the doctor to notify the nursing staff that a new set of orders has been written

e. a typed set of orders for a specific diagnosis or procedure that has been approved for use in the hospital

f. an entry of doctor's orders written on the doctors' order sheet, dated, notated for time, and signed by the doctor

2. a. electronically—EMR
   b. handwritten
   c. preprinted
   d. telephone

3. a. flagging by the doctor
   b. absence of symbols and by the absence of sign-off information

4. a. When CPOE is used, the HUC will not have the responsibility of transcribing written or preprinted doctors' orders but may still have to perform and document many of the tasks related to placement of telephone calls, patient discharges, transfers, and appointment scheduling.

b. Transcription of doctors' handwritten or preprinted orders is a process that is used to communicate doctors' orders to the nursing staff and other hospital departments. The transcription procedure includes Kardexing, ordering, using symbols, the signing-off process, and sometimes other steps. How the HUC goes about performing this procedure varies among health care facilities and from individual to individual.

5. a. ord
   b. M
   c. K
   d. example—Called to Joan 0900/ S.B. HUC
   e. example—PC sent, PC faxed, or PC scanned
   f. example—Pat notified 1900/ S.B. HUC
6. The correct answer is (a) after the step of transcription is completed
7. a. To indicate completion of the transcription procedure of a set of doctors' orders. To sign off, the HUC records the date, time, full name, and status (may use the abbreviation *SHUC* if a student HUC, or *CHUC* if certified) in black ink on the line directly below the doctor's signature.
   b. 1/5/2013 1000 Sharon Brown/SHUC
8. a. Read the complete set of doctors' orders.
   b. Send or fax the pharmacy copy of the doctors' order sheet to the pharmacy department.
   c. Complete stat orders.
   d. Place telephone calls as necessary to complete doctors' orders.
   e. Select the patient's name from the census on the computer screen, or collect all necessary forms.
   f. Order diagnostic tests, treatments, and supplies.
   g. Kardex all doctors' orders except medication orders.
   h. Write medication orders on MAR.
   i. Recheck your performance of each step for accuracy and thoroughness.
   j. Sign off the completed set of doctors' orders.
9. a. The purpose of Kardexing all the doctors' orders is to communicate new orders to the nursing staff and to update the patient's profile on the Kardex form.
   b. Activity, diet, vital sign frequency, treatment, diagnostic studies
10. Kardexing is usually done in pencil because new doctors' orders may involve changing or discontinuing an existing order.
11. Ordering by computer requires the HUC to select the patient's name from a computer screen and follow the steps to input the ordering information (according to the hospital computer program used).
12. Errors may cause serious harm or delay in treatment for the patient.
13. a.
    - errors of omission (missing written doctors' orders)
    - errors of interpretation (not understanding the written doctors' orders)
    - errors in the selection of the wrong patient on the computer screen or in labeling requisitions
    - errors in the selection of the patient's Kardex form
    - errors in reading the doctor's poor handwriting
    b. Refer to Table 9-1.
14. a. short order series
    b. prn
    c. stat
    d. standing
    e. standing
    f. short-series order
    g. one-time order
15. By the word *stat* (meaning "now") included in the order—*now* and *immediately* are usually considered to indicate stat orders that should receive urgent attention.

CHAPTER 10

Exercise 1

1. CBR
2. c̄
3. A&O
4. qid
5. °
6. BP
7. q
8. amb
9. ABR
10. ↑ or > should be arrow pointing up
11. BRP
12. RR
13. ad lib
14. q other day
15. bid
16. q day
17. tid
18. q hr
19. temp or T
20. as tol
21. rt or ®
22. lt or Ⓛ
23. D/C or DC
24. VS
25. I&O
26. OOB
27. min
28. wt
29. BR
30. R
31. ax
32. TPR
33. P
34. h, hr, hrs
35. prn
36. NVS or neuro ✓s
37. ↓ or <
38. HOB
39. BSC
40. q4h or q4°
41. CMS
42. SOB
43. CVP
44. Rout
45. CMT
46. x
47. assist
48. DBP
49. SBP
50. U/O
51. ac
52. hs
53. C/O

Exercise 2

1. left
2. right
3. discontinue or discharge
4. vital signs

5. blood pressure
6. three times a day
7. complete bed rest
8. with
9. temperature, pulse, and respiration
10. bed rest
11. minute
12. bathroom privileges
13. as desired
14. increase, above, or elevate
15. out of bed
16. alert and oriented
17. weight
18. ambulate
19. every other day
20. every day
21. two times a day
22. four times a day
23. every hour
24. absolute bed rest
25. temperature
26. as tolerated
27. intake and output
28. every
29. pulse
30. axillary or axilla
31. rectal
32. as necessary
33. respiratory rate
34. every 4 hours
35. hour, hours
36. neurologic vital signs or neurologic checks
37. decrease, below, or lower
38. routine
39. shortness of breath
40. head of bed
41. bedside commode
42. circulation, motion, and sensation
43. central venous pressure
44. routine
45. cardiac monitor technician
46. times
47. assistance
48. diastolic blood pressure
49. systolic blood pressure
50. urine output
51. before meals
52. hour of sleep
53. complains of

Review Questions

1. a. the patient may sit and hang (dangle) his feet over the edge of the bed
   b. elevated body temperature (fever)
   c. without fever
   d. vomit
   e. a scale used to measure temperature in which the freezing point of water is 0° and the boiling point is 100° (formerly called *Centigrade*)
   f. a scale used to measure temperature in which 32° is the freezing point of water and 212° is the boiling point

g. the discrepancy between the ventricular rate detected at the apex of the heart and the arterial rate at the radial pulse

2. a. complete bed rest
   b. bed rest with bathroom privileges when alert and oriented
   c. weight every other day
   d. vital signs every shift
   e. temperature, pulse, and respiration and blood pressure three times a day
   f. elevate head of bed 20 degrees
   g. check dressing for drainage every 2 hours
   h. temperature rectal or axillary only
   i. neurologic vital sign checks every 4 hours
   j. intake and output every shift
   k. out of bed as desired
   l. up as tolerated
   m. temperature every 4 hours
   n. ambulate today
   o. discontinue vital signs
   p. elevate head of bed 30 degrees
   q. may use bedside commode
   r. central venous pressure every hour
   s. check circulation, motion, and sensation in toes of left foot four times a day
   t. ACCU-CHEK four times a day, before meals and at bedtime
   u. call me if patient complains of shortness of breath
   v. call me if diastolic blood pressure over 90
   w. call me if urine output below 1000 milliliters

3. In 2001 TJC issued a Sentinel Event Alert on the subject of medical abbreviations, and 1 year later a National Patient Safety Goal (NPSG) requiring accredited organizations to develop and implement a list of abbreviations not to use. In 2004 TJC created the "do not use" list of abbreviations as part of the requirements for meeting that goal.

4. a. activity
   b. positioning
   c. observation
   d. observation
   e. observation
   f. observation
   g. activity
   h. positioning
   i. activity
   j. activity
   k. observation
   l. positioning
   m. activity
   n. observation

5. a. temperature
   b. pulse
   c. respiration
   d. blood pressure

6. a. oral
   b. rectal
   c. aural (ear)
   d. axillary
   e. temporal artery

7. The nurse would record the patient's blood pressure and pulse rate while the patient is supine (lying) and again while erect (sitting and/or standing).

8. a. blood glucose testing
   b. blood gases
   c. electrolytes analysis
   d. pulse oximetry
9. a. diabetic patients or patients who are receiving nutritional support (total parenteral nutrition)
   b. ACCU-CHEK Advantage, One Touch
10. a. recovery room, intensive care unit, pediatric unit, or any setting where a patient's oxygenation is considered unstable
    b. a noninvasive measurement of gas exchange and red blood cell oxygen-carrying capacity
11. oxygen saturation (pulse oximetry)
12. telemetry unit
13. a. The doctor may need this information to assist in diagnosing the patient's illness or interpreting the patient's progress.
    b. Any four of the following:
       • vital signs
       • orthostatics
       • observe for shortness of breath (SOB)
       • neurologic vital signs (NVS)
       • intake and output (I&O)
       • weight
       • circulation, motion, and sensation (CMS)
14. a. to monitor the patient's fluid balance
    b. *intake*—oral liquids, intravenous fluids
       output—urine, emesis, wound drainage (suction), liquid stool

CHAPTER 11

Exercise 1

1. SSE
2. KO
3. MR
4. sol'n
5. nec
6. cm
7. TWE
8. NG
9. NS
10. N/V
11. D/LR
12. DW
13. @
14. ORE
15. irrig
16. IV
17. cath
18. LR
19. st
20. SCD
21. stat
22. p
23. abd
24. TCDB
25. min
26. gtts
27. Δ
28. ASAP
29. /
30. H_2O_2
31. con't
32. CBI
33. TKO
34. mL
35. IVF
36. PVR or RV
37. ETS
38. WA or W/A
39. PICC
40. VAD
41. CVC
42. D_5W
43. $D_{10}W$
44. B/L
45. HL or heplock
46. before
47. drsg
48. LIS
49. KCL

Exercise 2

1. 1000 milliliters lactated Ringer's at 125 milliliters per hour, then discontinue
2. Soap suds enema hour of sleep (bedtime), may repeat times one
3. Give oil-retention enema; follow with tap water enema if necessary
4. Irrigate catheter three times a day with normal saline solution
5. 1000 milliliters 5% dextrose in water 0.9 normal saline to keep open
6. Insert nasogastric tube
7. Turn, cough, and deep breathe every 2 hours
8. Change intravenous tubing as soon as possible
9. Please obtain elevated toilet seat for patient
10. Start intravenous fluids of 10% dextrose in water at 120 milliliters per hour
11. Insert heparin lock
12. Shave bilateral inguinal groin area
13. Apply sequential compression device when in bed
14. Obtain postvoid residual urine volume today
15. Insert heparin lock immediately (urgent)

Review Questions

1. a. holding the incision area to provide support, promote a feeling of security, and reduce pain during coughing after surgery; a folded blanket or pillow is helpful for use as a splint
   b. a term that indicates that there are no clots at the tip of the needle or catheter and that the needle tip or catheter is not against the vein wall (open)
   c. the patient's own blood donated previously for transfusion as needed by the patient; use of this blood by the patient is also called *autotransfusion*
   d. blood donated by relatives or friends of the patient to be used for transfusion as needed
   e. insertion of a catheter into a body cavity or organ to inject or remove fluid
   f. catheter threaded through to the superior vena cava or the right atrium when used for the administration of intravenous therapy

g. elastic gauze used for temporary compression to various parts of the body to decrease swelling and reduce skin breakdown

h. a tight-fitting, custom-made garment that is used to put constant pressure on healed wounds to keep down scarring

i. process by which the tip of an IV catheter comes out of the vein or pokes through the vein and IV solution is released into surrounding tissue; can occur if the wall of the vein becomes permeable and leaks fluid

j. a disposable pad placed in areas where patients either lie or sit

k. an elevated seat that fits over a toilet and has handrails; used for patients who have difficulty sitting on a lower seat

l. the accidental administration of intravenously infused medicinal drugs into the surrounding tissue, by leakage (as with the brittle veins of elderly patients) or directly (by means of a puncture of the vein)

m. washing or flushing out of a body cavity, organ, or wound

2. a. The physical, emotional, social, economic, and spiritual needs of the patient; the patient's response to illness; and the effects of the illness on the ability to meet self-care needs

   b. Turning a comatose patient to avoid the development of decubitus ulcers (bedsores), or teaching insulin injection technique to a diabetic patient before the time of discharge. Interventions may include support measures, activity limitations, administration of medications, or treatments given to relieve the current condition or to prevent the development of further stress.

3. The central service department (CSD) distributes the supplies used for nursing procedures.

4. *Note:* Items may vary depending on type of nursing unit.
   a. Any five of the following:
   - chux
   - Fleet enema
   - rectal tube
   - irrigation trays
   - urinary catheter trays
   - IV solutions
   - IV catheters and needles
   - IV tubing
   - suction catheters and tubing
   - sterile gloves
   - exam gloves
   - masks
   - syringes and needles
   - disposable suture removal kits
   - dressings
   - abdominal pads
   - Telfa pads
   - gauze pads in various sizes
   - Kling
   - Vaseline gauze
   - tape (various types)
   - alcohol pads
   - glycerin swabs
   - irrigation solutions

b. Any five of the following:
   - adult disposable diapers
   - alternating pressure pad
   - egg-crate mattress
   - T.E.D. hose
   - pneumatic hose
   - colostomy kit
   - stoma bags
   - elastic abdominal binder
   - footboard
   - foot cradle
   - feeding pump and tubing
   - IV infusion pump
   - hypothermia machine
   - K-pad
   - restraints
   - sitz bath, disposable
   - sterile trays, including:
     - tracheostomy tray
     - bone marrow tray
     - paracentesis tray
     - lumbar puncture (spinal tap) tray
     - thoracentesis tray
     - central line tray

   Note: Some sterile trays may be found in C-locker or the floor supply closet.

5. If a rental charge has been assessed, it will be terminated, and the equipment will be readied for use by other patients.

6. Any three of the following:
   - Harris flush
   - oil retention
   - soap suds enema
   - tap water enema
   - Fleet enema
   - normal saline

7. a. The patient voids into a uroflowmeter that reads, measures, and computes the rate and amount of urine flow. The patient cannot urinate for at least 2 hours before the test.

   b. To evaluate the speed of urination, or amount voided per second, and the total time of urination—to evaluate bladder function

8. a. indwelling (retention catheter)—stays in place to drain urine from bladder on a continuous basis

   b. intermittent (straight) catheter—a single-use catheter that is removed after bladder is drained

9. a. bedside bladder ultrasound
   b. catheterization

10. a. continuously or intermittently
    b.
    - administer nutritional support such as total parenteral nutrition (TPN)
    - provide for intermittent or continuous administration of medication
    - transfuse blood or blood products
    - maintain or replace fluids and electrolytes

11. a. amount of solution
    b. name of solution
    c. rate solution is to run

12. Peripheral intravenous therapy is usually delivered via an intravenous injection into a vein (venipuncture) in the

arm or hand or, on rare occasions, in the foot (adult); a vein in the scalp or foot is often used when therapy is administered to infants. It is not threaded to the larger veins or to the heart as in central venous therapy.

A central line consists of a catheter inserted into the jugular or subclavian vein or a large vein in the arm and is threaded to the superior vena cava or the right atrium of the heart.

13. a. peripherally inserted central catheter (PICC or PIC)
    b. percutaneous CVC
    c. tunneled catheter
    d. implanted port
14. a. true
    b. false
    c. false
    d. true
    e. true
15. a. Any three of the following:
    - sodium chloride 0.45% (NaCl 0.45%, or half-strength NaCl)
    - sodium chloride 0.9% (NaCl 0.9%, or normal saline)
    - 5% dextrose in water (5% D/W, or D_5W)
    - 10% dextrose in water (10% D/W, or $D_{10}W$)
    - 5% dextrose in 0.2% sodium chloride (5% D/0.2% NaCl)
    - 5% dextrose in 0.45% sodium chloride (5% D/0.45% NaCl)
    - 5% dextrose in 0.9% sodium chloride (5% D/0.9% NaCl)
    - lactated Ringer's solution with 5% dextrose (LR/5%D)
    - 5% dextrose in 0.2% normal saline
    - 5% dextrose in 0.45% normal saline
    - lactated Ringer's solution
    b. Divide the number of milliliters in the IV bag by the rate of flow. In the doctor's order, 1000 mL 5% D/W @ 125 mL/hr, divide 1000 by 125. The answer is 8. The IV will run for 8 hours.
16. a. To maintain an intermittent line when IV fluids are no longer needed but IV entry is still required. It is commonly used for the administration of medication.
    b. With heparin or saline flushes ordered by the doctor to be administered at specific intervals
17. a. A
    b. B
    c. AB
    d. O
18. The laboratory would discard the blood, and the patient would need to have blood redrawn, causing additional discomfort and delaying treatment.
19. Return the unit of packed cells to the blood bank for proper storage (after confirming this with the nurse).
20. Make two trips to pick up each unit separately, or ask another person to pick up one unit while you pick up the other.
21. a. Swan Ganz—to monitor the heart's function and blood flow, usually in persons who are very ill
    b. arterial line—most commonly used in intensive care and anesthesia to monitor the blood pressure in real time (rather than by intermittent measurement), and to obtain samples for arterial blood gas measurements
22. a. Hemovac
    b. Jackson-Pratt (JP)
    c. Penrose drain

23. additional tubing or a specific type and/or size of catheter for a patient
24. Any two of the following:
    - aquathermia pad (K-pad)
    - hot compresses
    - warm soaks
    - sitz bath
25. Any two of the following:
    - alcohol sponge bath
    - ice bag
    - hypothermia mattress or bed
26. a. A doctor's order is usually required for the patient's insurance to pay for an item or equipment used.
    b. Any four of the following:
    - specialized beds
    - egg-crate mattress
    - sheepskin on bed
    - footboard
    - foot cradle
    - extended toilet seat (ETS)
    - immobilizer
    - sandbags to immobilize
    - elastic abdominal binder
    - sling
    - T.E.D. hose
    - jacket restraint for agitation and patient safety
    - may shampoo hair
    - change surgical dressing
    - pneumatic compression
    - TCDB splinting
    - ostomy nurse referral
27. Any four of the following:
    - acupressure
    - aromatherapy
    - imagery
    - journaling
    - magnets
    - massage
    - music therapy
    - tai chi
    - therapeutic touch

CHAPTER 12

Exercise 1

1. Na or Na^+
2. MN
3. NPO
4. reg
5. cl
6. cal
7. ADA
8. liq
9. chol
10. DAT
11. FF
12. CHO
13. NSA
14. FS
15. PEG
16. NAS
17. RD

18. K or K⁺
19. BMI
20. AHA
21. ADD

Exercise 2

1. sodium
2. nothing by mouth
3. regular
4. midnight
5. liquid
6. calorie
7. no salt added
8. American Diabetic Association
9. diet as tolerated
10. clear
11. cholesterol
12. carbohydrate
13. force fluids
14. full strength
15. percutaneous endoscopic gastrostomy
16. no added salt
17. registered dietitian
18. potassium
19. body mass index
20. American Heart Association
21. attention deficit disorder

Review Questions

1. a. a measurement of energy generated in the body by the heat produced after food is eaten
   b. excessive loss of body water; causes may include diseases of the gastrointestinal tract that cause vomiting or diarrhea, heat exposure, prolonged vigorous exercise
   c. inflammation of the stomach
   d. adequate water in the intracellular and extracellular compartments of the body
   e. a surgical procedure for inserting a tube through the abdominal wall and into the stomach; tube may be used for feeding or drainage
   f. adhering to the dietary laws of Judaism; the conventional meaning in Hebrew is "acceptable" or "approved"
   g. the taking in of food by mouth
   h. difficulty eating and swallowing
   i. an excess of body fat that threatens necessary body functions such as respiration
   j. a creation of an artificial opening into the jejunum that may be used for enteral feeding when it is necessary to bypass the upper gastrointestinal tract
   k. surgical formation of a permanent opening into the duodenum; may be for the purpose of introducing a tube for postpyloric feeding.
   l. having an excess amount of body fat, or the condition of having an excess amount of body fat, usually defined by body mass index
   m. feeding by means of a tube inserted into the stomach, duodenum, or jejunum through the nose or an opening in the abdominal wall; also called *tube feeding*
2. a. NPO p MN
   b. cl liq breakfast, then NPO
   c. 1000-cal ADA diet
   d. low-chol diet

   e. DAT
   f. reg diet
   g. low-Na diet
   h. NSA
3. a. computer
   b. telephone
4. a. anorexia and bulimia
   b. patient is obese, dehydrated, unable to swallow, unable to chew and/or ingest food
5. It is essential that all dietary information, including orders for nothing by mouth, tube feedings, allergies, limit fluids, force fluids, and calorie count, be sent to the nutritional care department so that necessary adjustments will be made when the patient's tray is prepared. All admitted patients require a diet order.
6. True food allergies such as allergies to tree nuts, fish, shellfish, and peanuts can produce life-threatening changes in circulation and bronchioles called *anaphylactic shock*.
7. a. standard diets
   b. therapeutic diets
   c. tube feedings
8. a. clear liquid—Clear liquids only, such as broth, bouillon, coffee, tea, carbonated beverages, clear fruit juices, gelatin, and popsicles.
   b. full liquid—Clear liquids with the addition of smooth-textured dairy products, custards, refined cooked cereals, vegetables, and all fruit juices.
   c. soft—Nonirritating, easily digestible foods and foods with modified fiber content, such as broiled chicken and boiled vegetables.
   d. mechanical soft—Addition of ground or finely diced meats, flaked fish, cottage cheese, cheese, rice, potatoes, pancakes, light breads, cooked vegetables, cooked or canned fruits, bananas, soups, or peanut butter.
   e. pureed—Most foods including meats, vegetables, and fruits can be processed (cooked and blended) to a pureed (smooth) consistency. No lumps or chunks, coarse textures, dried fruits, nuts, or seeds and no raw vegetables or fruits. Foods that require chewing are excluded from this diet. Some commercially prepared products are acceptable, including applesauce, pudding without rice, smooth custard, farina cereal, and stage 1 baby food.
9. a. full liquid, soft, mechanical soft, or regular diet
   b. the patient's nurse would evaluate the patient's status and determine what the patient can tolerate.
10. The nutritional care department will not know what the patient's condition is or what diet he or she can tolerate. The patient's nurse will know if the patient's diet should be advanced to full liquids or to solid food.
11. a. Kosher
   b. vegetarian
   (*Note:* Many other diets may be requested by patients.)
12. Any four of the following:
   - ADD diet
   - bland
   - BRAT
   - soft or low residue
   - low cholesterol
   - low sodium
   - low protein
   - high fiber

- diabetic (American Diabetic Association [ADA])
- calorie restricted
- renal
- prudent cardiac
- low fat
- high potassium
- potassium restricted
- hypoglycemic
- low carbohydrate
- dysphagia diets
- gastric bypass diets

13. a. Tube feedings are ordered for patients who have ingestion problems because of difficulty swallowing, are unable to eat sufficient nutrients, or who cannot absorb nutrients from the foods they eat.
    b. bolus, continuous, or cyclic manner
14. a. an enteral feeding set that includes bags and tubing
    b. a specific sized nasogastric tube
    c. formula and a feeding infusion pump, and if necessary an x-ray examination to verify placement
15. a. The doctor wants to encourage the patient to drink more fluids for hydration or rehydration purposes.
    b. To document the quantities and types of food consumed by the patient for further nutritional evaluation by the dietitian
16. a. to prepare a patient for surgery or treatment
    b. to prepare a patient for a diagnostic procedure
17. No: 2.5 g Na would be a modification to the soft diet and is not a diet change.
18. No: Limiting fluids to 1200 mL/day is a modification to the regular diet and is not a diet change.
19. Yes: All dietary orders need to be sent to the dietary department.
20. All orders pertaining to the patient's diets must be communicated to the nutritional care department so necessary adjustments will be made when the patient's trays are prepared. The dietitian also maintains a record (usually on computer) on each patient, which is updated with each order received.
21. TPN is very expensive and is customized for each patient, so if prepared before the changes are received, the already prepared formula must be discarded.

CHAPTER 13

Exercise 1

1. ASA
2. L
3. ADE
4. mg
5. KCL
6. PCN
7. G, gm, or g
8. mL or ml
9. mEq
10. gr
11. subling or sl
12. tinct or tr
13. PO
14. oz
15. amp
16. supp
17. SC, sq, or sub-q
18. mcg
19. noc
20. syr
21. IVPB
22. pr, R
23. PCA
24. IVP
25. LOC
26. prn
27. OTC
28. IV
29. BCOC
30. NTG
31. BS
32. cc
33. HA, H/A

Exercise 2

1. potassium chloride
2. adverse drug event
3. ampule
4. syrup
5. night
6. acetylsalicylic acid (aspirin)
7. microgram
8. ounce
9. subcutaneous
10. milliequivalent
11. penicillin
12. milliliter
13. per os (by mouth)
14. tincture
15. grain
16. milligram
17. suppository
18. gram
19. liter
20. sublingual (under tongue)
21. intravenous piggyback
22. patient-controlled analgesia
23. per rectum
24. *pro re nata* (as needed)
25. laxative of choice
26. intravenous push
27. over the counter
28. intravenous
29. bowel care of choice
30. nitroglycerin
31. bedside
32. cubic centimeters
33. headache

Review Questions

1. a. an injury or harmful reaction that results from the use of a drug
   b. a drug for which a prescription is not needed
   c. concentrated dose of medication or fluid, frequently given intravenously
   d. medications administered intravenously by means of a special infusion pump controlled by the patient within order ranges written by the physician
   e. by mouth

f. direct application of medication to the skin, eye, ear, or other parts of the body

g. injection of a medication into a muscle

h. pertaining to a medication administered by a route that bypasses the gastrointestinal (GI) tract, such as a drug given by injection, intravenously, or by skin patch

i. administration directly into a vein

j. a test given to determine the reaction of the body to a substance injected intradermally or applied topically to the skin; used to detect allergens, to determine immunity, and to diagnose disease

k. routes that bypass the gastrointestinal (GI) tract, such as by injection, intravenously, or by skin patch

l. method of giving concentrated doses of medication directly into the vein

m. a method of administering a medication in 50 to 100 mL of solution through an intravenous line that is inserted into a patient's vein and given on top of the main intravenous solution

n. injection given between the layers of the skin (used for skin tests)

2. Any of the following:
   - U (unit)
   - Q.D., QD, q.d., qd (daily)
   - Q.O.D, QOD, q.o.d., qod (every other day)
   - trailing zero (X.0 mg)
   - lack of leading zero (.X mg)
   - MS, MSO4 (can mean morphine sulfate or magnesium sulfate)
   - MgSO4 (magnesium sulfate)

3. a.
   - wrong drug
   - incorrect dose
   - administering at wrong time or not at all
   - administering by incorrect route

   Note: Illegible doctors' handwriting and transcription errors are responsible for as much as 61% of the medication errors. Drugs with similar names are also a common cause of error.

   b. When CPOE is used, the doctor enters orders directly into the patient's electronic medical record via computer, and the orders are automatically sent to the pharmacy, reducing the risk of errors in interpreting doctor's handwriting. The clinical decision support system (CDSS) provides the doctor with prompts that warn against the possibility of drug interaction, allergy, or overdose at the point of order entry.

4. *With EMR with CPOE:* The HUC no longer has the responsibility of interpreting doctors' handwritten medication orders. It is beneficial that the HUC recognize medication orders. The HUC will still have some responsibilities involving medications such as ordering stock medications for the nursing unit and printing required computerized medication pamphlets before a patient's discharge.

   Without EMR: The HUC is still transcribing medication orders in many hospitals. Transcription of medication orders varies among hospitals and may involve writing ordered medications on the patient's paper medication administration record (MAR) or entering medications into the patient's MAR.

5. a. Unit dose medicine cart—contains "unit doses" in separate drawers or bins specifically labeled for each patient as ordered by the doctor(s). The pharmacist fills these orders by reading the computerized orders written by the physician or by reading a hard or faxed copy of the physician's orders. The unit dose medication cart can be wheeled to the patient's bedside for administration of the medication.

   b. Computerized medication cart such as a Pyxis—requires the nurse to enter a confidential user identification (ID) and password to unlock the cart. The nurse always verifies the name of the medication, the dose, and the patient's name before removing the medication. The computerized medication carts remain in the medication room and are not taken from room to room.

6. Any two of the following:
   - aspirin
   - acetaminophen
   - mineral oil
   - milk of magnesia
   - many others

7. a. If an electronic medical record (EMR) is implemented in the facility, the medications are entered on the MAR when the doctor writes the order, and the registered or licensed practical nurse enters the time that the medications are administered into each patient's computerized MAR. The electronic MAR is a permanent part of the patient's EMR.

   b. If the EMR is not being used, the pharmacy prepares a printed medication record for each patient, which is sent to the nursing unit each morning. The registered nurse or the HUC adds to the MAR any new medications ordered, along with any changes to medication orders made during the day. The pharmacist, after receiving the faxed physician orders, makes those changes, and the printed medication administration record sent the following morning reflects those changes. When the patient is discharged, the printed MARs become a permanent part of the patient's chart.

   c. A handwritten MAR is used when CPOE or the printed MAR initiated by the pharmacy has not been implemented. Transcribing of medication orders may require the HUC to write the order on the MAR. In some hospitals, nurses are responsible for writing their assigned patients' medication orders on the MAR. Accuracy in copying the medication order from the physicians' order sheet onto the MAR is absolutely essential. The HUC initiates the record on the patient's admission. The record varies in the number of days (3 to 10 days) that medications may be entered. When the last date of the dated period on the MAR is reached, a new record with new dates is prepared, and all medications still in use are copied onto the new form. Handwritten MARs are also a permanent part of the patient's chart.

8. a. component 1: name of the drug
   b. component 2: dosage
   c. component 3: route of administration
   d. component 4: frequency of administration
   e. component 5: qualifying phrase

9. Any four of the following:
   - oral (PO)
   - sublingual (subling)
   - inhalation (nose, eye, rectal)
   - topical
   - parenteral (intradermal, intramuscular (IM), subcutaneous (SQ), intravenous (IV)

10. a. 2
    b. 6
    c. 7
    d. 14
    e. 11
    f. 9
    g. 13
    h. 5
    i. 3
    j. 4
    k. 12
    l. 15
    m. 1
    n. 8
    o. 16
    p. 10

11. a. narcotics
    b. analgesics with narcotics
    c. hypnotics
    d. sedatives (tranquilizers)

12. TPN solution is very expensive and is wasted if any change is ordered in the formula after it has been prepared.

13. a. stat
    b. prn
    c. standing
    d. one-time
    e. short-series order

14. a. PPD—test for tuberculosis
    b. cocci 1:100—test for coccidioidomycosis (valley fever)
    c. histoplasmin—test for histoplasmosis, a fungal disease

15. When EMR is in use, the drugs may be discontinued automatically and the nurse may leave a message via the computer for the doctor to renew the medication. When paper charts are used, the nurse may send a message via computer. Some hospitals use a renewal stamp as a reminder of the automatic stop date; the information is stamped on the physician's order sheet by the HUC or the patient's nurse before the expiration date of the medication. When the doctor checks the "yes" or "no" box indicating to renew or discontinue and signs his or her name, it is regarded as an order and is transcribed as such.

    Whenever a change is written, it is considered a new order and should be written as such on the MAR. It is illegal to erase or cross out parts of an order or to write over an order on the MAR. The old order must be discontinued according to the policy, and the new order written.

CHAPTER 14

Exercise 1

1. A1C
2. FBS
3. O&P
4. Hgb
5. ESR
6. K
7. AFB
8. RBC
9. PP
10. CSF
11. Fe
12. C&S
13. T&X-match or T&C
14. CBC
15. PAP
16. GTT
17. PC
18. PT/INR
19. Ua or U/A
20. ALP or alk phos
21. HBsAg
22. FS
23. HIV
24. Mg or Mg^+
25. hCG
26. WNL
27. PTT or APIT
28. T_3, T_4, T_7
29. TSH
30. S&A
31. Ag
32. BMP
33. CMV
34. HSV
35. T&S
36. Ab
37. Cx
38. RSV
39. CMP
40. lytes
41. Bx
42. POCT or PCT
43. PCV
44. RBS or BS
45. RPR
46. retics
47. PSA
48. Diff
49. WBC
50. PO_4 or phos
51. TIBC
52. Hct
53. LP
54. Na
55. NP
56. H&H
57. CO_2
58. ANA
59. HDL
60. BUN
61. Ca
62. CC, creat cl, or cr cl
63. Cl
64. CEA
65. BNP
66. LDL
67. ADH
68. CPK or CK
69. EBV
70. Ab
71. RDW
72. trig or TG
73. bili
74. STO

75. IgG/IgM
76. CRP
77. VRE
78. MRSA
79. XDR-TB
80. ACTH
81. C. diff
82. CRKP

Exercise 2

1. fasting blood sugar
2. ova and parasites
3. hemoglobin
4. erythrocyte sedimentation rate or sedimentation rate
5. potassium
6. acid-fast bacilli
7. red blood cells
8. postprandial
9. cerebrospinal fluid
10. iron
11. culture and sensitivity
12. type and crossmatch
13. complete blood cell count
14. prostatic acid phosphatase
15. glucose tolerance test
16. packed cells
17. prothrombin time, international normalized ratio
18. urinalysis
19. alkaline phosphatase
20. hepatitis B surface antigen
21. frozen section
22. human immunodeficiency virus
23. magnesium
24. human chorionic gonadotropin
25. within normal limits
26. partial thromboplastin time or activated partial thrombo-plastin time
27. thyroid tests
28. thyroid-stimulating hormone
29. sugar and acetone
30. antigen
31. basic metabolic chemistry panel
32. cytomegalovirus
33. herpes simplex virus
34. type and screen
35. antibody
36. culture
37. respiratory syncytial virus
38. comprehensive metabolic chemistry panel
39. electrolytes
40. biopsy
41. point-of-care testing
42. packed cell volume
43. random blood sugar or blood sugar
44. rapid plasma reagin
45. reticulocytes
46. prostatic specific antigen
47. differential
48. white blood cell count
49. phosphorus
50. total iron-binding capacity
51. hematocrit
52. lumbar puncture
53. sodium
54. nasopharynx
55. hemoglobin and hematocrit
56. carbon dioxide
57. antinuclear antibody
58. high-density lipoproteins
59. blood urea nitrogen
60. calcium
61. creatinine clearance
62. chloride
63. carcinoembryonic antigen
64. brain natriuretic protein
65. low-density lipoproteins
66. antidiuretic hormone
67. creatine phosphokinase or creatine kinase
68. Epstein-Barr virus
69. antibody
70. red cell distribution width
71. triglyceride
72. bilirubin
73. glycosylated hemoglobin
74. specimen to be obtained
75. immunoglobulin G and M
76. *Clostridium difficile*
77. carbapenem-resistant *Klebsiella pneumoniae*
78. extensively drug resistant tuberculosis
79. vancomycin-resistant *Enterococcus*
80. methicillin-resistant *Staphylococcus aureus*
81. adrenocorticotropic hormone
82. C-reactive protein

Review Questions

1. a. procedure to remove tissue from a living body for examination
    b. an immunoglobulin (protein) produced by the body that reacts with and neutralizes an antigen (usually a foreign substance)
    c. a microorganism that causes disease
    d. a procedure used to remove cerebrospinal fluid from the spinal canal
    e. a needle puncture into the uterine cavity to remove amniotic fluid, the liquid that surrounds the fetus
    f. blood that is undetectable to the eye
    g. after eating
    h. the mucous secretion from lungs, bronchi, or trachea
    i. the procedure to remove bone marrow from the breast-bone cavity for diagnostic purposes; also called a *bone marrow biopsy*
    j. the physical, chemical, and microscopic examination of the urine
    k. a surgical puncture and drainage of a body cavity
    l. the visual examination of urine using a special commercially treated stick
    m. the fluid portion of the blood in which the cells are suspended; it contains a clotting factor called *fibrinogen*
2. a. diagnostic purposes
    b. evaluation of a prescribed treatment
3. a. hematology, chemistry, microbiology
    b. toxicology, serology or immunology, pathology (including histology and cytology), blood bank, and urinalysis

4. a. Any five of the following:
  - blood
  - urine
  - stool
  - sputum
  - sweat
  - wound drainage
  - discharge from body openings
  - gastric washings (lavage)
  b. Any three of the following:
  - spinal fluid
  - bone marrow
  - abdominal fluid
  - pleural fluid
  - amniotic fluid
  - biopsy specimens
  - cervical smear

5. a. lumbar puncture
  b. sternal puncture or bone marrow biopsy
  c. abdominal paracentesis
  d. thoracocentesis or thoracentesis
  e. amniocentesis
  f. biopsy

6. The HUC should check to see that the specimen is labeled correctly. Call transport or personally take the specimen as soon as possible. Specimens that were collected by an invasive procedure (e.g., cerebrospinal fluid, cavity fluid, biopsy sample) cannot be sent through the tube system.

7. a. ordered routine—performed within a 4-hour period
  b. laboratory notified by phone or verbally or appropriate nursing personnel notified on the unit—performed immediately or ASAP
  c. requisitioned every day or entered into the computer for multiple days in advance—test would be performed every day until the doctor discontinues it
  d. the test would be ordered and performed at a specific time

8. a. guaiac
  b. Gastroccult
  c. Hemoccult

9. a. performs tests related to physical properties of the blood (including blood cells and their appearance), tests related to clotting and bleeding disorders, and coagulation (clotting studies done to monitor patients on anticoagulant therapy
  b. any six from Appendix F that have "hematology" listed in the "Laboratory Division" column

10. a. performs tests related to the study of chemical reactions that occur in living organisms
  b. any six from Appendix F that have "chemistry" listed in the "Laboratory Division" column.

11. a. urine glucose
    urine creatinine
    urine protein
    urine osmolality
  b. sodium (Na)
    potassium (K)
    chlorides (Cl)
    carbon dioxide (CO_2)

12. any three chemistry tests listed in Table 14-1

13. *Fasting* means that the patient may have water or other nonnutritional drinks. *NPO* means no food or liquid by mouth. In both cases, the patient's breakfast tray is held until the test is completed.

14. The HUC would ask the nurse to notify you of the time the patient has finished eating, and order the blood to be drawn. *Timed:* 2 hours after the patient finished eating

15. a. The study of poisons, their detection, their effects, and methods of treatment for conditions they produce; monitoring of drug use and detection of drug abuse
  b. The blood for peak levels is usually collected 15 minutes after IV infusion and 30 to 60 minutes after IM injection. The blood for trough levels is usually drawn 15 minutes before the next dose of medication is given to the patient. For peak-and-trough orders, the HUC must work closely with the laboratory, nursing staff, and pharmacist to ensure proper scheduling of collections.

16. a. Study of microorganisms that cause disease. Specimens are cultured (grown in a reproducing medium) and identified with the use of biochemical tests.
  b. Any six from Appendix F that have "bacteriology, virology, mycology, or parasitology" listed in the "Laboratory Division" column

17. a. study of immunologic substances
  b. Any three tests listed in Appendix F

18. a. Blood typing and cross-matching, storing blood and blood components for transfusion
  b. Before whole blood, packed cells, and some other blood components are administered, the patient must undergo a type and crossmatch, and a blood transfusion consent must be signed before blood or blood products are administered. The patient also may sign a refusal of blood transfusion form.

19. a. the study of urine
  b. voided, clean catch (or midstream), and catheterization

20. a. A sternal puncture would be performed to obtain pleural fluid, and a lumbar puncture would be performed to obtain CSF.
  b. These are nonretrievable specimens, meaning that the specimens were obtained by painful invasive procedures. If mislabeled, the specimen could be discarded; and if sent via pneumatic tube, the specimen could be lost or the tubes broken.

21. a. study of the nature and cause of disease, when changes in structure and function are noted
  b. *histology:* study of the microscopic structure of tissue
    cytology: study of cells obtained from body tissues and fluid

22. Read the laboratory values you have recorded back to the person in the laboratory.

CHAPTER 15

Exercise 1

1. IVP (also called IVU)
2. RLQ
3. KUB
4. BE
5. PA
6. UGI
7. lat
8. LS
9. LUQ
10. AP

11. GI
12. RUQ
13. CT
14. LLQ
15. GB
16. MRI
17. SBFT
18. CXR
19. DSA
20. PCXR
21. PTC or PTHC
22. Fx
23. H/O
24. F/U
25. CI
26. IVU (also called IVP)
27. US
28. PACS
29. PET
30. L&S
31. RIS
32. abd
33. mets
34. SNAT
35. SPECT or SPET
36. VQ

Exercise 2

1. barium enema
2. lumbosacral
3. kidneys, ureters, and bladder
4. ultrasound
5. abdominal, right lower quadrant, left upper quadrant
6. intravenous urogram and upper gastrointestinal
7. computed tomography
8. gastrointestinal
9. posteroanterior, lateral (x-ray examination)
10. magnetic resonance imaging
11. portable chest x-ray examination
12. upper gastrointestinal (x-ray examination), small bowel follow-through
13. liver and spleen
14. positron emission tomography
15. computed tomography, digital subtraction angiogram
16. suspected nonaccidental trauma, clinical indications

Review Questions

1. a. an agent that causes evacuation of the bowel (laxative)
   b. direct observation of deep body structures made visible through the use of a real-time viewing screen instead of film; contrast medium is required for this procedure
   c. method of application or employment of any therapeutic agent, limited usually to physical agents and devices
   d. process by which tumor cells spread to distant parts of the body
   e. alignment of the body on the x-ray table that is favorable for taking the best view of the part of the body being imaged
   f. medication prescribed by the doctor to be given before a diagnostic imaging procedure is performed; the department notifies the nursing unit of the time the medication is to be administered to the patient

2. The health unit coordinator, when using paper charts, would transcribe the handwritten doctors' orders, coordinate the preparation (write on MAR), or put a prep card in Kardex. When the electronic record is implemented, the health unit coordinator would coordinate the scheduling of procedures and the preparations but would not use the MAR or Kardex.

3. a. reason for procedure (clinical indication)
   b. transportation required
   c. whether patient is receiving intravenous fluids
   d. whether patient is receiving oxygen
   e. whether patient needs isolation precautions
   f. whether patient has a seizure disorder
   g. whether patient does not speak English
   h. whether patient is diabetic
   i. whether patient is sight or hearing impaired
   j. whether patient is pregnant or pregnancy test results are pending

4. a. radiographer—a person with special education in the area of radiography—performs x-ray studies
   b. radiologist—a doctor who is a specialist in radiology—interprets x-ray images

5. Benefits for the doctor include faster results, ability to compare an image with a previous image (if applicable), ability to share with other physicians, and reduced risk of lost film. Benefits for the patient include reduced delay in treatment, reduced risk of lost film, and protection of confidentiality. There is also a benefit for the environment in that X-ray photographic darkroom chemicals and toxins are eliminated from the process.

6. a. anteroposterior (AP)
   b. posteroanterior (PA)
   c. lateral (lat)
   d. oblique
   e. decubitus

7. Procedures that require the filming of bone structures or that are ordered to determine the position of other organs in relation to these structures can be performed by qualified radiology personnel without the need for preparation for the procedure.

8. a. Contrast medium is used to differentiate among soft tissue structures.
   b.
   - water
   - air
   - barium
   - iodinated contrast media
   - gas

9.
   - X-ray studies of the lower spine and pelvis should be ordered first, before a barium enema or an upper gastrointestinal study is done. The presence of barium in specific parts of the body may obscure the portion of the body that is being studied.
   - Abdominal studies that use ultrasound or CT should precede studies that use barium.
   - Liver and bone scans and nuclear medicine studies may conflict with barium studies and should be done first.
   - Three x-ray studies that require contrast media frequently are ordered at the same time for diagnostic reasons. Only one or sometimes two can be done on

the same day; thus studies may have to be scheduled 3 or more days in advance. The order of scheduling is as follows:
  a. intravenous urogram (IVU)
  b. barium enema (BE)
  c. upper gastrointestinal (UGI) or UGI and small bowel follow-through (SBFT)
10. a.
    BE
    Barium swallow
    IVU
    UGI
  b. For contrast medium to prove most effective, the patient must be prepared for the procedure before it is scheduled. If the patient is not properly prepared, the procedure will need to be canceled, causing a delay in diagnosis and treatment, perhaps a delay in discharge of the patient, and delays in the radiology department.
11. When it is an invasive procedure or when an injected contrast medium is used.
12. a. Special invasive x-ray and interventional radiology uses minimally invasive image-guided procedures to diagnose and treat diseases in nearly every organ system.
  b. Any three procedures listed in Table 15-2
13. a. with or without contrast media
  b. Any three procedures listed in Table 15-3
14. a. Ultrasonography is a technique that is used to visualize muscles, tendons, and many internal organs and to assess their size, structure, and the presence of pathologic lesions; it may also be used for therapeutic procedures.
  b. Any three procedures listed in Table 15-4
15. a. used to produce computer images (scans) of the interior of the body with the use of a powerful magnetic field and radiofrequency waves
  b. use of magnetic resonance to study blood vessels
16. a. The form lists any contraindications that may prevent the patient from having the procedure.
  b.
    pacemaker
    implanted port device
    neurostimulator
    intrauterine device (IUD)
    insulin pump
    older metal plates, pins, screws, or surgical staples
    ear implant
    older metal clips from aneurysm repair
    metal clips in eyes
    retained bullets
    pregnancy
17. a. uses radioactive materials called *radiopharmaceuticals* to determine the functioning capacity of organs
  b. Any three procedures listed in Table 15-6

CHAPTER 16

Exercise 1

1. EEG
2. EKG or ECG
3. EMG
4. RA
5. LOC
6. ABG
7. CBG
8. ERCP
9. EGD
10. EPS
11. NCS
12. OSA
13. BAER
14. ENG
15. SEP
16. VEP
17. DVT
18. TEE
19. PFT
20. IPG
21. ICG
22. TTT
23. QEEG
24. ABI
25. ASI

Exercise 2

1. arterial blood gases
2. electrocardiography
3. electroencephalography
4. leave on chart
5. electromyography
6. room air
7. esophagogastroduodenoscopy
8. endoscopic retrograde cholangiopancreatography
9. electrophysiologic study
10. capillary blood gases
11. nerve conduction studies
12. obstructive sleep apnea
13. brainstem auditory evoked response
14. electronystagmography
15. somatosensory evoked potential
16. visual evoked potential
17. deep vein thrombosis
18. transesophageal echocardiography
19. pulmonary function test
20. impedance plethysmography
21. impedance cardiography
22. tilt table test
23. ankle brachial index
24. arterial stiffness index
25. quantitative electroencephalography

Review Questions

1. a. a catheter placed in an artery that continuously measures the patient's blood pressure
  b. test used to evaluate the function of the vestibular portion of the eighth cranial nerve (CN VIII) to evaluate the function of cranial nerve VIII; can indicate disease in the temporal portion of the cerebrum
  c. a noninvasive endoscopic study; a small capsule that is swallowed by the patient transmits and records pictures of the esophagus and small intestine
  d. reflection of an ultrasound wave back to the transducer from a structure in the plane of the sound beam
  e. a tubular instrument (rigid or flexible) with a light source and a viewing lens for observation that can be inserted through a body orifice or through a small incision

f. cessation of breathing

g. visualization of the interior of organs and cavities of the body with an endoscope; biopsies may be performed during an endoscopy

h. portable device that records the heart's electrical activity and produces a continuous ECG tracing over a specified period

i. diagnostic or therapeutic technique that requires an incision and/or entry into a body cavity and/or interruption of normal body functions

j. a chronic ailment that consists of recurrent attacks of drowsiness and sleep during the daytime

k. a diagnostic or therapeutic technique that does not require the skin to be broken or a cavity or organ of the body to be entered

l. the cessation of breathing during sleep

m. a blockage in a canal, vessel, or passage of the body

n. ultrasound procedure that displays a rapid sequence of images (like a movie) instantaneously while an object is being examined

o. a cardiac study that demonstrates the waveform produced by electrical impulses from the electrocardiograph

p. the transmission of data electronically to a distant location

2. a. Electrodiagnostic procedures are used to evaluate the cardiovascular, nervous, and muscular systems to diagnose conditions and diseases.

   b. Indications include numbness, tingling, weakness, muscle cramping, or pain.

3. A noninvasive procedure is a diagnostic or therapeutic technique that does not require the skin to be broken or a cavity or organ of the body to be entered.

   An invasive procedure is a diagnostic or therapeutic technique that requires an incision and/or entry of a body cavity and/or interruption of normal body functions. Some invasive procedures require a routine preparation and/or an on-call medication and/or an NPO order or other dietary restriction orders, and some require sedation.

4. a. visual evoked potentials (VEPs)—Abnormal results may be seen in patients with neurologic disease; used to detect lesions of the eye, disorders of neurologic development, and eyesight problems or blindness in infants or may be used during eye surgery to provide a warning of possible damage to the optic nerve.

   b. brainstem auditory-evoked response (BAER) or auditory brainstem-evoked potential (ABEP)—used to detect lesions in the brainstem, used in low-birthweight newborns to screen for hearing disorders, and may be effective in the early detection of brain tumors of the posterior fossa.

   c. somatosensory evoked potentials (SEPs)—used to assess patients with spinal cord injury, to monitor spinal cord functioning during spinal surgery, to monitor treatment of diseases (e.g., multiple sclerosis), to evaluate the location and extent of areas of brain dysfunction after head injury, and to pinpoint tumors at an early stage.

5. a. An electroencephalography (EEG) is performed to identify and assess patients with seizures and to study brain function; may be used to diagnose brain tumors, epilepsy, other brain diseases, or injuries, and to confirm brain death or cerebral silence.

   b. A quantitative electroencephalogram (QEEG) uses digital pattern recognition to identify functional problems such as attention-deficit/hyperactivity disorder (ADHD) (brain mapping).

6. Anticonvulsant medications—**examples:** phenobarbital (Luminal) and phenytoin (Dilantin).

7. a. A caloric study is performed to evaluate the function of cranial nerve VIII; also can indicate disease in the temporal portion of the cerebrum.

   b. An electromyogram (EMG) used in the assessment of patients with diffuse or localized muscle weakness; often combined with electroneurography; can be used to identify primary muscle diseases and to differentiate them from primary neurologic pathologic conditions.

   c. A nerve conduction study (NCS) is used to identify peripheral nerve injury in patients with localized or diffuse weakness, to differentiate primary peripheral nerve disease from muscular injury, and to document the severity of injury in legal cases; also is used to monitor nerve injury and response to treatment.

8. Electrodiagnostic tests of the cardiovascular system include procedures involving the heart and the vascular system. The results of electrodiagnostic tests and other cardiovascular studies aid the physician in making a diagnosis and prescribing treatment.

9. Specific cardiac medications, such as digoxin (Lanoxin), diltiazem (Cardizem), and nitroglycerin (Nitro-Bid, Nitro-Dur, Nitrostat, Transderm-Nitro)

10. Any three of the following:
    - electrocardiogram (EKG or ECG)
    - impedance cardiography (IPG)
    - Holter monitor
    - cardiac stress test (exercise electrocardiogram or treadmill stress test)
    - thallium or sestamibi stress test
    - echocardiogram
    - plethysmography vascular studies
    - vascular ultrasound studies—arterial and venous Doppler studies
    - vascular duplex scans

11. a. thallium and sestamibi stress tests
    b.
    - echocardiogram
    - plethysmography vascular studies
    - vascular ultrasound studies—arterial and venous Doppler studies
    - vascular duplex scans

12. a. A cardiac catheterization is performed to visualize the heart chambers, arteries, and great vessels, most often to evaluate chest pain or abnormalities detected in a cardiac stress test; also used to locate the region of coronary occlusion (blockages) and to determine the effects of valvular heart disease

    b. Measurements revealed by the use of a Swan-Ganz catheter are used to guide and evaluate therapy.

    c. An arterial line continuously measures the patient's blood pressure. It is most commonly used in intensive care and anesthesia to monitor the blood pressure in real time (rather than by intermittent measurement). The arterial line may also be used to obtain samples for arterial blood gas measurements.

13. a. venous plethysmography—a noninvasive method of determining venous thrombosis and deep vein thrombophlebitis
    b. arterial plethysmography—performed to rule out occlusive disease of the lower extremities; may also be used to identify arteriosclerotic disease in the upper extremity
    c. impedance plethysmography (IPG)—performed to estimate blood flow and quantify blood volumes

14. a. Arterial Doppler ultrasound—used to evaluate the blood flow to and through the upper extremities (arms) and the lower extremities (legs); records the patient's blood pressure of the arteries in the arms or legs along with taking ultrasound images. Used for the following:
    • to evaluate numbness and tingling sensations in the hands, arms, feet, and legs
    • to evaluate sensation of fatigue and heaviness in the arms and legs
    • to investigate the possibility of thoracic outlet syndrome
    b. Vascular Doppler ultrasound—provides real-time imaging that displays how the patient's blood is flowing through the arteries; makes it easier to detect narrowing of the arteries, blockages, and blood clots; also helps with monitoring the progression of arterial disease in a patient.
    c. Vascular ultrasound and vascular duplex scanning, including:
    • *carotid Doppler flow analysis:* used to detect the flow of blood in the major neck artery
    • *carotid duplex scan:* used in the extracranial carotid artery to directly detect occlusive disease
    • *vascular ultrasound studies (Doppler flow studies) on lower extremities:* show flow changes caused by changes within the blood vessels

15. Any six listed in Table 16-1
16. a. The presence of stool would obscure visualization of the intestinal walls.
    b. Barium also would obscure visualization of the intestinal walls.
    Note: Gastrointestinal endoscopic studies cannot be done if the patient is not properly prepared.
17. a. gastric analysis
    b. esophageal manometry
    c. secretin test
18. Evaluates, treats, and cares for patients with breathing or other cardiopulmonary (pertaining to the heart and lungs) disorders. The cardiopulmonary department also may perform presurgical evaluations.
19. a. Any four of the following:
    • oximetry (pulse oximetry, ear oximetry, oxygen saturation)
    • arterial blood gases (ABGs)
    • arterial blood gases with lytes
    • capillary blood gases (CBGs)
    b. anticoagulants—enoxaparin (Lovenox), heparin (Heparin), warfarin (Coumadin)
20. a. the sleep study department performs studies to assess a patient's sleep patterns
    b. narcolepsy (excessive daytime sleepiness); insomnia—motor spasms while sleeping documented cardiac rhythm disturbances limited to sleep time

CHAPTER 17

Exercise 1

1. LUL
2. OT
3. PT
4. L/min
5. O_2
6. IPPB
7. RUL
8. ROM
9. RLL
10. ADLs
11. CABG
12. RML
13. USN
14. SVN
15. LLL
16. lb or #
17. NWB
18. WP
19. HP
20. TENS
21. EPC
22. ES
23. CPM
24. IS
25. MDI
26. CPT
27. AA
28. BiW
29. AKA
30. STM
31. LEs
32. HD
33. THR or THA
34. ORIF
35. Tx
36. TT
37. ISOM
38. BKA
39. ET
40. HA
41. PEP
42. PDPV
43. O_2 SAT
44. UD
45. >
46. TKR or TKA
47. <
48. CP
49. CPR
50. HBOT
51. TTOT
52. CPAP
53. BUE
54. BLE
55. RUE
56. LUE
57. RLE
58. LLE
59. PTA

60. RT
61. PROM
62. WBAT
63. FWW
64. PD
65. ICD
66. ADS
67. DPI
68. SIDS
69. NC/NP
70. SaO$_2$
71. CBNT
72. PTCA
73. BiPAP
74. SpO$_2$

Exercise 2

1. oxygen
2. left upper lobe
3. right lower lobe
4. occupational therapy, occupational therapist
5. physical therapy, physical therapist
6. sudden infant death syndrome
7. activity of daily living
8. pounds
9. right upper lobe
10. right middle lobe
11. non–weight bearing
12. range of motion
13. liters per minute
14. small volume nebulizer
15. left lower lobe
16. intermittent positive-pressure breathing
17. ultrasonic nebulizer
18. hot packs
19. whirlpool
20. continuous passive motion
21. electrical stimulation
22. electronic pain control
23. transcutaneous electrical nerve stimulation
24. incentive spirometry
25. chest physiotherapy
26. metered-dose inhaler
27. open reduction, internal fixation
28. tilt table
29. arterial oxygen concentration
30. above-the-knee amputation
31. unit dose
32. heated aerosol
33. isometric
34. lower extremities
35. soft tissue massage
36. hemodialysis
37. traction
38. postural drainage, percussion and vibration
39. greater than
40. total knee replacement or arthroplasty
41. total hip replacement or arthroplasty
42. endotracheal tube
43. below-the-knee amputation
44. less than
45. twice a week

46. positive expiratory pressure
47. cold packs
48. active assisted
49. cardiopulmonary resuscitation
50. hyperbaric oxygen therapy
51. transtracheal oxygen therapy
52. continuous positive airway pressure
53. both or bilateral upper extremities
54. both or bilateral lower extremities
55. right upper extremity
56. left upper extremity
57. right lower extremity
58. left lower extremity
59. physical therapist assistant
60. respiratory therapy, respiratory therapist
61. passive range of motion
62. weight bearing as tolerated
63. front-wheel walker
64. coronary artery bypass graft
65. dry powder inhaler
66. adult distress syndrome
67. implantable cardioverter-defibrillator
68. peritoneal dialysis
69. nasal cannula or nasal prongs
70. continuous bronchodilator nebulizer therapy
71. percutaneous transluminal coronary angioplasty
72. O$_2$ SAT
73. bilevel positive airway pressure
74. oxygen concentration via pulse oximetry

Review Questions

1. a. a high-pitched harsh sound heard during inspiration that is caused by obstruction of the upper airway and is a sign of respiratory distress and therefore requires immediate attention
   b. of equal dimensions; holding ends of contracting muscle fixed so that contraction produces increased tension at a constant overall length
   c. exercise that causes the heart and lungs to work harder to benefit the cardiovascular and circulatory systems
   d. a room where hydrotherapy is performed
   e. the process of removing dirt, foreign objects, damaged tissue, and cellular debris from a wound or a burn to prevent infection and to promote healing
   f. a common, abnormal respiratory sound that consists of discontinuous bubbling noises caused by fluid in the small airways or atelectasis and is heard on auscultation of the chest during inspiration
   g. the act of listening for sounds within the body to evaluate the condition of the heart, blood vessels, lungs, pleura, intestines, or other organs, or to detect fetal heart sounds
   h. difficult or labored breathing
   i. removal of a previously inserted tube (such as an endotracheal tube)
   j. a tiny metal or plastic tube that is placed into an artery, blood vessel, or other duct to hold the structure open
   k. a gas-driven device that produces an aerosol
   l. sounds that are heard continuously during inspiration or expiration or both and are caused by

air moving through airways narrowed by constriction or swelling of airways or partial airway obstruction

m. application of an electric shock to the myocardium through the chest wall to restore normal cardiac rhythm; external defibrillators deliver the shock through the chest wall, whereas internal defibrillators (ICDs) deliver the shock via implanted electrodes within the heart

n. insertion and placement of a tube within the trachea (may be endotracheal or tracheostomy)

o. exercise that involves strengthening muscles by forcing them to work very hard for a brief time

2. a. medication, surgery, and/or placement of various therapeutic cardiac instruments

b. cardiovascular laboratory (CV lab or cardiac cath lab), the special x-ray division of radiology, or surgery

3. a. coronary artery bypass graft (CABG) or off-pump coronary artery bypass (OPCAB)

b. placement of stents

c. angioplasty

4. a. a vein from the leg, called the *saphenous vein*

b. the internal mammary artery (IMA)

5. a. Used in most cases to increase the heart rate in severe bradycardia by electrically stimulating the heart muscle

b. Monitors and restores proper rhythm by sending low-energy shocks to the heart when the heart begins to beat rapidly or erratically. Most ICDs are also capable of pacing the heart in response to bradycardia.

6. a. Because of the invasive nature and associated risks, it is expected that any treatment or intervention would occur in conjunction with the test itself.

7. Any two of the following:
- embolization
- biliary drainage and stenting
- brachytherapy
- chemoembolization
- hemodialysis access maintenance
- stent insertion
- infection and abscess drainage
- needle biopsy
- radiofrequency ablation
- endograft insertion
- thrombolysis
- transjugular intrahepatic portosystemic shunt (TIPS)
- percutaneous nephrostomy tube insertion
- varicocele embolization
- varicose vein treatment
- vena cava filter
- vertebroplasty

Note: The interventional radiology department performs many other procedures.

8. a. to evaluate patients with respiratory conditions and perform treatments to maintain or improve function of their respiratory system

b.
- oxygen therapy
- aerosol treatment (SVN, USN, IPPB, inhalers, and so on)
- incentive spirometry
- chest percussion therapy or chest physiotherapy
- mechanical ventilator

9. a. It is important for the respiratory therapist to be aware of the entire doctor's order so he or she can bring all of the supplies and equipment to the patient's room, saving the therapist time and reducing delay in the patient's treatment.

10. the amount of oxygen (flow rate and/or concentration) how oxygen is to be administered (delivery device or mode of delivery)

11. a. metered-dose inhaler (MDI)
small-volume nebulizer (SVN) (handheld nebulizer [HHN])
dry powder inhaler (DPI)
hypertonic ultrasonic nebulizer (USN)

b. Any two of the following:
- nasal decongestants
- bronchodilators
- antiasthmatics
- corticosteroids
- intranasal corticosteroids
- mucolytics
- antimicrobials

12. A small-volume nebulizer or hypertonic ultrasonic nebulizer treatment is given by a respiratory therapist to loosen lung secretions. A Lukens trap often is used by a respiratory therapist to collect a sterile sputum specimen.

13. a. Incentive spirometry is often used postoperatively to encourage the patient to take protracted, slow, deep breaths and to reinforce such breathing; improves inspiratory muscle performance, thereby reestablishing or simulating the normal pattern of pulmonary hyperinflation.

b. CPT is used to loosen secretions in the area underlying the percussion via the air pressure that is generated by the cupped hand on the chest wall.

c. NIPPV enhances the breathing process by giving the patient a mixture of air and oxygen from a flow generator through a tightly fitted facial or nasal mask.

d. Mechanical ventilation is indicated when the patient's spontaneous ventilation is inadequate to maintain life. It also is indicated to prevent imminent collapse of other physiologic functions or ineffective gas exchange in the lungs.

14. a. Specializes in the treatment of nonhealing, or slow-healing, wounds such as pressure sores caused by sitting or lying in one position and foot and leg ulcers connected to diabetes and burns; provides educational, medical, and supportive services to patients and their caregivers.

b. Hyperbaric oxygen therapy delivers oxygen systemically to injured areas quickly and in high concentrations. The increased pressure changes the normal cellular respiration process and causes oxygen to dissolve in the plasma. This stimulates the growth of new blood vessels, resulting in a substantial increase in tissue oxygenation that can arrest certain types of infections and enhance wound healing.

15. a. skin traction and skeletal traction

b. overhead frame and trapeze

16. a. physical therapy

b. occupational therapy

c. speech therapy

17. a. Physical therapy is the division within the hospital that treats patients to improve and restore their functional mobility.
   b. gait training, exercise, water therapy, and heat and ice treatments

18. a. works toward rehabilitation of patients, in conjunction with other health team members, to return the patient to the greatest possible independence
   b. Any three of the following:
   • occupational therapy for evaluation and treatment if needed daily
   • training in activities of daily living (ADLs)
   • supply and train in adaptive equipment such as button hooks and feeding utensils for ADLs
   • occupational therapy to increase mobility
   • fabrication of cock-up splint for left upper extremity

19. a. the evaluation and treatment of oral, motor, swallowing, cognitive-linguistic, speech and language disorders
   b. patients with developmental problems related to the ability to speak and be understood as well as deficiencies that are a result of stroke, seizures, cancer, and other brain injuries

20. a. When the kidneys fail to remove those wastes, medical intervention is necessary to sustain life.
   b. *hemodialysis (extracorporeal dialysis)*—the removal of waste products from the blood via use of a machine through which the blood flows
      peritoneal dialysis—the introduction of a fluid (dialyzing fluid) into the abdominal cavity that absorbs the wastes from the blood through the lining of the abdominal cavity, or peritoneum; the dialysate is then emptied from the abdominal cavity

21. a. Procedures may be performed in a division of the diagnostic imaging department or a totally separate department; some new treatments are performed in the interventional radiology department.
   b. Many of those who undergo radiation therapy are outpatients; however, the HUC may be called on to schedule an appointment (by requisition or telephone) for an inpatient requiring treatment for a malignant neoplasm (cancer).

CHAPTER 18

Exercise 1

1. wk
2. NINP
3. DME
4. DNR
5. Rx
6. appt

Exercise 2

1. appointment
2. durable medical equipment
3. do not resuscitate/do not intubate
4. no information, no publication
5. week
6. take (e.g., treatment, medication) prescription

Review Questions

1. a. A request by the patient's attending physician for the opinion of a second physician with respect to diagnosis and treatment of the patient
   b. A film that contains a greatly reduced photo image of printed or graphic matter
   c. Many pediatric hospitals and/or units have a patient room with a bed so a parent can stay with the child 24 hours a day.

2. a. hospital name
   b. patient's name and age
   c. patient's location (unit and room number)
   d. name of the doctor requesting the consultation
   e. patient's diagnosis
   f. urgency of consultation and any additional information provided in the order
   g. patient's insurance information, located on the patient's face sheet

3. The health unit coordinator, on receiving a request (electronic or handwritten doctor's order) for a patient medical record from another facility, would:
   • prepare a release of information form for the patient's nurse to have the patient sign
   • place a call to the HIMS department of the health care facility to request records
   • fax the signed information release form to the HIMS department of the health care facility
   The requested records are then faxed to the nursing unit.

4. The faxed records are scanned into the patient's electronic medical record or placed in the patient's current chart if paper charts are used. After the records have been scanned into the patient's EMR, the original documents are stamped as "scanned" with the date and time and are placed in a bin or a box to be picked up by HIMS.

5. If the HUC is responsible and the EMR is used, the HUC would print the specified documents from the patient's EMR; if paper charts are used, the HUC would photocopy the specified documents from the patient's paper chart. The HUC would prepare an information release form for the patient's nurse to have the patient sign. If sending hard copies of the medical record, the copied records would be placed in an envelope, labeled with the patient's ID label, and handed to the transport person who arrives to transport the patient. The records could also be faxed to the receiving facility. When paper charts are used, the original documents are returned to their proper order in the patient's paper chart.

6. a. coordinates the patient's care to improve quality of care while reducing costs; interacts on a daily basis with the patient, the patient's family, health care team members, and payer representatives; acts as the patient's advocate in getting home health services that best suit the patient's needs; coordinates financial coverage through private insurers such as Medicare
   b. usually is requested for chronically ill, seriously ill, or injured patients, as well as for long-term high-cost cases

7. a. financial assistance for patients
   b. transportation home
   c. arrangement of meals for families staying at hospital or for patients for home after discharge
   d. support for abuse victims (call protective services if necessary)

e. assistance in planning custodial care

f. arrangement of homebound teacher or in-hospital teacher

g. evaluation of home care providers

h. arrangement of living assistance for families of patients when necessary

8. Notify the department or facility that performs the test or examination; schedule a time convenient for the involved department and the patient; advise the patient's nurse to inform the patient and/or patient's family; record the scheduled time on the patient's Kardex form.

9. a. Arrange with the pharmacy for medications the patient is taking.

b. Note on the census when the patient leaves and returns.

c. Cancel meals for the length of the absence.

d. Cancel any hospital treatments for the length of the absence.

e. Arrange for any special equipment that the patient may need.

f. Provide the nurse with a temporary absence release to have the patient sign.

10. Any six of the following examples:
- Call patient's family to come to the hospital
- Diabetic nurse to do diabetic teaching with patient
- Have ostomy nurse work with and train patient in colostomy care
- Transfer patient to the parent teaching or transition room, and teach mother to change dressings; also, train in feeding tube care and feeding technique
- Cardiopulmonary (resp care) to do preop and postop teaching
- Preop teaching
- No visitors, limited number of visitors, or have visitors speak $\bar{c}$ nurse before seeing pt
- DNR/DNI (do not resuscitate/do not intubate) or no code
- NINP (no information, no publication)
- Notify Dr. John Sinclair of pt.'s adm to ICU
- Notify hospitalist if systolic BP >190

11. A do not resuscitate/do not intubate (DNR/DNI) order may be requested by a patient on admission. This order is not a complete refusal of care; it simply states that a resuscitation code should not be performed in the event of cardiac or respiratory arrest. A verbal request by a patient or a patient's family member is not legal.

12. A room with a bed where a parent can stay with his or her child so that after training he or she can assume full care of the child. The child then may be discharged to the parent's care.

Note: DNR/DNI must be a written doctor's order to be legal.

13. Many pediatric hospitals and/or units have a patient room with a bed for a parent to stay 24 hours a day with his or her child. The parent, after training, will assume full care of the child. The child then may be discharged to the parent's care.

CHAPTER 19

Exercise 1

1. MSSU
2. postop
3. OBS
4. Dx
5. preop
6. OPS
7. SSU
8. BIBA
9. DOA
10. IVDU

Exercise 2

1. outpatient surgery
2. before surgery
3. diagnosis
4. observation
5. after surgery
6. medical short stay unit
7. short stay unit
8. brought in by ambulance
9. dead on arrival
10. intravenous drug user

Review Questions

1. a. the number assigned to the patient on or before admission; it is used for records identification and for all subsequent admissions to that hospital (also may be called *health* or *medical record number*)

b. a number assigned to the patient to access insurance information; usually a unique number is assigned each time the patient is admitted to the hospital

c. surgery on part of the GI tract performed as a treatment for morbid obesity

d. pertaining to the time of surgery

e. a list of all occupied (including patient name, age, acuity, and doctor's name) and unoccupied hospital beds

f. the process of entering personal information into the hospital information system to enroll a person as a hospital patient and create a patient record; patients may be registered as inpatients, outpatients, or observation patients

g. signature of permission obtained after the patient has been given a description of the procedure, alternatives, risks, probable results, and anything else that is generally disclosed to patients

h. one or more disorders (or diseases) in addition to a primary disease or disorder, or the effect of such additional disorders or diseases

i. surgery that is not emergency or mandatory and can be planned at the patient's convenience

j. the process of obtaining information and partially preparing admitting forms before the time of the patient's arrival at the health care facility

k. an example of an alarm system that includes monitoring software and an ankle bracelet that contains a tiny radio transmitter designed to prevent infants from being removed from a health care facility without authorization

l. a viewing screen located in the surgical waiting areas and the hospital cafeteria designed to keep family and friends updated on the status of a surgical patient

m. a form used to record daily admissions, discharges, and transfers for quick reference and to assist in tracking empty beds.

n. a book used for a long-term record of admissions, discharges, and transfers for future reference. A patients' ID label is placed in the book with the date of admission entered next to it

o. a whiteboard located in the nurses' station area on which to record census information such as unit room numbers, admitting doctors' names, and the name of the nurse assigned to each patient. The patient's name intentionally may be omitted to maintain patient confidentiality.

2. a.
   - scheduled
   - direct
   - urgent
   - emergency
   b.
   - inpatient
   - observation patient
   - outpatient

3. a. A doctor with admitting privileges to the hospital must authorize a patient's admission.
   b. The admitting diagnosis and/or patient age usually determines the type of nursing unit that is suitable, and the nursing staff usually decides on the specific bed.

4. a. Copy insurance cards.
   b. Verify insurance (may be done in advance when admission is scheduled).
   c. Ask patient or patient guardian to sign appropriate insurance forms.
   d. Interview patient or family to obtain personal information.
   e. Prepare admission forms (admission service agreement and face sheet) and obtain signatures.
   f. Ask patient whether he or she has an advance directives document or would like to create one (required in most states).
   g. Prepare patient's identification bracelet and, if necessary, identification labels—patients may be asked to read and initial information on bracelet.
   h. Secure patient valuables if necessary.
   i. Supply and explain required information, including a copy of the Patients' Bill of Rights and hospital privacy laws (required by The Joint Commission [TJC]).
   j. Include any test results, prewritten orders, or consents that were previously sent to the admitting department in the packet that accompanies the patient to the nursing unit.

5.
   - Protect confidentiality.
   - Ensure privacy when asking for personal information.
   - Be proficient and professional.
   - Asking whether the patient was hospitalized previously can hasten the registration process and reduce the risk of error in assignment of health information management and patient account numbers (demographics would have to be verified in case of possible changes).
   - Treat each patient as an individual.
   - Listen carefully.
   - Project a friendly, courteous attitude.
   - Include family or significant other in the process.

6. a. A form initiated by the admitting department and included in the inpatient medical record that contains personal and demographic information, usually computer generated at the time of admission (also may be called the *information sheet* or *front sheet*).
   b. A form signed on the patient's admission that sets forth the general services that the hospital will provide; also may be called *conditions of admission, contract for services,* or *treatment consent.*
   c. A plastic band with a patient identification label affixed to it that is worn by the patient throughout hospitalization. In the obstetrics department, the mother and the baby would share the same identification label affixed to their ID bracelets.
   e. Self-adhesive labels used on the patient's identification bracelet to identify forms, requisitions, specimens, and so forth.
   f. When a patient chooses to have valuable items placed in the safe, the items are put into a numbered valuables envelope and the patient is given a numbered claim check. The number is entered electronically or handwritten in the patient's chart, and the envelope is placed in the hospital safe.

7. a.
   - allergy alert—red
   - fall risk—yellow
   - DNR/DNI—purple
   b.
   - seizure alert
   - diabetic
   - extremity restriction
   - isolation

8. a. a legal document that indicates a patient's wishes in the event that the patient becomes incapacitated and unable to make decisions regarding medical care
   b. living will and a power of attorney for health care

9. a. admitting diagnosis
   b. diet
   c. activity
   d. diagnostic tests and procedures
   e. medications
   f. treatment orders
   g. request for old records
   h. patient care category or code status

10. a. Greet the patient on his or her arrival to the nursing unit. Also applicable when EMR is used.
   b. Inform the patient that the nurse will be notified of his or her arrival; notify the nurse who will be caring for the patient of the arrival. Also applicable when EMR is used.
   c. Notify the attending doctor and/or hospital resident or the hospitalist of the patient's arrival. Also applicable when EMR is used.
   d. Move the patient's name from the admission screen on the computer to the correct bed on the nursing unit. Also applicable when EMR is used.
   e. Record the patient's admission on the admission, discharge, and transfer log sheet (ADT log sheet) and the census board. Also applicable when EMR is used.
   f. Check the patient's signature on the admission service agreement form.
   g. Complete the procedure for preparation of the paper chart.

h. Prepare any other labels or identification cards used by the facility. Also applicable when EMR is used.

i. Place the patient identification labels in the correct place in the patient's paper chart, or place in the nursing unit patient label book if EMR is used.

j. Fill in all the necessary information on the patient's Kardex form, or enter it into the computer if Kardex is computerized (if paper charts used); place the Kardex form in the proper place in the Kardex file (if paper charts used).

k. Enter appropriate required data into the computer (if this is a HUC responsibility), or scan required forms into the patient's EMR if the EMR is used.

l. Place the allergy information in all the designated areas, or write "NKA" (if paper charts used); prepare an allergy bracelet with allergies written on it to be placed on the patient's wrist if necessary.

m. Note code status on front of chart if necessary (if paper charts used).

n. Place a label or a piece of red tape stating "name alert" on the spine of the chart if there is a patient on the unit with the same or a similar name (if paper charts used).

o. Transcribe the admission orders according to hospital policy (if paper charts used); monitor the patient's EMR if EMR is used.

11. a. A surgical patient's admission is basically the same as a medical patient's admission, except that the preop tests, x-ray studies, and so on should be performed as soon as possible.

b. Surgeries may be performed on an inpatient basis (patient admitted before surgery day), on an outpatient basis (in the outpatient department of the hospital or an off-campus surgicenter), or as a same-day surgery (patient is admitted the day surgery is to be performed).

12. a. This is the area where a patient is prepared for surgery. It is also a waiting area for surgical patients.

b. Procedures may include shaving the surgical area, insertion of a saline lock, starting of IV fluids, and/or insertion of a catheter (may be done in the operating room). Preoperative breathing treatments may also be administered in this area. If the patient is a same-day surgery admission, the surgical consent form will also be signed and witnessed here. The anesthesiologist and surgeon will visit the patient; the patient will be asked to repeat his or her name and a second identifier such as birth date by both doctors. The anesthesiologist will ask the patient to again state the last time he or she had anything to eat or drink and whether the patient has any allergies (even though this information has been documented by the nurse). The surgeon will ask the patient to state the surgery that is to be performed and will usually mark the operative area with a black marker.

13. a. description of surgery for surgery consent

b. laxatives or enemas

c. shaves, scrubs, or showers

d. name of anesthesiologist or anesthesiology group

e. miscellaneous orders

f. diet (anesthesiologist usually writes this order)

g. preoperative medication (anesthesiologist usually writes this order)

14. a. current history and physical record (H&P)

b. accurate, signed, and dated surgery consent

c. blood consent or refusal

d. signed admission service agreement (also called *conditions of admission*)

e. completed nursing preoperative checklist

f. MAR

g. all preoperative diagnostic test results

15. a. Label the surgery forms with the patient's identification labels, and place them within the patient's paper chart (if paper charts used).

b. Check the patient's electronic or paper chart for the history and physical report (H&P); check the patient's electronic or paper chart for the required signed consent forms.

c. Check the patient's electronic or paper chart for any previously ordered diagnostic studies such as laboratory tests, x-ray examinations, and so forth.

d. File the current medication administration record in the patient's chart (if paper charts used).

e. Print at least five face sheets to place in the paper chart. If the EMR is used, maintain five face sheets in a notebook to provide to consulting doctors and other health care providers as requested.

f. Place at least three sheets of patient identification labels in the patient's paper chart. If the EMR is used, maintain three sheets of labels in a notebook to label specimens as necessary.

g. Notify the appropriate nursing personnel when surgery calls for the patient.

16.
- diet
- intake and output
- intravenous fluids
- vital signs
- catheters, tubes, and drains
- activity
- positioning
- observation of the operative site
- medications

17. 1. a. Inform the patient's nurse of the patient's arrival to the PACU as soon as possible.

b. Inform the patient's nurse of the expected arrival of the patient from the recovery room. (Also applicable when EMR is used).

2. Place all operating records behind the proper divider in the patient's chart.

3. Write the date of surgery and the surgical procedure in the designated places on the patient's Kardex form or in the computer.

4. Transcribe the doctors' postoperative orders. Notify the nurse who is caring for the patient of stat doctors' orders. (All preoperative orders are automatically discontinued postoperatively. The HUC usually starts a new Kardex form for the patient).

18. a. It is designed to keep family and friends updated on the status of a surgical patient.

b. It keeps the family and friends of the surgery patient informed and allows them the ability to leave the waiting area to get a meal or cup of coffee in the cafeteria without worrying about missing information about the patient.

19. It is important that the HUC monitor the patient's electronic medical record (EMR) consistently, including admission, preoperative, and postoperative orders, for tasks that may need to be performed. The surgical consent is usually entered into the patient's EMR so the HUC can prepare the consent for the patient's nurse to have the patient sign.

20. It is equally important that the HUC scan signed consent forms, handwritten progress notes, and/or records faxed, sent, or brought in with the patient from other facilities.

CHAPTER 20

Exercise 1

1. AMA
2. Disch
3. ECF
4. SNF
5. Trans

Exercise 2

1. against medical advice
2. discharge
3. extended care facility
4. skilled nursing facility
5. transfer

Review Questions

1. a. examination of a body after death; it may be performed to determine the cause of death or for medical research purposes
    b. occurs when no brain function is present
    c. an illness ending in death
    d. death
    e. after death
    f. care and services of a nonmedical nature, which consist of feeding, bathing, watching, and protecting the patient
    g. the process of removing donated organs; may also be referred to as *harvesting*
    h. donating or giving one's organs and/or tissues after death; one may designate specific organs (e.g., only cornea) or may donate any needed organs
    i. a signed consent that authorizes a specific funeral home or agency to remove the deceased from a health care facility
    j. a death that occurs because of sudden, violent, or unexplained circumstances, or a patient who expires unexpectedly within the first 24 hours after admission to the hospital; deaths investigated by a coroner
    k. a medical facility for patients who require expert nursing care or custodial care; may also be referred to as a *skilled nursing facility*
    l. a meeting that includes the doctor or doctors caring for the patient, the primary nurses, the case manager or social worker, and other caregivers (may include family) involved in the patient's care
    m. centralized, coordinated, multidisciplinary process that ensures that the patient has a plan for continuing care after leaving the hospital

2.
    a. To review and evaluate the goals and outcomes of the patient's recovery progress and to modify the care plan as needed. Often a patient care conference is scheduled before the time of a patient's discharge so that a post hospitalization care plan can be developed.
    b. The case manager or social worker works with the patient and the patient's family, nurses, and physician(s).

3. a.
    - discharge home
    - discharge to another facility
    - discharge home with assistance
    - discharge against medical advice (AMA)
    - expiration
    b. often there are patients waiting to be admitted, some for hours in the emergency department. Withholding notification of a discharge order will cause a delay in a patient's admission and treatment.

4. a. Read the entire order carefully when transcribing the discharge order.
    b. Notify the discharged patient's nurse when a discharge order has been written (when the EMR with CPOE is implemented, the HUC may print out the medication information sheets for medications that the patient will be taking after discharge).
    c. Enter a "pending discharge" with the expected departure time into the computer.
    d. Explain the procedure for discharge to the patient and/or the patient's relatives.
    e. If necessary, notify other departments that may be giving the patient daily treatments.
    f. Arrange for any appointments requested by the doctor.
    g. Arrange transportation if required.
    h. Prepare credit slips for medications returned to the pharmacy or equipment and supplies returned to the central services department (CSD).
    i. Notify nursing personnel or transportation service to transport the patient to the discharge area when the patient is ready to leave.
    j. Write the patient's name on the admission, discharge, and transfer sheet, and erase the patient's name from the unit census board.
    k. Notify environmental services to clean the discharged patient's room.
    l. Prepare the patient's paper chart for the health information management services (HIMS) department.

5. a.
    - Notify case management or social service of the doctor's orders to discharge to another facility.
    - Transportation usually will be arranged by the case manager or social worker.
    - Complete the continuing care or transfer form (the case worker or social worker may complete the form).
    - Print from the computer or photocopy patient chart forms as requested in the doctor's orders. Once the copies have been made, it is important to place the *original* paper chart forms back into the patient's chart in proper sequence.
    - Place the continuing care form and requested chart form *copies* in a sealed envelope with the patient's identification label affixed on the outside of the envelope.
    - Complete the procedures for a routine discharge.

b.
- Notify case management or social service of the doctor's discharge to home with assistance order.
- Prepare the continuing care form.
- Obtain a release of information signature from the patient.
- Print from the computer or photocopy the chart forms as indicated in the doctor's order; replace *originals* in patient's chart.
- Place the continuing care form and *copies* of chart forms as required and give to appropriate family member.
- Complete the procedures for a routine discharge.

6.
- Check the summary or DRG worksheet for the doctor's summation and the patient's final diagnosis. It is important to have this information on patient discharge so that coding of diagnosis-related groups may be placed on the chart by HIMS personnel.
- Check for the correct patient identification labels on chart forms.
- Shred all chart forms that have been labeled and have no documentation on them.
- Check for old records or split records and send with the chart to HIMS.
- Arrange chart forms in discharge sequence according to hospital policy.
- Send the discharged patient's chart to HIMS, along with any old records of the patient (must be sent the same day as discharge).

7. Ask the patient to be seated until the nurse is advised. The hospitalist, resident, or admitting doctor may be called to speak with the patient. The patient may be advised that insurance may not cover the hospital bill if the patient leaves against medical advice. Everything possible is done to encourage the patient to remain in the hospital until treatment has been completed; however, if the patient insists on leaving, a release form would be prepared.

8. a.
- The HUC may be asked to call a member of the clergy from a specific religion to speak with the patient or to perform final rites.
- A notation should be made on the patient's Kardex form of any final rites that have been performed. It is important to remind clergy that a lighted candle may not be used when oxygen is in use in the patient's room.
- The HUC may be asked to call family.
- He or she may be asked to call the morgue.
- He or she may prepare required forms for family to sign.

b. The hospitalist, resident, or doctor must be notified to pronounce the patient dead and record the time of death. The patient's doctor must complete a death certificate, and a report of the death must be filed with the Bureau of Vital Statistics.

9. a. Most hospitals have a stretcher with a lower compartment that may be covered with a sheet to transport a deceased patient, making it unnecessary to close the doors to patient rooms on the unit when the patient is being transported to the morgue.

b. The HUC would prepare forms for the family to sign and make necessary calls if and when requested to do so.

10. In most cases, in order to be an organ donor the patient must be declared brain dead (referred to as *clinical death*) and be connected to a ventilator.

11. a. The law gives the coroner permission to study the body by dissection to determine whether evidence of foul play is present.

b. A coroner's case is one in which the patient's death is a result of sudden, violent, or unexplained circumstances, such as an accident, a poisoning, or a gunshot wound. Deaths that occur less than 24 hours after the start of hospitalization may also be called coroner's cases.

12. a. Contact the attending doctor, hospitalist, or resident when asked by the nurse to do so, to verify the patient's death. The HUC will notify the attending or other doctors involved in patient's care when requested to do so.

b. Notify the hospital operator of the patient's death.

c. Prepare any forms that may be needed. Check the chart for a signed autopsy consent form.

d. Notify the mortuary that has been requested by the family.

e. Check the chart or ask the patient's nurse to determine whether the body is to be taken to the morgue or is to remain there until the mortuary arrives.

f. The nurse or CNA will gather the clothes of the deceased and will place them in a patient belongings bag to be labeled with the patient's name, the room number, and the date.

h. Obtain the mortuary book from the nursing office, or have a mortuary form prepared when the mortician arrives.

i. Complete the procedures for a routine discharge.

13. a. a change in status of acuity (for nursing care)

b. the need for an isolation room

14. a. Transcribe the order for a transfer from one unit to another unit.

b. Notify the nurse who is caring for the patient of the transfer order. Notify the admitting department of the transfer order to obtain a new room assignment.

c. Communicate new unit and room assignment to the nurse who is caring for the patient.
Notify the receiving unit of the transfer by telephone or by computer.

d. Record the transfer on the unit admission, discharge, and transfer log sheet (ADT log sheet).

e. Send the patient's chart, Kardex form, and current MAR with the patient to the receiving unit (if paper charts are used). Send all thinned records, old records, (if paper charts are used), and x-ray films with the patient to the receiving unit.

f. Erase the patient's name from the census board.

g. Notify all departments that perform regularly scheduled treatments on the patient via computer. Notify the nutritional care department of the transfer via computer.

h. Notify environmental services to clean the room.

i. Notify the attending doctor and all other doctors involved with the patient's care.

15. a. Transcribe the order for the transfer to another room on the same unit.

b. Notify the nurse who is caring for the patient of the request for transfer.

c. Place the patient's chart in the correct slot in the chart rack after correcting the labels on the patient's chart and replacing patient ID labels with corrected labels, and place the Kardex form in its new place in the Kardex form file (if paper charts are used).

d. Move the patient's name to the correct bed on the computer census screen; send the change to the nutritional care department (if paper charts are used).

e. Record the transfer on the unit admission, discharge, and transfer log sheet (ADT log sheet).

f. Notify environmental services to clean the room (when EMR is used, the request will be sent to environmental services automatically).

g. Notify the switchboard and the information center of the change (may not be necessary when EMR is used).

16. a. Notify the nurse who is caring for the patient of the expected arrival of a transferred patient.

b. Introduce yourself to the transferred patient on his or her arrival to the unit, and notify the nurse who is caring for the patient of the transferred patient's arrival.

c. Place the patient's chart in the correct slot in the chart holder, print corrected patient ID labels, label the patient's chart, and place the Kardex form in the proper place (if paper charts are used).

d. Record the receiving of a transfer patient on the unit admission, discharge, and transfer log sheet, and write the patient's name on the census board.

e. Notify the nutritional care department of the patient's transfer.

f. Move the patient's name from the unit the patient came from and place it in the correct bed on the computer census screen.

g. Transcribe any new doctors' orders (if paper charts are used).

17. Discharge or transfer orders may include orders to be carried out before the time of a patient's discharge or information such as instructions for the patient to follow after leaving the hospital, requests for appointments for the patient, and so forth.

18. Additional tasks include monitoring the patient's EMR, printing forms from the computer, and scanning consents, handwritten progress notes, and other records or reports into the patient's EMR.

CHAPTER 21

Exercise 1

1. Occupational Safety and Health Administration
2. methicillin-resistant *Staphylococcus aureus*
3. AIDS-related complex
4. Centers for Disease Control and Prevention
5. personal protective equipment
6. Rescue individuals in danger; Alarm—Sound the alarm; Confine the fire by closing all doors and windows; Extinguish the fire with the nearest suitable fire extinguisher
7. acquired immunodeficiency syndrome
8. hepatitis C virus
9. tuberculosis
10. human immunodeficiency virus
11. hepatitis B virus

Exercise 2

1. OSHA
2. MRSA
3. ARC
4. CDC
5. PPE
6. RACE
7. AIDS
8. HCV
9. TB
10. HIV
11. HBV

Review Questions

1. a. condition in which the patient's heart contractions are absent or insufficient to produce a pulse or blood pressure (may also be referred to as *code arrest*)

b. condition in which the patient ceases to breathe or respirations are so depressed that the blood cannot receive sufficient oxygen and therefore the body cells die (also may be referred to as *code arrest*)

c. disease that may be transmitted from one person to another

d. cart stocked by the nursing and pharmacy staff with emergency medication, advanced breathing supplies, intravenous solutions and appropriate tubing, needles, a heart monitor and defibrillator, an oxygen tank, and a suction machine (used in emergency situations)

e. disease-carrying organisms too small to be seen with the naked eye

f. an emergency that is life-threatening

g. placement of a patient apart from other patients for the purpose of preventing the spread of infection, or protecting a patient whose immune system is compromised

h. an episode that does not normally occur within the regular hospital routine and may involve patients, visitors, physicians, hospital staff, or students

i. coordinates with health officials when it comes to reporting and monitoring incidents of infectious diseases that may lead to epidemic outbreaks

j. a department in the hospital that addresses the prevention and containment of liability regarding patient care incidents

k. a planned procedure that is carried out by hospital personnel when a large number of people may have been injured or exposed to hazardous materials

l. infections that are acquired within the health care facility

2. a.
   • accidents
   • thefts from persons on hospital property
   • errors of omission of patient treatment or errors in administration of patient treatment, including medication
   • exposure to blood and body fluids, as may be caused by a needle stick

b. Documentation of all incidents is important in identifying hazards and preventing continuing problems and in the case of a lawsuit that may arise from them.

3. a.
   - infectious agent or pathogen (bacteria)
   - reservoir or source in which pathogen can live and grow (e.g., human body, contaminated water or food, animals, insects)
   - means of escape (e.g., blood, urine, feces, wound drainage)
   - route of transmission (e.g., air, contact, body excretions)
   - point of entrance (e.g., mouth, nostrils, breaks in the skin)
   - susceptible host (individual who does not have adequate resistance to the invading pathogen)

   b.
   - gloves
   - gown—moisture-resistant gowns
   - mask—pocket masks with one-way valves
   - goggles or glasses

4. a. active tuberculosis (TB)
   b. measles
   c. chicken pox
   d. meningitis

5. A culture is the most common way to confirm and identify microorganisms; sensitivity testing determines which antibiotics will destroy the identified microbes.

6. a. Hands should be washed when one arrives at work, before and after personal breaks, and after any patient specimen is handled (even if bagged).
   b. Clean the telephone receiver with an antiseptic wipe on arrival and periodically throughout the day.
   c. Use antiseptic solution frequently throughout the day.
   d. Avoid putting your hands on your face, in your eyes, or in your mouth while at the nursing station.

7. a. organ transplant recipients
   b. burn victims
   c. those receiving chemotherapy

8. a.
   - sexual contact
   - use of needles that were previously injected into someone who carried the AIDS virus
   - from an infected mother to her infant during pregnancy, birth, or breast feeding
   - through blood transfusions

   b. *Pneumocystis jiroveci* pneumonia (PCP), pneumonia caused by *P. jiroveci* , and Kaposi sarcoma (KS), an otherwise rare skin cancer

9. a. hepatitis B virus (HBV)
   b. *Mycobacterium tuberculosis*

10. *Streptococcus*, *Staphylococcus*, Clostridium, Enterococcus, and *Pseudomonas*. Methicillin-resistant *Staphylococcus aureus* (MRSA) is a variation of the common bacterial species *S. aureus*.

11. Excellent hand-washing technique is the best way for health care workers to stop the spread of nosocomial infection.

12.

   Provide accurate information to inquiring visitors.
   Order PPE and isolation packs as needed.
   Wear gloves when handling or transporting specimen
   Practice good hand-washing technique throughout the working day.
   Eating, drinking (open cups), and handling of contact lenses should not be done at the nursing station.
   Food should not be stored in refrigerators with specimens.

13. a. code red (fire)
    b. code blue (cardiac or respiratory arrest)
    c. code orange (hazardous material spill)
    d. code pink or amber alert (infant or child abduction)
    e. code gray (combative person)
    f. code silver (person with a weapon or hostage situation)

14. A material safety data sheet (MSDS) is a communication tool that provides details on chemical dangers and safety procedures.

15. *R*—Rescue individuals in danger.
    A—Alarm: Sound the alarm.
    C—Confine the fire by closing all doors and windows.
    E—Extinguish the fire with the nearest suitable fire extinguisher.

16. a. The HUC may be expected to assist with the evacuation of patients who are endangered by the fire. If the fire is not on the unit, the HUC may help nursing personnel to close the doors to patient rooms. All hospital units or sections of the hospital are separated by fire doors. These doors are constructed to help contain the fire in one area.
    b. The HUC usually is designated to handle communication and to call off-duty health care personnel to assist in caring for hospital patients and disaster victims and in handling communications. The role of the HUC varies among hospitals.

17.
   - Avoid the use of extension cords.
   - Do not overload electrical circuits.
   - Inspect cords and plugs for breaks and fraying.
   - Unplug equipment when servicing.
   - Unplug equipment that has liquid spilled in it.
   - Unplug and do not use equipment that is malfunctioning.

18.
   - Notify the hospital telephone operator to announce the code.
   - Direct the code arrest team to the patient's room.
   - Remove the patient information sheet from the patient's chart, and take or send the chart to the patient's room.
   - Notify all doctors connected with the patient's case (attending doctor, consultants, and residents).
   - Notify the patient's family of the situation if requested to do so.
   - Label laboratory specimens with the patient's ID label; enter the test ordered in the computer, and send the specimen to the laboratory stat.
   - Call the appropriate departments for treatments and supplies as needed.
   - Alert the admissions department and the intensive care unit (ICU) about the possibility of a transfer to ICU.
   - For a successful code, follow the procedure regarding transfer to another unit.

   (For an unsuccessful code procedure, follow Procedure 20-4 regarding postmortem care).

19. Multiple injury car accident
    Train or airplane accident
    A bombing
    An earthquake
    Infectious disease outbreak
    A group of people exposed to hazardous chemicals

20. a. In larger hospitals the task of delivering flowers to patients may be assigned to a hospital volunteer. In this case the HUC may need only to direct the volunteer to the correct room. In hospitals in which the representative from the florist delivers the flowers directly to the unit, the HUC should ascertain that the patient is still on the unit or within the hospital before signing for and accepting the flowers. After signing the delivery slip, the HUC may deliver the flowers to the patient's room. The HUC must be aware of any restrictions—for example, flowers are not allowed on some nursing units, such as intensive care or cardiopulmonary (respiratory care) units, and latex balloons are not allowed in most hospitals (especially not on pediatric units). If family members are present, flowers and balloons may be sent home with them.

b. Mail is delivered to the nursing unit daily. The mail is checked, and the patient's room and bed numbers are written on each envelope. In the event that the patient has been discharged, the HUC would write "Discharged" in pencil on the envelope and return it to the mailroom. The mail may be distributed to patients as time allows, or the task may be designated to a hospital volunteer.

CHAPTER 22

Unit 1

Exercise 1

1.

WR	CV	S
cyt /	o /	logy
cell		study of

2.

WR	S
gastr /	ectomy
stomach	excision, surgical removal of

3.

P	WR	S
sub /	hepat/	ic
under	liver	pertaining to

4.

WR	CV	WR	CV	S
electr /	o /	cardi /	o /	gram
electricity		heart		record of

5.

WR	CV	S
cardi /	o /	logy
heart		study of

6.

P	WR	S
trans /	hepat/	ic
across	liver	pertaining to

Exercise 2

1. cardiology
2. cytology
3. gastrectomy
4. gastroenteritis
5. gastric
6. intragastric
7. nephrectomy

Review Questions

1. a. languages past and present: Greek (example: *nephrology*), Latin (example: *maternal*), and modern languages, such as French (example: *lavage*).

b. eponyms—generally named after discoverer (example: *Papanicolaou [Pap] smear*)

c. acronyms—words formed from first letter of a descriptive phrase (example: *laser*)

2. a. word root: the basic part of a word (example: *gastr/ic*)

b. prefix: the part of the word placed before the word root to alter its meaning (example: *intra/gastric*)

c. suffix: the part of the word added at the end of the word to alter its meaning (Example: gastr/ic)

d. combining vowel: usually an *o* used between word roots or between a word root and a suffix (example: *gastr/o/enteritis*)

3. a. A combining vowel is not used when a prefix and a word root are connected.

b. When two word roots are connected, the combining vowel usually is used even if the second root begins with a vowel.

c. When a word root is connected to a suffix, a combining vowel usually is not used if the suffix begins with a vowel.

4. a. dividing medical terms into word parts and identifying each word part

b. when given a definition of a medical condition, using word parts to build corresponding medical terms

Unit 2

Review Questions

1.
- The cell is the basic unit of all living things—the human body is made up of trillions of cells.
- The cell membrane (eggshell), the boundary of the cell, actively or passively regulates the movement of a substance into and out of the cell. The cell membrane keeps the cell intact. The cell dies if the cell membrane can no longer carry out these functions.
- The cytoplasm (egg white) is the main body of the cell in which are found various organelles, such as the mitochondria, which are specialized structures that carry out activities necessary for the cell's survival.
- The nucleus (egg yolk), a small structure, is located near the center of the cell. It is the control center of the cell and plays an important role in reproduction. Chromosomes located in the nucleus contain the genes that determine hereditary characteristics.

2.
- Epithelial tissue: Epithelial tissue forms a protective covering (skin) and lines body cavities (e.g., digestive, respiratory, and urinary tracts).
- Connective tissue: The main functions of connective tissue are to connect and hold tissues together, to transport substances, and to protect against foreign invaders. Connective tissue forms and protects bones, fat, blood cells, and cartilage and provides immunity.
- Muscle tissue: Muscle tissue makes up the muscles of the body that contract and relax to produce movement.
- Nerve tissue: Nerve tissue forms parts of the nervous system, which conducts electrochemical impulses and helps to coordinate body activities.

3. a. An organ is made up of two or more types of tissues that perform one or more common functions.

b. A system is made up of a group of organs that work closely together with a common purpose to perform complex body functions.

4.
- Cranial cavity—brain
- Spinal cavity—spinal core
- Thoracic cavity—any one of the following: heart, lungs, trachea, esophagus, thymus gland, and major blood vessels
- Abdominal cavity—any one of the following: stomach; most of the intestines; and the kidneys, ureters, liver, pancreas, gallbladder, and spleen
- Pelvic cavity—any one of the following: bladder, urethra, reproductive organs, part of the large intestine (sigmoid colon), and the rectum

5. a. right upper quadrant (RUQ), left upper quadrant (LUQ), right lower quadrant (RLQ), and left lower quadrant (LLQ)

b. right hypochondriac region, epigastric region, left hypochondriac region, right lumbar region, umbilical region, left lumbar region, right iliac region, hypogastric region, left iliac region

6. The anatomical position is the point of reference that ensures proper description: body erect, face and feet forward, arms at side, and palms facing forward.

7. 1. e
2. d
3. h
4. c
5. a
6. b
7. g
8. f
9. k
10. i
11. l
12. j
13. n
14. m
15. p
16. o

8. a. protects the underlying tissues
b. assists in regulating body temperature
c. passes messages of pain, cold, and touch to the brain
d. synthesis of vitamin K

9. a. epidermis
b. dermis, or true skin
c. subcutaneous tissue (or hypodermis)

10. a. melanin
b. albinism

11. oil glands (sebaceous glands)

12. sweat glands (sudoriferous glands)

13. a. Change in bowel or bladder habits
A sore that does not heal
Unusual bleeding or discharge
Thickening or lump in the breast, testes, or elsewhere
Indigestion or difficulty in swallowing
Obvious change in a wart or mole
Nagging cough or hoarseness
b. First-degree burns damage the epidermis.
Second-degree burns damage the epidermis and the dermis.

Third-degree burns destroy the epidermis, dermis, and subcutaneous tissue.

14. 1. b
2. a or h
3. e
4. f
5. d
6. c
7. h
8. g

Exercise 1

1. internal organs
2. skin
3. cell
4. tissue
5. skin
6. hair
7. disease
8. cancer
9. connective tissue, flesh
10. epithelium
11. fat
12. tumor
13. skin
14. cancer
15. nail
16. life

Exercise 2

1. pertaining to
2. study of
3. one who specializes in the diagnosis and treatment of (specialist, physician)
4. resembling
5. inflammation
6. tumor
7. producing, originating, causing
8. through, across, beyond
9. pertaining to
10. under or below
11. to view

Exercise 3

Word Part	Type of Word Part
1. cyt / o	WR/CF
2. a. derm / o,	WR/CF
b. dermat / o	WR/CF
c. cutane / o	WR/CF
3. , -logist	S
4. , -oid	S
5. viscer / o	WR/CF
6. hist / o	WR/CF
7. a. -al	S
b. –ous	S
8. , -logy	S
9. trans-	P
10. a. carcin / o,	WR/CF
b. cancer / o	WR/CF
11. sub-	P
12. onc/o	WR/CF

Exercise 4

1.	WR	CV	S		
	cyt /	o /	logy		study of cells
2.	WR	S			
	trich /	oid			resembling hair
3.	WR	CV	S		
	path /	o /	logy		study of (body changes caused by) disease
4.	WR	CV	S		
	path /	o /	genic		producing disease
5.	WR	S			
	derm /	al			pertaining to skin
6.	WR	S			
	cyt /	oid			resembling a cell
7.	WR	S			
	viscer /	al			pertaining to internal organs
8.	WR	CV	S		
	hist /	o /	logy		study of tissue
9.	WR	CV	S		
	dermat /	o /	logist		one who specializes in the diagnosis and treatment of skin (diseases)
10.	WR	S			
	dermat /	itis			inflammation of the skin
11.	WR	CV	S		
	carcin /	o /	genic		producing cancer
12.	WR	S			
	epitheli/	al			pertaining to epithelium
13.	WR	S			
	carcin /	oma			cancerous tumor
14.	WR	S			
	epitheli /	oma			tumor composed of epithelial (cells)
15.	WR	S			
	sarc /	oma			tumor composed of connective tissue
16.	WR	S			
	lip /	oma			tumor (containing) fat
17.	WR	CV	S		
	path /	o /	logist		one who specializes in the diagnosis and treatment of disease
18.	WR	S			
	dermat /	oid			resembling skin
	WR	S			
	derm/	oid			resembling skin
19.	WR	CV	S		
	dermat /	o /	logy		study of skin (branch of medicine that deals with skin diseases)
20.	P	WR	S		
	trans /	derm /	al		pertaining to (entering) through the skin
21.	WR	CV	S		
	onc /	o /	logy		study of tumors (cancer)
22.	P	WR	S		
	sub /	ungu /	al		pertaining to under the nail
23.	P	WR	S		
	sub /	cutane/	ous		pertaining to under the skin
24.	P		S		
	bi/		opsy		view of life
25.	WR	CV	S		
	onc/	o/	logist		One who specializes in the diagnosis and treatment of tumors (cancer)

Exercise 5

1. cytoid
2. trichoid
3. a. dermoid
   b. dermatoid
4. pathologist
5. dermatologist
6. a. dermal
   b. cutaneous
7. visceral
8. histology
9. pathology
10. dermatology
11. pathogenic
12. cytology
13. dermatitis
14. lipoma
15. epithelioma
16. epithelial
17. carcinogenic
18. sarcoma
19. carcinoma
20. a. transdermal
    b. transcutaneous
21. oncology
22. subungual
23. subcutaneous
24. biopsy
25. oncologist

Exercise 6

Spelling exercise

Exercise 7

- posteroanterior
- right upper quadrant
- anteroposterior
- right lower quadrant
- subcutaneous
- lateral
- cancer
- left lower quadrant
- left upper quadrant
- biopsy

Unit 3

Review Questions

1. a. protects the internal organs
   b. provides the framework for the body
   c. acts with muscles to produce movement

d. produces blood cells

e. stores calcium and phosphorus

2. periosteum

3. a. long, short, flat, and irregular

b. Bones have their own system of blood vessels and nerves.

Bones contain *red bone marrow* (produces red blood cells, white blood cells, and platelets) and yellow *bone marrow* (consists mostly of adipose tissue, or fat).

Bones are covered with a thin membrane called *periosteum*, which is necessary for growth and repair and is the attachment point for ligaments and tendons.

4. a. skull, hyoid bone, vertebral column, and rib cage

b. the limbs that have been appended to the axial skeleton

5. *cranium* (8 bones):

a. frontal, 1

b. parietal, 2

c. temporal, 2

d. ethmoid, 1

e. sphenoid, 1

f. occipital, 1

face (14 bones):

a. maxilla, 2

b. mandible, 1

c. nasal, 2

d. lacrimal, 2

e. zygomatic, 2

f. vomer, 1

g. inferior nasal concha (2)

h. palatine (2)

6. hyoid (1 bone)

7. a. malleus (2)

b. incus (2)

c. stapes (2)

8. a. cervical (7)

b. thoracic (12)

c. lumbar (5)

d. sacrum (1)

e. coccyx (1)

9. a. scapula

b. clavicle

c. humerus

d. radius

e. ulna

f. carpals

g. metacarpals

h. phalanges

10. a. ilium

b. ischium

c. pubis

11. a. femur

b. patella

c. tibia

d. fibula

e. tarsal

f. metatarsal

g. phalanges

12. a. A joint is that place in the skeleton where two or more bones meet. Joints allow for movement and hold bones together.

b. A ligament is a tough band of tissue that connects one bone with another bone at a joint.

13. a. enable movement of body parts

b. maintain posture

c. stabilize joints

d. generate heat

14. a. Skeletal muscles enable the body to move.

Smooth muscles generally make up the walls of hollow organs and serve to propel substances through body passageways and to adjust the body

Cardiac muscle, which is found only in the heart, is an involuntary muscle.

b. Muscles are attached to the bones by tendons.

15. a. osteoarthritis—The most common form of arthritis, usually occurs in weight-bearing joints, such as the hips or knees, as chronic inflammation of the bone and joints caused by degenerative changes in the cartilage covering the surfaces of the joints. It occurs most often in older individuals.

b. rheumatoid arthritis—Rheumatoid arthritis, which is thought to be an autoimmune disease, usually manifests between the ages of 35 and 50 years, more commonly in women.

16. a. laminectomy

b. diskectomy

17. osteoclasts, osteoblasts

18. osteoporosis

19. Any of the following:

• calcium supplements and vitamin D

• weight-bearing exercise

• hormonal replacement therapy (if appropriate)

• correct posture

• drugs to slow down the dissolving process of the osteoclasts

20. a. headaches

b. ringing in the ears

c. hearing loss

d. dizziness

21. a. broken bone, no open wound

b. broken bone, open wound

c. bone has been twisted apart

d. bone is splintered or crushed

e. bone is partially bent and partially broken

f. occurs when the vertebrae collapse by trauma or pathology

22. a. arthroplasty

b. performed to replace an arthritic or damaged joint. An artificial joint, or *prosthesis*, is used to replace the patient's hip or knee joint.

Exercise 1

(*Note:* Not all of the combining forms will be labeled on the diagram.)

1. crani / o

2. clavic / o

3. clavicul / o

4. scapul / o

5. cost / o

6. humer / o

7. stern / o

8. vertebr / o

9. phalang / o

10. femor / o

11. patell / o

12. phalang / o

Exercise 2

1. joint
2. bone
3. rib
4. skull
5. femur
6. muscle
7. humerus
8. patella
9. sternum
10. clavicle
11. scapula
12. phalange
13. vertebra(e)
14. clavicle
15. electrical activity, electricity
16. lamina
17. cartilage
18. meniscus
19. curved (laterally)

Exercise 3

1. phalang / o
2. arthr / o
3. oste / o
4. femor / o
5. patell / o
6. scapul / o
7. vertebr / o
8. a. clavic / o
   b. clavicul / o
9. crani / o
10. stern / o
11. humer / o
12. cost / o
13. a. my / o
    b. myos / o
14. lamin / o
15. chondr / o
16. menisc / o

Exercise 4

1. -plasty
2. -algia
3. a. -ar
   b. -ic
   c. -al
   d. -ous
4. -tomy
5. -ectomy
6. -graph
7. -graphy
8. -gram
9. -trophy
10. -osis
11. -scope
12. -scopy
13. -centesis
14. -pathy

Exercise 5

1. pain
2. instrument to record

3. record, x-ray image
4. process of recording, x-ray imaging
5. surgical incision or to cut into
6. development, nourishment
7. pertaining to
8. surgical repair
9. surgical removal
10. pertaining to
11. abnormal condition
12. visual examination
13. instrument used for visual examination
14. surgical puncture to aspirate fluid
15. disease of

Exercise 6

1. intra-
2. dys-
3. sub-
4. a. a-
   b. an-
5. inter-
6. supra-

Exercise 7

1. within
2. above
3. below
4. difficult, painful, labored, abnormal
5. without
6. between

Exercise 8

1. WR   CV WR CV S
   electr /o /my /o /gram   record of electrical activity of muscle

2. WR S
   my/oma   a tumor (formed of) muscle (tissue)

3. WR   CV WR   S
   stern/o /clavicul /ar   pertaining to the sternum and clavicle

4. WR   S
   crani/al   pertaining to the cranium

5. WR   CV WR   S
   vertebr /o /cost /al   pertaining to the vertebrae and ribs

6. WR   S
   arthr/itis   inflammation of a joint

7. P   WR   S
   inter/vertebr / al   pertaining to between the vertebrae

8. WR   S
   humer / al   pertaining to the humerus

9. P S/WR
   dys/trophy   abnormal development

10. P   WR   S
    sub/scapul /ar   pertaining to below the scapula

11. WR   S
    arthr/osis   abnormal condition of a joint

12. WR   CV WR CV S
electr / o / my / o /
graph y   process of recording the
electrical activity of
muscle

13. WR   CV S
arthr/o/gram   x-ray image of a joint

14. WR   CV WR CV S
electr /o/my/o/graph   instrument to record the
electrical activity of
muscle

15. WR CV WR   S
stern/o/cost/al   pertaining to the sternum
and ribs

16. WR   S
arthr/algia   pain in a joint

17. P WR S
sub/cost/al   pertaining to below a rib (or
ribs)

18. WR   S
femor/al   pertaining to the femur

19. WR   CV S
clavic/o/tomy   surgical incision into the
clavicle

20. WR CV S
arthr/o/tomy   surgical incision of a
joint

21. P   WR S
intra/crani/al   pertaining to within the
cranium

22. P WR
a/trophy   without development (or
decrease in size of a
normally developed
organ)

23. WR CV S
arthr/o/plasty   surgical repair of a joint

24. WR S
oste/oma   tumor (composed of) bone

25. WR S
cost/ectomy   excision of a rib cranium

26. WR CV S
crani/o/plasty   surgical repair of the

27. WR   S
patell/ectomy   excision of the patella

28. WR   S
vertebr/ectomy   excision of a vertebra

29. WR CV S
crani/o/tomy   surgical incision into the
cranium

30. P   WR S
supra/scapul/ar   pertaining to above the
scapula

31. WR   S
myos/itis   inflammation of muscle

32. WR   CV S
chondr/o/genic   producing cartilage

33. WR CV S
arthr/o/scopy   visual examination of the
inside of a joint

34. WR   S
chondr/itis   inflammation of the
cartilage

35. WR CV S
arthr/o/scope   instrument used to visualize
a joint

36. WR   S
chondr/ectomy   excision of cartilage

37. WR   S
lamin/ectomy   excision of the lamina

38. WR S
stern/al   pertaining to the sternum

39. WR   S
menisc/ectomy   excision of the meniscus

40. WR CV S
arthr/o/centesis   surgical puncture to
aspirate fluid from a
joint

41. WR   S
menisc/itis   inflammation of the
meniscus

Exercise 9

1. cranial
2. myositis
3. subscapular
4. femoral
5. arthrotomy
6. chondrectomy
7. arthralgia
8. arthritis
9. arthrosis
10. humeral
11. atrophy
12. vertebrocostal
13. craniotomy
14. costectomy
15. subcostal
16. arthrogram
17. vertebrectomy
18. electromyogram
19. clavicotomy
20. electromyography
21. dystrophy
22. myoma
23. electromyograph
24. sternoclavicular
25. intervertebral
26. intracranial
27. sternocostal
28. patellectomy
29. cranioplasty
30. osteoma
31. clavicotomy
32. chondrogenic
33. arthroscopy
34. arthroscope
35. chondritis
36. chondrectomy
37. laminectomy
38. sternal
39. arthrocentesis
40. meniscectomy
41. meniscitis

Exercise 10

1. branch of medicine dealing with the diagnosis and treatment of diseases, fractures, or abnormalities of the musculoskeletal system
2. doctor specializing in orthopedics
3. progressive, crippling disease of the muscles
4. insertion of a hollow needle into the sternum to obtain bone marrow sample for laboratory study

Exercise 11

Spelling exercise

Exercise 12

1. orthopedics, orthopedist
2. sternal puncture
3. electromyography
4. a. lower inner leg bone
   b. upper arm bone
   c. neck bone
   d. pelvic bone
   e. collarbone
   f. arm bone, thumb side
5. a. costectomy
   b. (correct)
   c. laminectomy
   d. clavicotomy
   e. (correct)
   f. patellectomy
   g. osteoarthrotomy
   h. (correct)
6. arthrogram, arthrocentesis

Exercise 13

1. above-the-knee amputation
2. below-the-knee amputation
3. fracture
4. open reduction, internal fixation
5. herniated nucleus pulposus
6. nonsteroidal antiinflammatory drugs
7. electromyogram, electromyography
8. total hip arthroplasty
9. total hip replacement

Unit 4

Review Questions

1. a. central nervous system (CNS)—consists of the brain and spinal cord
   b. peripheral nervous system (PNS)—consists of the nerves of the body (12 pairs of cranial and 31 pairs of spinal nerves
2. monitors, regulates, and controls the functions of body organs and body systems by using nerve impulses to transmit information from one part of the body to another
3. neuron, sensory, motor
4. a. cerebrum: contains sensory, motor, sight, and hearing centers; memory, judgment, and emotional reactions also take place in the cerebrum
   b. cerebellum: assists in coordination of voluntary muscles and maintains balance
   c. brainstem: contains the control centers for blood pressure, respiration, and heartbeat

5. extends from the brainstem passing through the spinal cavity to between the first and second lumbar vertebrae; the pathway for conducting sensory and motor impulses to and from the brain
6. dura mater, arachnoid, pia mater
7. 1. a
   2. f
   3. d
   4. e
   5. b
   6. c
8. a. preictal
   b. interictal
   c. postictal

Exercise 1

(*Note:* Not all of the combining forms will be labeled on the diagram.)
1. cerebell / o
2. cerebr / o
3. encephal / o
4. mening / o
5. myel / o
6. neur / o

Exercise 2

1. cerebrum
2. brain
3. nerve
4. gray matter
5. meninges
6. dura mater
7. spinal cord or bone marrow
8. cerebellum
9. speech
10. mind
11. four

Exercise 3

1. neur / o
2. cerebr / o
3. mening / o
4. myel / o
5. cerebell / o
6. encephal / o
7. dur / o
8. poli / o
9. phas / o
10. psych / o
11. quadr/i

Exercise 4

1. -oma
2. -plasty
3. -ar, -al, -ic, -ous
4. -rrhaphy
5. -rrhea
6. -itis
7. -logist
8. -gram
9. -logy
10. -rrhagia

11. -cele
12. -ectomy
13. -tomy
14. -algia
15. -ia

Exercise 5

1. record, x-ray image
2. inflammation
3. the study of
4. discharge
5. rapid discharge
6. to suture
7. herniation, protrusion
8. pertaining to, pertaining to
9. surgical removal
10. surgical repair
11. surgical incision
12. pain
13. abnormal condition
14. abnormal condition
15. paralysis, stroke
16. half
17. beside, beyond, around
18. pertaining to, pertaining to

Exercise 6

1. WR CV S
   neur/o/logy
   study of nerve (branch of medicine that deals with the nervous system)

2. WR CV WR S
   cerebr /o /spin /al
   pertaining to the brain and spine

3. WR S
   neur/algia
   pain in a nerve

4. WR CV WR S
   poli/o/myel/itis
   inflammation of the gray matter and the spinal cord

5. WR CV S
   neur/o/plasty
   surgical repair of a nerve

6. WR S
   encephal /itis
   inflammation of the brain

7. WR S
   mening/itis
   inflammation of the meninges

8. WR CV S
   neur/o/pathy
   disease of a nerve

9. WR CV S
   neur/o/logist
   one who specializes in the diagnosis and treatment of nerves

10. WR CV S
    encephal/o/cele
    herniation of brain tissue through (a gap in) the skull

11. WR   CV   WR   CV S
    electr / o / encephal / o / gram   recording of electrical activity of the brain

12. WR   CV WR CV S
    mening /o / myel / o / cele   protrusion of the spinal cord and meninges through the vertebral column

13. WR   S
    cerebell/itis   inflammation of the cerebellum

14. WR   S
    cerebr/osis   abnormal condition of the brain

15. WR   S
    neur/oma   tumor of nerve (cells)

16. WR CV S
    myel/o/rrhagia   hemorrhage into the spinal cord

17. WR CV S
    myel/o/gram   x-ray image of the spinal cord with the use of dye

18. WR   S
    neur/itis   inflammation of a nerve

Exercise 7

1. a disease characterized by hardening patches along the brain and the spine
2. convulsive disorder of the nervous system marked by recurrent or chronic seizures
3. partial paralysis and lack of muscle coordination from a defect, injury, or disease of the brain present at birth or shortly after
4. impaired blood supply to parts of the brain
5. process of recording brain structures with the use of sound recorded on a graph
6. paralysis of the right or left side of the body
7. paralysis of the legs and/or lower part of the body
8. paralysis that affects all four limbs
9. removal of cerebrospinal fluid for diagnostic purposes (in the lumbar area of the spine)
10. accumulation of blood in the subdural space
11. radiologic imaging that produces images of "slices" of the body with the use of x-rays
12. a noninvasive procedure for imaging tissues that uses a magnetic field
13. loss of expression or understanding of speech or writing

Exercise 8

1. neuritis
2. encephalitis
3. meningitis
4. neuroplasty
5. neurologist
6. neuropathy
7. neuroma
8. neuralgia
9. cerebrospinal
10. meningomyelocele
11. cerebellitis

12. encephalocele
13. myelorrhagia
14. electroencephalogram
15. myelogram

Exercise 9

Spelling exercise

Exercise 10

Spelling exercise

Exercise 11

1. neurology, neurologist
2. cerebrovascular accident, CVA, hemiplegia
3. meningitis, spinal puncture (lumbar puncture), spinal puncture (lumbar puncture)
4. a. electroencephalography
   b. myelography
   c. pneumoencephalography
   d. echoencephalography

Exercise 12

1. central nervous system
2. cerebrospinal fluid
3. computed tomography
4. cerebrovascular accident
5. electroencephalogram
6. evoked potentials
7. lumbar puncture
8. multiple sclerosis
9. peripheral nervous system
10. positron emission tomography
11. magnetic resonance imaging
12. transient ischemic attack

Unit 5

Review Questions

1. The eye is the organ of vision. It is divided into three layers: the sclera, choroid, and retina.
2. a. skull bones
   b. eyelashes
   c. eyelids
   d. lacrimal apparatus
   e. conjunctiva
3. 1. f
   2. h
   3. j
   4. i
   5. b
   6. d
   7. k
   8. a
4. a. cones; adaptation to bright light and color vision
   b. rods; adaptation to dim light
5. a. The small anterior cavity in front of the lens is divided into an anterior and a posterior chamber and is filled with aqueous humor, and the large posterior cavity behind the lens is filled with vitreous humor.
   b. The functions of these fluids are to maintain the shape of the eyeball with proper intraocular pressure and to assist in bending the light rays to focus on the retina.

6. a. conjunctiva
   b. cornea
   c. aqueous humor
   d. pupil
   e. lens
   f. vitreous humor
   g. retina
7. cloudiness of the lens of the eye
8. abnormal increase in intraocular pressure
9. the separation of the retina from the choroid
10. a. photocoagulation
    b. cryosurgery
    c. scleral buckling
12. hearing and equilibrium (sense of balance)
13. a. pinna and auditory canal
    b. tympanic membrane, eustachian tube, malleus, incus, stapes
    c. oval window, cochlea, semicircular canals
14. Sound enters the pinna, travels through the auditory canal, and strikes the tympanic membrane, which sends the ossicles into motion. The stapes vibrate the oval window, and the waves continue to travel via the fluid in the cochlea to the auditory nerve and on to the brain.
15. a. chronic infections
    b. head injuries
    c. prolonged exposure to environmental noise
    d. hypertension
    e. cardiovascular disease
    f. ototoxic drugs
16. a. masking the noise with the use of music
    b. biofeedback

Exercise 1

1. 1. blephar / o
   2. conjunctiv / o
   3. irid / o
   4. kerat / o
   5. ophthalm / o
   6. retin / o
   7. scler / o
2. 1. myring / o
   2. ot / o
   3. staped / o

Exercise 2

1. Retina
2. Cornea
3. Sclera
4. Eye
5. Conjunctiva
6. Ear
7. Tympanic membrane
8. Eyelid
9. Iris
10. Stapes

Exercise 3

1. Ophthalm / o
2. Blephar / o
3. Retin / o
4. Ot / o
5. Myring / o

6. Scler / o
7. Conjunctiv / o
8. Irid / o
9. Kerat / o
10. Staped / o

Exercise 4

1. WR   CV   S   instrument used for visual examination of the eye

    ophthalm/o/scope
2. WR   CV   S   one who specializes in the diagnosis and treatment of the eye

    ophthalm/o/logist
3. WR   S   excision of the eye
    ophthalm/ectomy
4. WR CV S   discharge from the ear
    ot   /o   /rrhea
5. WR CV S   instrument used for visual examination of the ear

    ot   /o   /scope
6. WR CV WR CV S   incision into the iris and sclera

    irid / o / scler / o / tomy
7. WR   S   excision of (part of) the iris

    irid/ectomy
8. WR   CV   S   surgical repair of the eyelid

    blephar/o/plasty
9. WR   CV   S   suture of an eyelid
    blephar/o/rrhaphy
10. WR CV   WR   S   inflammation of the cornea and conjunctiva

    kerat / o / conjunctiv / itis
11. WR CV S   herniation of (a layer of the) cornea

    kerat/o/cele
12. WR   S   inflammation of the conjunctiva

    conjunctiv/itis
13. WR   CV   S   incision of the tympanic membrane

    myring /o /tomy
14. WR   CV   S   surgical repair of the tympanic membrane

    myring /o /plasty
15. WR CV S   incision into the cornea
    kerat /o /tomy
16. WR CV WR CV WR   CV   S   specialist of ear, nose, and throat

    ot / o/ rhin/ o/ laryng/ o/ logist

Exercise 5

1. otitis media
2. ophthalmoscope
3. blepharorrhaphy
4. otorrhea

5. iridosclerotomy
6. scleroplasty
7. iridectomy
8. keratocele
9. otoscope
10. ophthalmectomy
11. sclerotomy
12. blepharoplasty
13. myringotomy
14. myringoplasty
15. keratoconjunctivitis
16. conjunctivitis
17. keratotomy
18. otorhinolaryngologist

Exercise 6

1. cloudiness of the lens of the eye
2. removal of the clouded lens of the eye
3. separation of the retina from the choroid
4. surgical removal of the eyeball
5. weakness of the eye muscle (crossed eyes)
6. eye disease caused by increased pressure from within the eye
7. a professional person trained to examine the eyes and prescribe glasses
8. transplantation of a donor cornea into the eye of a recipient

Exercise 7

Spelling exercise

Exercise 8

1. ophthalmoscope, otoscope
2. otitis media, myringotomy
3. cataract, cataract extraction
4. enucleation, ophthalmectomy
5. strabismus

Exercise 9

1. pupils equal, round, reactive to light and accommodation
2. otitis media
3. photorefractive keratectomy
4. radial keratotomy
5. oculus dexter (right eye)
6. oculus sinister (left eye)
7. oculus uterque (both eyes)
8. ear, nose, and throat

Unit 6
Review Questions

1. a. transportation of nutrients, oxygen, and hormones to cells and removal of wastes
   b. protection by white blood cells and antibodies to defend the body against foreign invaders
   c. regulation of body temperature, fluids, and water volume of cells
2. See Fig. 22-20 for labeled diagram.
3. See Fig. 22-20 for labeled diagram.
4. a. arteries: carry blood away from heart (except for the pulmonary artery)
   b. arterioles: connect arteries to capillaries

c. capillaries: exchange of substances between the blood and the body cells

d. venules: connect capillaries to veins

e. veins: carry blood back to the heart (except for the pulmonary vein)

5. a. The systolic pressure (upper number) represents the pressure in the aorta and other large arteries during ventricular contraction.

b. The diastolic pressure (lower number) represents the pressure during relaxation of the heart.

6. a. plasma

b. transports nutrients and waste material
transports hormones
assists in blood clotting

7. a. erythrocytes: carry oxygen

b. leukocytes: fight against pathogenic microorganisms

c. platelets: aid in blood clotting

8. a. O

b. A

c. B

d. AB

9. maintenance of fluid balance and immunity

10. 1. g
2. b
3. c
4. a
5. d
6. h
7. e
8. j
9. f
10. i

Exercise 1

	Type	Meaning
1.	P	below normal
2.	P	without
3.	WR	blood
4.	WR	spleen
5.	WR	cell
6.	S or WR	narrowing
7.	P	inside
8.	WR	white
9.	WR	red
10.	WR	blood vessel
11.	WR	heart
12.	WR	artery
13.	P	surrounding (outer)
14.	P	between
15.	P	within
16.	S or WR	hardening
17.	S or WR	condition of the blood
18.	S	enlargement
19.	WR	vein
20.	WR	aorta
21.	WR	clot
22.	P	above normal
23.	P	fast, rapid
24.	P	slow

Exercise 2

	Type	Word Elements
1.	WR/CF	aort / o
2.	S	-megaly
3.	S or WR	-sclerosis or sclerosis
4.	P	inter-
5.	WR/CF	arteri / o
6.	WR/CF	angi / o
7.	WR/CF	leuk / o
8.	S or WR	-stenosis or stenosis
9.	WR/CF	splen / o
10.	P	a-, an-
11.	S	-pexy
12.	P	endo-
13.	WR/CF	hem / o
14.	WR/CF	cyt / o
15.	P	hypo-
16.	WR/CF	erythr / o
17.	WR/CF	cardi / o
18.	P	peri-
19.	S or WR	-emia, emia
20.	WR/CF	phleb / o
21.	WR/CF	thromb / o
22.	P	tachy
23.	P	brady

Exercise 3

1. WR   S
   aort /ic   pertaining to the aorta

2. WR   CV   S
   splen /o /megaly   enlargement of the spleen

3. WR   CV   S
   hem /o /rrhage   rapid flow of blood (from a blood vessel)

4. WR   S
   thromb /osis   abnormal condition (formation) of a blood clot

5. WR   CV   WR
   leuk /o /cyte   white blood cell

6. WR   CV   WR
   erythr /o /cyte   red blood cell

7. WR   CV   S
   cardi /o /logist   one who specializes in the diagnosis and treatment of the heart

8. WR   CV   S
   cardi /o /megaly   enlargement of the heart

9. WR   CV   S
   phleb/o /tomy   incision into the vein (to withdraw blood)

10. WR   CV   S
    angi /o /rrhaphy   suturing of a blood vessel

11. WR   S
    splen/ectomy   excision of the spleen

12. WR   CV   S
    splen /o /pexy   surgical fixation of the spleen

13. P   WR   S
    endo/card/itis   inflammation of the inner (lining) of the heart

14. WR CV S
arteri /o /sclerosis — hardening of the arteries

15. WR CV S
arteri /o /stenosis — constriction (narrowing) of the arteries

16. WR CV WR S
thromb/o/phleb/itis — inflammation of a vein caused by a clot

17. WR S
hemat/oma — tumor-like mass formed from blood in the tissues

18. WR CV S
hemat/o/logy — study of blood

19. WR S
leuk/emia — blood condition of white (disease characterized by rapid, abnormal production of white blood cells)

20. PS (WR)
an /emia — blood condition of without (deficiency of erythrocytes)

21. WR CV WR CV S
electr / o / cardi / o / gram — record of electrical activity of the heart

22. WR CV WR CV S
electr / o / cardi / o / graph — machine used to record electrical activity of the heart

23. WR CV WR CV S
electr / o / cardi / o / graphy — process of recording electrical activity of the heart

24. WR CV S
angi /o /gram — x-ray image of blood vessels

25. WR CV S
arteri /o /gram — x-ray image of an artery

26. WR CV S
aort /o /gram — x-ray image of the aorta

27. P WR S
peri /card /itis — inflammation of the outer (sac) of the heart

28. P WR S
tachy /card /ia — condition of rapid heart (rate)

29. P WR S
brady /card /ia — condition of slow heart (rate)

30. WR CV S
angi /o /plasty — surgical repair of a blood vessel

Exercise 4

1. aortogram
2. arteriogram
3. angiogram
4. electrocardiogram
5. endocarditis
6. arteriosclerosis
7. thrombophlebitis
8. hematology
9. cardiology
10. cardiologist
11. cardiomegaly
12. phlebotomy
13. splenectomy
14. splenopexy
15. hemorrhage
16. leukocyte
17. erythrocyte
18. pericarditis

Exercise 5

1. laboratory test that measures the volume percentage of red blood cells in whole blood
2. laboratory procedure that measures the oxygen-carrying pigment of the red blood cells
3. sudden stopping of the heartbeat
4. pertaining to the heart and blood vessels
5. excision of hemorrhoids
6. heart attack (damage of the heart muscle from insufficient blood supply to the area)
7. enlarged veins in the rectal area
8. Pertaining to within a vein
9. diagnostic procedure to visualize the heart and to determine the presence of heart disease or heart defects
10. dilation of a weak area of the arterial wall
11. floating mass that blocks a blood vessel
12. high blood pressure
13. low blood pressure
14. inability of the heart to pump enough blood to the body parts
15. blood vessels that supply blood to the heart
16. abnormal accumulation of fluid in the intercellular spaces of the body
17. variation from a normal rhythm
18. condition of rapid heart rate

Exercise 6

Spelling exercise

Exercise 7

1. a. hematology b. hematocrit, hemoglobin
2. a. myocardial infarction
   b. coronary occlusion
   c. coronary thrombosis
3. splenectomy, hemorrhoidectomy
4. cardiovascular
5. cardiologist
6. a. cardiac arrest b. cardiac arrest (or "code")
7. electrocardiography, electrocardiograph
8. a. cardiac catheterization b. angiography
9. a. WBC
   b. RBC
   c. platelets
10. plasma

Exercise 8

1. blood pressure
2. atherosclerotic heart disease
3. coronary artery bypass graft
4. coronary artery disease

5. congestive heart failure
6. electrocardiogram
7. echocardiogram
8. electrocardiogram
9. human immunodeficiency virus
10. hypertension
11. ventricular fibrillation
12. myocardial infarction
13. percutaneous transluminal coronary angioplasty
14. peripheral vascular disease
15. red blood cell (erythrocyte)
16. white blood cell (leukocyte)
17. deep vein thrombosis
18. extracorporeal membrane oxygenation
19. abdominal aortic aneurysm

Unit 7

Review Questions

1. a.
   - Mouth
   - Pharynx
   - Digestive sphincter muscles
   - Esophagus
   - Stomach
   - Small intestine
   - Large intestine
   b.
   - Salivary glands
   - Teeth and tongue
   - Liver
   - Gallbladder
   - Pancreas
2. a. taking nutrients into the digestive tract through the mouth
   b. the chemical and mechanical breakdown of food for use by the body cells
   c. transfer of digested food from the small intestine to the bloodstream
   d. the removal of solid waste from the body
3. a. The chewing of food, or mastication, starts the mechanical breakdown of food necessary for metabolism, the utilization of digested food by body cells.
   b. The tongue helps guide the food to the teeth, where mechanical digestion begins and the salivary glands produce saliva that contains the enzyme amylase.
4. a. upper esophageal, lower esophageal (cardiac), pyloric, ileocecal, and anal sphincters
   b. Sphincters are circular muscles that close or open a natural body opening to regulate the passage of substances.
5. peristalsis
6. a. Gastric glands located in the mucous membrane lining of the stomach secrete enzymes (lipase and pepsin) and hydrochloric acid and mix and churn the food to a liquid consistency. The process of mixing and churning continues the mechanical breakdown of food into a liquid referred to as *chyme*.
   b. After about 30 minutes the food begins to leave the stomach at 30-minute intervals. It takes 2 to 4 hours for the stomach to empty completely.
7. the small intestines

8. absorption of water and the elimination of solid wastes
9. mouth; pharynx; esophagus (upper and lower esophageal sphincter); stomach (pyloric sphincter); small intestine—duodenum, jejunum, ileum (ileocecal sphincter between small and large intestine); large intestine—cecum, colon (ascending colon, transverse colon, descending colon, sigmoid colon); rectum (anal sphincter)
10. 1. e
    2. a
    3. b
    4. f
    5. d

Exercise 1

(*Note:* Not all of the combining forms will be labeled in the diagram.)
1. appendic / o
2. chol / o or chol / e
3. col / o
4. duoden / o
5. esophag / o
6. gastr / o
7. gloss / o or lingu / o
8. hepat / o
9. ile / o
10. pancreat / o
11. stomat / o
12. cheil / o
13. sigmoid / o
14. proct / o

Exercise 2

1. mouth
2. tongue
3. stomach
4. rectum
5. pancreas
6. intestine
7. liver
8. lip
9. esophagus
10. condition of / S
11. bile, gall
12. bladder
13. duodenum
14. colon
15. ileum
16. abdomen
17. appendix
18. abdomen
19. stone or calculus
20. creation of an artificial opening into / S
21. hernia
22. sigmoid colon

Exercise 3

1. -tomy—incision into a body part; *laparotomy:* incision into the abdomen
2. -ectomy—surgical removal (of a body part); *appendectomy:* surgical removal of the appendix
3. -stomy—creation of an artificial opening into; *colostomy:* creation of an artificial opening into the colon

Exercise 4

1. WR CV S
   gloss /o /plegia   paralysis of the tongue
2. WR   S
   append /ectomy   surgical removal of the
                           appendix
3. R   CV WR   S
   chol / e / cyst / ectomy   surgical removal of the
                           gall bladder
4. WR CV S
   gastr /o /stomy   creation of an artificial
                           opening into the
                           stomach (for feeding
                           purposes)
5. WR   CV S
   hepat /o /megaly   enlargement of the liver
6. WR CV S
   ile /o /stomy   creation of an artificial
                           opening into the ileum
7. WR   CV S
   pylor /o /plasty   surgical repair of the
                           pyloric sphincter
8. WR   CV S
   proct /o /rrhea   excessive discharge from
                           the rectum
9. WR CV WR S
   chol /e /cyst /itis   inflammation of the
                           gallbladder
10. WR   S
    gastr /itis   inflammation of the
                           stomach
11. P   WR S
    sub /lingu /al   pertaining to under the
                           tongue
12. WR S
    ile /itis   inflammation of the
                           ileum
13. WR CV WR CV S
    chol / e / cyst / o / gram   x-ray image of the
                           gallbladder
14. WR   CV S
    sigmoid /o /scopy   visual examination of the
                           sigmoid colon
15. WR   S
    gastr /ectomy   surgical removal of the
                           stomach
16. WR CV S
    gastr /o /scopy   visual examination of the
                           stomach
17. WR CV S
    gastr /o /scope   instrument used for visual
                           examination of the
                           stomach
18. WR   S
    col /itis   inflammation of the
                           colon
19. WR   S
    hepat /itis   inflammation of the liver
20. WR CV S
    col /o /stomy   creation of an artificial
                           opening into the colon

21. WR CV S
    herni/o /rrhaphy   surgical repair of a hernia
                           (by suturing of the con-
                           taining structure)
22. WR   CV S
    colon /o /scope   instrument used for visual
                           examination of the
                           colon
23. WR   CV S
    colon /o /scopy   visual examination of the
                           colon
24. WR   CV WR CV
    esophag /o /gastr/o/
    WR   CV S
    duoden/o /scopy   visual examination of the
                           esophagus, stomach,
                           and duodenum

Exercise 5

1. stomatitis
2. cholecystitis
3. cholelithiasis
4. cholecystogram / D
5. cholecystectomy / S
6. pancreatitis
7. proctoscope
8. proctoscopy / D
9. abdominocentesis / D
10. colostomy / S
11. ileostomy / S
12. esophagoscopy / D
13. gastroscope
14. esophagoenterostomy / S
15. gastritis
16. glossorrhaphy / S
17. cheiloplasty / S
18. colectomy / S
19. glossoplegia
20. stomatogastric
21. sublingual
22. proctorrhea
23. hepatomegaly
24. hepatoma
25. pancreatic
26. appendicitis
27. appendectomy / S
28. colonoscopy / D
29. colonoscope
30. esophagogastroduodenoscopy / D

Exercise 6

1. condition of painful intestines accompanied by diarrhea
2. x-ray image of the esophagus and the stomach
3. examination (fasting x-ray—barium is used as the contrast medium) of the colon
4. x-ray image of the gallbladder
5. yellowness of the skin and eyes
6. inflammation of the colon with the formation of ulcers
7. ulcer in the stomach
8. chronic inflammatory disease that can affect any part of the bowel

Exercise 7

Spelling exercise

Exercise 8

1. b. ileostomy: *Ile* is the word root for the small intestine; *-stomy* is the suffix that means artificial opening.
2. cholelithiasis, cholecystogram, cholecystectomy
3. sublingual
4. a. esophagoscopy, esophagoscope
   b. gastroscopy, gastroscope
   c. proctoscopy, proctoscope
5.
   a. gastrectomy
   b. pyloroplasty
   c. vagotomy
6. a. laparotomy
   b. (correct)
   c. herniorrhaphy
   d. colectomy
   e. (correct)

Exercise 9

1. barium enema
2. gastrointestinal
3. gastroenterology, gastroenterologist
4. gastroesophageal reflux
5. esophagogastroduodenoscopy
6. peptic ulcer disease
7. upper gastrointestinal

Unit 8

Review Questions

1. a. to exchange gases—Oxygen is taken into the body and carbon dioxide is removed; also helps to regulate the acid-base balance and enables the production of vocal sounds.
   b. The *upper respiratory system* refers to the nose, nasal cavities, sinuses, pharynx, and larynx. The *lower respiratory system* refers to the trachea, bronchi, alveoli, and lungs.
2. oxygen, carbon dioxide
3. oxygen, carbon dioxide
4. a. nose—warms and moistens the air, removes pathogenic microorganisms, and removes foreign particles, such as dust, from the air
   b. pharynx—both air and food travel through the pharynx (throat); food passes from the pharynx to the esophagus, whereas air passes from the pharynx into the larynx
   c. larynx—a passageway for both food and air; a flap of cartilage, called the *epiglottis*, automatically covers the larynx during the act of swallowing to prevent the passage of food from the pharynx into the larynx
   d. trachea—the passage of air
   e. bronchus—the passage of air
   f. bronchioles—at the end of each bronchiole is a grapelike cluster of air sacs called *alveoli*
   g. alveoli—the walls of the alveoli are single celled, which allows for an exchange of gases to take place between the alveoli and the capillaries
5. air → nose → pharynx → larynx → trachea → bronchi → bronchioles → alveoli, where the exchange of carbon dioxide and oxygen takes place

6. larynx
7. a. hemothorax
   b. pneumothorax
   c. atelectasis
   d. pulmonary embolism
8. chronic obstructive pulmonary disease (COPD)
9. a. cigarette smoking
   b. environmental pollution
   c. occupational hazards
   d. chronic infections
10. acute respiratory distress syndrome (ARDS)

Exercise 1

1. bronch / o
2. laryng / o
3. pharyng / o
4. pleur / o
5. pulmon/o
6. pneum / o
7. pneumon / o
8. nas/o
9. rhin / o
10. trache / o

Exercise 2

1. pneum / o, pneumon / o, pulmon / o
2. pharyng / o
3. laryng / o
4. trache / o
5. tonsill / o
6. bronch / o
7. pleur / o
8. rhin / o
9. pnea / o
10. thorac / o

Exercise 3

1.	P	WR	
	dys /pnea		difficulty breathing
2.	WR	CV S	
	pharyng /o /cele		abnormal protrusion in the pharynx
3.	P	S	
	a /pnea		without breathing (temporary stopping of breathing)
4.	WR	CV WR S	
	bronch /o /trache /al		pertaining to the bronchi and trachea
5.	WR	CV WR S	
	trache /o /esophag /eal		pertaining to the trachea and esophagus
6.	P	WR S	
	endo /trache /al		pertaining to within the trachea
7.	WR	CV S	
	pharyng /o /plegia		paralysis of the pharynx
8.	WR CV WR	S	
	rhin /o /pharyng /itis		inflammation of the nose and throat

9. | WR | CV | S |
   rhin /o /rrhagia   rapid flow of blood from the nose (nosebleed)

10. | WR | CV | S |
   bronch /o /scope   instrument used for visual examination of the bronchi

11. | WR | CV | S |
   bronch /o /scopy   visual examination of the bronchi

Exercise 4

1. bronchitis
2. laryngitis
3. tracheostomy
4. pneumonectomy or pneumectomy
5. lobectomy
6. pleuropexy
7. rhinoplasty
8. thoracotomy
9. thoracentesis or thoracocentesis
10. tonsillitis
11. adenoiditis

Exercise 5

1. pneumothorax
2. emphysema
3. pneumonia
4. pleuropexy
5. pharyngitis

Exercise 6

1. tissue in the nasopharynx
2. excision of a lobe of the lung
3. disease of the alveoli of the lung
4. (infection or) inflammation of a lung
5. (infection or) inflammation of the pharynx, larynx, or bronchi
6. without breathing (temporary stopping of breathing)
7. difficulty breathing
8. abnormal protrusion in the pharynx
9. excision of the larynx
10. air in pleural cavity (that causes lung to collapse)
11. rapid flow of blood from the nose (nosebleed)
12. x-ray image of the lung and bronchi
13. instrument used for visual examination of the larynx
14. chronic disease characterized by attacks of dyspnea, wheezing, and coughing
15. chronic obstruction of the airway
16. chronic infectious disease that commonly affects the lungs

Exercise 7

Spelling exercise

Exercise 8

1. thoracocentesis
2. laryngoscope, endotracheal
3. dyspnea, tracheostomy, tracheostomy, tracheostomy
4. bronchoscopy, bronchoscope
5. pneumothorax, dyspnea, thoracotomy, thoracotomy
6. tonsillectomy, adenoidectomy

Exercise 9

1. acute (adult) respiratory distress syndrome
2. chronic obstructive pulmonary disease
3. endotracheal
4. nasopharyngeal
5. pulmonary embolism
6. respiratory syncytial virus
7. severe acute respiratory syndrome
8. tuberculosis
9. upper respiratory infection

Unit 9

Review Questions

1. to monitor and regulate extracellular fluids and to remove some of the waste material from the blood and excrete it from the body
2. Kidneys—to remove waste from the blood, to balance the water and electrolytes in the body by removing and retaining water, and to assist in RBC production by releasing erythropoietin.

   Ureters—have muscular walls that contract to keep urine moving toward the bladder. A backup of urine into the kidney is prevented by a flap fold of mucous membrane at the entrance of the ureters into the bladder.

   Urinary bladder—a temporary reservoir for the urine it receives from the ureters.

   Urethra—a tube through which urine passes from the bladder to the outside of the body.
3. nephrons
4. 95% water and 5% waste material (urea, uric acid, creatinine, and ammonia)
5. to produce and eject the male reproductive cell (sperm, or spermatozoa) and to secrete the hormone testosterone
6. Testes—produce sperm (sex cells) and testosterone (hormone)
   Scrotum—contains the testes and their accessory organs
   Vas deferens—carries sperm to the urethra
   Urethra—a passageway for both semen and urine
   Seminal vesicles—produces and ejects the male reproductive cell (sperm, or spermatozoa) and secretes the hormone testosterone
   Prostate gland—secretes a fluid that aids in the motility of sperm and aids in ejaculation (expulsion of semen from the male urethra)
   Penis—deposits sperm in the female vagina during ejaculation after erection (stiffening) of the penis, produced by an increased blood supply to the spongelike tissue of the penis
7. sperm travels from the seminiferous tubules (production) → epididymis (sperm matures and becomes motile) → vas deferens (passageway) → seminal vesicles (add nourishing secretions) → prostate (add motility secretions) → urethra (passageway) → to the outside
8. 1. c
   2. e
   3. b
   4. g

Exercise 1

1. a. 1. cyst / o
2. nephr / o

3. pyel / o
4. ren / o
5. ureter / o
6. urethr / o
   b. 1. ureter / o
      2. urethr / o
      3. orchi / o
      4. orchid / o
      5. prostat / o
      6. vas / o

Exercise 2

1. ur / o, urin / o
2. pyel / o
3. ren / o, nephr / o
4. ureter / o
5. cyst / o
6. orchi / o, orchid / o
7. vas / o
8. urethr / o
9. prostat / o

Exercise 3

1. WR   S
   ur /emia   urine in the blood
2. WR CV S
   ur /o /logist   doctor who specializes
                               in the diagnosis and
                               treatment of diseases
                               of the urinary tract
                               and of the male repro-
                               ductive organs
3. WR   CV WR CV S
   nephr / o / lith / o / tomy   incision into the kidney
                               to remove a stone
4. WR   S
   prostat /ectomy   surgical removal of the
                               prostate gland
5. WR   S
   nephr /itis   inflammation of the
                               kidney
6. WR CV S
   ur /o /logy   study of urine (branch
                               of medicine that
                               deals with the urinary
                               system and the male
                               reproductive system)
7. WR   S
   orchi /ectomy   excision of a testis
8. WR   CV WR S
   nephr /o /lith /iasis   condition of kidney
                               stone
9. WR   CV S
   cyst /o /cele   herniation of the urinary
                               bladder
10. WR CV S
    cysts /o /scopy   visual examination of
                               the bladder
11. WR   S
    nephr /ectomy   excision of a kidney

12. WR   CV S
    nephr /o /pexy   surgical fixation of a
                               kidney
13. WR CV WR   S
    pyel /o /nephr /itis   inflammation of the kid-
                               ney and renal pelvis
14. WR   S
    ureter /algia   pain in the ureter
15. WR   S
    urethr /al   pertaining to the urethra
16. WR   CV WR CV S
    ureter / o / lith / o / tomy   incision into the ureter
                               to remove a stone
17. WR   S
    cyst /itis   inflammation of the
                               bladder
18. WR   CV S
    urethr /o /plasty   surgical repair of the
                               urethra
19. WR   CV   S
    urethr /o /rrhaphy   suture of a urethral tear

Exercise 4

1. cystoscopy
2. nephritis
3. nephrectomy
4. urologist
5. hematuria
6. uremia
7. urethrorrhaphy
8. vasectomy
9. prostatectomy
10. ureteralgia
11. cystocele
12. cystogram
13. pyelonephritis
14. nephrolithotomy
15. urethroplasty
16. nephropexy
17. urology
18. orchiectomy or orchidectomy

Exercise 5

1. a laboratory test to analyze urine to assist in the diagnosis of disease
2. kidney stone
3. swelling of the scrotum caused by the collection of fluid
4. removal of part of the prostate gland through the urethra
5. surgical removal of the foreskin of the penis
6. pertaining to the urine
7. passage of urine from the body

Exercise 6

Spelling exercise

Exercise 7

1. urinary catheterization, urinalysis
2. cystitis
3. KUB, blood urea nitrogen, BUN
4. urologist
5. cystoscopy, the patient may be anesthetized

Exercise 8

1. antidiuretic hormone
2. benign prostatic hyperplasia
3. benign prostatomegaly
4. blood urea nitrogen
5. creatinine
6. intravenous pyelogram
7. intravenous urogram
8. kidneys, ureters, and bladder
9. urinary tract infection
10. urinalysis
11. transurethral resection of the prostate

Unit 10

Review Questions

1. The functions of the female reproductive system are to produce the female reproductive cell (ovum), to produce hormones, and to provide for conception and pregnancy.
2. Uterus—in pregnancy, functions to contain and nourish the fetus; rhythmic myometrial contractions during labor assist in the birthing process; also plays a role in menstruation.

    Ovaries—produce two hormones: estrogen and progesterone.

    Fallopian tubes—fertilization, the union of the sperm and the ovum, usually takes place within the fallopian tube.

    Vagina—receives the penis during sexual intercourse and is the lower part of the birth canal through which the baby passes from the uterus to the outside of the body.

    Mammary and Bartholin's glands—secrete lubricating substances.
3. a. estrogen and progesterone
   b. Estrogen is responsible for the development of the female reproductive organs and the development of female secondary sex characteristics, such as breasts and pubic hair.
4. perineum
5. pelvic inflammatory disease
6. ectopic pregnancy
7. endometriosis

Exercise 1

1. cervic / o
2. colp / o
3. vagin / o
4. hyster / o
5. metr / o
6. uter / o
7. oophor / o
8. salping / o

Exercise 2

1. men / o
2. gynec / o
3. colp / o or vagin / o
4. perine / o
5. salping / o
6. oophor / o
7. hyster / o, metr / o, or uter / o
8. cervic / o
9. mast / o or mamm / o

Exercise 3

1.	WR CV S		
	gynec /o /logy		study of women (branch of medicine that deals with female reproductive organs)
2.	WR CV S		
	colp /o /rrhaphy		suture of the vagina
3.	WR S		
	oophor /ectomy		surgical removal of an ovary
4.	WR S		
	oophor /itis		inflammation of an ovary
5.	WR CV WR S		
	salping / o / oophor / ectomy		excision of a fallopian tube and an ovary
6.	WR CV S		
	salping /o /pexy		surgical fixation of a fallopian tube
7.	WR S		
	hyster /ectomy		surgical removal of the uterus
8.	P WR CV S		
	dys /men /o /rrhea		painful menstrual discharge
9.	WR CV S		
	colp /o /scope		instrument used for visual examination of the vagina (and cervix)
10.	WR CV S		
	mamm /o /plasty		surgical repair of the breast(s)
11.	P WR CV S		
	a /men /o /rrhea		without menstrual discharge
12.	WR CV S		
	mamm /o /gram		x-ray image of the breast
13.	WR CV WR CV S		
	hyster / o / salping / o / gram		x-ray image of the uterus and fallopian tubes
14.	WR CV S		
	colp /o /scopy		visual examination of the vagina and cervix

Exercise 4

1. oophorectomy
2. gynecology
3. salpingopexy
4. oophoritis
5. colposcope
6. metrorrhea
7. cervicectomy
8. hysterosalpingo-oophorectomy
9. salpingocele
10. ureterovaginal
11. cervicitis

12. hysterectomy
13. colporrhaphy
14. perineoplasty
15. vaginal
16. mastectomy
17. salpingo-oophorectomy
18. dysmenorrhea
19. hysterosalpingogram
20. amenorrhea
21. mammogram
22. mammoplasty
23. colposcopy

Exercise 5

1. physician who specializes in the diagnosis and treatment of women
2. pertaining to the uterus
3. instrument used for expanding the vagina to allow for visual examination of the vagina and cervix
4. excessive uterine bleeding during and between periods
5. surgical procedure to scrape the uterus and the inner walls
6. female reproductive cell

Exercise 6

a. dilation and curettage
b. hysterosalpingo-oophorectomy
c. perineoplasty
d. colporrhaphy
e. salpingopexy

Exercise 7

Spelling exercise

Exercise 8

1. f
2. a
3. b
4. c
5. g
6. h
7. d
8. e

Exercise 9

1. a doctor who practices obstetrics
2. source of nourishment for the fetus
3. fluid that surrounds the fetus
4. incision into the uterus through the abdominal wall to deliver the fetus

Exercise 10

1. gynecology, obstetrics
2. vaginal speculum, cervical Pap smear

Exercise 11

1. cesarean section
2. dilation and curettage
3. follicle-stimulating hormone
4. obstetrics, obstetrical
5. pelvic inflammatory disease
6. postpartum
7. term—premature—abortions—living

8. estimated date of delivery
9. bilateral salpingo-oophorectomy

Unit 11

Review Questions

1. Much the same as those of the nervous system—communication, integration, and control; however, endocrine functions are carried out in a much different manner.
2. Iodine is necessary in the body for the production of thyroxine by the thyroid gland.
3. Endocrine glands are ductless glands that do not have tubes to carry their secretions to other parts of the body, whereas exocrine glands have tubes that carry their secretions from the producing gland to other parts or organs of the body.
4. 1. b, c, d, f, j
   2. g
   3. k
   4. e, l
   5. a
   6. i
   7. h
5. islets of Langerhans, pancreas
6. necessary for the metabolism of carbohydrates in the body
7. a. polyuria
   b. polydipsia
   c. glycosuria
   d. hyperglycemia
   e. polyphagia
8. hyperthyroidism

Exercise 1

1. aden / o
2. thyr / o, thyroid / o
3. adren / o, adrenal / o
4. parathyroid / o

Exercise 2

1. adenitis
2. thyroidectomy
3. parathyroidectomy
4. adenoid
5. adenoma
6. adenosis
7. adrenalitis

Exercise 3

1. islets of Langerhans (pancreas)
2. thyroid gland
3. adrenal gland
4. thyroid gland
5. adrenal gland
6. pituitary gland

Exercise 4

1. diabetes insipidus
2. Addison disease
3. Cushing disease
4. hypothyroidism
5. secretions

Exercise 5

Spelling exercise

Exercise 6

1. diabetes mellitus, islets of Langerhans, Ua, FBS, GTT, HbA$_{1c}$, blood glucose monitoring
2. a. pituitary
   b. adrenal cortex
   c. islets of Langerhans
   d. adrenal medulla
   e. ovary
   f. testes
   g. thyroid gland
3. a. protein-bound iodine
   b. T$_3$, T$_4$, T$_7$ uptake
   c. thyroid scan

Exercise 7

1. adrenocorticotropic hormone
2. diabetes mellitus
3. follicle-stimulating hormone
4. glycohemoglobin (glycosylated hemoglobin)
5. luteinizing hormone
6. prolactin
7. parathyroid hormone
8. thyroid-stimulating hormone

Glossary

Following is a list of terms that are discussed throughout the book. After each definition is the number of the chapter in which the term is introduced. Additional terms may be found in content-specific chapter vocabulary lists. Page numbers for all terms may be located in the Index.

2-D (2-dimensional) M-mode Echocardiogram A technique used to "see" actual heart structures and their motions (16)

Accepting Assignment Providers of medical services agreeing that the receipt of payment from Medicare for a professional service will constitute full payment for that service (2)

Accountability Taking responsibility for ones actions; being answerable to someone for something one has done (6)

Accreditation Recognition that a health care organization has met an official standard (2)

Ace Wraps Elastic gauze used for temporary compression to various parts of the body to decrease swelling and reduce skin breakdown (11)

Active Exercise Exercise performed by the patient without assistance as instructed by physical therapist (17)

Activities of Daily Living Tasks that enable individuals to meet basic needs (eating, bathing, and so forth) (17)

Activity Order A doctor's order that defines the type and amount of activity a hospitalized patient may have (10)

Acuity Level of care patients would require on the basis of their medical condition; used to evaluate staffing needs (3)

Acupuncture originated in China more than 5,000 years ago and is based on a belief that all living things have a vital energy, called "qi" (3)

Acute Care Level of health care, generally provided in hospitals or emergency departments, for sudden, serious illnesses or trauma (3)

Admission Day Surgery Surgery scheduled on the day of the patient's arrival to the hospital; may be called *same-day surgery (SDS)* or *save-a-day surgery (SAD)* (19)

Admission Orders Electronic or handwritten instructions provided by the doctor for the care and treatment of the patient upon entry into the hospital (19)

Admission Packet A preassembled packet of standard chart forms to be used on admission of a patient to the nursing unit (8)

Admission Service Agreement or Conditions of Admission Agreement (COA or C of A) A form signed upon the patient's admission that sets forth the general services that the hospital will provide; also may be called conditions of admission, contract for services, or treatment consent (19)

Admission, Discharge, and Transfer Log Book (ADT Log Book) A book used for a long term record of admissions, discharges, and transfers for future reference. A patients' ID label is placed in the book with the date of admission entered next to it. (19)

Admission, Discharge, and Transfer Log Book (ADT Log Book) Book used to record all admissions, discharges, and transfers on a nursing unit for future reference (7)

Admission, Discharge, and Transfer Log Sheet (ADT Log Sheet) A form used to record daily admissions, discharges, and transfers for quick reference and to assist in tracking empty beds (19)

Admission, Discharge, and Transfer Sheet (ADT Sheet) Form used to record daily admissions, discharges, and transfers for quick reference and to assist in tracking empty beds (7)

Admixture The result of adding a medication to a bag of intravenous solution (13)

Adult Disposable Diapers An absorbent garment worn by patients who are incontinent (11)

Advance Directives Legal Documents that indicate a patient's wishes in the event that the patient becomes incapacitated and unable to make decisions regarding medical care (19)

Adverse Drug Event (ADE) Injuries or harmful reactions that result from the use of a drug

Aerobic Exercise Causes the heart and lungs to work harder to benefit the cardiovascular and circulatory system (17)

Aerosol Liquid suspension of particles in a gas stream for inhalation purposes (17)

Afebrile Without fever (10)

Ageism (Age Discrimination) Stereotyping of and discrimination against individuals or groups because of their age (5)

Aggressive A behavioral style in which a person attempts to be the dominant force in an interaction. Aggressive behavior may escalate into a physical and/or verbal act. (5)

Airborne Precautions (Isolation) Transmission-based precautions -requires use of a mask and a private room with monitored negative air pressure and high-efficiency filtration, in conjunction with standard precautions (21)

Allergy Bracelet A plastic bracelet (usually red) that is worn by a patient that indicates allergies they may have (8)

Allergy Identification Bracelet A plastic band with an insert on which allergy information is printed, or a red plastic band that has allergy information written directly on it, that the patient wears throughout the hospitalization (19)

Allergy Information Information obtained from the patient regarding sensitivities to medications, food, and/or other substances (e.g., wool, tape) (19)

Allergy Labels Labels affixed to the front cover of a patient's paper chart that indicate a patient's allergies (8)

Allergy An acquired, abnormal immune response to a substance that does not normally cause a reaction; may include medications, food, tape, and many other items (8)

Alternative Medicine Any practice not generally recognized by the medical community as standard or conventional medical approaches and used instead of standard treatments (3)

American Nurses Association (ANA) The national professional association of registered nurses in the United States founded in 1896 to improve standards of health and the availability of health care (3)

American Recovery and Reinvestment Act (ARRA) commonly referred to as **the Stimulus** or **the Recovery Act**, is an economic stimulus package enacted in 2009. The act significantly expanded HIPAA requirements affecting group health plans. (6)

Amniocentesis A needle puncture into the uterine cavity to remove amniotic fluid, the liquid that surrounds the unborn baby (14)

Anaerobic Exercise Involves strengthening muscles by forcing them to work very hard for a brief time (17)

Angioplasty A medical procedure in which a balloon is used to open narrowed or blocked blood vessels of the heart (coronary arteries) (17)

Ankle Brachial Index A non-invasive study to measure the difference in blood pressure between the upper and lower extremities (16)

Anorexia Nervosa Intense fear of gaining weight or becoming fat, although underweight (12)

Antibody An immunoglobulin (protein) produced by the body that reacts with and neutralizes an antigen (usually a foreign substance) (14)

Antigen Any substance that induces an immune response (14)

Apical Rate Heart rate obtained from the apex of the heart (10)

Apnea The cessation of breathing (16)

Aquathermia Pad A waterproof plastic or rubber pad used to apply heat or cold that is connected by hoses to a bedside control unit that contains a temperature regulator, a motor for circulating the water, and a reservoir of distilled water (also called a K-pad or a water flow pad) (11)

Arterial Blood Gases A diagnostic study to measure arterial blood oxygen, carbon dioxide and pH (acidity) to attain information needed to assess and manage a patient's respiratory status (16)

Arterial Doppler Ultrasound Uses the same method as the vascular Doppler except that it is designed specifically for testing outer extremities such as arms and legs (16)

Arterial Line (Art line or A line) A catheter placed in an artery that measures the patient's blood pressure continuously and/or to obtain samples for arterial blood gas measurements (11)

Arterial Line (Art or A line) A catheter placed in an artery that continuously measures the patient's blood pressure (16)

Arterial Plethysmography Usually performed to rule out occlusive disease of the lower extremities, or may identify arteriosclerotic disease in the upper extremity (16)

Arterial Stiffness Index A non-invasive test that determines the flexibility and health of the arterial wall (16)

Ascom 914T Pocket Receiver A wireless voice- and message-transmission system, and customized alarm and positioning applications (4)

Assertive A behavioral style in which a person stands up for their own rights and feelings without violating the rights and feelings of others (5)

Assignment Sheet A form completed at the beginning of each work shift that indicates the nursing staff member(s) assigned to each patient on that nursing unit (3)

Assistant Nurse Manager A registered nurse who assists the nurse manager in coordinating activities on the nursing unit (3)

Attending Physician Term applied to a physician who admits and is responsible for a hospital patient (3)

Attitude A manner of thought or feeling expressed in a person's behavior (6)

Auscultation The act of listening for sounds within the body to evaluate the condition of the heart, blood vessels, lungs, pleura, intestines, or other organs, or to detect fetal heart sounds (17)

Autologous Blood The patient's own blood donated previously for transfusion as needed by the patient; also called *autotransfusion* (11)

Autonomy state of functioning independently, personal liberty (6)

Autopsy Examination of a body after death; it may be performed to determine the cause of death or for medical research purposes (20)

Axillary Temperature The temperature reading obtained by placing the thermometer in the patient's axilla (armpit) (10)

Bariatric Surgery Surgery on part of the GI tract performed as a treatment for morbid obesity (19)

Bedside Commode A chair or wheelchair with an open seat, used at the bedside by the patient for the passage of urine and stool (10)

Binder A cloth or elastic bandage that is usually used for abdominal or chest support (11)

Biometric Authentication Methods for uniquely recognizing humans based upon one or more intrinsic physical or behavioral traits (4)

Biopsy Tissue removed from a living body for examination (14)

Bladder Ultrasound A noninvasive method of assessing bladder volume and other bladder conditions using ultrasonography to determine the amount of urine retention or post-void residual urine. A portable, ultrasound device, called a **bladder scanner** is used. (11)

Blood Pressure The measurement of the pressure of blood against the artery walls (10)

Blood Transfusion Consent A patient's written permission to receive blood or blood products (19)

Blood Transfusion Refusal A patient's written permission to refuse blood or blood products (19)

B-mode scanning An image made up of a series of dots, each indicating a single ultrasonic echo. The position of a dot corresponds to the time elapsed, and the brightness of a dot corresponds to the strength of the echo (16)

Body Mass Index Body weight in kilograms divided by height in square meters; this is the usual measurement to define overweight and obesity (12)

Bolus Rounded mass of food formed in the mouth and ready to be swallowed; also defined as a concentrated dose of medication or fluid, frequently given intravenously (discussed in Chapter 13) (12)

Brainstorming Structured group activity that allows three to ten people to tap into the creativity of the group to identify new ideas. Typically in quality improvement, the technique is used to identify probable causes and possible solutions for quality problems (7)

Broken Record Technique An assertiveness technique that consists of just repeating your requests or your refusals every time you are met with resistance (5)

Browser A software program that allows one to search for and view various kinds of information on the Web, such as web sites, video, audio, etc (1)

Bulimia Nervosa Recurrent episodes of binge eating (rapid consumption of a large amount of food in a discrete period of time) and self-induced vomiting, along with use of laxatives or diuretics (12)

Bulletin Boards There may be two or more boards on a nursing unit including one for education and policy changes and one for personal information for nursing staff (4)

Census Board White boards usually in the nurses' station area on which to record census information including unit room numbers, admitting doctors' names, and the name of the nurse assigned to each patient (4)

Caloric Study A test performed to evaluate the function of cranial nerve VIII. It also can indicate disease in the temporal portion of the cerebrum (16)

Calorie A measurement of energy generated in the body by the heat produced after food is eaten (12)

Capillary Blood Gases A diagnostic study performed primarily on infants. Blood is obtained from the infant's capillary arterial vessel, usually from the heel (16)

Capitation Payment method whereby the provider of care receives a set dollar amount per patient, regardless of services rendered (2)

Capsule Endoscopy A non-invasive endoscopic study. A small capsule which is swallowed by the patient transmits and records pictures of the esophagus and small intestine (16)

Cardiac Arrest The patient's heart contractions are absent or insufficient to produce a pulse or blood pressure (may also be referred to as code arrest) (21)

Cardiac Monitor Technician A person who observes the cardiac monitors; health unit coordinators may be cross-trained to this position (10)

Cardiac Monitor is a device that shows the electrical and pressure waveforms of the cardiovascular system for measurement and treatment. Monitors heart function, providing visual and audible record of heartbeat. (10)

Cardiac Pacemaker An electronic device, temporary or permanent, that regulates the pace of the heart when the heart is incapable of doing it (17)

Cardiac Stress Test A noninvasive study that provides information about the patient's cardiac function (16)

Cardiopulmonary Resuscitation (CPR) The basic life-saving procedure of artificial ventilation and chest compressions done in the event of a cardiac arrest (TJC requires all health care workers to be certified in CPR) (6)

C-Arm A mobile fluoroscopy unit used in surgery or at the bedside (15)

Case Manager Health care professional and expert in managed care who assists patients in assessing health and social service systems to ensure that all required services are obtained; coordinates care with doctor and insurance companies (2)

Catastrophic Coverage Coverage a Medicare beneficiary has after reaching a certain amount of "out of pocket" monies paid for their medications during the temporary coverage gap. The beneficiary will pay a coinsurance amount (like 5% of the drug cost) or a copayment ($2.15 or $5.35 for each prescription) for the rest of the calendar year. (2)

Cathartic An agent that causes evacuation of the bowel (laxative) (15)

Catheterization Insertion of a catheter into a body cavity or organ to inject or remove fluid (11)

Celsius (C) A scale used to measure temperature in which the freezing point of water is 0° and the boiling point is 100° (formerly called *Centigrade*) (10)

Census Board A white board located in the nurses' station area on which to record census information such as; unit room numbers, admitting doctors' names, and the name of the nurse assigned to each patient. The patient's name intentionally may be omitted to maintain patient confidentiality. (19)

Census Sheet A list of patients including room and bed numbers and other relevant information that may be printed from a computer menu

Census Worksheet Form used on a nursing unit that includes a list of patient's names, room and bed numbers, with blank spaces next to each name. This may be used by the HUC to record patient activities (May also be called a Patient Information Sheet or a Patient Activity Sheet) (7)

Census A list of all occupied (including patient name, age, acuity, and doctor's name) and unoccupied hospital beds (19)

Centers for Disease Control and Prevention (CDC) Division of the U. S. Public Health Service that investigates and controls diseases that have epidemic potential (21)

Central Line A catheter inserted into the jugular or subclavian vein or a large vein in the arm and is threaded to the superior vena cava or the right atrium of the heart (11)

Central Service Department (CSD) Charge Slip Form that is initiated to charge a discharged patient for any items used during their hospital stay that were not charged to the patient at the time of use (7)

Central Service Department (CSD) Credit Slip Form that is used to credit a patient for items found in the room unused after the patient's discharge, or if a patient was mistakenly charged for an item that was not used (7)

Central Service Discrepancy Report List of items that are missing from the nursing unit patient supply cupboard or closet that were not charged to a patient. A discrepancy report is sent to the nursing unit each day from the central service department. (7)

Certification The process of testifying to or endorsing that a person has met certain standards (1)

Certified Health Unit Coordinator A health unit coordinator who has passed the national certification examination sponsored by the National Association of Health Unit Coordinators (NAHUC) (1)

Certified Nursing Assistant A certified health care giver who performs basic nursing tasks (3)

Certified Respiratory Therapist (CRT) After completion of an approved respiratory therapy program, graduates may become credentialed by taking an entry level examination to become a CRT (17)

Change-of-Shift Report A communication process between shifts, in which nursing personnel who are going "off duty" report nursing unit activities to personnel coming "on duty" (report may be provided in person or may be tape-recorded). HUCs may give the report to each other or may listen to the nurse's report). (7)

Chemical Code A term used when medical intervention only (such as medication) will be used in a cardiac or respiratory arrest (21)

Chief Executive Officer Individual in direct charge of a hospital who is responsible to the governing board (2)

Chiropractic Medicine Complementary and alternative health care profession with the purpose of diagnosing and treating mechanical disorders of the spine and musculoskeletal system with the intention of affecting the nervous system and improving health (3)

Chronic Long-lasting: describes an illness or medical condition that lasts over a long period and sometimes causes a long-term change in the body (3)

Chux A disposable pad placed in areas where patients either lie or sit (11)

Compression Garment A tight-fitting, custom-made garment that is used to put constant pressure on healed wounds to keep down scarring (11)

Clean Catch A method of obtaining a urine specimen using a special cleansing technique; also called a midstream urine (14)

Client Server Based EMR System The software is hosted on the hospital internal server and the licenses are purchased outright. (2)

Clinical Death Occurs when no brain function is present (20)

Clinical Decision Support System (CDSS or CDS) An interactive decision support system (DSS) computer software designed to assist physicians at the point of order entry (1)

Clinical Indications Notations recorded when diagnostic imaging is ordered that indicates the reason for doing the procedure (15)

Clinical Pathway A method of outlining a patient's path of treatment for a specific diagnosis, procedure, or symptom (3)

Clinical Tasks Tasks performed at the bedside or in direct contact with the patient (direct patient care) (1)

Cloud or Web-Based EMR (Virtualization of Computer Function) An Internet site hosts data and programs instead of keeping them on an internal computer (2)

Code Blue (Code Arrests) A term used in hospitals to summon additional help for a patient who has stopped breathing and/or whose heart has stopped beating (cardiac arrest) (21)

Code of Ethics A set of rules and procedures for professional conduct based on the values and ethical standards of an organization or profession (6)

Code or Crash Cart A cart stocked by the nursing and pharmacy staff with emergency medication, advanced breathing supplies, intravenous solutions and appropriate tubing, needles, a heart monitor and defibrillator, an oxygen tank, and a suction machine (used in emergency situations) (21)

Color Doppler A form of sonography or echocardiology: colorization is used to identify the direction and speed (velocity) of blood flow (16)

Color-coded Alert Wristbands Alert wristbands are used in many hospitals to quickly communicate a certain health care status or an "alert" that a patient may have. States have standarized colors. The three colors that are standard in most states include red meaning "allergy alert," yellow meaning "fall risk," purple meaning "DNR (do not resuscitate), other alerts that may have varying colors from state to state include seizure alert, diabetic, extremity restricted, and isolation." (19)

Communicable Disease A disease that may be transmitted from one person to another (21)

Communication The process of transmitting feelings, images, and ideas from the mind of one person to the mind of another person or persons by the use of speech, signals, writing, or behavior. (5)

Community Health Concerned with the members of a community with emphasis on prevention and early detection of disease (2)

Comorbidity The presence of one or more disorders (or diseases) in addition to a primary disease or disorder, or the effect of such additional disorders or diseases (19)

Complementary Medicine Nonstandard treatments that may be used along with standard treatments. (3)

Computed Radiology Use of a digital imaging plate rather than film (15)

Computed Tomography A radiographic process that uses ionizing radiation to create computerized images (scans) of body organs in sections or that can be coronal, saggital or three dimensional (referred to as a CT scan) (15)

Computer Physician Order Entry A computerized program into which physicians directly enter patient orders; replaces handwritten orders on an order sheet or prescription pad (1)

Computerized Medication Cart Storage cart that requires confidential user ID and a password to gain access to medications (example: Pyxis Medstatons) (13)

Confidence Belief in oneself and one's abilities; self-confidence; self-reliance, assurance — usually comes with knowledge (6)

Confidentiality The legally protected right afforded to all patients of having personal and medical information (written or spoken) protected (6)

Conflict A disagreement or clash between ideas, values, principles, or people (5)

Constraint Induced (Movement) Therapy (CI Therapy) A therapy to treat a dysfunctional upper extremity that involves constraining the functional arm in a sling to improve the movement and use of the affected arm (17)

Consultation Order A request by the patient's attending physician for the opinion of a second physician with respect to diagnosis and treatment of the patient (18)

Continuous Quality Improvement (CQI) The practice of continuously improving quality of each function at each level of every department of the health care organization (also called *total quality management*—or *TQM*) (7)

Contrast Media Substances (solids, liquids, or gases) used in diagnostic imaging procedures that permit the radiologist to distinguish between various body soft tissue structures; may be injected, swallowed, inhaled, or introduced by rectum (15)

Coroner A public officer whose primary function is to investigate by inquest any death thought to be of other than natural causes (20)

Coroner's Case A death that occurs because of sudden, violent, or unexplained circumstances, or a patient who expires unexpectedly within the first 24 hours after admission to the hospital (deaths investigated by a coroner) (20)

Coverage Gap (Donut Hole) A temporary coverage gap in Medicare that occurs after the beneficiary and their Medicare Part D Drug Plan have spent a set amount of money in total prescription drug expenses. The beneficiary pays 100% of drug costs while in the donut hole until another set amount is reached then the beneficiary receives catastrophic coverage. (2)

Crackles (Rales) A common, abnormal respiratory sound that consists of discontinuous bubbling noises caused by fluid in the small airways or atelectasis and heard on auscultation of the chest during inspiration (17)

Crisis Stress A profound effect experienced by individuals and resulting from common, uncontrollable, often unpredictable life experiences (7)

Critical (Panic) Value Messages A message usually involving a laboratory value of such variance with normal as to be life-threatening unless some intervention was done by the physician, and for which there were interventions that were possible (4)

Cultural Differences Factors such as age, gender, race, religion, socioeconomic status, etc (5)

Culturally Sensitive Care Care that involves understanding and being sensitive to a patient's cultural background. Also called **Cultural Competence.** (5)

Culture and Sensitivity The growth of microorganisms in a special media (culture), followed by a test to determine the antibiotic to which they best respond (sensitivity) (14)

Culture A set of values, beliefs, and traditions that are held by a specific social group (5)

Custodial Care Care and services of a nonmedical nature, which consist of feeding, bathing, watching, and protecting the patient (20)

Custodial Care Unskilled care given for the primary purpose of meeting personal needs, such as bathing and dressing (2)

Cytology The study of cells (14)

Daily Laboratory Test A test that is ordered once by the doctor and is performed every day until the doctor discontinues the order (14)

Daily TPRs Taking each patient's temperature, pulse, and respiration at certain times each day (10)

Damages Monetary compensation awarded by a court for an injury caused by the act of another (6)

Dangle The patient sits and dangles their feet over the edge of the bed (10)

Débridement The process of removing dirt, foreign objects, damaged tissue, and cellular debris from a wound or a burn to prevent infection and to promote healing (17)

Decoding The process of translating verbal and nonverbal symbols received from the sender to determine the message (5)

Defendant Refers to the person against whom a civil or criminal action is brought (6)

Defibrillation Application of an electric shock to the myocardium through the chest wall to restore normal cardiac rhythm. External defibrillators deliver the shock through the chest wall, while internal defibrillators (ICD) deliver the shock via implanted electrodes within the heart. (17)

Dehydration Excessive loss of body water. Causes may include; diseases of the gastrointestinal tract that cause vomiting or diarrhea, heat exposure, prolonged vigorous exercise (e.g., in a marathon), kidney disease, and medications (diuretics). (12)

Deposition Pretrial statement of a witness under oath, taken in question-and-answer form, as it would be in court, with opportunity given to the adversary to be present to cross-examine (6)

Desk Top a non-mobile personal computer (PC) intended to be used at the same dedicated location day after day for use by one computer operator at any given moment (4)

Diagnosis-Related Group Classification system used to determine payments from Medicare by assigning a standard flat rate to major diagnostic categories. This flat rate is paid to hospitals regardless of the full cost of the services provided. (2)

Dialysis A mechanical process to remove toxic wastes from the blood, which would normally be filtered out by the kidneys (17)

Diastolic Blood Pressure The minimum level of blood pressure measured between contractions of the heart; in blood pressure readings, it is the lowest, lower number of the two measurements (10)

Diet Manual Hospitals are required to have available in the dietary office and on all nursing units an up-to-date diet manual that has been jointly approved by the medical and nutritional care staffs. May also be called the **Diet Formulary** (may be available on computer). (12)

Diet Order A doctor's order that states the type and quantity of food and liquids the patient may receive (12)

Dietary Reference Intake (DRI) The framework of nutrient standards now in place in the United States; this provides reference values for use in planning and evaluating diets for healthy people (12)

Dietary Supplements A product (other than tobacco) taken by mouth that contains a "dietary ingredient" intended to supplement the diet; dietary supplements come in many forms, including extracts, concentrates, tablets, capsules, gel caps, liquids, and powders (12)

Differential (DIFF) Identification of the types of white cells found in the blood (14)

Dipstick Urine The visual examination of urine using a special chemically treated stick (14)

Direct Admission A patient who was not scheduled to be admitted and is admitted from the doctor's office, clinic, or emergency room (19)

Director of Nursing A registered nurse in charge of nursing services (may be called director of patient services, nursing administrator, vice president of nursing services, or chief nursing officer [CNO]) (3)

Disaster Procedure A planned procedure that is carried out by hospital personnel when a large number of people may have been injured or exposed to hazardous materials (21)

Discharge Order A doctor's order that states that the patient may leave the hospital – a doctor's order is necessary for a patient to be discharged from the hospital (20)

Discharge Planning Centralized, coordinated, multidisciplinary process that ensures that the patient has a plan for continuing care after leaving the hospital (20)

Diversity Social inclusiveness: ethnic variety, as well as socioeconomic and gender variety, in a group, society, or institution (5)

Doctor A person licensed to practice medicine (used interchangeably with the term *physician* throughout this textbook) (1)

Doctors' Orders The health care that a doctor prescribes in writing for a hospitalized patient (1)

Doctors' Roster Alphabetic listing of names, telephone numbers, and directory telephone numbers of physicians on staff (most hospitals have made this available via computer) (4)

Document Management System Computer system (or set of computer programs) used to track and store electronic documents and/or images of paper documents (4)

Document Scanner Device used to transmit images of paper documents/pictures to be entered into the patient's electronic record (4)

Document Shredder A machine located in hospitals that shreds confidential material — most hospitals have bins located in each nursing unit that is emptied periodically and taken to an area where the contents are shredded in the shredder (4)

Donor-Specific or Donor-Directed Blood Blood donated by relatives or friends of the patient to be used for transfusion as needed (11)

Doppler Ultrasound A procedure used to monitor moving substances or structures, such as flowing blood or a beating heart (16)

Downtime Requisition A paper order form (requisition) that is used to process information when the computer is not available for use (4)

Drug Enforcement Administration (DEA) A U.S. Department of Justice law enforcement agency tasked with suppressing the sale of recreational drugs by enforcing the Controlled Substances Act of 1970. It shares concurrent jurisdiction with the FBI in narcotics enforcement matters. (13)

Dumbwaiter A mechanical device for transporting food or supplies from one hospital floor to another (4)

Duodenostomy Surgical formation of a permanent opening into the duodenum. May be for the purpose of introducing a tube for post-pyloric feeding. (12)

Dysphagia Difficulty eating and swallowing (12)

Dyspnea Difficult or labored breathing (17)

Echo The reflection of an ultrasound wave back to the transducer from a structure in the plane of the sound beam (16)

Egg-Crate Mattress A foam rubber mattress (11)

Elective Surgery Surgery that is not emergency or mandatory and can be planned at the patient's convenience (19)

Electrocardiogram (EKG or ECG) A graphic recording of the electrical impulses that the heart generates during the cardiac cycle (16)

Electroencephalogram (EEG) A graphic recording of the electrical activity of the brain (16)

Electrolytes A group of tests done in chemistry, which usually includes sodium, potassium, chloride, and CO_2 (14)

Electromyogram (EMG) A record of muscle contraction produced by electrical stimulation. Used in the assessment of patients with diffuse or localized muscle weakness. (16)

Electronic Intensive Care Unit (eICU) An intensive care unit with a highly advanced electronic clinical information system, and a consolidated treatment Unit (also called *Advanced Intensive Care Unit or tele ICU*) (3)

Electronic Medical Record An electronic record of patient health information generated by one or more encounters in any care delivery setting (1)

Electronic Patient Status Tracking Board A viewing screen located in the surgical waiting areas, the hospital cafeteria and other areas in the hospital designed to keep family and friends updated on the status of a surgical patient. Displays the status of surgical patients through the perioperative process from the patient's arrival in the perioperative suite through discharge from PACU. (19)

Electronystagmography (ENG) A test used to evaluate nystagmus (involuntary rapid eye movement) and the muscles that control eye movement (16)

Electrophysiologic Study (EPS) A method of studying evoked potentials within the heart (16)

Elevated Toilet Seat (ETS) An elevated seat that fits over a toilet and has handrails; used for patients who have difficulty sitting on a lower seat (11)

Elitism A belief or attitude that a selected group of persons whose personal abilities, specialized training or other attributes place them at the top of any field and are the people whose views on a matter are to be taken most seriously (5)

Email (electronic mail) is used to send and receive messages and is frequently used for communication between the HUC and hospital personnel and departments within the hospital (4)

Emergency Admission An admission necessitated by accident or a medical emergency; such an admission is processed through the emergency department (19)

Emesis Vomit (10)

Empathy The ability to identify with and understand somebody else's feelings or difficulties (6)

Empathy The ability to understand and to enter into another's feelings or the ability to "put one's self into another's shoes (5)

Encoding Translating mental images, feelings, and ideas into verbal and nonverbal symbols to communicate them to the receiver (5)

Endoscope A tubular instrument (rigid or flexible) with a light source and a viewing lens for observation that can be inserted through a body orifice or through a small incision (16)

Endoscopy The visualization of the interior of organs and cavities of the body with an endoscope. Biopsies may be obtained during an endoscopy. Endoscopic surgeries are discussed in Chapter 17. (16)

Endotracheal Tube A tube inserted through the mouth that supplies air to the lungs and assists breathing. The ET tube is connected to a ventilator. (17)

Enema The introduction of fluid and/or medication into the rectum and sigmoid colon (11)

Enteral Feeding Set Equipment needed to infuse tube feeding; includes plastic bag for feeding solution and may be ordered with or without pump (12)

Enteral Nutrition The provision of liquid formulas into the gastrointestinal (GI) tract by tube or by mouth (12)

Epidemiologist Coordinates with health officials when it comes to reporting and monitoring incidents of infectious diseases that may lead to epidemic outbreaks. *Epidemiology* is the branch of medicine that deals with the study of the causes, distribution, and control of disease in populations. (21)

Hepatitis B Virus An infectious blood-borne disease that is a major occupational hazard for health care workers (21)

E-prescribing (electronic prescribing) The electronic transmission of prescription information from the prescriber's computer (hospital or doctor's office) to a pharmacy computer (1)

Ergonomics Branch of ecology that is concerned with human factors in the design and operation of machines and the physical environment (7)

Erythrocyte A red blood cell (14)

Esophageal Manometry (Esophageal Function Study, Esophageal Motility Study) Performed in the endoscopy department and is used to identify and document the severity of disease that affects the swallowing function of the esophagus and to document and quantify gastroesophageal reflux. (16)

Esteem Needs A person's need for self-respect and for the respect of others (5)

Ethics A system of moral principles (beliefs) that determine how we make judgments in regard to right and wrong (6)

Ethnocentrism The inability to accept other cultures, or an assumption of cultural superiority (5)

Evidence All the means by which any alleged matter of fact, the truth of which is submitted to investigation at trial, is established or disproved; evidence includes the testimony of witnesses and the introduction of records, documents, exhibits, objects, or any other substantiating matter offered for the purpose of inducing belief in the party's contention by the judge or jury (6)

Evoked Potential (EPs) Tests used to evaluate specific areas of the cortex that receive incoming stimuli from the eyes, ears, and lower or upper extremities or sensory nerves (16)

Expert Witness A person who has special knowledge of the subject about which they are to testify; this knowledge must generally be such as is not normally possessed by the average person (6)

Expiration A death (20)

Extended Care Facility A medical facility for patients who require expert nursing care or custodial care; may also be referred to as a skilled nursing facility (20)

Extravasation The accidental administration of intravenously infused medicinal drugs into the surrounding tissue, by leakage (as with the brittle veins of elderly patients) or directly (by means of a puncture of the vein) (11)

Extubation Removal of a previously inserted tube (such as an endotracheal tube) (17)

Face Sheet A form initiated by the admitting department and included in the inpatient medical record that contains personal and demographic information, usually computer generated at the time of admission (also may be called the *information form* or *front sheet*) (19)

Fahrenheit (F) A scale used to measure temperature in which 32° is the freezing point of water and 212° is the boiling point (10)

Fasting No solid foods by mouth and no fluids containing nourishment (e.g., sugar, milk) (14)

Fax Machine A telecommunication device that transmits copies of written material over a telephone wire from one site to another (4)

Febrile Elevated body temperature (fever) (10)

Feedback Verbal or nonverbal response to a message (5)

Feeding Tube A small flexible plastic tube that is usually placed in the patient's nose and that goes down to the stomach or small intestine to provide and/or increase nutritional intake (12)

Fidelity Reliability, trustworthiness, dependability, doing what one promises (6)

Five-Step Problem Solving Model A step by step process designed to solve problems (7)

Flagging A method used by the doctor to notify the nursing staff that a new set of orders has been written (9)

Fluoroscopy The direct observation of deep body structures made visible through the use of a real time viewing screen instead of film; contrast medium is required for this procedure (15)

Fogging Assertive skill in which a person responds to a criticism by making noncommittal statements that cannot be argued against (5)

Foley Catheter A type of indwelling catheter (tube) that is inserted into the bladder for urine collection and measurement (11)

Food Allergy A negative physical reaction to a particular food that involves the immune system (people with food allergies must avoid offending foods) (12)

Food and Drug Administration (FDA) U.S. government agency whose purpose is to ensure that foods, drugs, cosmetics, and medical devices are safe and properly labeled (13)

Food Intolerance Non-allergic food hypersensitivity — a more common problem than food allergies, involving digestion (people with food intolerance can eat some of the offending foods without suffering symptoms) (12)

Fowler's Position A semi-sitting position (10)

Gastric Suction Used to remove gastric contents (11)

Gastritis Inflammation of the stomach (12)

Gastroenteritis Inflammation of the stomach and intestines (12)

Gastrointestinal (GI) Study A diagnostic study related to the gastrointestinal system. GI studies often are performed in the endoscopy department. (16)

Gastrostomy A surgical procedure for inserting a tube through the abdominal wall and into the stomach. The tube may be used for feeding or drainage. (12)

Gavage Feeding by means of a tube inserted into the stomach, duodenum, or jejunum through the nose or an opening in the abdominal wall; also called *tube feeding* (12)

Governing Board Group of community citizens at the head of the hospital organizational structure (2)

GPS Tracking Systems Used for tracking patients, hospital personnel, equipment, controlling temperatures and for reducing hospital theft prevention identification purposes (4)

Guaiac A method of testing stool for hidden (occult) blood using guaiac as a reagent (may also be called a Hemoccult Slide Test) (14)

Handheld Computer a kind of portable computer that is intended to be held and used in a hand (4)

Harris Flush or Return Flow Enema A mild colonic irrigation that helps expel flatus (11)

Health Information Technology for Economic and Clinical Health (HITECH) Act Created to stimulate the adoption of electronic health records (EHR) and supporting technology in the United States (6)

Health Insurance Portability and Accountability Act (HIPAA) A U.S. law designed to provide privacy standards to protect patients' medical records and other health information provided to health plans, doctors, hospitals and other health care providers (6)

Health Maintenance Organization Organization that has management responsibility for providing comprehensive health care services on a prepayment basis to voluntarily enrolled persons within a designated population (2)

Health Unit Coordinator Preoperative Checklist A checklist used by the health unit coordinator to ensure that the patient's paper chart is ready for surgery (19)

Health Unit Coordinator The health care team member who performs nonclinical patient care tasks for the nursing unit (also may be called *unit clerk* or *unit secretary*) (1)

Hemodialysis (Extracorporeal Dialysis) The removal of waste products from the blood as attained by the utilization of a machine through which the blood flows (17)

Hemovac A disposable suction device (evacuator unit) connected to a drain that is inserted into or close to a surgical wound (11)

Heparin Lock A vascular access device (also called *intermittent infusion device, heplock,* or *saline lock*) that is placed on a peripheral intravenous catheter when used intermittently (11)

Hepatitis C Virus Another hepatitis infection that is bloodborne and that may also be an occupational hazard for health care workers (21)

Holistic Nursing Care A modern nursing practice that expresses the philosophy of total patient care that considers the physical, emotional, social, economic, and spiritual needs of the patient (also called *comprehensive care*). (3)

Holter Monitor A portable device that records the heart's electrical activity and produces a continuous EKG tracing over a specified period (16)

Home Health Equipment and services provided to patient in-home to ensure comfort and care (2)

Homeopathy A natural medicine that treats the whole person with natural medicines. It is good therapy for mood swings, depression, anxiety, obsessive-compulsive disorder, and also attention-deficit/hyperactivity disorder. (3)

Hospice Supportive care for terminally ill patients and their families (2)

Hospital Departments Divisions within the hospital that specialize in services, such as the nutritional care department, which plans and prepares meals for patients, employees, and visitors (1)

Hospital Robots Used to make up for nursing and staff shortages. Robots used to dispense medication, make deliveries, visit patients and help doctors reach patients across distance. (4)

Hospitalist Full-time, acute care specialist who focuses exclusively on hospitalized patients (3)

Hostile Working Environment A threatening or sexually oriented atmosphere or pattern of behavior that is determined to be a form of harassment (6)

HUC Clinical Experience The time the HUC student spends on a nursing unit (after completing the classroom portion of an educational program) with a working HUC to acquire hands-on work experience (5)

HUC Preceptor An experienced working HUC who is selected to train/teach an HUC student or a new employee (5)

HUGS Infant Protection System An example of an alarm system that includes monitoring software and an ankle bracelet that contains a tiny radio transmitter designed to prevent infants from being removed from a health care facility without authorization (19)

Human Immunodeficiency Virus (HIV) The virus that causes acquired immunodeficiency syndrome (21)

Hydration Adequate water in the intracellular and extracellular compartments of the body (12)

Hydrotherapy The use of water—including continuous tub baths, wet sheet packs, or shower sprays—to soothe pains and treat various conditions and diseases (17)

Hyperbaric Oxygen Therapy A treatment that involves breathing 100% oxygen while in an enclosed system pressurized to greater than one atmosphere (sea level) (17)

Hypertonic A concentrated salt solution (>0.9%) (17)

Hypnotics Drugs that induce sleep (13)

Hypotonic A dilute salt solution (<0.9%) (17)

Identification Labels Labels that contain individual patient information for identifying patient records or other personal items (8)

Impedance Cardiography A flexible and fast-acting noninvasive monitoring system that measures total impedance (resistance to the flow of electricity in the heart) (16)

Impedance Plethysmography (IPG) A noninvasive study that is performed to estimate blood flow and quantify blood volumes. (16)

Incident An episode that does not normally occur within the regular hospital routine and may involve patients, visitors, physicians, hospital staff, or students (21)

Incontinence Inability of the body to control the elimination of urine and/or feces (11)

Indigent A person who is living in extremely poverty — lacking the necessities of life, such as food, clothing, etc (2)

Induced Sputum Specimen A sputum specimen obtained by performing a respiratory treatment to loosen lung secretions (17)

Indwelling or Retention Catheter A catheter that remains in the bladder for a longer period until a patient is able to void completely and voluntarily, or as long as hourly accurate measurements are needed (11)

Infiltration The tip of the IV catheter comes out of the vein or pokes through the vein, and IV solution is released into surrounding tissue. This also could occur if the wall of the vein becomes permeable and leaks fluid (11)

Informed Consent Doctrine that states that before patients are asked to consent to a risky or invasive diagnostic or treatment procedure, they are entitled to receive certain information: (1) a description of the procedure, (2) any alternatives to it and their risks, (3) risks of death or serious bodily disability from the procedure, (4) probable results of the procedure, including any problems with recuperation and anticipated time of recuperation, and (5) anything else that is generally disclosed to patients who are asked to consent to a procedure. (6)

Informed Consent The duty to inform a patient (description of the procedure, alternatives, risks, probable results, and anything else that is generally disclosed to patients) before a signature of permission is obtained (19)

Ingest or Ingestion The taking in of food by mouth (12)

Inhalation Liquid medications are most commonly administered by the respiratory care department as part of their treatment procedure (13)

Injectables Medications that are given by forcing a liquid into the body by means of a needle and syringe (intra-arterial, intradermal, intramuscular, intravenous, and subcutaneous) (13)

Inpatient Surgery Surgery performed that requires the patient to stay overnight or longer in the hospital (19)

Inpatient Patient to receive medical or surgical care whose doctor has written an admission order (3)

Instillation To slowly introduce fluid into a cavity or a passage of the body to remain for a specific length of time before it is drained or withdrawn. (The purpose is to expose tissues of the area to the solution, to hot or cold, or to a drug or substance in the solution.) (13)

Intake and Output The measurement of the patient's fluid intake and output (10)

Intensivist Specializes in the care of critically ill patients, usually in an intensive care unit (ICU) (3)

Interdisciplinary Teamwork Well-coordinated collaboration across health care professionals toward a common goal (improved, efficient patient care) (3)

Intermittent (Straight) Catheter A single-use catheter that is introduced long enough to drain the bladder (5 to 10 minutes) and is then removed (11)

International Statistical Classification of Diseases (ICD) system A detailed description of known diseases and injuries. Each disease (or group of related diseases) is described with its diagnosis and is given a unique code, up to six characters long. Published by the World Health Organization. (2)

Internet Service Provider A company that provides Internet connections and services to individuals and organizations for a monthly fee (1)

Interpreter A person who facilitates oral communication between or among parties who are conversing in different languages (5)

Intervention Synonymous with treatment (17)

Intradermal Injection Injected between the layers of the skin (used for skin tests) (13)

Intramuscular Injection (IM) Medication is injected directly into the muscle. (13)

Intraoperative Pertaining to the period during a surgical procedure (19)

Intravenous Hyperalimentaion The administration of nutrients by intravenous feeding, especially to individuals unable to take in food through the alimentary tract (12)

Intravenous Infusion Administered directly into a vein (13)

Intravenous Infusion The administration of fluid through a vein (11)

Intravenous or IV Piggyback (IVPB) A method of administering a medication in 50 to 100 mL of solution through an intravenous line that is inserted into a patient's vein and given by hanging it above level of primary fluid bag (13)

Intravenous or IV Push (IVP) Method of giving concentrated doses of medication directly into the vein (13)

Intubation Insertion and placement of a tube within the trachea (may be endotracheal or tracheostomy) (17)

Invasive Procedure A diagnostic or therapeutic technique that requires an incision and/or entry of a body cavity and/or interruption of normal body functions (16)

Irrigation Washing or flushing out of a body cavity, organ, or wound (11)

Isolation The placement of a patient apart from other patients for the purpose of preventing the spread of infection, or protecting a patient whose immune system is compromised (21)

Isometric Of equal dimensions. Holding ends of contracting muscle fixed so that contraction produces increased tension at a constant overall length (17)

IV Infusion Pump A device used to regulate the flow or rate of intravenous fluid; more commonly called an *IV pump* (11)

Jackson-Pratt (JP) A disposable suction device (evacuator unit) that is connected to a drain that is inserted into or close to a surgical wound (11)

Jejunostomy A creation of an artificial opening into the jejunum that may be used for enteral feeding when it is necessary to bypass the upper gastrointestinal tract (12)

Kangaroo Pump A brand name of a feeding pump used to administer tube feeding (12)

Kardex File A portable file that contains and organizes the Kardex forms for each patient on the nursing unit (9)

Kardex Form A form on which the health unit coordinator records doctors' orders; it is used by the nursing staff for a quick reference of the patient's current orders (9)

Kardexing The process of recording and updating doctors' orders on the Kardex form (many hospitals have eliminated the paper Kardex form in favor of entering all patient orders into the computer) (9)

Kosher To adhere to the dietary laws of Judaism; the conventional meaning in Hebrew is "acceptable" or "approved" (12)

Label Printer Machine that prints patient labels from information entered into the computer; located near the health unit coordinator's area (4)

Laptop or Notebook A portable computer. Some laptops are actually in a tablet form. Tablets are essentially just laptops with a touch screen and possibly a pen for input. (4)

Liability Condition of being responsible for damages resulting from an injurious act or from discharging an obligation or debt (6)

Licensed Practical Nurse A graduate of a 1-year school of nursing who is licensed in the state in which he or she is practicing; provides direct care and functions under the direction of the registered nurse (3)

Living Will A declaration made by the patient to family, medical staff, and all concerned with the patient's care, stating what is to be done in the event of a terminal illness; it directs the withholding or withdrawing of life-sustaining procedures (19)

Locator Communication Tracking System A device worn by nursing personnel, including health unit coordinators, so their location may be detected on the interactive console display when necessary; also used for communication between nursing unit personnel and the nursing station (4)

Long-Term Care (LTC) A variety of services often provided in nonhospital settings which help meet both the medical and non-medical needs of people with a chronic illness or disability who cannot care for themselves for long periods of time (2)

Love and Belonging Needs A person's need to have affectionate relationships with people and to have a place in a group (5)

Lumbar Puncture A procedure used to remove cerebrospinal fluid from the spinal canal (14)

Magnet Status Award given by the American Nurses' Credentialing Center to hospitals that satisfy a set of criteria designed to measure their strength and quality of nursing (2)

Magnetic Resonance Angiography (MRA) Use of magnetic resonance to study blood vessels (15)

Magnetic Resonance Imaging A technique used to produce computer images (scans) of the interior of the body with the use of a powerful magnetic field and radiofrequency waves (15)

Managed Care The use of a planned and systematic approach to providing health care, with the goal of offering quality care at the lowest possible cost (2)

Manipulation Attempts at influencing or controlling other's actions or behaviors to one's own advantage (5)

Mass Communication System A system that in an emergency can quickly and efficiently deliver messages to tens, hundreds, or thousands of recipients (4)

Material Safety Data Sheet (MSDS) A basic hazard communication tool that gives details on chemical dangers and safety procedures (21)

Meaningful Use (EMR) use of certified EMR technology in ways that can be measured significantly in quality and in quantity (1)

Medicaid Federal and state program that provides medical assistance to the indigent (2)

Medical Emergency An emergency that is life threatening (21)

Medical Malpractice Professional negligence of a health care professional; failure to meet a professional standard of care, resulting in harm to another, for example, failure to provide "good and accepted medical care" (6)

Medical Savings Account (MSA) A tax exempt bank account that is *owned by an individual* and managed by a financial institution. The individual must have a qualified a high deductible health plan. An individual cannot use the tax benefit of an MSA until the qualified health plan is in place. Also called a **Health Savings Account (HSA)**. (2)

Medicare Government insurance; enacted in 1965 for individuals older than age 65 and any person with a disability who has received Social Security benefits for 2 years (some disabilities are covered immediately) (2)

Medication Administration Record (MAR) Computerized list of medications that each individual patient is currently taking; it is used by the nurse to administer and document medications (13)

Memory Sheet A note pad kept by the telephone and used to write down messages that need to be relayed and tasks that need to be completed (7)

Message Images, feelings, and ideas transmitted from one person to another (5)

Metastasis The process by which tumor cells spread to distant parts of the body (15)

Methicillin-Resistant *Staphylococcus Aureus* (MRSA) A variation of the common bacteria, *Staphylococcus aureus*. It has evolved the ability to survive treatment with beta-lactam antibiotics, including penicillin and methicillin (21)

Microfilm A film that contains a greatly reduced photo image of printed or graphic matter (18)

M-mode Echo Image obtained with M-mode echocardiography shows the motion (M) of the heart over time. 2-D M-mode would be a two-dimensional study. (16)

Modality A method of application or employment of any therapeutic agent, limited usually to physical agents and devices (15)

Morbid Obesity An excess of body fat that threatens necessary body functions such as respiration (12)

Name Alert A method of alerting staff when two or more patients with the same or similarly spelled last names are located on a nursing unit (8)

Narcolepsy A chronic ailment that consists of recurrent attacks of drowsiness and sleep during the daytime (16)

Narcotic Controlled drug that relieves pain or produces sleep (13)

Nasogastric Tube (NG Tube) A tube that is inserted through the mouth or nose into the stomach and is used to feed the patient, or to drain stomach contents to prevent vomiting (11)

Native American Healing The practices and healing beliefs of hundreds of indigenous tribes of North America. Native American Healing is a combination of religion, spirituality, herbal medicine, and rituals. (3)

Naturopathic Medicine Alternative medical system that proposes that there is a healing power in the body that establishes, maintains, and restores health. Treatments include nutrition and lifestyle counseling, nutritional supplements, medicinal plants, exercise, homeopathy, and treatments from traditional Chinese medicine. (3)

Nebulizer A gas-driven device that produces an aerosol (17)

Needleless Heplock or Saline Lock A safe, sharp device that is placed on a peripheral intravenous catheter when used intermittently (11)

Negative Assertion An assertive skill in which a person verbally accepts having made an error without letting it reflect on their worth as a human being (5)

Negative Inquiry An assertive skill in which a person requests clarification of a criticism to get to the real issue (5)

Negligence Failure to satisfactorily perform one's legal duty, such that another person incurs some injury (6)

Nerve Conduction Studies (NCS) Performed to identify peripheral nerve injury in patients with localized or diffuse weakness, to differentiate primary peripheral nerve disease from muscular injury, and to document the severity of injury in legal cases. (Often performed with an EMG.) (16)

Neurologic Vital Signs (Neuro checks) The measurement of the function of the body's neurologic system; includes checking pupils of the eyes, verbal response, and so forth (10)

Nonassertive (Passive) A behavioral style in which a person allows others to dictate her or his self-worth (5)

Nonclinical Tasks Tasks performed away from the bedside (indirect patient care) (1)

Noninvasive Procedure A diagnostic or therapeutic technique that does not require the skin to be broken or a cavity or organ of the body to be entered (16)

Non-teaching Service The delivery of patient care without the involvement of providing clinical education and training to future and current doctors, nurses, and other health professionals (19)

Nonverbal Communication Communication that is not written or spoken but creates a message between two or more people through eye contact, body language, or symbolic and facial expression (5)

Nosocomial Infection An infection that is obtained by the patient while in the hospital. Also known as a *hospital acquired infection (HAI)*. (14)

Nosocomial Infections Infections that are acquired from within the health care facility (21)

Nuclear Medicine A technique that uses radioactive materials to examine anatomy and functional capacity of an organ (15)

Nurse Manager A registered nurse who assists the director of nursing in carrying out administrative responsibilities and is in charge of one or more nursing units (may also be called *unit manager, clinical manager,* or *patient care manager*) (3)

Nurse Practitioner (NP) A registered nurse (RN) who has completed advanced education (a minimum of a master's degree) and training in the diagnosis and management of common medical conditions, including chronic illnesses (3)

Nurses' Station The desk area of a nursing unit (1)

Nursing Intervention Nursing interventions are actions undertaken by a nurse to further the course of treatment for a patient (3)

Nursing Observation Order A doctor's order that requests the nursing staff to observe and record certain patient signs and symptoms (10)

Nursing Preoperative Checklist A checklist used to ensure that the paper or electronic chart and the patient are properly prepared for surgery (19)

Nursing Service Department Hospital department responsible for all nursing care administered to patients (3)

Nursing Team A group of nursing staff members who care for patients on a nursing unit (1)

Nursing Unit Administration Division within the hospital responsible for non-clinical patient care (3)

Nursing Unit An area within the hospital that includes equipment and nursing personnel available for the care of a given number of patients (also may be referred to as a wing, floor, pod, strategic business unit, ward, or station) (1)

Nutrients Substances derived from food that are used by body cells, for example, carbohydrates, fats, proteins, vitamins, minerals, and water (12)

Obese or Obesity An excess amount of body fat usually defined by body mass index (12)

Observation Patient A patient who is assigned to a bed on the nursing unit to receive care for a period of less than 24 hours; also may be referred to as a *medical short-stay* or *ambulatory patient* (19)

Obstructive Sleep Apnea The cessation of breathing during sleep (16)

Occlusion A blockage in a canal, vessel, or passage of the body (16)

Occult Blood Blood that is undetectable to the eye (14)

Occupational Safety and Health Administration (OSHA) A U.S. governmental regulatory agency that is concerned with the health and safety of workers (21)

Old Record A patient's paper record from previous admissions stored in the health information management department that may be retrieved for review when a patient is admitted to the emergency room, nursing unit, or outpatient department; older microfilmed records also may be requested by the patient's doctor (8)

"On Call" Medication Medication prescribed by the doctor to be given before the diagnostic imaging procedure is performed; the department notifies the nursing unit of the time the medication is to be administered to the patient (15)

One-Time or Short-Series Order A doctor's order that is executed according to the qualifying phrase, and then is automatically discontinued (9)

Oral Temperature The temperature reading obtained by placing the thermometer in the patient's mouth under the tongue (10)

Oral By mouth (13)

Ordering The process of ordering diagnostic procedures, treatments, or supplies from hospital departments other than nursing (9)

Organ Donation Donating or giving one's organs and/or tissues after death; one may designate specific organs (e.g., only cornea) or may donate any needed organs (20)

Organ Procurement The process of removing donated organs; may also be referred to as harvesting (20)

Orthostatic Hypotension A temporary lowering of blood pressure (hypotension) usually due to suddenly standing up; also called postural hypotension (10)

Orthostatic Vital Signs Measurement (Orthostatics) Recording the patient's blood pressure and pulse rate while the patient is supine (lying) and again while erect (sitting and/or standing)

Outpatient A patient receiving medical or surgical care while registered as an outpatient and whose doctor has not written an admission order. The patient's doctor may order the patient to stay overnight for observation without writing an admitting order. (3)

Outpatient Surgery Surgery performed that does not require an overnight hospital stay. (Also called *ambulatory surgery, same day surgery (SDS), save a day surgery (SAD)*. (19)

Over-the-Counter Drugs A drug for which a prescription is not needed. The FDA defines OTC drugs as safe and effective for use by the general public without a doctor's prescription (13)

Oxygen Saturation A noninvasive measurement of gas exchange and red blood cell oxygen-carrying capacity (10)

Pap Smear A test performed to detect cancerous cells in the female genital tract; the Pap staining method also can study body secretions, excretions, and tissue scrapings (14)

Paracentesis A surgical puncture and drainage of a body cavity (14)

Paraphrase Repeating a message back to the sender in your own words to clarify meaning (5)

Parent Teaching or Transition Room Many pediatric hospitals and/or units have a patient room with a bed so a parent can stay with the child 24 hours a day. Parents, after training, will assume full care of the child while they still have the support of the nursing staff. The child may then be discharged home to the parents' care. (18)

Parenteral Nutrition A mode of feeding that does not use the GI tract, instead providing nutrition by intravenous delivery of nutrient solutions (12)

Parenteral Routes Pertaining to a medication administered by a route that bypasses the gastrointestinal (GI) tract, such as a drug given by injection, intravenously, or by skin patch (13)

Partial Parenteral Nutrition (PPN) A solution, containing some essential nutrients, is injected into a vein to supplement other means of nutrition, usually a partially normal diet of food (12)

Passive Aggressive A type of aggressive behavior characterized by an indirect expression of negative feelings, resentment, and aggression in an unassertive way (as through sullenness, obstructionism, stubbornness, and unwillingness to communicate) (5)

Passive Exercise Exercise in which the patient is submissive and the physical therapist moves the patient's limbs (17)

Patent or Patency A term that indicates that there are no clots at the tip of the needle or catheter, and that the needle tip or catheter is not against the vein wall (open) (11)

Pathogen A microorganism that causes disease (14)

Pathogenic Microorganisms Disease-carrying organisms too small to be seen with the naked eye (21)

Pathology The study of body changes caused by disease (14)

Patient (pt) A person who receives health care, including preventive, promotional, acute, chronic, and all other services in the continuum of care (1)

Patient Account Number A number assigned to the patient to access insurance information; usually, a unique number is assigned each time the patient is admitted to the hospital (19)

Patient Call System Intercom Device used to communicate between the nurses' station and patient rooms on the nursing unit (4)

Patient Care Conference A meeting that includes the doctor or doctors caring for the patient, the primary nurses, the case manager or social worker, and other caregivers (may include family) involved in the patient's care (20)

Patient Care Conference Meeting of a patient's doctor or resident, primary nurse, case manager or social worker, and other health care professionals for the purpose of planning the patient's care (3)

Patient Health Information Management Number The number assigned to the patient on or before admission; it is used for records identification and is used for all subsequent admissions to that hospital (also may be called health or medical records number) (19)

Patient Identification Bracelet A plastic band with a patient identification label affixed to it that is worn by the patient throughout hospitalization. In the obstetrics department, the mother and the baby would share the same identification label affixed to their ID bracelets (19)

Patient identification labels are self-adhesive labels used on the patient's identification bracelet to identify forms, requisitions, specimens, and so forth (19)

Patient Label Book Book used to store labels for patients when CPOE has been implemented; it is also used to store labels for discharged patients for a short time after the time of their discharge (7)

Patient Portal An online application that allows a patient to register for an appointment, schedule an appointment, request prescription refills, send and receive secure patient-physician messages, view lab results, or pay bills electronically (2)

Patient Support Associate Nursing unit staff member whose duties may include some patient-admitting responsibilities, coding, or stocking of nursing units; job description and title may vary among hospitals (3)

Patient-Controlled Analgesia (PCA) Medications administered intravenously by means of a special infusion pump controlled by the patient within order ranges written by the physician (13)

Pedal Pulse The pulse rate obtained on the top of the foot (10)

Pen Tab or Tablet PC Computer that may be removed from its base, or a portable computer that can be taken into patient rooms, with a stylus used to enter information directly into a patient's electronic record, as in a notebook (4)

Penrose Drain A drain that is inserted into or close to a surgical wound; it may lie under a dressing, extend through a dressing, or be connected to a drainage bag or suction device (11)

Percutaneous Endoscopic Gastrostomy Insertion of a tube through the abdominal wall into the stomach under endoscopic guidance (12)

Perennial Stress The wear and tear of day-to-day living, with the feeling that one is a square peg trying to fit into a round hole (7)

Perioperative Services Department of the hospital that provides care before (preoperative), during (intraoperative), and after (postoperative) surgery. It encompasses total care of the patient during the surgical experience (3)

Perioperative Pertaining to the time of surgery (19)

Peripheral Intravenous Therapy An infusion of a liquid prepared solution directly into a vein intermittently or continuously (11)

Peripherally Inserted Central Catheter (PICC or PIC) A catheter inserted into the arm and advanced until the tip lies in the superior vena cava and placement is checked with an X-ray (11)

Peritoneal Dialysis The introduction of a fluid (dialyzing fluid) into the abdominal cavity that then absorbs the wastes from the blood through the lining of the abdominal cavity, or peritoneum then the dialysate is emptied from the abdominal cavity. (17)

Personal Data Assistant (PDA) A handheld mobile device that functions as a personal information manager (Also called a *personal digital assistant* or *palmtop computer*) (4)

Philosophy Guiding or underlying principles — attitude toward life (6)

Physician extender a health care provider who is not a physician but who performs medical activities typically performed by a physician (3)

Physician's Assistant (PA) One who practices medicine under the supervision of physicians and surgeons (3)

Physiologic Needs A person's physical needs, such as the need for food and water (5)

Picture Archiving and Communication Systems Computers or networks dedicated to the storage, retrieval, distribution, and presentation of images. Full PACS handle images from various modalities, such as ultrasonography, magnetic resonance imaging, positron emission tomography, computed tomography, endoscopy, mammography, and digital radiography. (15)

Plaintiff Person who brings a lawsuit against another (6)

Plasma The fluid portion of the blood in which the cells are suspended; it contains a clotting factor called fibrinogen (14)

Pneumatic Hose Stockings that promote circulation by sequentially compressing the legs from ankle upward, promoting venous return (also called *sequential compression devices* or *pneumo boots*) (11)

Pneumatic Tube System System in which air pressure transports tubes carrying supplies, *some* lab specimens, and some medications to and from hospital units or departments (4)

Pocket Pager Small electronic device that when activated by entering a series of numbers into a telephone delivers a digital or voice message to the carrier of the pager (4)

Point-of-care testing (POCT) Medical testing at or near the site of patient care (10)

Policies and Procedures (online or manual) Information such as guidelines for practice and hospital regulations found on line or in a book (1)

Polycom SpectraLink A wireless telephone system that allows hospital workers to have immediate access to each other, and most importantly, to patients (4)

Portable X-ray An X-ray taken by a mobile X-ray machine that is moved to the patient's bedside (15)

Position Alignment of the body on the X-ray table that is favorable for taking the best view of the part of the body being imaged (15)

Positioning Order A doctor's order that requests that the patient be placed in a specified body position (10)

Positive Pressure Pressure greater than atmospheric pressure (17)

Post Residual Urine Volume The measurement of urine left in the bladder after urination (11)

Postmortem After death (a postmortem examination is the same as an autopsy) (20)

Postoperative Orders Orders electronically or handwritten immediately after surgery. Postoperative orders cancel preoperative orders. (19)

Postprandial After eating (14)

Power of Attorney for Health Care The patient appoints a person (called a *proxy* or *agent*) to make health care decisions should the patient be unable to do so (19)

Pre-admit The process of obtaining information and partially preparing admitting forms before the time of the patient's arrival at the health care facility (19)

Precept To train or teach (a student or a new employee) (5)

Preoperative and Postoperative Patient Care Plan A plan that includes preoperative teaching, goals, and outcomes. This plan is reviewed and modified during the intraoperative and postoperative periods (19)

Preoperative Care Unit A unit within the surgery area where a patient is prepared for surgery (19)

Preoperative Orders Orders electronically or handwritten by the doctor before the time of surgery to prepare the patient for the surgical procedure (19)

Pre-printed Orders A typed set of orders for a specific diagnosis or procedure that has been approved for use in the hospital (9)

Primary Care Physician A general practitioner or internist, chosen by an individual to serve as his or her health-care professional (Sometimes referred to as *gatekeepers*) (3)

Primary Insurance Insurance coverage that is responsible for paying claims first and protects against medical expenses up to the policy's limit, regardless of whatever other insurance you hold

Principles Basic truths; moral code of conduct (6)

Proprietary For profit (2)

Pulse Deficit The discrepancy between the ventricular rate detected at the apex of the heart and the arterial rate at the radial pulse (10)

Pulse Oximeter A device that measures gas exchange and red blood cell oxygen-carrying capacity by attaching a probe to either the ear or the finger (also called an *oxygen saturation monitor*) (10)

Pulse Oximetry A noninvasive method of measuring gas exchange and red blood cell oxygen-carrying capacity (considered to be the fifth vital sign) (10)

Pulse Rate The number of times per minute the heartbeat is felt through the walls of the artery (10)

Quantitative Electroencephalogram (QEEG) (Brain-mapping) Uses digital pattern recognition to identify *functional problems*, such as attention deficit hyperactivity disorder (ADHD) (16)

Quid Pro Quo (Latin) Involves making conditions of employment (hiring, promotion, retention) contingent on the victim's providing sexual or other favors (6)

Radial Pulse Pulse rate obtained on the wrist (10)

Random Specimen A specimen that can be collected at any time (14)

Range of Motion The range in which a joint can move (17)

React Saying or doing the first thing that comes to you and allowing negative emotions to take over in response to another person or event (a negative choice) (7)

Real-Time Imaging An ultrasound procedure that displays a rapid sequence of images (like a movie) instantaneously while an object is being examined (16)

Receiver The person who receives the message (5)

Recertification A process by which certified health unit coordinators exhibit continued personal and professional growth and current competency to practice in the field (1)

Recommended Dietary Allowance (RDA) The average daily intake of a nutrient that meets the requirements of nearly all (97% to 98%) healthy people of a given age and gender. Also commonly known as **Recommended Daily Allowance**. (12)

Rectal Instillation Medications prepared specifically for insertion into the rectum. Enemas are also instilled into the rectum. (13)

Rectal Temperature The temperature reading obtained by placing the thermometer in the patient's rectum (10)

Rectal Tube A plastic or rubber tube designed for insertion into the rectum; when written as a doctor's order, *rectal tube* means the insertion of a rectal tube into the rectum to remove gas and relieve distention (11)

Reference Range Range of normal values for a laboratory test result (14)

Reflex Testing Additional tests done on a specimen subsequent to initial test results, and used to further identify significant diagnostic information required for appropriate patient care (14)

Registered Dietitian One who has completed an educational program, served an internship, and passed an examination sponsored by the American Dietetic Association (12)

Registered Nurse Graduate of a 2- or 4-year college–based school of nursing or a 3-year hospital–based program who is licensed in the state in which they are practicing; may provide direct patient care or may supervise patient care given by others (3)

Registrar The admitting personnel who registers a patient to the hospital (19)

Registration The process of entering personal information into the hospital information system to enroll a person as a hospital patient and create a patient record; patients may be registered as inpatients, outpatients, or observation patients (19)

Regular Diet A diet that consists of all foods and is designed to provide good nutrition (12)

Rehydration Restoration of normal water balance in a patient through the administration of fluids orally or intravenously (12)

Release of Remains A signed consent that authorizes a specific funeral home or agency to remove the deceased from a health care facility (20)

Remote Patient Monitoring Uses new wireless technologies to remotely collect and send data to medical professionals for interpretation (3)

Requisition A paper form used to order diagnostic procedures, treatments, or supplies from hospital departments other than nursing when the computer is down (also called a *downtime requisition*) (9)

Resident A graduate of a medical school who is gaining experience in a hospital (3)

Resistive Exercise Exercise that uses opposition. A T band or water may be used to provide resistance for patient exercises. (17)

Respect Holding a person in esteem or honor; having appreciation and regard for another (6)

Respiration Rate The number of times a patient breathes per minute (10)

Respiratory Arrest When the patient ceases to breathe, or when respirations are so depressed that the blood cannot receive sufficient oxygen, and therefore, the body cells die (also may be referred to as *code arrest*) (21)

Respond A positive approach to a person or event putting distance between you and the event (a positive choice) (7)

Respondeat Superior **(Latin)** "Let the master answer:" Legal doctrine that imposes liability upon the employer as a result of the action of an employee. *Note:* The employee is also liable for their own actions. (6)

Restraints Devices used to control patients who exhibit dangerous behavior or to protect the patient (11)

Retaliation Revenge; payback (6)

Reverse or Protective Isolation A precautionary measure taken to prevent a patient with low resistance to disease from becoming infected (21)

Rhythm Strip A cardiac study that demonstrates the waveform produced by electrical impulses from the electrocardiogram (16)

Risk Management A department in the hospital that addresses the prevention and containment of liability regarding patient care incidents (21)

Robotic Surgery The use of robots in performing surgery (2)

Role Fidelity Requires that healthcare professionals remain their scope within their scope of legitimate practice (6)

Routine Preparation The standard preparation suggested by the radiologist to prepare the patient for a diagnostic imaging study (15)

Safety and Security Needs The need to be sheltered, to be clothed, to feel safe from danger, and to feel secure about their job and financial future (5)

Scan An image produced with the use of a moving detector or a sweeping beam; image is produced by computed tomography, magnetic resonance imaging, nuclear medicine, and ultrasonography (15)

Scheduled or Planned Admission A patient admission planned in advance; it may be urgent or elective (19)

Scope of Practice Legal description of what a specific health professional may and may not do (6)

Search Engine A website that collects and organizes content (1)

Secondary Insurance Insurance coverage used to supplement existing policies or to cover any gaps in insurance coverage – billed after primary insurance has paid (also called *supplemental insurance*) (2)

Skilled Nursing Facility (SNF) A medical institution that provides medical, nursing, or custodial care for an individual over a prolonged period (2)

Sedative An agent given to reduce or relive anxiety, stress, excitement. **Sedative-hypnotic** is given to induce sleep and to relieve anxiety. (13)

Self-Actualization Needs The need to maximize one's potential (5)

Self-Esteem Confidence and respect for oneself (5)

Sender The person who transmits the message (5)

Serology The study of blood serum or other body fluids for immune bodies, which are the body's defense when disease occurs (14)

Serum Plasma from which fibrinogen, a clotting factor, has been removed (14)

Server or Application Server Provides network services to other computers on a network (4)

Set of Doctor's Orders An entry of doctor's orders written on the doctor's order sheet, dated, notated for time, and signed by the doctor (9)

Sexual Harassment Unwanted, unwelcome behavior; sexual in nature (6)

Sheepskin A pad made out of lamb's wool or synthetic material; used to prevent pressure sores (used frequently in long-term care) (11)

Shift Manager Registered nurse who is responsible for one or more units during their assigned shift (also may be called *nursing coordinator* or *charge nurse*) (3)

Signing Off A process by which the health unit coordinator records data (date, time, name, and status) on the doctor's order sheet to indicate the completion of transcription of a handwritten set of doctor's orders (9)

Sitz Bath Application of warm water to the pelvic area (11)

Skin Test A test given to determine the reaction of the body to a substance injected intradermally or applied topically to the skin. Skin tests are used to detect allergens, to determine immunity, and to diagnose disease (13)

Smart Phone A high-end mobile phone built on a mobile computing platform with more advanced computing ability (4)

Social Network An online community of people with a common interest who use a website or other technologies to communicate with each other and share information, resources, etc (4)

Special Invasive X-ray and Interventional Procedures Diagnosing and treating patients using the least invasive techniques currently available in order to minimize risk to the patient and improve health outcomes (15)

Spica Cast A cast which begins at the chest and includes one or both lower limbs (17)

Spirometry A study conducted to measure the body's lung capacity and function (16)

Splint An orthopedic device for immobilization, restraint, or support of any part of the body; may be rigid (metal, plaster, or wood) or flexible (felt or leather) (17)

Splinting Holding the incision area to provide support, promote a feeling of security; and reduce pain during coughing after surgery; a folded blanket or pillow is helpful for use as a splint (11)

"Split" or Thinned Chart Portions of the patient's current paper chart that are removed when the chart becomes so full that it is unmanageable (8)

Sputum The mucous secretion from lungs, bronchi, or trachea (14)

Staff Development Department responsible for orientation of new employees and continuing education of employed nursing service personnel (also may be called *educational services*) (3)

Standard Chart Forms Forms included in all inpatient paper charts that are used to regularly enter information about patients (8)

Standard of Care The legal duty one owes to another according to the circumstances of a particular case; it is the care that a reasonable and prudent person would have exercised in the given situation (6)

Standard Precautions The creation of a barrier between the health care worker and the patient's blood and body fluids (also may be called *universal precautions*) (21)

Standard Supply List A computerized or written record of the quantity of each item that the nursing unit currently needs to last until the next supply order date (separate lists are found inside cabinet doors, in supply drawers, and on the code or crash cart) (7)

Standing Order A doctor's order that remains in effect and is executed as ordered until the doctor discontinues or changes it (9)

Standing prn Order Similar to a standing order, except that it is executed according to the patient's needs (9)

Stat Order A doctor's order that is to be executed immediately, then automatically discontinued (9)

Statute of Limitations Time within which a plaintiff must bring a civil suit; this limit varies with the type of suit, and it is set by the various state legislatures

Statute Law passed by the legislature and signed by the governor at the state level and the president at the federal level (6)

Stent A tiny metal or plastic tube that is placed into an artery, blood vessel, or other duct to hold the structure open (17)

Stereotyping The assumption that all members of a culture or ethnic group act in the same way (generalizations that may be inaccurate) (5)

Sternal Puncture The procedure to remove bone marrow from the breastbone cavity for diagnostic purposes; also called a bone marrow biopsy (14)

Straight Catheter see Intermittent (Straight) Catheter (11)

Stress A physical, chemical, or emotional factor that causes bodily or mental tension and may cause disease (7)

Stridor A high-pitched harsh sound heard during inspiration that is caused by obstruction of the upper airway, is a sign of respiratory distress and thus requires immediate attention (17)

Stuffing Charts Placing extra chart forms in patients' paper charts so they will be available when needed (8)

Subculture Subgroup within a culture; people with a distinct identity but who have specific ethnic, occupational, or physical characteristics found in a larger culture (5)

Subcutaneous Injection (sq or sub-q) Injection of a small amount of a medication under the skin into fatty or connective tissue (13)

Sublingual (Subling) under the tongue (13)

Superbugs Pathogens that have become resistant to most of the antibiotics currently available, and often result in life-threatening infections that are extremely difficult to treat (14)

Supplemental Chart Forms Patient chart forms used only when specific conditions or events dictate their use (8)

Supply Needs List A sheet of paper used by all nursing unit personnel to jot down items that need reordering (7)

Suppository Medicated substance mixed in a solid base that melts when placed in a body opening; suppositories are commonly used in the rectum, vagina, or urethra (13)

Surfing the Web Using different search engines on the Web to locate information (1)

Surfing the Web Using different websites on the Internet to locate information (2)

Surgery Consent A patient's written permission for an operation or invasive procedure (19)

Surgery Schedule A list of all the surgeries to be performed on a particular day; the schedule may be printed from the computer or sent to the nursing unit by the admitting department (19)

Swan-Ganz Catheter placed in the neck or the chest that measures pressures in the patient's heart and pulmonary artery (11)

SWAT HUC, Nurse, or SWAT Team A health unit coordinator, a nurse, or a group of health care workers that are on call for all units in the hospital to provide assistance as needed (3)

Symbols Notations written in black or red ink on the doctor's order sheet to indicate completion of a step of the transcription procedure (9)

Systolic Blood Pressure The blood pressure measured during the period of ventricular contraction; in blood pressure readings, it is the higher, upper number of the two measurements (10)

Tactfulness Sensitivity to what is proper and appropriate in dealing with others; use of discretion regarding the feelings of others (6)

Tank Room A room where hydrotherapy is performed (17)

Teaching Service The delivery of patient care while providing clinical education and training to future and current doctors, nurses, and other health professionals (19)

Team Leader Registered nurse who is in charge of a nursing team (also may be called *pod leader* or *charge nurse*) (3)

Team Patient Care Model Consists of a charge nurse and two to three team leaders, along with four to five team members who are working under the supervision of each team leader (3)

TED Hose (Thrombo-Embolic-Deterrent) A brand name for an antiembolism (AE) hose

Telecommunication The transmission, emission or reception of data or other information, in the form of signs, signals, writings, images and sounds or any other form, via wire, radio, visual or other electromagnetic systems *(from the American Nurses Association)* (3)

Telelift Usually located in a small room between nursing units—consists of a small boxcar that is carried on a conveyor belt to designated locations. A keypad is used to program the car to go to a specific unit or department. (4)

Telemedicine The combined use of telecommunications and computer technologies to improve the efficiency and effectiveness of healthcare services by eliminating the traditional constrains of place and time (2)

Telemetry The transmission of data electronically to a distant location (16)

Telephoned Order/s Order/s for a patient called into a health care facility (usually to the patient's nurse) by the doctor (9)

Telepresence (Virtual Presence) The virtual presence of somebody whose actions are transmitted by electronic signals to a physically remote site. (2)

Temperature The quantity of body heat, measured in degrees—Fahrenheit or Celsius (10)

Terminal Illness An illness ending in death (20)

Therapeutic Diet A diet with modifications or restrictions (also called a *special diet*) that must be ordered by the doctor (12)

Thoracentesis A needle puncture into the pleural space in the chest cavity to remove pleural fluid for diagnostic or therapeutic reasons (14)

Tilt Table Test (TTT) A cardiovascular study done with the use of a "tilt table" to test for syncope (16)

Timed Specimen A specimen that must be collected at a specific time (14)

Tissue Typing Identification of tissue types to predict acceptance or rejection of tissue and organ transplants (14)

Titer The quantity of substance needed to react with a given amount of another substance—used to detect and quantify antibody levels (14)

Topical Direct application of medication to the skin, eye, ear, or other parts of the body (13)

Total Care Nursing Model One nurse provides total care to assigned patients (also called **Primary Care Model** or **Case Nursing Model**) (3)

Total Parenteral Nutrition (TPN) The provision of all necessary nutrients via veins (discussed in detail in Chapter 13) (12)

Toughbook A brand of laptop designed to withstand vibration, drops, spills, extreme temperature, and other rough handling used in many hospitals (4)

Traction A mechanical pull to part of the body to maintain alignment and facilitate healing; traction may be static (continuous) or intermittent (17)

Transcription A process used to communicate the doctors' orders to the nursing staff and other hospital departments; computers or handwritten requisitions are used (1)

Transesophageal Echocardiogram (TEE) A procedure used to assess the heart's function and structures. A probe with a transducer on the end is inserted down the throat. (16)

Transfer Order A doctor's order that requests that a patient be transferred to another hospital room, another nursing unit or to another facility (20)

Trendelenburg Position A position in which the head is low and the body and legs are on an inclined plane (sometimes used in pelvic surgery to displace the abdominal organs upward, out of the pelvis, or to increase the blood flow to the brain in hypotension and shock (10)

Triage Nursing interventions. Classification defined as establishing priorities of patient care, usually according to a three-level model: emergent, urgent, and non-urgent. (3)

Tube Feeding Administration of liquids into the stomach, duodenum, or jejunum through a tube (12)

Tuberculosis (TB) A disease caused by *Mycobacterium tuberculosis*, an airborne pathogen (21)

Tympanic Temperature The temperature reading obtained by placing an aural (ear) thermometer in the patient's ear (10)

Type and Crossmatch The patient's blood is typed, then is tested for compatibility with blood from a donor of the same blood type and Rh factor (14)

Type and Screen The patient's blood type and Rh factor are determined, and a general antibody screen is performed (14)

Ultrasonography A technique that uses high-frequency sound waves to create an image (scan) of body organs (also may be referred to as sonography or echography) (15)

Ultrasound Therapy A deep heating modality using high-energy sound waves that is most effective for heating tissues or deep joints and is performed by a physical therapist (17)

Unit Dose Medicine Cart Contains "unit doses" in separate drawers or bins specifically labeled for each patient as ordered by the doctor(s) (13)

Unit Dose Any premixed or prespecified dose; often administered with small volume nebulizer or intermittent positive-pressure breathing treatments (17)

Urgent Admission A patient not scheduled to be admitted, sent from doctor's office or another facility and needing immediate care (19)

Urinalysis The physical, chemical, and microscopic examination of the urine (14)

Urinary Catheterization A tube is placed in the body to drain and collect urine from the bladder (11)

Urine Flow Test A test that evaluates the speed of urination, or amount voided per second, and the total time or urination (11)

Urine Reflex Urine is tested; if certain parameters are met, a culture is performed (14)

Urine Residual Urine that remains in the bladder after urination (11)

Uroflowmeter a funnel-shaped device that reads, measures, and computes the rate and amount of urine flow (11)

Valuables Envelope A container for storing the patient's jewelry, money, and other valuables that is placed in the hospital safe for safekeeping (19)

Values Clarification A method of determining and accessing one's values and how those values affect personal decision making (6)

Values Personal beliefs about the worth of a principle, standard, or quality; what one holds as most important—values reflect a person's sense of right and wrong (6)

Vascular Doppler Ultrasound Takes real time video that displays how the patient's blood is flowing through the arteries. This makes it easier to detect narrowing of the arteries, blockages, and blood clots. It also helps with monitoring the progression of arterial disease in a patient (16)

Vascular Duplex Scanning Called "duplex" because it combines the benefits of Doppler with B-mode scanning (16)

Venipuncture Needle puncture of a vein (11)

Venous Plethysmography Measures changes in the volume of an extremity; usually performed on a leg to exclude DVT (deep vein thrombosis) (16)

Ventilator A machine that is used to give the patient breaths through the ET or tracheostomy tube (17)

Verbal Communication The use of language or actual spoken words (5)

Vital Signs Measurements of body functions, including temperature, pulse, respiration, and blood pressure (10)

Vocera Mobile Applications Allows users to leverage the benefits of Vocera instant voice communication anytime, anywhere on any device (Apple iPhone, Blackberry, or Android) (4)

Vocera 802.11 Voice Device A device that can be integrated with data event notification and escalation applications, critical alert and alarm systems, and patient monitoring (4)

Vocera B2000 Communications Badge A wearable device that weighs less than two ounces and can easily be clipped to a shirt pocket or worn on a lanyard. It enables instant two-way voice conversation without the need to remember a phone number or use a handset. (4)

Vocera Smartphone Supports traditional phone dialing as well as the Vocera badge capabilities with one touch instant communication and voice system interface and is compatible with the Vocera system (4)

Voice Activated Transcription A local, PC-based large vocabulary voice-recognition engine that generates reports, often using macros and templates to make the process more efficient and reduce recognition errors (2)

Voice Paging System System by which the hospital telephone operator pages a message for a doctor or makes other announcements; the system reaches all hospital areas (used only when absolutely necessary to keep noise level down) (4)

Void (micturate or urinate) To empty, especially the urinary bladder (11)

Voluntary Not for profit (nonprofit) (2)

WALLaroo A locked workstation that is located on the wall outside a patient's room; it stores the patient's paper chart or a laptop computer, and when unlocked, it forms a shelf to write upon (8)

Web Address (URL, or uniform resource locator) Keywords that when entered after "http://www..."on the Web will take the user to a specified location, referred to as a *Website* (1)

Wheezes Sounds that are heard continuously during inspiration or expiration, both and are caused by air moving through airways narrowed by constriction or swelling of airway or partial airway obstruction (17)

Work Ethics Moral values regarding work (6)

Workable Compromise Dealing with conflict in such a way that the solution is satisfactory to all parties (5)

Workplace Behavior A pattern of actions and interactions of an individual that directly or indirectly affects their effectiveness while at work; the attitude and amount of enthusiasm that one brings to their job (6)

Workstation A relatively powerful kind of desktop with a faster processor, more memory and other advanced features, when compared to a more basic desktop (4)

Workstation on Wheels (WOW) A mobile computer that can be taken to a patient's bedside, allowing nurses and other healthcare providers the ability to access and enter information into patient records (4)

Index

Page numbers followed by *f,* indicates figures; *t,* indicates tables; and *b,* indicates boxes.